Recent Studies in Clinical Neurology

Recent Studies in Clinical Neurology

Editor: Samuel Armstrong

MURPHY & MOORE
www.murphy-moorepublishing.com

www.murphy-moorepublishing.com

MURPHY & MOORE

Cataloging-in-Publication Data

Recent studies in clinical neurology / edited by Samuel Armstrong.
p. cm.
Includes bibliographical references and index.
ISBN 978-1-63987-485-9
1. Neurology. 2. Nervous system--Diseases. 3. Clinical neuropsychology. I. Armstrong, Samuel.
RC346 .R43 2021
616.8--dc23

Murphy & Moore Publishing,
1 Rockefeller Plaza,
New York City, NY 10020, USA

ISBN 978-1-63987-485-9 (Hardback)

Contents

Preface

The branch of science that is concerned with the study of disorders of the nervous system is known as neurology. It deals with the diagnosis and treatment of all the conditions and diseases of peripheral and central nervous system as well as their blood vessels, coverings and all effector tissues such as muscles. Neurology is a non-surgical specialty and its specialists can be involved in clinical trials, clinical research and translational research. Symptoms that may require medical attention within this field are confusion, dizziness, change in sensation, muscle weakness and coordination problems. Patients with multiple sclerosis, stroke, neuromuscular disorders, seizure disorders, infections of the nervous system such as encephalitis or brain abscesses, etc., are also treated within this field. The various sub-fields of neurology and their clinical aspects are glanced at in this book. It provides significant information of this discipline to help develop a good understanding. Students, researchers, experts and all associated with neurology will benefit alike from this book.

This book is a result of research of several months to collate the most relevant data in the field.

When I was approached with the idea of this book and the proposal to edit it, I was overwhelmed. It gave me an opportunity to reach out to all those who share a common interest with me in this field. I had 3 main parameters for editing this text:

1. Accuracy – The data and information provided in this book should be up-to-date and valuable to the readers.
2. Structure – The data must be presented in a structured format for easy understanding and better grasping of the readers.
3. Universal Approach – This book not only targets students but also experts and innovators in the field, thus my aim was to present topics which are of use to all.

Thus, it took me a couple of months to finish the editing of this book.

I would like to make a special mention of my publisher who considered me worthy of this opportunity and also supported me throughout the editing process. I would also like to thank the editing team at the back-end who extended their help whenever required.

Editor

1

"Studying injured minds" – the Vietnam head injury study and 40 years of brain injury research

Vanessa Raymont[1,2,3], Andres M. Salazar[2], Frank Krueger[2] and Jordan Grafman[2,4]*

[1] Vietnam Head Injury Study, Henry M. Jackson Foundation, National Naval Medical Center, Bethesda, MD, USA
[2] Cognitive Neuroscience Section, National Institute of Neurological Disorders and Stroke, National Institutes of Health, Bethesda, MD, USA
[3] Department of Radiology, Johns Hopkins University, Baltimore, MD, USA
[4] Traumatic Brain Injury Research Laboratory, Kessler Foundation, West Orange, NJ, USA

Edited by:
Ibolja Cernak, Johns Hopkins University, USA

Reviewed by:
Jeffrey J. Bazarian, University of Rochester, USA
Vassilis E. Koliatsos, Johns Hopkins University School of Medicine, USA
Harvey S. Levin, Baylor College of Medicine, USA

***Correspondence:**
Jordan Grafman, Traumatic Brain Injury Research Laboratory, Kessler Foundation, 1199 Pleasant Valley Road, West Orange, NJ 07052, USA.
e-mail: jgrafman@kesslerfoundation.org

The study of those who have sustained traumatic brain injuries (TBI) during military conflicts has greatly facilitated research in the fields of neuropsychology, neurosurgery, psychiatry, neurology, and neuroimaging. The Vietnam Head Injury Study (VHIS) is a prospective, long-term follow-up study of a cohort of 1,221 Vietnam veterans with mostly penetrating brain injuries, which has stretched over more than 40 years. The scope of this study, both in terms of the types of injury and fields of examination, has been extremely broad. It has been instrumental in extending the field of TBI research and in exposing pressing medical and social issues that affect those who suffer such injuries. This review summarizes the history of conflict-related TBI research and the VHIS to date, as well as the vast range of important findings the VHIS has established.

Keywords: brain imaging, brain injury, brain lesion, neuropsychology

THE RECENT HISTORY OF COMBAT-RELATED TBI RESEARCH

Traumatic brain injury (TBI) is the principal cause of death and disability in those under 35 in the USA. Each year TBI leads to approximately 55,000 deaths, as well as 50,000 cases of associated physical, cognitive, behavioral, and social deficits (Kraus and McArthur, 1996). TBI remains extremely prevalent in combat situations, with nearly two-thirds of injured US soldiers sent from Iraq to Walter Reed Army Medical Center sustaining TBI (Warden, 2006). As recently as 2009, it was quoted that "Head injury has always been, and remains, an unpopular subject with British neurologists, presumably because they tend to see it as a surgical rather than a medical disorder." (van Gijn, 2009). Fortunately this has not been the case for all neurologists. Much of what is known about TBI (e.g., the clinical course, cognitive changes, incidence of post-traumatic epilepsy, PTE) is in fact as a result of neurological studies in military populations. The First World War was the first conflict that led to a major move forward in the study of TBI because of the sheer quantity of casualties, the extent of trench warfare (and so vulnerability to head injuries), the unprecedented use of artillery, and a change to small, low velocity ammunition, which tended to create focal injuries. In addition, advances in the field of neurosurgery meant penetrating head wounds were no longer inevitably fatal. Gordon Holmes, a London neurologist described several groups of First World War veterans, including 23 cases of occipital lesions (Lepore, 1994). This led to what became the standard illustration of the cortical map of the retina (Holmes and Lister, 1916). Henry Head, another English neurologist, had conducted pioneering work into the somatosensory system prior to the First World War, and he expanded this work with George Riddoch by testing reflex activities of isolated portions of the spine subjected to gunshot wounds (Holmes, 1941). Across the channel, brain injury rehabilitation units in Frankfurt and Cologne were responsible for major innovations in neuropsychological assessments and rehabilitation techniques (Boake and Diller, 2005).

During the Second World War, the Russian psychologist Aleksandr Luria examined psychological dysfunctions in patients with brain lesions, and his work gave impetus to the emerging field of neuropsychology. Luria's early work with Zazetsky (Luria, 1972), an ex-soldier who tried to make sense of his "shattered world" predated interest by others in the personal experience of those with TBI. Hans-Lukas Teuber and Morris Bender focused on visual deficits (Bender and Teuber, 1948) and long-term outcome from TBI (Teuber, 1975). Teuber was the first to report on the role of preinjury intelligence in cognition post-TBI (Weinstein and Teuber, 1957), and he also introduced was that of double dissociation of function, which has since become essential to functional localization (Lackner, 2009). Suzanne Corkin started assessing Second World War veterans while working for Teuber. She subsequently commented on the long-term prognosis of TBI, and developed the concept of exacerbated decline in intelligence post-TBI (Corkin et al., 1984, 1989). Her work with conflict-associated TBI was continued by Newcombe and Marshall in Second World War veterans, and later, in Korean War veterans. They focused on language difficulties post-TBI (Newcombe et al., 1971), long-term outcome, and rehabilitation (Newcombe et al., 1980). Their research helped develop a new classification for acquired alexias and lead to the conceptualization of the dual routes of visual processing that Ungerleiter and Mishkin later formalized in their theory (Mishkin, 1972). The neuropsychiatrist, Lishman (1992), was another early proponent of TBI research, and was amongst the first who examined social behavior changes following TBI.

HISTORY OF THE VIETNAM HEAD INJURY STUDY

SET UP AND PHASE 1

The Vietnam Head Injury Study (VHIS) was set up by William F. Caveness, a neurologist and retired Naval Reserve captain who had served in the Korean War, who was chief of the Laboratory of Experimental Neurology at the National Institute of Neurological and Communicative Disorders and Stroke from 1965. He designed the VHIS registry, which gathered information on 1,221 Vietnam veterans who sustained a TBI between 1967 and 1970 (Caveness et al., 1979). Of the 58,000 US combat fatalities in the Vietnam War, about 40% were due to head and neck wounds. The Vietnam conflict was the first that involved large scale helicopter evacuations and early treatment by neurosurgical teams close to the battlefield, so that most patients received definitive treatment with hours of their injuries, allowing a much higher rate of survival than in previous conflicts (Carey et al., 1982; Rish et al., 1983). In addition, the low velocity penetrating fragment wounds typically sustained resulted in relatively focal defects, and so these subjects provided a particularly large and informative group for study. It should be noted, therefore, that the data from this cohort addresses issues predominantly affecting those with penetrating TBI. This may contrast with closed injuries, which are considerably commoner in the civilian population and especially in mild cases lack some of the frequent, significant sequelae of penetrating TBI, such as impaired consciousness. Caveness requested that field neurosurgeons complete registry forms on those they anticipated would survive, detailing wound characteristics and neurological status immediately post-injury. Although he received around 2,000 registry forms, addresses could only be found for 1,221. Phase 1 (PH1) of the VHIS was a retrospective review of those subjects' military and veterans affairs (VA) medical records from the 5-years post-injury (e.g., Caveness et al., 1979; Weiss et al., 1983, 1986). Patients were excluded if they had a spinal cord injury or if insufficient medical records were available. Caveness set up the VHIS to primarily study the causes of PTE but unfortunately died before the beginning of Phase 2 (PH2; e.g., Caveness et al., 1979; Rish et al., 1979, 1980, 1981; Mohr et al., 1980). The team of investigators that inherited the VHIS subsequently expanded the scope of the study well beyond his original focus.

PHASE 2 – 15 YEARS ON

Phase 2 evaluated 520 head-injured subjects from the original registry who responded to mailings, as well as 85 uninjured Vietnam veteran control subjects, matched by age. Of those who did not come to PH2, some had died, some declined, and some did not respond; 92% had penetrating head injuries (e.g., Grafman et al., 1986a, 1988, 1992; Salazar et al., 1987). Analysis of subjects who did and did not participate in PH2 showed no significant differences in terms of demographics or lesion type (Jonas et al., 1987). Subjects attended Walter Reed Army Medical Center, Washington, DC, USA for a 1-week evaluation, which consisted of neuropsychological, neurological, language, and brain imaging assessments. Specific subgroups and individual patients have returned more often for selected studies between each phase following PH2.

PHASE 3 – 35 YEARS POST-TBI

Of the 520 head-injured subjects assessed at PH2, 484 were still alive, and 182 attended Phase 3 (PH3). Additionally, 17 head-injured subjects identified in PH1 that did not attend PH2 were assessed. Of the original 80 control subjects recruited in PH2, 32 attended and a further 23 were recruited. Subjects were assessed at the National Naval Medical Center, Bethesda, MD, USA, with a broad battery of neuropsychological, neurological, psychiatric, and imaging assessments. Brain lesions were identified by CT scan, and the data were reconstructed with a 3-mm overlapping slice thickness and a 1-mm interval. MRI scans were not used as a large number of the subjects had retained metal in their brains. Lesions were processed using "analysis of brain lesions" software (ABLe; Makale et al., 2002; Solomon et al., 2007). Within ABLe, the lesions were drawn manually in native space on each 1 mm thick slice by Vanessa Raymont (a psychiatrist with clinical experience of reading CT scans), and reviewed by Jordan Grafman, enabling a consensus decision to be reached regarding the limits of each lesion. Normalized lesion volume was calculated, and the percentage of brain lobes and regions involved determined. This methodology is explained further in our earlier paper (Raymont et al., 2008). However, this meant that the assessment of these lesions was to some extent dependent on subjective measurements.

PHASE 4 – 40+ YEARS LATER

Subjects from PH3 were invited to attend for Phase 4 (PH4) of the VHIS, approximately 40–45 years post-injury. PH4 is currently in progress at the National Institute of Neurological Disorders and Stroke in Bethesda, MD, USA, and contains a core set of tasks that are similar to those previously administered in PH2 and PH3, so longitudinal assessments can be completed. In addition, further molecular genetic studies are planned that examine the role of genetic polymorphisms in recovery of function from TBI and in predicting various kinds of outcomes. Experimental cognitive neuroscience studies in PH4 will expand upon previous work in social neuroscience, examining the brain areas associated with certain forms of economic decision-making, human belief systems and moral thinking, social status, and aggression. In addition, PH4 will examine the role of caregiver personality in outcome after combat-related TBI. We hope that these studies contribute to the emerging fields of social neuroscience and behavioral genetics, and lead to improved management and outcome of the patient with a TBI. Although there was no evidence of Alzheimer's disease (AD) in this cohort at PH3, given the evidence of links between AD and TBI (Lindsay et al., 2002), Ann McKee, a neuropathologist from Boston University has also agreed to conduct autopsies on the brains of all VHIS subjects who consent. This will provide yet another dimension to the study by examining the causes and effects of long-term pathological changes following TBI, including the development of abnormal Tau deposits.

The advantages of studying this population have included their uniformity of age, gender, and education at time of injury, as well as the availability of preinjury intelligence data, making this a unique population for longitudinal assessment.

SELECTED FINDINGS FROM THE VHIS

One great advantage of the VHIS is that it has allowed the collection of a vast amount of data from a large cohort, which can subsequently be used to help answer basic neuropsychological questions (e.g., Rueckert and Grafman, 1996, 1998; Dimitrov et al., 1999; Lee et al., 1999). Over 80 papers have been published using VHIS data to date, and many more are expected. Here we describe some selected findings from each phase in order to give the reader a sense of the breadth and depth of our findings.

NEUROSURGICAL FINDINGS

A number of clinical questions regarding acute neurosurgical management were addressed at PH1, and are reviewed elsewhere (Grafman and Salazar, 1999). These include the use of improved protocols for evacuation and triage of large numbers of casualties, aggressive procedures for definitive surgical debridement close to the front, the issues of dural closure, retained metal and bone fragments, incidence and management of brain abscesses, use of antibiotics and anticonvulsants, and the timing of cranioplasty, among others. For example, it was reported that 491 cranioplasties were performed in 1,030 subjects from the registry, with a morbidity rate of 5.5% and a mortality rate was 0.2%, largely associated with surgical outcome (Rish et al., 1979). From these findings it was suggested that cranioplasty after penetrating TBI should be deferred for a minimum of 1 year, to control morbidity. Skull defects or cranioplasty were not found to predict tendency to post-traumatic seizures. In summary, the neurosurgical experience of the Vietnam War marked a turning point in the approach to emergency evacuation and management of severe TBI.

Research at PH2 further investigated the associations of traumatic unconsciousness post-TBI. Surprisingly, only 15% of the 342 subjects who survived severe penetrating TBI had prolonged loss of consciousness. Over half had no or only momentary unconsciousness after injury, and some even remained in battle and received citations for bravery. Over 40% had good recollection of injury events and were also alert at first examination, sometimes in spite of large lesions, further illustrating the largely focal nature of these wounds. The areas most associated with traumatic unconsciousness post-TBI in this cohort included the posterior limb of the left internal capsule, left basal forebrain, midbrain, and hypothalamus (Salazar et al., 1986).

EPILEPSY

Previous studies of World War Two (Walker and Jablon, 1961) and Korean War veterans (Weiss and Caveness, 1972) had confirmed the association between post-traumatic seizures and penetrating TBI. At PH2, of the 421 veterans who had sustained a TBI, 53% had a history of PTE, which had started within a year of TBI in the majority of cases (Salazar et al., 1985). About one-half of the group were still experiencing seizures 15 years after injury. The relative risk of developing PTE dropped from about 580 times higher than the general age-matched population in the first year, to 25 times higher after 10 years, and the frequency of seizures in the first year predicted subsequent severity of seizures. Anticonvulsant therapy with phenytoin in the first year after injury did not prevent later seizures. Patients with focal neurological signs or large lesions had an increased risk of developing PTE. PTE was also associated with the presence of hematoma or retained metal fragments (Weiss et al., 1986). Only five affected brain areas significantly predicted seizure occurrence: right vertex gray matter, left convexity cortex, left temporal gray matter, right frontal white matter, and right corona radiate. Lesions in the left hippocampus correlated with increased seizure frequency, whereas insula and splenium lesions correlated with lower seizure frequency. Lesions of the posterior callosum and caudate nucleus were associated with less persistent seizures. From these data, the authors were able to develop a predictive formula (incorporating data from previous, shorter term studies of risk factors for seizures, all of which suggested that the time between injury and onset of PTE is independent of injury characteristics) for the time between injury and first seizure (**Figure 1**).

$$Q_n = 0.7304 \exp(-0.0915n) + 0.2359 \exp(-0.0001n^2)$$

(Where Q_n=probability of surviving n months after a TBI without developing PTE)

FIGURE 1 | Predictive formula for the risk of developing PTE.

At PH3, the prevalence of seizures in the 199 TBI veterans who attended was 43.7%, similar to that 20 years earlier (Raymont et al., 2010). Remarkably 12.6% reported initial onset of PTE more than 14 years post-injury. These subjects were not different from earlier onset PTE subjects in any of the clinical measures examined. Within this cohort, the most common seizure type last experienced was complex partial seizures (31.0%), with increasing frequency post-injury. Eighty-eight percentage of subjects with PTE were receiving anticonvulsants. Left parietal lobe lesions and retained ferric metal fragments were associated with PTE and total brain volume loss predicted seizure frequency, although it should be emphasized that there is not substantial evidence in the general literature for lesion location being predictive of PTE.

MOTOR DISORDERS

Motor impairments following TBI are a common problem, which are very limiting to patient functioning. Within the first few months following a unilateral brain lesion affecting the motor cortex, therapeutic efforts are aimed primarily at the restoration of motor function on the hemiplegic side. Following on from the localization work conducted at the time of World War One, research carried out at PH1 reported that parietal wounds were particularly associated with hemiparesis, and that regardless of the features of the hemiparesis initially, the severity of the final syndrome was greatest in the hand and arm and least in the face (Mohr et al., 1980). At PH2, 90 subjects were found to have hemiparesis (Schwab et al., 1993), and in 32% of these subjects this prevented them from working. The relationship of preinjury left-hand dominance to post-injury distal motor skills was examined at PH2 (Grafman et al., 1985a). No persistent deficits were seen on distal motor tasks in left-handed adults who suffered a penetrating TBI, compatible with the previously reported relative sparing of persistent neuropsychological deficits in left-handed subjects following brain damage. In addition, other results indicated similar long-term functional outcome in right and left hemisphere-damaged subjects, despite more severe contralateral functional motor deficits following lesions of the left hemisphere. These results demonstrated that unilateral TBI involving the motor areas of either hemisphere has detrimental effects on ipsilateral upper extremity motor function, suggesting that the left hemisphere has greater neuronal representation for bilateral motor processes (Smutok et al., 1989).

FATIGUE

Fatigue is a common and disabling symptom following TBI, and studies have suggested that the ventromedial prefrontal cortex (vmPFC) could play a significant role in fatigue pathophysiology. At PH3 it was found that individuals with vmPFC lesions were significantly more fatigued than individuals with dorsolateral prefrontal cortex (dlPFC) lesions, individuals with non-frontal lesions, or healthy controls (Pardini et al., 2010). The larger the lesion volume, the higher the fatigue score. This demonstrated that the vmPFC plays a critical role in penetrating brain injury-related fatigue, and possibly provides a rationale to link fatigue to different vmPFC functions, such as effort and reward perception. In contrast, also at PH3, insomnia was found to be associated with left dorsomedial PFC lesions, presumably due to a disruption of the brain systems sustaining the sleep control mechanisms that are associated with brain stem and other midline structures (Koenigs et al., 2010).

NEUROPSYCHOLOGICAL ASSOCIATIONS

One vital issue that was examined at PH2 was the link between preinjury intelligence (as measured by the Armed Forces Qualification Test, AFQT-7A, 1960; DoD) and lesion characteristics, as well as preservation of cognitive function long-term post-TBI. Grafman et al. (1986a, 1988) reported that post-injury overall intelligence was most predicted by preinjury intelligence, followed by size of lesion, with some controls and a few TBI subjects showing an increase in AFQT score from preinjury to PH2 (**Figure 2**), probably secondary to maturation of the educational abilities tested in the AFQT. Lesion location was least important in predicting overall intelligence 15 years post-injury. For subtest scores of intelligence, lesion location assumed much greater predictive value. Specifically, left temporal and occipital lesions impaired performance on subtests assessing vocabulary and object-function matching ability.

Both cognitive change and return to work at PH2 were significantly related to total brain volume loss, third ventricle width, and septum caudate distance (Groswasser et al., 2002), with volume loss and third ventricle width being the most predictive. This suggests that quantity of brain disruption post-TBI influences long-term recovery of day-to-day functioning.

The same issues were revisited at PH3, via examination of past and current performance on the AFQT and current performance on the Wechsler Adult Intelligence Scale (WAIS-III). Raymont et al. (2008) reported that those with TBI showed a greater degree of overall cognitive decline overall during the years following injury compared with controls, which became increasingly significant

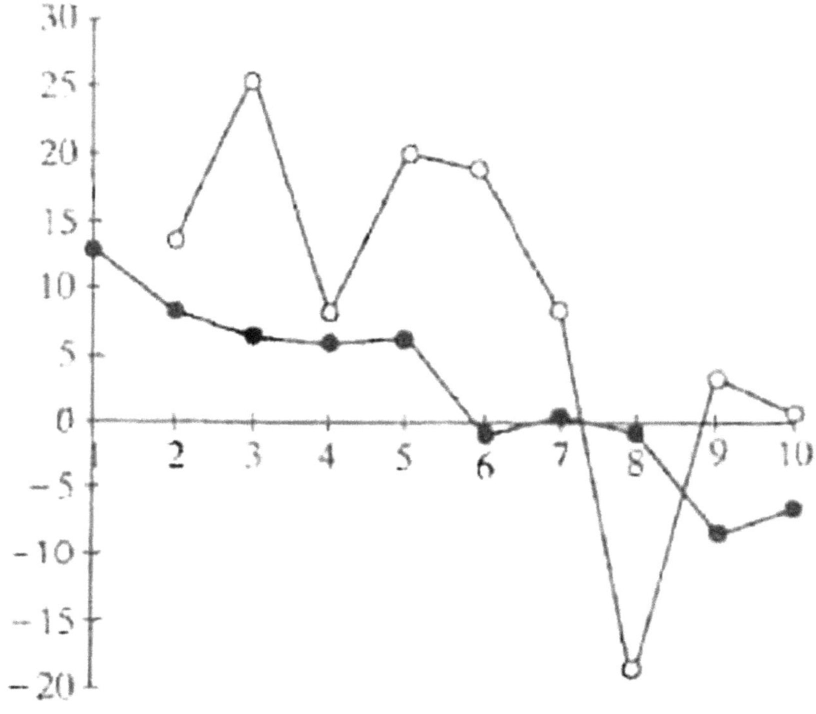

FIGURE 2 | Pre- and PH2 Armed Forces Qualification Test (AFQT) scores in head injured subject (filled circles, $r = -0.32$) and controls (open circles, $r = -0.44$). Plot of pre- to PH2 AFQT differences (D-AFQT) by preinjury AFQT deciles.

later in life. Preinjury intelligence was the most consistent predictor of cognitive outcome and while laterality of lesion was not a factor, there were some predictable associations between atrophy and specific regions of tissue loss and long-term cognitive functioning (see **Figure 3**, which represents the change in intelligence seen in subjects with TBI only).

The VHIS has thus produced some important contributions in terms of theories of neuroplasticity following TBI (Romero et al., 2002). Recent research has emphasized that this takes place via both local restitution, as well as reorganization and compensatory reassignment; processes which may vary at different points in the lifespan. The VHIS has been important in terms of highlighting how these changes may alter with aging, and how they may be impacted by a variety of factors, such as genetic make up (Raymont and Grafman, 2006).

Phase 2 included a review of the long-term outcome of post-TBI aphasia. At PH2, it was reported that aphasia occurred in 244 of the 1,030 patients with TBI, correlating with cause of injury and initial loss of consciousness. The aphasia disappeared within 10 years in 34% of cases. Sensorimotor aphasia usually changed to motor aphasia; motor aphasia disappeared; and sensory aphasia persisted. These improvements continued years after any accompanying hemiparesis stabilized, and were not related to wound site, depth, or whether the wound was caused by gunshot or fragment (Mohr et al., 1980). Chronic non-fluent aphasics demonstrated syntactic processing deficits in all language modalities, with greater posterior extension of their lesions in Wernicke's area, with some involvement of the underlying white matter and basal ganglia in the left hemisphere (Ludlow et al., 1986). This paper also highlighted that that deeper lesions involving the white matter may be the key factor associated with lack of recovery and persistence of language deficits. One PH2 case study also reflected on the localization of calculation knowledge (Grafman et al., 1989). Despite an almost totally destroyed left hemisphere and a severe linguistic disorder, the subject retained the ability to read and write single and two-place digits, perform simple addition and subtraction, accurately judge magnitudes and quantities, and recognize arithmetic operational symbols. This supported the hypothesis of right hemisphere participation in selected aspects of number processing.

Besides more descriptive findings, detailed experiments on the functions of suppression of context-inappropriate meanings

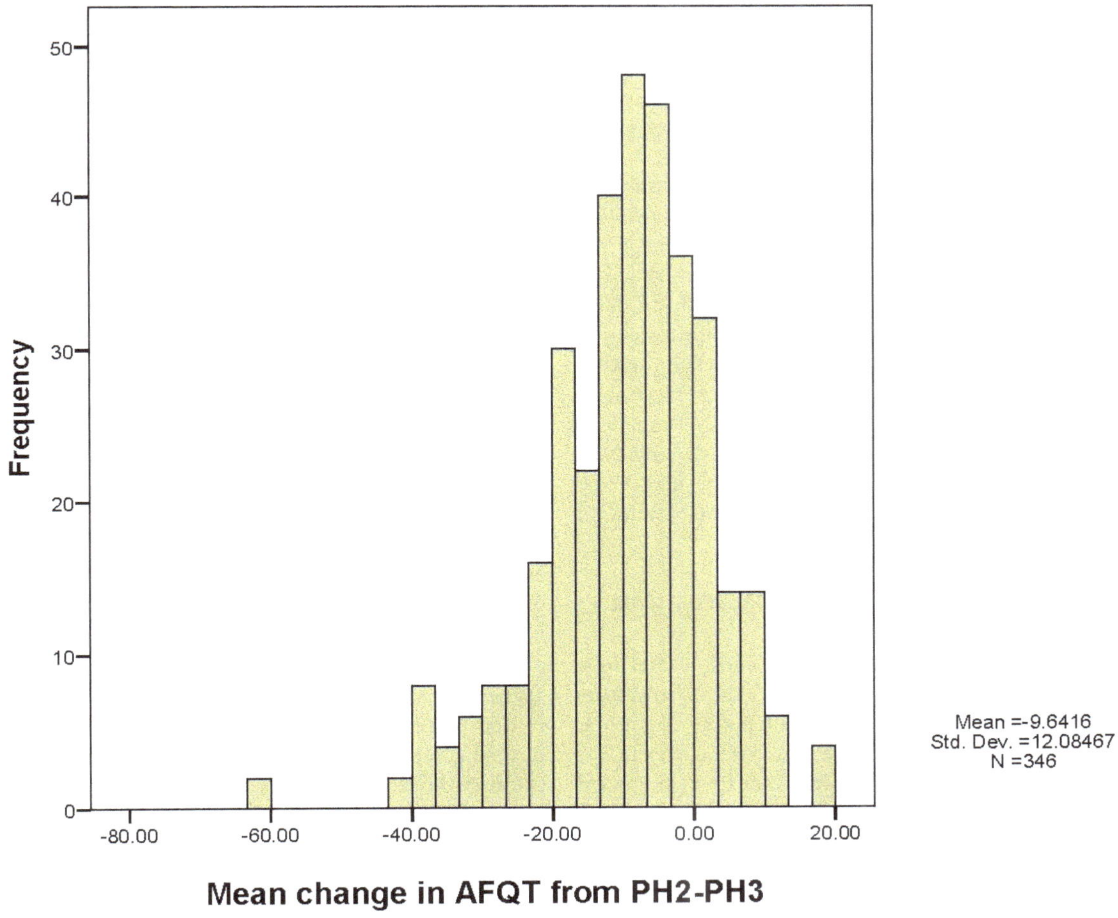

FIGURE 3 | Mean change in AFQT scores from Phase 2 to Phase 3 in subjects with TBI.

during lexical ambiguity resolution were conducted in PH3. Those with prefrontal lesions were found to have significantly lower accuracy rates for context-inappropriate conditions, suggesting a loss of the control aspects of inhibitory processes in lexical ambiguity resolution following prefrontal cortex damage (Frattali et al., 2007).

MEMORY DISORDERS

At PH2, deficits in semantic memory, verbal episodic memory, and visual episodic memory were found to be associated with lesion location, in a manner roughly consistent with the existing neuropsychological literature (Salazar et al., 1986). The advantage of being able to examine isolated brain lesions was vital in enabling the VHIS to identify possible site-specific sources of memory impairment. One case study demonstrated that the fornix cerebri has a role in the maintenance of information accessibility to both encoding and recall during post-working memory processing, as well as in the organization of verbal information (Grafman et al., 1985b). Another explored the basis of facial recognition memory, finding that impairment on tests of face memory was most associated with bilateral lesions and with unilateral lesions of the temporal lobe (Grafman et al., 1986b).

Schooler et al. (2008) used a specific modeling technique; mixture modeling (Muthén and Muthén, 1998–2004), to classify VHIS lesion groups and explore associations with subtypes of memory performance. One striking finding was that marked short term memory deficits were found in all classes of individuals with TBI, regardless of lesion location, and any concomitant effects of depressive symptomatology and substance dependence.

Theories of posterior parietal lobe involvement in memory have evolved over the years. However, definitive neuropsychological evidence supporting the superior parietal lobe's purported role in working memory has been lacking. At PH3, subjects with superior parietal lesions were compared to those with no damage in this region and with control subjects with no history of TBI. Superior parietal damage was associated with deficits on tests involving the manipulation and rearrangement of information in working memory, but not on working memory tests requiring only rehearsal and retrieval processes, nor on tests of long-term memory. These results indicated that the superior parietal cortex is critically important for the manipulation of information in working memory (Koenigs et al., 2009a).

REASONING, DECISION-MAKING, MOOD, AND SOCIAL BEHAVIORAL PLANNING

The large number of subjects with circumscribed frontal lobe lesions in the VHIS enabled both PH2 and PH3 to investigate altered performance on standardized tests of higher cognition. One study of patients with lesions in the prefrontal cortex utilizing the Tower of Hanoi task (Goel and Grafman, 1995) suggested that both subjects with frontal lesions and controls use the same general strategy to solve problems, and that patients' difficulties have little to do with planning deficits (as is generally assumed in the neuropsychology literature). Patient performance was rather explained in terms of an inability to see or resolve a goal–subgoal conflict, which is compatible with several other accounts of frontal lobe dysfunction. In a study of subjects with frontal lobe damage, their performance on the Tower of London task suggested impairment in execution-related processes (Carlin et al., 2000). Such analyses of data collected as part of the VHIS led to further conclusions on the regional contribution of planning and representations, which ultimately lead to novel theories of how the brain represents knowledge and responds to complex events (Goel and Grafman, 2000; Goel et al., 2001; Rattermann et al., 2001; Wood and Grafman, 2003; Wood et al., 2003).

Reasoning

While the role of left prefrontal cortex in reasoning tasks has long been recognized, the role of right prefrontal cortex remains unclear. One study undertaken at PH2 (Goel et al., 2007) found that the right prefrontal cortex plays an essential role in resolving indeterminate relations with no belief-bias cues, a fact that was later confirmed by a fMRI study in healthy control subjects (Goel et al., 2009). In addition, studies of decision-making and social behavior at PH2 provided new insight into these deficits, and helped define appropriate modes of assessing such difficulties in subjects with frontal lesions.

Many VHIS subjects had been previously dishonorably discharged from the military, when personality changes seen after frontal lobe injuries were less recognized. Thus, the VHIS was vital in establishing improvements in the assessment of those with frontal lobe syndrome. It was found that there may be subgroups of patients with specific social deficits even within groups whose lesion encompasses a larger region, e.g., vmPFC lesions (Sanfey et al., 2003; Goel et al., 2004; Mah et al., 2004, 2005). Administration of the Everyday Problem Solving Inventory (EPSI) suggested that some patients with prefrontal lobe lesions may have impaired social judgment that can be directly revealed only through the use of such relatively novel neuropsychological tests (Dimitrov et al., 1996).

Mood disorders

As well as examining the impact of TBI on executive functioning, the VHIS reported on effects in terms of mood and other psychological disorders. At PH2, subjects with TBI were compared with controls in terms of anxiety and aggressive symptoms, to explore the hypotheses regarding the regulation of anxiety by frontal cortical mechanisms (Grafman et al., 1986c). Results indicated that patients with right orbitofrontal lesions were prone to abnormally increased anxiety and depressive symptoms, whereas patients with left dorsofrontal lesions were prone to abnormally increased anger and hostility. These data suggested that mood symptoms are subject to influence by locality of brain damage. These theories were expanded during PH3, when the correlates of depressive disorder were studied in greater detail, in particular whether damage to either the vmPFC or dlPFC is related to the pathogenesis of depression. Bilateral vmPFC lesions were associated with low levels of depression, whereas bilateral dorsal PFC lesions (involving dorsomedial and dorsolateral areas in both hemispheres) were associated with substantially higher levels of depression. These findings suggested both the vmPFC and dorsal PFC are critical to depression, with vmPFC damage offering some resistance to depression, and dorsal PFC damage conferring vulnerability (Koenigs et al., 2008).

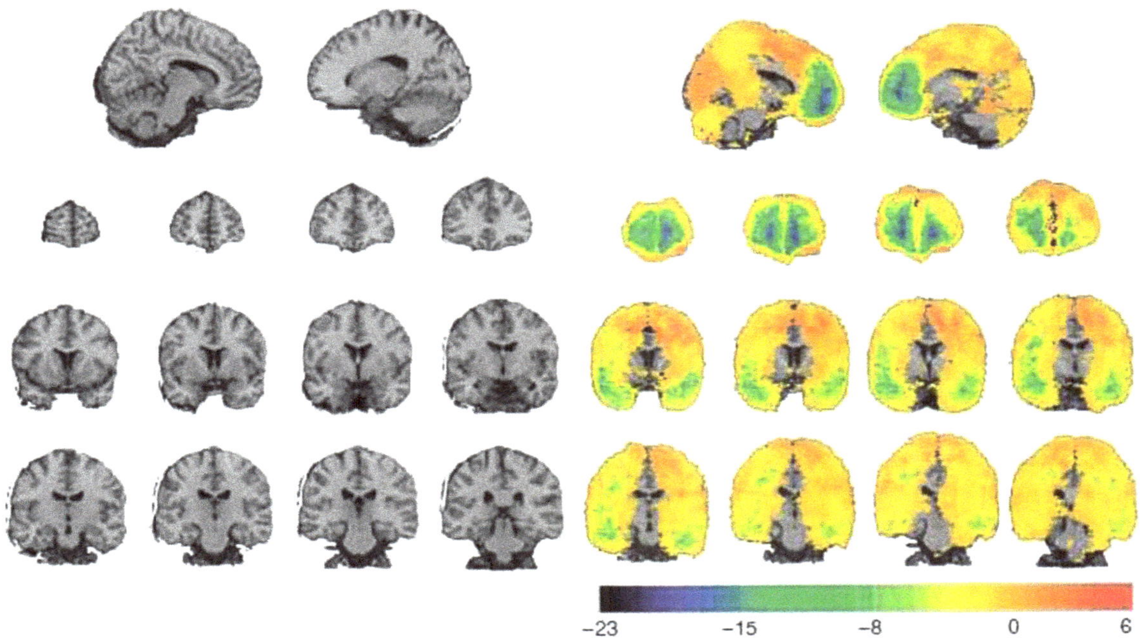

FIGURE 4 | Lesion difference analysis. A healthy adult brain is shown on the left. The lesion difference analysis for the corresponding slices is shown on the right. The color of each voxel indicates the difference between the number of veterans with damage to that voxel that developed PTSD and did not develop PTSD. The colors blue and green indicate the most negative values – areas where damage was relatively infrequently associated with PTSD. Top row, sagittal views of negative value clusters in prefrontal cortex. The left hemisphere ($x = -10$) is on the left and the right hemisphere ($x = 16$) is on the right. Second row, coronal views of negative value clusters in bilateral prefrontal cortex. Slices are arranged with the anterior most slice on the left ($y = 66$, $y = 56$, $y = 36$, respectively). In each coronal slice, the right hemisphere is on the reader's left (radiological convention). Third row, coronal views of negative value clusters in bilateral anterior temporal lobe ($y = 14$, $y = 8$, $y = 2$, $y = -4$, respectively). Fourth row, coronal views of posterior temporal lobe ($y = -10$, $y = -16$, $y = -22$, $y = -28$, respectively).

Post-traumatic stress disorder (PTSD) was specifically assessed at PH3, in particular the causal contribution of specific brain areas to PTSD symptoms. There was a substantially reduced occurrence of PTSD among those individuals with damage to one of two regions of the brain: the vmPFC and an anterior temporal area (that included the amygdala; **Figure 4**). The decreased prevalence of PTSD following vmPFC or amygdala damage appeared to be related to an overall reduction of symptom intensity or number, rather than a complete abolishment of all symptoms, suggesting that treatments aimed at selectively inhibiting vmPFC and/or amygdala function could be used to treat PTSD (Koenigs et al., 2009b).

Personality

Phase 2 investigators sought to establish more concrete evidence for the postulated associations between interictal personality traits and complex partial epilepsy (Swanson et al., 1995). An association between interictal psychopathology and complex partial, partial generalized, and generalized seizures was found, but there were no significant between group differences.

Social cognition

In 1999, PH2 reported a single VHIS case very similar to the famous nineteenth-century patient Phineas Gage (Dimitrov et al., 1999). Phineas Gage's case was described by his physician (Harlow, 1848, 1868), after he sustained a discrete but severe prefrontal cortex lesion during a railroad accident. Not only did Gage regain full consciousness and survive the incident, but he also demonstrated intact speech, learning, memory, and intelligence. However, his personality was profoundly changed, and he lost his "sense of responsibility" and respect for social conventions (Dimitrov et al., 1999). The subject described at PH2 was a 50-year-old male patient with a right frontal ventromedial lesion who showed preserved general cognitive, abstract thinking, and problem-solving abilities, in contrast to gross impairment in his social competence, social decision-making, and social conduct. He also demonstrated diminished sensitivity to socially relevant stimuli and situational nuances, impairment in sexual behavior, lost sense of responsibility, and disinhibition. This was cited as evidence for the regulation of emotion and social conduct by the vmPFC.

It is well reported that those with frontal lobe lesions may present with aggressive behavior. At PH2 family observations and self-reports were collected using scales and questionnaires that assessed a range of aggressive attitudes and behavior (Grafman et al., 1996). Patients with vmPFC lesions consistently demonstrated aggression scores significantly higher than controls and patients with lesions in other brain areas. However, the presence of aggressive and violent behavior was not associated with lesion size or history of seizures. The genotyping that was carried out as part of PH3 demonstrated an association between prefrontal cortex lesions and MAO-A in modulating aggression (Pardini et al., in press).

Results from a wealth of imaging and lesion studies have highlighted the involvement of the PFC in social cognition. Accumulating evidence demonstrates that representations within the lateral PFC enable people to coordinate their thoughts and actions with their intentions to support goal-directed social behavior. Despite the importance of this region in guiding social interactions, remarkably little is known about the functional organization and forms of social inference processed by the lateral PFC. Evidence from PH2 introduced a framework for understanding the inferential architecture of the PFC; "structured event complex theory" (Barbey et al., 2009). Data from both PH2 and PH3 have subsequently added to the evidence that regions of the PFC that are critical for both implicit and explicit social cognitive, as well as moral judgment processing. It seems there is considerable overlap between regions utilized when individuals engage in social cognition or assess moral appropriateness of behaviors, underscoring the similarity between social cognitive and moral judgment processes. The structured event complex theory emphasizes the dynamic flexibility in neural circuits involved in both implicit and explicit processing, and the likelihood that neural regions thought to uniquely underlie both processes in fact heavily interact (Forbes and Grafman, 2010).

Emotional intelligence (EI) has been referred to a set of competencies that are essential features of human social behavior (Krueger et al., 2009). At PH3 two components of this were assessed; (1) Strategic EI – the competency to understand emotional information and to apply it to management of yourself and others and, (2) Experiential EI – the competency to perceive emotional information and to integrate it into thinking. It was found that vmPFC damage diminishes strategic EI and dlPFC damage diminished experiential EI in subjects with frontal lobe damage.

An aspect of normal social cognition development is the development of stereotypical attitudes. At PH2, subjects with PFC lesions and controls were administered the Implicit Association Task (IAT) that measured the degree of association between male and female names and their stereotypical attributes of strength and weakness. Patients with dlPFC lesions and controls showed a strong association, whereas patients with vmPFC lesions had a significantly lower association, between the stereotypical attributes of men and women and their concepts of gender. This finding provided support for the hypothesis that patients with vmPFC lesions have a deficit in automatically accessing certain aspects of overlearned associated social knowledge (Milne and Grafman, 2001). At PH3, clinical observations of patients with ventral frontal and anterior temporal lesions revealed marked abnormalities in social attitudes. Gozzi et al. (2009) used the IAT to determine the differential effects of the vmPFC, ventrolateral prefrontal (vlPFC), and superior anterior temporal lobe (aTL) cortical lesions on attitudes. It was found that larger lesions in either the vmPFC or the superior aTL were associated with increased stereotypical attitudes, whereas larger lesions in the vlPFC were associated with decreased stereotypical attitudes.

FUNCTIONAL OUTCOME

In PH2, the relationship between neurological, neuropsychological, and social interaction impairments to work status was examined (e.g., Schwab et al., 1993; Salazar et al., 1995). Only 56% of the subjects with TBI were working at PH2, compared to 82% of the uninjured controls. Seven impairments correlated with work status; PTE, paresis, visual field loss, verbal memory loss, visual memory loss, psychological problems, and violent behavior. These disabilities had a cumulative and surprisingly equipotent affect upon the likelihood of work, suggesting that patients find it harder to compensate for increasing amounts of disabilities, whatever the disability. The authors suggested that a simple summed score of the number of these seven disabilities can yield a residual "disability score" which may prove to be a practical tool for assessing the likelihood of return to work post-TBI (**Figures 5** and **6**).

Additionally, 82% had used VA educational benefits to return to school (Kraft et al., 1993), and 64% had achieved associate or bachelor's degrees. Return to work was strongly related to level of educational achievement, particularly among the most severely disabled. Though only 56% of the TBI group were employed at PH2, the occupational distribution of those who were working differed little from uninjured controls, or the male labor force (Kraft et al., 1993). Thus severity of injury appears to affect educational achievement and return to work, but not the occupational distribution of those who do manage to return, implying some level of plasticity may occur which can overcome loss or brain tissue, but may still be restrained by other psychological or social factors.

GENETICS

It has been established that that recovery of function after brain damage results from complex interactions between both environmental effects and genetic factors (Lindsay et al., 2002). In recent years, there has also been increasing evidence of links of between-specific genotypes and risk for accelerated cognitive decline or dementia following TBI. Any associations found between genetic information and outcome following TBI may also aid the acute triage of brain-injured patients as well as help to target future treatments.

One of the major advances at PH3 was the assessment of a large number of the genetic markers and their relation to various outcome measures. Raymont et al. (2008) reported the links with cognition. All subjects were both healthy and physically fit before their injury, yet preinjury intelligence was found to be significantly predicted by the following genotypes; GRIN2C rs689730, GAD2 rs2839670, and DBH444. It was suggested that the presence of all of these markers could account for 15.5% of the variability in preinjury intelligence. However, only GRIN2A rs968301 was found to be able to predict current intelligence and change in intelligence from preinjury to PH3. Experimental animal studies have revealed impaired plasticity following TBI, even in the absence of significant anatomical damage (Giza et al., 2006), evidenced by examining *N*-methyl-D-aspartate (NMDA). NMDA consists of a number of subunits, including the GRIN glutamate receptor, which seems to be specifically involved in the pathophysiology of CHI, including acting as a marker of neuronal death (Parton et al., 2005). There was a trend for dominant homozygotes to have a greater level of decline in intelligence from PH2 to PH3.

	R	Model chi square	Degree of freedom	*p*
Model 1 Work = preinjury intelligence	0.17	21.50	1 *df*	0.001
Model 2 Work = preinjury intelligence + volume loss	0.39	99.66	2 *df*	0.001
Model 3 Work = postinjury intelligence	0.38	90.44	1 *df*	0.001
Model 4 Work = postinjury intelligence + volume loss	0.48	141.58	2 *df*	0.001
Model 5 Work = postinjury intelligence + volume loss + disability score*	0.50	111.43	3 *df*	0.001
Model 6 Work = disability score	0.42	83.68	1 *df*	0.001

* Residual disability score: Number of residual impairments (1-7)

FIGURE 5 | Logistic regression analysis outcomes for predictive factors of variation in work status.

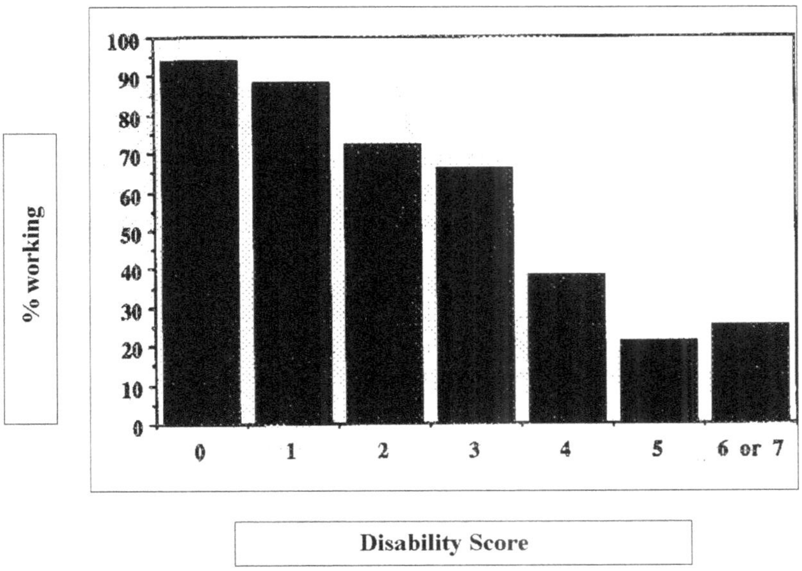

FIGURE 6 | Vietnam Head Injury Study, percent working by disability score. The disability score represents the number of disabilities present (1–7).

Neurotrophins such as brain-derived neurotrophic factor (BDNF) have an impact on neuronal function and synaptic plasticity in the brain (Varon et al., 1991). Recent evidence has shown functional differences between the proteins coded for by the val66 and met66 BDNF alleles in healthy subjects and patients with neurological or psychiatric disorders (Krueger et al., 2011). PH3 reported a functional relationship between the BDNF val66met genotype and recovery of executive function in subjects with frontal lobe lesions. Individuals carrying one or two copies of the BDNF met allele performed significantly better on cognitive tests measuring executive functions of the frontal cortex compared with individuals carrying the val/val homozygotes, suggesting that the val66met BDNF polymorphism may act differently in the injured and healthy brain.

OVERALL SIGNIFICANCE AND CONSEQUENCES OF THE VHIS

The US military population offers a number of advantages for the study of the effects of TBI; its size, relative uniformity, the fact that all subjects are initially healthy, and the potential for long-term follow-up. Additionally, preinjury intelligence and aptitude testing is available on most military recruits, and the VA medical system allows them to be tracked over a long follow-up period. Given this, and the timing of its initiation coinciding with greater survival from conflict-related TBI, means the VHIS has been and continues to be instrumental in gathering long-term data about subjects with TBI. Results from the VHIS have suggested that penetrating TBI carries a high risk of long-term sequelae, such as PTE and cognitive impairment, which may occur decades after injury, so has provided solid evidence that such patients may require long-term medical follow up. It should be emphasized, however, that these results may not always be generalizable to closed TBI, and therefore the type of injuries seen in the civilian population. Our findings are probably compatible with focal lesions secondary to a variety of causes (e.g., stroke, tumor, etc.), but closed TBI may have additional white matter shearing and pathology that is more extensive than that seen in penetrating TBI. Penetrating TBI also crosses traditional vascular boundaries and does not generally respect different neuronal susceptibilities to disease, so does have a unique signature or profile of impairments in any individual patient, but by interpreting our results by lesion site, we have tried to make our results generalizable by location. However, the ability to maintain a longitudinal assessment of a large sample of subjects from preinjury, through acute injury and many years of follow up is fraught with difficulties. The VHIS has only been able to review the long-term clinical, neuropsychological, and genetic characteristics in a subset of the original cohort, and we may well have seen differing results if we had been able to examine the entire sample throughout the length of the study.

Besides a core clinical evaluation, each phase of the VHIS has tried to address emerging issues within cognitive neuroscience, neurology, and psychiatry. For instance, the need for an accurate assessment of the brain lesions in PH3 lead to the development of the ABLe software program (Makale et al., 2002; Solomon et al., 2007), which characterizes lesions in terms of volume and intersection with Brodmann areas and allows for correlations between subjects with overlapping lesions and behavioral deficit.

In addition, PH2 of the VHIS led directly to the establishment of the Defense and Veterans Head Injury Program (DVHIP). Such TBI units and programs at major Military and VA Hospitals continue to operate to this day, now as Defense and Veterans Brain Injury Centers (DVBIC). Until the creation of the DVHIP, there had been no national systematic program providing TBI-specific care and rehabilitation within the VA (Salazar et al., 2000). The DVHIP was created initially as an interagency clinical program oriented to treatment, rehabilitation, and care management. It was formed by collaboration between the Department of Defense, the Department of Veteran Affairs, the Brain Injury Association (BIA), and the International Brain Injury Association (IBIA). The principal goals of the program now are to ensure that military and veteran TBI patients receive standardized TBI-specific evaluation, treatment, and follow-up, while at the same time helping to define optimal acute and chronic care for victims of TBI nationwide, as well as conducting rehabilitation and clinical treatment trials. The DVHIP also included a simple, updated Head and Spinal Combat Injury Registry form similar to that used by in the original VHIS registry, which is now used within the military and VA via the DVBIC. This has been approved by the Joint Committee of Military Neurosurgeons of the American Association of Neurological Surgeons (AANS) and Congress of Neurological Surgeons (CNS) for deployment in time of war. Thus not only has the VHIS been vital in its contribution to our understanding of TBI and neuropsychology, it has helped produce a system that will facilitate the early identification of future injured soldiers and their long-term management – a worthy legacy for Dr. Caveness and the many victims of TBI studied in the last 40 years. The unique breadth and length of follow up of this cohort makes the future prospects

Table 1 | Five key findings of the VHIS.

PHASE 1
Predictors of brain infection.
Defer cranioplasty until 1 year post-TBI.
Incidence of motor deficits – parietal wounds associated with hemiparesis.
Aphasia occurred in about 25%, correlating with gunshot cause and initial loss of consciousness.
Skull defects and cranioplasty did not predict tendency to PTE.
PHASE 2
Greatest predictor of cognitive decline is premorbid IQ.
Incidence of PTE can be predicted by and left hippocampus lesions correlate with seizure frequency.
Deficits in semantic memory, verbal episodic memory, and visual episodic memory were found to be associated with lesion location.
Right orbitofrontal lesions were prone to anxiety and depression, whereas patients with left dorsofrontal lesions were prone to anger and hostility. Such studies lead to further conclusions on the regional contribution of planning and representations, which ultimately lead to theories of how the brain represents knowledge and responds to complex events.
Seven impairments correlated with work status; PTE, paresis, visual field loss, verbal memory loss, visual memory loss, psychological problems, and violent behavior.
PHASE 3
Greatest predictor of cognitive decline is premorbid IQ.
GRIN2A rs968301 may predict current intelligence and change in change in intelligence after TBI.
Short term memory deficits were found in all classes of brain-injured individuals, regardless of lesion location pattern.
Bilateral ventromedial PFC lesions were associated with low levels of depression, whereas bilateral dorsal PFC lesions (involving dorsomedial and dorsolateral areas in both hemispheres) were associated with substantially higher levels of depression.
Left parietal lobe lesions and retained ferric metal fragments were associated with PTE and total brain volume loss predicted seizure frequency.

Table 2 | Possible future goals for studies of military TBI patients.

1. Further longitudinal studies to explore long-term cognitive impairment post-TBI, and its interaction with normal aging, dementias and other diseases.
2. Comparison of current blast injuries with prior data on closed and penetrating injuries.
3. Combine functional and structural studies to compare functional and connectivity changes, to improve research and clinical imaging of penetrating and closed TBI.
4. Extend genotyping and proteomic research to assess inheritable factors for brain damage response and neuroplasticity, and using such knowledge to help triage types of TBI acutely and target future treatments.
5. Further examination of the role of psychological and psychiatric pathology in cognitive outcome.
6. Additional pathological and imaging correlates of clinical outcome.
7. Addressing emerging cognitive neuroscience issues.
8. Development of neuroprotection as well as cell-based rehabilitation strategies to enhance plasticity.

for information to be collected from PH4 very exciting, and the VHIS has provided a model for subsequent longitudinal studies of TBI (**Tables 1** and **2**). Given the increasing numbers of both civilian patients and military casualties suffering TBI, which will certainly require care in the future, expanding such research seems long overdue.

ACKNOWLEDGMENTS

We are grateful to our research participants whose dedicated, selfless, long-term commitment to the Vietnam Head Injury Study enabled us to carry out our research and change the way the United States military diagnoses and treats traumatic brain injury. We also thank all of the associated principal investigators and collaborators who have helped insure the success of our research program. In particular we want to single out Herbert Brown, Max Hoyt, Karen Schwab, and William F. Caveness for their efforts in helping establish and sustain the Vietnam Head Injury Study. Finally, one of us (Jordan Grafman) benefited from the wise consul of Freda Newcombe, Charles G. Matthews, Herbert Weingartner, and Alwyn Lishman in the early stages of the Vietnam Head Injury Study.

REFERENCES

AFQT-7A. (1960). Department of Defense Form 1293. March 1.

Barbey, A. K., Krueger, F., and Grafman, J. (2009). An evolutionarily adaptive neural architecture for social reason- ing. *Trends Neurosci.* 32, 603–610.

Bender, M. B., and Teuber, H. L. (1948). Spatial organization of visual per- ception following injury to the brain. *Arch. Neurol. Psychiatry* 59, 39–62.

Boake, C., and Diller, L. (2005). "History of rehabilitation for traumatic brain injury," in *Rehabilitation for Trau- matic Brain Injury*, eds W. M. High, A. M. Sander, M. A. Struchen, and K. Hart (Oxford: Oxford University Press), 3–13.

Carey, M. E., Sacco, W., and Merkler, J. (1982). An analysis of fatal and non- fatal head wounds incurred dur- ing combat in Vietnam by U.S. forces. *Acta Chir. Scand. Suppl.* 508, 351–356.

Carlin, D., Bonerba, J., Phipps, M., Alexander, G., Shapiro, M., and Graf- man, J. (2000). Planning impair- ments in frontal lobe dementia and frontal lobe lesion patients. *Neu- ropsychologia* 38, 655–665.

Caveness, W. F., Meirowsky, A. M., Rish, L., Mohr, J. P., Kistler, J. P., Dil- lon, D., and Weiss, G. H. (1979). The nature of posttraumatic epilepsy. *J. Neurosurg.* 50, 545–553.

Corkin, S., Rosen, T. J., Sullivan, E. V., and Clegg, R. A. (1989). Pene- trating head injury in young adult- hood exacerbates cognitive decline in later years. *J. Neurosci.* 9, 3876–3883.

Corkin, S., Sullivan, E. V., and Carr, F. A. (1984). Prognostic factors for life expectancy after penetrating head injury. *Arch. Neurol.* 41, 975–977.

Dimitrov, M., Grafman, J., and Holl- nagel, C. (1996). The effects of frontal lobe damage on every- day problem solving. *Cortex* 32, 357–366.

Dimitrov, M., Phipps, M., Zahnl, T. P., and Grafman, J. (1999). A thor- oughly modern gage. *Neurocase* 5, 345–354.

Forbes, C. E., and Grafman, J. (2010). The role of the human prefrontal cortex in social cognition and moral judgment. *Annu. Rev. Neurosci.* 33, 299–324.

Frattali, C., Hanna, R., McGinty, A. S., Gerber, L., Wesley, R., Grafman, J., and Coelho, C. (2007). Effect of pre- frontal cortex damage on resolving lexical ambiguity in text. *Brain Lang.* 102, 99–113.

Giza, C. C., Maria, N. S., and Hovda, D. A. (2006). N-methyl-D-aspartate receptor subunit changes after trau- matic brain injury to the developing brain. *J. Neurotrauma* 23, 950–961.

Goel, V., and Grafman, J. (1995). Are the frontal lobes implicated in "plan- ning" functions? Re-interpreting data from the tower of Hanoi. *Neu- ropsychologia* 33, 623–642.

Goel, V., and Grafman, J. (2000). Role of the right prefrontal cortex in Ill-structured planning. *Cogn. Neu- ropsychol.* 17, 415–436.

Goel, V., Pullara, S. D., and Grafman, J. (2001). A computational model of frontal lobe dysfunction: work- ing memory and the tower of Hanoi task. *Cogn. Sci.* 25, 287–313.

Goel, V., Shuren, J., Sheesley, L., and Grafman, J. (2004). Asymmetrical involvement of frontal lobes in social reasoning. *Brain* 127, 783–790.

Goel, V., Stollstorff, M., Nakic, M., Knut- son, K., and Grafman, J. (2009). A Role for right ventromedial pre- frontal cortex in reasoning about indeterminate relations. *Neuropsy- chologia* 47, 2790–2797.

Goel, V., Tierney, M., Sheesley, L., Bar- tolo, A., Vartanian, O., and Graf- man, J. (2007). Hemispheric spe- cialization in human prefrontal cor- tex for resolving certain and uncer- tain inferences. *Cereb. Cortex* 17, 2245–2250.

Gozzi, M., Raymont, V., Solomon, J., Koenigs, M., and Grafman, J. (2009). Dissociable effects of prefrontal and anterior temporal cortical lesions on stereotypical gender attitudes. *Neu- rology* 74, 749–754.

Grafman, J., Jonas, B., and Salazar, A. (1992). Epilepsy following penetrat- ing head injury to the frontal lobes. Effects on cognition. *Adv. Neurol.* 57, 369–378.

Grafman, J., Jonas, B. S., Martin, A., Salazar, A. M., Weingartner, H., Lud- low, C., Smutok, M. A., and Vance, S. (1988). Intellectual function fol- lowing penetrating head injury in Vietnam veterans. *Brain* 111(Pt 1), 169–184.

Grafman, J., Kampen, D., Rosenberg, J., Salazar, A., and Boller, F. (1989). Calculation abilities in a patient with a virtual left hemispherectomy. *Behav. Neurol.* 2, 183–194.

Grafman, J., and Salazar, A. (1999). The William Fields Caveness Viet- nam head injury study: past and future. *Brain Inj. Source* 3, 12–14.

Grafman, J., Salazar, A., Weingartner, H., Vance, S., and Amin, D. (1986a). The relationship of brain-tissue loss vol- ume and lesion location to cognitive deficit. *J. Neurosci.* 6, 301–307.

Grafman, J., Salazar, A. M., Weingart- ner, H., and Amin, D. (1986b). Face memory and discrimination: a pre- liminary analysis of the persistent effects of penetrating brain wounds. *Int. J. Neurosci.* 29, 125–139.

Grafman, J., Vance, S. C., Weingart- ner, H., Salazar, A. M, and Amin, (1986c). The effects of lateralized frontal lesions on mood regulation. *Brain* 109(Pt 6), 1127–1148.

Grafman, J., Smutok, M., Sweeney, J., Vance, S. C., Salazar, A. M., and Weingartner, H. (1985a). Effects of left-hand preference on postinjury measures of distal motor ability. *Per- cept. Mot. Skills* 61, 615–624.

Grafman, J., Salazar, A. M., Weingart- ner, H., Vance, S. C., and Lud- low, C. (1985b). Isolated impairment of memory following a penetrating lesion of the fornix. *Arch. Neurol.* 42, 1162–1168.

Grafman, J., Schwab, K., Warden, D., Pridgen, A., Brown, H. R., and Salazar, A. M. (1996). Frontal lobe injuries, violence, and aggression: a report of the Vietnam head injury study. *Neurology* 46, 1231–1238.

Groswasser, Z., Reider-Groswasser, I. I., Schwab, K., Ommaya, A. K., Prid- gen, A., Brown, H. R., Cole, R., and Salazar, A. M. (2002). Quantitative imaging in late TBI. Part II: cogni- tion and work after closed and pen- etrating head injury: a report of the Vietnam head injury study. *Brain Inj.* 16, 681–690.

Harlow, J. M. (1848). Passage of an iron rod through the head. *Boston Med. Surg. J.* 39, 389–393.
Harlow, J. M. (1868). *Recovery After Severe Injury to the Head.* Boston: Massachusetts Medical Society.
Holmes, G. (1941). Henry Head. *Obit. Not. Fell. R. Soc.* 3, 665–689.
Holmes, G., and Lister, W. T. (1916). Disturbances of vision from cere- bral lesions, with special reference to the cortical representation of the macula. *Brain* 39, 34.
Jonas, B. S., Schwab, K., and Salazar, A. M. (1987). "Factors influencing participation in a multi-stage study of head injury: potential biases in the Vietnam head injury study," in *Proceedings of the Section on Survey Research Methods of the Association for Statistical Analysis.*
Koenigs, M., Barbey, A., Postle, B. R., and Grafman, J. (2009a). Supe- rior parietal cortex is critical for the manipulation of information in working memory. *J. Neurosci.* 29, 14980–14986.
Koenigs, M., Huey, E. D., Raymont, V., Cheon, B., Solomon, J., Wassermann, E. M., and Grafman, J. (2009b). Focal brain damage protects against post- traumatic stress disorder in combat veterans. *Proc. Natl. Acad. Sci. U.S.A.* 106, 22486–22491.
Koenigs, M., Holliday, J., Solomon, J., and Grafman, J. (2010). Left dorso- medial frontal brain damage is asso- ciated with insomnia. *J. Neurosci.* 30, 16041–16043.
Koenigs, M., Huey, E. D., Calamia, M., Raymont, V., Tranel, D., and Graf- man, J. (2008). Distinct regions of prefrontal cortex mediate resistance and vulnerability to depression. *Nat. Neurosci.* 11, 232–237.
Kraft, J. F., Schwab, K. A., Salazar, A. M., and Brown, H. R. (1993). Occupa- tional and educational achievements of head injured Vietnam veterans at 15-year follow-up. *Arch. Phys. Med. Rehabil.* 74, 596–601.
Kraus, J. F., and McArthur, D. L. (1996). Epidemiologic aspects of brain injury. *Neurol. Clin.* 14, 435–450.
Krueger, F., Barbey, A. K., McCabe, K., Strenziok, M., Zamboni, G., Solomon, J., Raymont, V., and Grafman, J. (2009). The neural bases of key competencies of emotional intelligence. *Proc. Natl. Acad. Sci. U.S.A.* 106, 22486–22491.
Krueger, F., Pardini, M., Huey, E. D., Raymont, V., Solomon, J., Lipsky, R. H., Hodgkinson, C. A., Gold- man, D., and Grafman, J. (2011). The role of the Met66 brain-derived neurotrophic factor allele in the recovery of executive functioning after combat-related traumatic brain injury. *J. Neurosci.* 31, 598–606.
Lackner, J. R. (2009). Hans-Lukas Teu- ber: a remembrance. *Neuropsychol. Rev.* 19, 4–7.
Lee, S. S., Wild, K., Hollnagel, C., and Grafman, J. (1999). Selective visual attention in patients with frontal lobe lesions or Parkinson's disease. *Neuropsychologia* 37, 595–604.
Lepore, F. E. (1994). Harvey Cushing, Gordon Holmes, and the neurolog- ical lessons of World War I. *Arch. Neurol.* 51, 711–722.
Lindsay, J., Laurin, D., Verreault, R., Hebert, R., Helliwell, B., Hill, G. B., and McDowell, I. (2002). Risk factors for Alzheimer's disease: a prospective analysis from the Cana- dian study of health and aging. *Am. J. Epidemiol.* 156, 445–453.
Lishman, W. A. (1992). What is neu- ropsychiatry? *J. Neurol. Neurosurg. Psychiatr.* 55, 983–985.
Ludlow, C. L., Rosenberg, J., Fair, C., Buck, D., Schesselman, S., and Salazar, A. (1986). Brain lesions asso- ciated with nonfluent aphasia fifteen years following penetrating head injury. *Brain* 109(Pt 1), 55–80.
Luria, A. R. (1972). *The Man with a Shattered World: The History of a Brain Wound.* New York: Basic Books.
Mah, L., Arnold, M. C., and Grafman, J. (2004). Lesions of prefrontal cor- tex impair social perception. *Am. J. Psychiatry* 161, 1247–1255.
Mah, L. W. Y., Arnold, M. C., and Graf- man, J. (2005). Deficits in social knowledge following lesions of ven- tromedial prefrontal cortex. *J. Neu- ropsychiatry Clin. Neurosci.* 17, 66–74.
Makale, M., Solomon, J., Patronas, N. J., Danek, A., Butman, J. A., and Graf- man, J. (2002). Quantification of brain lesions using interactive auto- mated software. *Behav. Res. Methods Instrum. Comput.* 34, 6–18.
Milne, E., and Grafman, J. (2001). Ven- tromedial prefrontal cortex lesions in humans eliminate implicit gender stereotyping. *J. Neurosci.* 21, 1–6.
Mishkin, M. (1972). "Cortical visual areas and their interactions," in *Brain and Human Behavior*, eds G. Kar- czmar and J. C. Eccles (Berlin: Springer), 178–208.
Mohr, J. P., Weiss, G. H., Caveness, W. F., Dillon, J. D., Kistler, J. P., Meirowsky, A. M., and Rish, B. L. (1980). Language and motor disor- ders after penetrating head injury in Vietnam. *Neurology* 30, 1273–1279.
Muthén, L. K., and Muthén, B. O. (1998– 2004). Mplus User's Guide, 3rd Edn. Los Angeles: Muthén & Muthén.
Newcombe, F., Brooks, N., and Badde- ley, A. (1980). Rehabilitation after brain damage: an overview. *Int. Rehabil. Med.* 2, 133–137.
Pardini, M., Krueger, F., Hodgkinson, C., Raymont, V., Ferrier, C., Gold- man, D., Strenziok, M., Guida, S., and Grafman, J. (in press). Prefrontal cortex lesions and MAO-A modulate aggression in penetrating traumatic brain injury.
Pardini, M., Krueger, F., Raymont, V., and Grafman, J. (2010). Ventro- medial prefrontal cortex modulates fatigue after penetrating traumatic brain injury. *Neurology* 74, 749–754.
Parton, A., Coulthard, E., and Husain, M. (2005). Neuropharmacological modulation of cognitive deficits after brain damage. *Curr. Opin. Neu- rol.* 18, 675–680.
Rattermann, M. J., Spector, L., Grafman, J., Levin, H., and Howard, H. (2001). Partial and total-order planning: evi- dence from normal and prefrontally damaged populations. *Cogn. Sci.* 25, 941–975.
Raymont, V., and Grafman, J. (2006). Cognitive neural plasticity dur- ing learning and recovery from brain damage. *Prog. Brain Res.* 157, 199–206.
Raymont, V., Greathouse, A., Red- ing, K., Lipsky, R., Salazar, A., and Grafman, J. (2008). Demographic, structural and genetic predictors of late cognitive decline after penetrat- ing head injury. *Brain* 131(Pt 2), 543–558.
Raymont, V., Salazar, A. M., Lipsky, R., Goldman, D., Tasick, G., and Graf- man, J. (2010). Correlates of post- traumatic epilepsy 35 years follow- ing combat brain injury. *Neurology* 75, 224–229.
Rish, B. L., Caveness, W. F., Dillon, J. D., Kistler, J. P., Mohr, J. P., and Weiss, G. H. (1981). Analysis of brain abscess after penetrating cran- iocerebral injuries in Vietnam. *Neu- rosurgery* 9, 535–541.
Rish, B. L., Dillon, J. D., Caveness, W. F., Mohr, J. P., Kistler, J. P., and Weiss, G. H. (1980). Evolu- tion of craniotomy as a debridement technique for penetrating cranio- cerebral injuries. *J. Neurosurg.* 53, 772–775.
Rish, B. L., Dillon, J. D., Meirowsky, A. M., Caveness, W. F., Mohr, J. P., Kistler, J. P., and Weiss, G. H. (1979). Cranioplasty: a review of 1030 cases of penetrating head injury. *Neuro- surgery* 4, 381–385.
Rish, B. L., Dillon, J. D., and Weiss, G. H. (1983). Mortality following pen- etrating craniocerebral injuries. An analysis of the deaths in the Vietnam head injury registry population. *J. Neurosurg.* 59, 775–780.
Romero, S. G., Manly, C. F., and Graf- man, J. (2002). Investigating cogni- tive neuroplasticity in single cases: Lessons learned from applying func- tional neuroimaging techniques to the traditional neuropsychological case study framework. *Neurocase* 8, 355–368.
Rueckert, L., and Grafman, J. (1996). Sustained attention deficits in patients with right frontal lesions. *Neuropsychologia* 34, 953–963.
Rueckert, L., and Grafman, J. (1998). Sustained attention deficits in patients with lesions of poste- rior cortex. *Neuropsychologia* 36, 653–660.
Salazar, A., Grafman, J., Jabbari, B., Vance, S. C., and Amin, D. (1987). "Epilepsy and cognitive loss after penetrating head injury," in *Advances in Epileptology*, eds P. Wolf, W. Dam, M. Janz and F. Dreifuss (New York: Raven Press), 627–631.
Salazar, A. M., Grafman, J., Vance, S. C., Weingartner, H., Dillon, J. D., and Ludlow, C. (1986). Conscious- ness and amnesia following pene- trating head injury. *Neurology* 36, 178–187.
Salazar, A. M., Jabbari, B., Vance, S. C., Grafman, J., Amin, D., and Dillon, J. D. (1985). Epilepsy after penetrating head injury. I. Clinical correlates: a report of the Vietnam head injury study. *Neurology* 35, 1406–1414.
Salazar, A. M., Schwab, K., and Grafman, J. H. (1995). Penetrating injuries in the Vietnam war. Traumatic uncon- sciousness, epilepsy, and psychoso- cial outcome. *Neurosurg. Clin. N. Am.* 6, 715–726.
Salazar, A. M., Zitnay, G. A., Warden, D. L., and Schwab, K. A. (2000). Defense and Veterans Head Injury Program: background and overview. *J. Head Trauma Rehabil.* 15, 1081–1091.
Sanfey, A. G., Hastie, R., Colvin, M. K., and Grafman, J. (2003). Phineas Gauged: decision-making and the human prefrontal cortex. *Neuropsy- chologia* 41, 1218–1229.
Schooler, C., Caplan, L. J., Revell, A. J., Salazar, A. M., and Grafman, J. (2008). Brain lesion and memory functioning: short-term memory deficit is independent of lesion location. *Psychon. Bull. Rev.* 15, 521–527.
Schwab, K., Grafman, J., Salazar, A. M., and Kraft, J. (1993). Residual impair- ments and work status 15 years after penetrating head injury: report from the Vietnam head injury study. *Neu- rology* 43, 95–103.
Smutok, M. A., Grafman, J., Salazar, A. M., Sweeney, J. K., Jonas, B. S., and DiRocco, P. J. (1989). Effects of uni- lateral brain damage on contralateral and ipsilateral upper extremity func- tion in hemiplegia. *Phys. Ther.* 69, 195–203.
Solomon, J., Raymont, V., Braun, A., Butman, J. A., and Grafman, J. (2007). User-friendly software for the analysis of brain lesions (ABLe). *Comput. Methods Programs Biomed.* 86, 245–254.

Teuber, H. L. (1975). Recovery of func- tion after brain injury in man. *Ciba Found. Symp.* 34, 159–190.

van Gijn, J. (2009). From the archives. Cerebral involvement in head injury. A study based on the examination of two hundred cases. By W. Ritchie Russell, MD. 1932; 55: 549–603.*Brain* 132, 565–567.

Varon, S., Hagg, T., and Manthorpe, M. (1991). Nerve growth factor in CNS repair and regeneration. *Adv. Exp. Med. Biol.* 296, 267–276.

Warden, D. J. (2006). Military TBI during the Iraq and Afghanistan wars. *Head Trauma Rehabil.* 21, 398–402.

Weinstein, S., and Teuber, H. L. (1957). The role of pre-injury education and intelligence level in intellectual loss after brain injury. *J. Comp. Physiol. Psychol.* 50, 535–539.

Weiss, G. H., and Caveness, W. F. (1972). Prognostic factors in the persistence of posttraumatic epilepsy. *J. Neuro- surg.* 37, 164–169.

Weiss, G.H., Feeney, D.M., Caveness, W.F., Dillon, D., Kistler, J. P., Mohr, J. P., and Rish, B. L. (1983). Prognostic factors for the occurrence of posttraumatic epilepsy. *Arch. Neurol.* 40, 7–10.

Weiss, G. H., Salazar, A. M., Vance, S. C., Grafman, J., and Jabbari, B. (1986). Predicting posttraumatic epilepsy in penetrating head injury. *Arch. Neu- rol.* 43, 771–773.

Walker, A. E., and Jablon, S. (1961). *A Follow up Study of Head Wounds in World War II.* Washington, DC: Veterans Administration.

Wood, J. N., and Grafman, J. (2003). Human prefrontal cortex: pro- cessing and representational per- spectives. *Nat. Rev. Neurosci.* 4, 139–147.

Wood, J. N., Romero, S. G., Makale, M., and Grafman, J. (2003). Category- specific representations of social and non-social knowledge in the human prefrontal cortex. *J. Cogn. Neurosci.* 15, 236–248.

2

Before it is too late: professional responsibilities in late-onset Alzheimer's research and pre-symptomatic prediction

Silke Schicktanz[1]*, Mark Schweda[1,2], Jesse F. Ballenger[3], Patrick J. Fox[4], Jodi Halpern[5], Joel H. Kramer[6], Guy Micco[5], Stephen G. Post[7], Charis Thompson[8,9], Robert T. Knight[10,11] and William J. Jagust[5,11]

[1] Department of Medical Ethics and History of Medicine, University Medical Center Göttingen, Göttingen, Germany
[2] Lichtenberg Kolleg, University of Göttingen, Göttingen, Germany
[3] Health Administration Department, Drexel University, Philadelphia, PA, USA
[4] Institute for Health & Aging, University of California, San Francisco, San Francisco, CA, USA
[5] UC Berkeley-UCSF Joint Medical Program, School of Public Health, University of California, Berkeley, Berkeley, CA, USA
[6] Memory and Aging Center, Sandler Neurosciences Center, University of California, San Francisco, San Francisco, CA, USA
[7] Compassionate Care & Bioethics, Stony Brook Medicine, Stony Brook, NY, USA
[8] Department of Gender and Women's Studies, University of California, Berkeley, Berkeley, CA, USA
[9] Department of Sociology, London School of Economics, London, UK
[10] Department of Psychology, University of California, Berkeley, Berkeley, CA, USA
[11] Helen Wills Neuroscience Institute, University of California, Berkeley, Berkeley, CA, USA

Edited by:
Aron K. Barbey, University of Illinois at Urbana-Champaign, USA

Reviewed by:
Jim M. Monti, Beckman Institute for Advanced Science and Technology, USA
Edward Huey, Columbia University, USA

***Correspondence:**
Silke Schicktanz, Department of Medical Ethics and History of Medicine, University Medical Center Göttingen, Humboldtallee 36, 37073 Göttingen, Germany
e-mail: Silke.schicktanz@medizin.uni-goettingen.de

The development of a wide array of molecular and neuroscientific biomarkers can provide the possibility to visualize the course of Alzheimer's disease (AD) at early stages. Many of these biomarkers are aimed at detecting not only a preclinical, but also a pre-symptomatic state. They are supposed to facilitate clinical trials aiming at treatments that attack the disease at its earliest stage or even prevent it. The increasing number of such biomarkers currently tested and now partly proposed for clinical implementation calls for critical reflection on their aims, social benefits, and risks. This position paper summarizes major challenges and responsibilities. Its focus is on the ethical and social problems involved in the organization and application of dementia research, as well as in healthcare provision from a cross-national point of view. The paper is based on a discussion of leading dementia experts from neuroscience, neurology, social sciences, and bioethics in the United States and Europe. It thus reflects a notable consensus across various disciplines and national backgrounds. We intend to initiate a debate on the need for actions within the researchers' national and international communities.

Keywords: late-onset Alzheimer's dementia, medical ethics, recommendations, biomarker, public health policy, research participation, cultural diversity, public engagement

INTRODUCTION

Alzheimer's disease (AD) is a substantial individual threat and a major public-health challenge (WHO, 2012). Until now, there is no preventive measure or curative therapy for late-onset AD (LOAD), and symptom relief is limited (Daviglus et al., 2010). New research approaches aim at delaying onset of LOAD through treatment of "at-risk individuals". This mirrors a general shift from pathological diagnosis to assessment of risk factors: Prediction and the start of treatment are now considered plausible approaches at the pre-symptomatic phase (Sperling et al., 2011, 2013; Shim and Morris, 2011).

Biomarkers for the identification of at-risk healthy individuals include genetic testing of APOE ε4 (Keage et al., 2010) as well as vascular risk factors (Kivipelto et al., 2005). Neurological biomarkers comprise positron emission tomography (PET) measures of beta-amyloid plaques (Aβ) (Nordberg et al., 2013), cerebrospinal fluid (CSF levels of Aβ and of total-and phosphorylated-tau) (Visser et al., 2009; Landau and Frosch, 2014), functional and structural magnetic resonance imaging (MRI), e.g., hippocampal volume (Filippi et al., 2012), and biomarkers reflecting metabolic or inflammatory changes associated with LOAD (Mapstone et al., 2014). Several of these biomarkers might predict LOAD even at the mild cognitive impairment (MCI) (Petrella et al., 2011; Prestia et al., 2013) or pre-MCI stage (Parra et al., 2010). Since some examinations are invasive, time-consuming, expensive, or ethically problematic, neuro-psychological and cognitive tests (e.g., MiniMental-State (MMSE)) (Jessen et al., 2011; Palmqvist et al., 2012) or blood tests (Mapstone et al., 2014) are also explored as low-cost-low-risk tests for potential public screening. The likely dynamic of different biomarkers during the pathophysiological process of LOAD is a major challenge (Jack et al., 2013) and still requires extensive validation of the various markers (Albert et al., 2011).

In summary, the stages discussed include a long asymptomatic stage where healthy or minimally symptomatic individuals have different (genetic, physiological, or molecular) risk factors, followed by a pre-dementia stage with mild symptoms that can be differentiated into subjective cognitive impairment (SCI) or MCI, and, finally, a symptomatic clinical dementia stage. For each of these different stages, biomarkers like the ones mentioned above are being explored and need to be validated in view of their use for dementia prevention. Three major levels are distinguished that parallel the three stages of disease development (Wright et al., 2009; Kryscio, 2014): *Primary prevention* addresses the healthy public; *secondary prevention* aims at early detection of disease by screening biomarkers to apply treatment that can stop progression. *Tertiary prevention* follows the clinical diagnosis with the aim of slowing down progression or reducing complications. The biomarkers as well as the diagnosis of the prodromal stage need to be validated, reproduced, standardized, and tested for predictive value in longitudinal studies. However, the potential for biomarkers to identify individuals who are asymptomatic and could benefit from therapies (not yet available) has revolutionized thinking about the approach to dementia care and changed the landscape of clinical trials for dementia.

This trend towards pre-symptomatic prediction has recently evoked strong ethical and sociological criticism (Le Couteur et al., 2013; Lock, 2013). Thus, David Le Couteur and his colleagues argue that it will mainly lead to overdiagnosis of AD and will therefore rather harm people. It is important to note that the development of biomarkers for LOAD occurs in an environment that, so far, largely lacks systematic ethical reflection. There is not even a specific ethical framework that could help politicians, public health decision makers, healthcare professionals, and families to deal with people at risk for developing dementia. Since biomarker research for dementia is still in its infancy, this is a critical point in time for developing an appropriate ethical framework in view of current research and future clinical implementation. The potential of current biomarker research to challenge understandings and clinical practices regarding LOAD should not be underestimated (Waldemar et al., 2007). In addition to the above mentioned future aim of primary, secondary, and tertiary prevention, some biomarkers have been approved by regulatory agencies and are, at least theoretically, available for clinical application. Such biomarkers could theoretically be used for predictive and screening purposes. This could occur if patients request these tests or if these tests were publicly promoted, e.g., as part of a so-called national dementia strategy.

Important questions that have not found sufficient consideration, so far, are related to the value and risk of knowing for different actors such as potentially affected persons, their families, the medical profession, and the various national healthcare systems (Karlawish, 2011). Furthermore, the current scholarly debate has to expand its scope beyond the setting of Western, industrialized countries. While healthcare policies and legal frameworks are contextualized in national settings, the research community is increasingly globalized. The resulting tensions have not received sufficient consideration, so far. They pose new problems and emphasize our responsibility as professionals and scientists to act as mediators between local contexts and global developments.

The following interdisciplinary considerations identify four different ethical and social dimensions, thus systematizing the current debate around central problems, controversies, and open questions in order to promote future research initiatives and open a more cross-cultural perspective: 1. healthcare and research policy balancing between research for early diagnosis and care provision for existing patients, 2. ethical issues related to participation in dementia research and disclosure of information on pre-dementia stages such as MCI, 3. long-term implications of dealing with predictive information on a personal and social level in different cultures and healthcare systems, and 4. enhancing the dialog between scientists, the public, and persons being directly affected.

PUBLIC POLICY GOALS AND CONCERNS

RATIONALE

Late-onset AD has become the target of many national action plans worldwide, e.g., in Australia, France, the Netherlands, Norway, and England. The challenge of the research lies in the complexity of progressive, multi-dimensional dementing syndromes: First, the aging brain can show multiple forms of pathological change causing dementia progression. Second, even in LOAD, different neuropathological factors, such as amyloid plaques, neurofibrillary tangles, and synaptic alterations, have been identified, but the contribution of each to the clinical picture is controversial. Third, LOAD often shows mixed etiology with vascular diseases. Finally, relationships between the genetic and neuronal level on the one hand and the cognitive and behavioral level on the other have not been established.

A variety of approaches are employed to diagnose LOAD (Waldemar et al., 2007). Genetic ApoE-tests are not recommended due to their low predictive value (Goldman et al., 2011). The major paradigm shift is to identify brain changes as biomarkers for predicting cognitive decline at preclinical stages (Albert et al., 2011; Hampel et al., 2014). Even among AD researchers, the concept of pre-symptomatic AD is being debated and requires validation. Although methods of neuroimaging to detect disease specific pathological brain changes might offer better prediction than genetic testing, they also raise important public health concerns regarding resource allocation.

RECOMMENDATIONS

In the framework of democratic regulation of research and healthcare, shifts in agenda and priority setting require public information and debate. If early diagnosis is to be clinically employed, there is a need to validate the biomarkers and to identify possible co-factors explaining variation between pathological and symptomatic levels. However, an exclusive focus of public policy in dementia research on early detection raises concerns. First, it is not clear whether efficient treatment with acceptable side-effects will be available in the immediate future. It is an ethical requirement to avoid premature success reports and ill-founded claims that may undermine the legitimacy of biomedical research. Second, scientific and public policy communities should be transparent regarding uncertainties and potential financial and social costs of early diagnosis and treatments in order to foster informed public deliberation and adequate consideration of benefits and concerns.

KEY QUESTIONS FOR FURTHER DEBATES AND RESEARCH

- Is there a socially accepted wish to know or share knowledge about dementia predisposition? Is there social and cultural diversity about this?
- Given the heterogeneous structure of public healthcare in various countries, what is the overarching professional responsibility in organizing a transnational strategy for care and prevention of dementia?
- What is the responsibility of a nation to promote primary prevention of dementia targeting the healthy population, especially if evidence for effectiveness remains uncertain?

ETHICAL ISSUES OF RESEARCH PARTICIPATION

RATIONALE

Research into LOAD depends on the participation of large numbers of affected persons at different stages of neuronal decline. Informed consent is considered a necessary precondition. It includes sufficient information, assessment of capacity and understanding, as well as voluntary authorization (Appelbaum, 2007). Since affected persons display different levels of capacity, their involvement poses a range of ethical problems (Kim et al., 2011).

Pre-symptomatic persons are usually considered competent. However, they will often not be aware of being in an "at-risk state". Therefore, their identification as research subjects cannot rely solely on self-recruitment, but requires antecedent measures. As a result, persons might be confronted with information causing psychological distress, posing difficult questions of disclosure, and leading to social stigmatization (Illes et al., 2007). Out of fear, pre-symptomatic persons may also be more vulnerable to therapeutic misconception (Fisher et al., 2012) and might falsely expect a therapeutic benefit of biomarker research. Research subjects should understand the difference between biomarker research and clinical trials. Of course, the value of participating in biomarker research may change over time from primarily altruistic to more personal benefit, as standardization and knowledge improve.

Involving persons with *early stages* of LOAD is important for investigating the standard course of disease and testing the predictive value of biomarkers as well as the efficacy of new therapeutic approaches. However, including these persons poses the problem of assessing decision-making capacity. Depending on type and stage of dementia, this capacity may not be stable but rather fluctuating, and usually declines over time (Karlawish, 2003; Kim et al., 2011). Finally, the assessment of capacity depends on emotional factors, interests, and expectations, and varies between socio-cultural contexts. It requires not only understanding risks and benefits, but also appreciating how research participation will affect one's own life. People with early LOAD may have deficits that could make it difficult to meet this criterion (Karlawish, 2003).

Involving persons in *advanced stages* of LOAD poses the problems of research with incompetent subjects. Higher safeguards such as minimal-risk conditions and alternative procedures to protect personal integrity and best interest are applied, especially in potentially non-therapeutic research. Notably, there is no international consensus on the definition of minimal-risk conditions and the acceptability of proxy decisions (Kopelman, 2004).

RECOMMENDATIONS

Furthering research constitutes an honorable objective. However, there are still substantial national differences regarding the development and implementation of ethical guidelines for research with cognitively impaired participants (American College of Physicians, 1989; Council of Europe, 1997; National Bioethics Advisory Commission, 1998). Regardless of the national research setting, the different stages of the potential subjects' LOAD have to be taken into account. As affected persons' capacity to consent can change over time, it has to be re-evaluated on a regular basis to decide which informed consent conditions apply.

Studies involving *pre-symptomatic persons* have to observe high standards when dealing with potentially problematic predictive and diagnostic information. Special attention should be paid to questions of disclosing, storing, and passing on this information. Suitable measures should be taken to minimize the risks of psychological distress, familial issues, and social discrimination.

Studies addressing persons with *early stages* of dementia will include many individuals who are clearly capable of providing informed consent and there are existing methods for assessing this and documenting it (Marson et al., 1995). Such methods should be sensitive to cultural differences. Instead of generalizing incapacity of affected persons, supportive tools should be implemented in unclear cases to maintain or enhance decision-making capacity. The informed consent procedure should meet requirements such as use of simple language, repetition of explanation, rehearsals by affected persons and family members, and visual presentations for increasing the understanding of risks and benefits. Furthermore, family members can function as mediators (not as legal proxies) where this is suitable to increase the affected persons' capacity. Continuing supervision and re-assessment of decision-making capacity appears advisable to detect episodic variation and long-term decline.

Studies involving persons with *advanced forms* of LOAD have to protect the personal integrity and best interest of incompetent subjects. They require careful assessment of risks and benefits to meet minimal risk conditions for non-therapeutic research. Proxy decision-making can involve ethical problems regarding authorization, presumed will, and psychological burden. Alternatively, research advance directives allow the determination of a person's will with regard to research participation in the case of cognitive incapacity. This necessitates sufficient deliberation and consultations with trained professionals to avoid misunderstandings, as well as a professional and legal framework that ensures adherence. Also, opt-out models should be clarified. Manifestations of assent, continuing self-identity, and "natural will" should be taken into account (Karlawish, 2003; Kim et al., 2011).

LOAD research also offers an opportunity to explore new, innovative models of informed consent. Thus, the realization of a model of "gradual informed consent transfer" could emphasize the development of sustained relationships among subjects/patients, physicians and caregivers, and (an)other significant person(s)/proxy medical decision maker(s). This allows for gradual transfer of consent-giving capacity from the research subject to accompanying others, e.g., during a longitudinal study, and makes it more likely that these "companion proxies" will know and implement the subject's wishes (Overton et al., 2013).

KEY QUESTIONS FOR FURTHER DEBATES AND RESEARCH

- How can we detect and overcome potential loopholes such as therapeutic misunderstanding in existing informed consent practices given a high risk of fear and psychological distress in connection with a diagnosis of (pre-)dementia?
- Given the complexity of information on biomarkers and dementia, how can subjects' understanding of information regarding research, diagnostics, and treatment be improved?
- How can we overcome a narrow focus on individual autonomy and consider ethically and legally the role of the family and the social practice of knowledge-sharing in pre-dementia research?

INDIVIDUAL AND SOCIAL CONSEQUENCES

RATIONALE

Predictive and diagnostic information on LOAD can open possibilities of adapting life plans and making provisions. It may also provide psychological relief and social exoneration. On the other hand, it can pose difficult ethical problems:

On the *individual level*, this information can lead to psychological distress and irreversible decisions, even up to pre-emptive suicide, particularly when no efficacious therapies are available. It can affect persons' perceptions of themselves and their families, leading to negative self-images. The REVEAL-study on ApoE-genetic testing actually suggests that impacts might be less severe (Green et al., 2009). However, some studies indicate that lay people consider genetic information as less decisive than, e.g., family history (Chilibeck et al., 2011). Others point at considerable cultural or even national differences regarding peoples' interests to pursue genetic risk assessment for AD (Alzheimer Europe, 2011). Similar studies for neuro-biomarkers are needed to assess whether genetic and neuroscientific information differ from a lay person's perspective. If the predictive value of biomarkers is better than ApoE-genetic tests, their individual and social implications might differ.

In the *family context*, prognostic information can cause serious disruptions, especially when inheritable risk-factors may be involved. This poses the question of who else might be concerned, directly or indirectly. Thus, the affected person is confronted with disclosure dilemmas between privacy, protection, and family responsibilities (Rehmann-Sutter and Müller, 2009).

On a *societal level*, an increasing gap between prognosis/diagnosis and treatment can be accompanied by stigmatization. This can lead to the classification of pre-symptomatic risk-bearers, overburden them with responsibilities, and result in their medicalization. It can also promote their discrimination (e.g., with regard to legal status, job positions, or access to health insurance) and commercial exploitation, e.g., through dubious direct-to-consumer testing (Garand et al., 2009).

RECOMMENDATIONS

In dealing with predictive information, highest professional and legal standards should be observed to protect subjects from psychological distress, moral dilemmas, and social stigmatization. This information should be used to empower affected persons and optimize their treatment and care. Attempts to exclude them from social participation, healthcare, or other resources must be inhibited. Professional guidelines should be based on more empirical, cross-cultural studies on how lay people actually deal with LOAD risk prediction.

In a future scenario of clinical implementation of research results, the subjects would have to be informed in advance about all relevant possible research outcomes and their potential implications. Their right not to know would have to be respected (e.g., by offering an option to waive claims to be informed). However, this presents practical and ethical challenges for clinical drug trials. Subjects would need to agree before entering the study that they would find out their biomarker status as it may be unethical to expose participants who do not express the targeted biomarkers to drugs. If information were disclosed, professional counseling would have to be provided. This should include a critical revision of the information's reliability, significance, and implications for family members in order to prevent rash and inconsiderate reactions such as pre-emptive suicides. Furthermore, practical coping strategies and concrete problem solutions have to be delineated. To avoid stigmatization and discrimination, restrictive standards of confidentiality and data protection for any biomarker test including imaging techniques would be needed. Professional practice should take into account cultural diversity in dealing with such information. Given the globally diverse population and differences in legal systems, attempts are needed to foster a dialog between science and law. In countries with low levels of informed consent, counseling, or data protection, the scientific community should promote high standards for clinical application. Finally, scientists and policy makers investing in profit seeking biomedical industries gaining from this research should avoid conflicts of interest. Legal regulations are needed to preclude an unhampered market of direct-to-consumer testing without sufficient evidence-base or adequate supervision and counseling.

KEY QUESTIONS FOR FURTHER DEBATES AND RESEARCH

- How can ethical and clinical guidelines be respectful and sensitive to diverse ethnic populations having often very different understandings of family hierarchy, gender, and age norms?
- How can international consensus about data protection and anti-stigmatization strategies be ensured (e.g., by international associations)?
- How do we gain a minimum international ethics standard for research to ensure ethically acceptable transnational cooperation and to avoid "ethics dumping" (i.e., outsourcing of research into countries with lowest ethics standards or missing control)?

EXPLORING DIVERSITY AND PROMOTING PUBLIC DIALOG

RATIONALE

While the neuroscience community is increasingly globalized, cross-national comparison reveals significant differences in images, practices, and policies regarding LOAD. Some national policies emphasize individual suffering and public health burden, others dignity, quality of life of affected persons, and societal solidarity. Correspondingly, the focus of public discourses, interest group strategies, and governmental policies can be on supporting biomarker research or rather on providing adequate care for patients in advanced stages. Diversity presents a practical and economic challenge in dealing with research subjects from different cultural backgrounds. At the same time, it constitutes a resource for problem solving of complex human issues (Illes et al., 2007).

RECOMMENDATIONS

Since biomarker research still is in an early phase, it is a critical point in time to envision the spectrum of implications for dealing with LOAD. An intensified dialog between neuroscience, social sciences, and humanities will increase the understanding of the diversity and intersectionality (cross-influences of cultural categories such as gender, class, religion) of cultural attitudes towards LOAD and healthcare. Researchers and clinicians should be careful not to impute their own attitudes without critical consideration. Deliberative participatory processes in setting research and healthcare policy priorities should be strengthened to include the different perspectives and to benefit from the abundance of approaches.

The involvement of those affected is a constitutive feature of modern science governance that recognizes the right to self-determination but also aims at empowering patients and their families to take a more active role in shaping science (Schicktanz et al., 2012). Patient associations are important mediators, but a balanced plurality of advocacy groups should be included in order to avoid a one-sided perspective (e.g., by over-representing or neglecting either patients or their care-givers). Overall, framing dementia only as a threat to social and healthcare systems should be avoided, since this increases the stigmatization of patients and their families. Further research into causes, prevention, and treatment of LOAD, as well as adequate and respectful care for those affected, are necessary. Both constitute morally justified and valuable concerns that should not be pitted against each other. More national and international scientific societies should function as mediators and dialog platforms to foster an interdisciplinary and socially engaged discourse on the aims of LOAD research.

KEY QUESTIONS FOR FURTHER DEBATES AND RESEARCH

- How can we organize public deliberation that adequately involves the perspectives of those already affected by LOAD?
- How can we foster a dialog between various experts from bioscience, clinical care, social gerontology, ethics, and public health research in each country?
- How can the dominance of one-sided negative images and metaphors of dementia (e.g., "threat", "epidemic", "loss of self", "public burden", "living death") be overcome?

AUTHOR STATEMENT

All authors made substantial contributions to the conception or design of the work, drafted the work or revised it critically for important intellectual content, and gave their final approval of the version to be published. They agree to be accountable for all aspects of the work in ensuring that questions related to the accuracy or integrity of any part of the work are appropriately investigated and resolved.

ACKNOWLEDGMENTS

The authors would like to thank the International Office, University of Göttingen, and the Center for Science, Technology, Medicine, and Society, UCB, the Center on Aging, UCB, and the Helen Wills Neuroscience Institute, UCB, for funding the Workshop "Bioethics and Sciences of Aging: The Case of Dementia" at the University of California, Berkeley, as well as the Alexander von Humboldt-Foundation, the German Federal Ministry for Education and Research (Grant No. 01GP1004A), and the German Academic Exchange Service (DAAD) for funding the research stays of Silke Schicktanz and Mark Schweda. We acknowledge support by the German Research Foundation and the Open Access Publication Funds of the Göttingen University.

REFERENCES

Albert, M. S., DeKosky, S. T., Dickson, D., Dubois, B., Feldman, H. H., Fox, N. C., et al. (2011). The diagnosis of MCI due to AD. Recommendations from NIA and AAWG. *Alz. Dement.* 3, 1–10. doi: 10.1016/j.jalz.2011.03.008

Alzheimer Europe. (2011). *The Value of Knowing.* Luxembourg: Alzheimer Europe.

American College of Physicians. (1989). Cognitively impaired subjects. *Ann. Int. Medicine* 111, 843–848. doi: 10.7326/0003-4819-111-10-843

Appelbaum, P. S. (2007). Assessment of Patients' competence to consent to treatment. *N Engl. J. Med.* 357, 1834–1840. doi: 10.1056/NEJMcp074045

Chilibeck, G., Lock, M., and Sehdev, M. (2011). Postgenomics, uncertain futures and the familiarization of susceptibility genes. *Soc. Sci. Med.* 72, 1768–1775. doi: 10.1016/j.socscimed.2010.01.053

Council of Europe. (1997). *Convention on Human Rights and Biomedicine.* Oviedo: Council of Europe.

Daviglus, M. L., Bell, C. C., Berrettini, W., Bowen, P. E., Connolly, E. S. Jr., Cox, N. J., et al. (2010). National institutes of health state-of-the-science conference statement: preventing alzheimer's disease and cognitive decline. *Ann. Intern. Med.* 153, 176–181. doi: 10.7326/0003-4819-153-3-201008030-00260

Filippi, M., Agosta, F., Barkhof, F., Dubois, B., Fox, N. C., Frisoni, G. B., et al. (2012). EFNS task force: the use of neuroimaging in the diagnosis of dementia. *Eur. J. Neurol.* 19, 1487–1501. doi: 10.1111/j.1468-1331.2012.03859.x

Fisher, C. E., Dunn, L. B., Christopher, P. P., Holtzheimer, P. E., Leykin, Y., Mayberg, H. S., et al. (2012). The ethics of research on deep brain stimulation for depression: decisional capacity and therapeutic misconception. *Ann. N Y Acad. Sci.* 1265, 69–79. doi: 10.1111/j.1749-6632.2012.06596.x

Garand, L., Lingler, J. H., Conner, K. O., and Dew, M. A. (2009). Diagnostic labels, stigma and participation in research related to dementia and mild cognitive impairment. *Res. Gerontol. Nurs.* 2, 112–121. doi: 10.3928/19404921-2009 0401-04

Goldman, J. S., Hahn, S. E., Catania, J. W., LaRusse-Eckert, S., Butson, M. B., Rumbaugh, M., et al. (2011). Genetic counseling and testing for Alzheimer disease: joint practice guidelines of the American college of medical genetics and the national society of genetic counselors. *Genet. Med.* 13, 597–605. doi: 10. 1097/GIM.0b013e31821d69b8

Green, R. C., Roberts, J. S., Cupples, L. A., Relkin, N. R., Whitehouse, P. J., Brown, T., et al. (2009). Disclosure of APOE genotype for risk of Alzheimer's disease. *N. Engl. J. Med.* 361, 245–254. doi: 10.1056/NEJMoa0809578

Hampel, H., Lista, S., Teipel, S. J., Garaci, F., Nisticò, R., Blennow, K., et al. (2014). Perspective on future role of biological markers in clinical therapy trials of Alzheimer's disease: a long-range point of view beyond 2020. *Biochem. Pharmacol.* 88, 426–449. doi: 10.1016/j.bcp.2013.11.009

Illes, J., Rosen, A., Greicius, M., and Racine, E. (2007). Prospects for prediction: ethics analysis of neuroimaging in Alzheimer's disease. *Ann. N Y Acad. Sci.* 1097, 278–295. doi: 10.1196/annals.1379.030

Jack, C. R., Knopman, D. S., Jagust, W. J., Petersen, R. C., Weiner, M. W., Aisen, P. S., et al. (2013). Tracking pathophysiological processes in Alzheimer's disease:

an updated hypothetical model of dynamic biomarkers. *Lancet Neurol.* 12, 207–216. doi: 10.1016/s1474-4422(12)70291-0

Jessen, F., Wiese, B., Bickel, H., Eiffländer-Gorfer, S., Fuchs, A., Kaduszkiewicz, H., et al. (2011). Prediction of dementia in primary care patients. *PLoS One* 6:e16852. doi: 10.1371/journal.pone.0016852

Karlawish, J. H. (2003). Research involving cognitively impaired adults. *N. Engl. J. Med.* 348, 1389–1392. doi: 10.1056/NEJMsb030172

Karlawish, J. H. (2011). Addressing the ethical, policy and social challenges of preclinical Alzheimer disease. *Neurology* 77, 1487–1493. doi: 10.1212/WNL.0b013e318232ac1a

Keage, H. A. D., Matthews, F. E., Yip, A., Gao, L., McCracken, C., McKeith, I., et al. (2010). APOE and ACE polymorphisms and dementia risk in the older population over prolonged follow-up: 10 years of incidence in the MRC CFA study. *Age Ageing* 39, 104–111. doi: 10.1093/ageing/afp210

Kim, S. Y. H., Karlawish, J. H., Kim, H. M., Wall, I. F., Bozoki, A. C., and Appelbaum, P. S. (2011). Preservation of the capacity to appoint a proxy decision maker: implications for dementia research. *Arch. Gen. Psychiatry* 68, 214–219. doi: 10.1001/archgenpsychiatry.2010.191

Kivipelto, M., Ngandu, T., Fratiglioni, L., Viitanen, M., Kåreholt, I., Winblad, B., et al. (2005). Obesity and vascular risk factors at midlife and the risk of dementia and Alzheimer disease. *Arch. Neurol.* 62, 1556–1560. doi: 10.1001/archneur.62.10.1556

Kopelman, L. M. (2004). Minimal risk as an international ethical standard in research. *J. Med. Philos.* 29, 351–378. doi: 10.1080/03605310490500545

Kryscio, R. J. (2014). Secondary prevention trials in Alzheimer disease: the challenge of identifying a meaningful end point. *JAMA Neurol.* 71, 947–949. doi: 10.1001/jamaneurol.2014.1120

Landau, S. M., and Frosch, M. P. (2014). Tracking the earliest pathologic changes in Alzheimer disease. *Neurology* 82, 1576–1577. doi: 10.1212/wnl.0000000000000392

Le Couteur, D. G., Doust, J., Creasey, H., and Brayne, C. (2013). Political drive to screen for predementia: not evidence based and ignores the harms. *BMJ* 347:f5125. doi: 10.1136/bmj.f5125

Lock, M. (2013). *The Alzheimer Conundrum.* Princeton: Princeton University Press.

Mapstone, M., Cheema, A. K., Fiandaca, M. S., Zhong, X., Mhyre, T. R., MacArthur, L. H., et al. (2014). Plasma phospholipids identify antecedent memory impairment in older adults. *Nat. Med.* 20, 415–418. doi: 10.1038/nm.3466

Marson, D. C., Cody, H. A., Ingram, K. K., and Harrell, L. E. (1995). Neuropsychologic predictors of competency in Alzheimer's disease. Using a rational reasons legal standard. *Arch. Neurol.* 52, 955–959. doi: 10.1001/archneur.1995.00540340035011

National Bioethics Advisory Commission. (1998). *Research Involving Persons with Mental Disorders That May Affect Decisionmaking Capacity. Volume I Report and Recommendations of the National Bioethics Advisory Commission.* Rockville, MD: NBAC.

Nordberg, A., Carter, S. F., Rinne, J., Drzezga, A., Brooks, D. J., Vandenberghe, J., et al. (2013). A European multicentre PET study of fibrillar amyloid in Alzheimer's disease. *Eur. J. Nucl. Med. Mol. Imaging* 40, 104–114. doi: 10.1007/s00259-012-2237-2

Overton, E., Appelbaum, P. S., Fisher, S. R., Dohan, D., Roberts, L. W., and Dunn, L. B. (2013). Alternative decision makers' perspectives on assent and dissent for dementia research. *Am. J. Geriatr. Psychiatry* 21, 346–354. doi: 10.1016/j.jagp.2013.01.027

Palmqvist, S., Hertze, J., Minthon, L., Wattmo, C., Zetterberg, H., Blennow, K., et al. (2012). Comparison of brief cognitive tests and CSF biomarkers in predicting Alzheimer's disease in mild cognitive impairment: six-year follow-up study. *PLoS One* 7:e38639. doi: 10.1371/journal.pone.0038639

Parra, M. A., Abrahams, S., Logie, R. H., Méndez, L. G., Lopera, F., and Della Sala, S. (2010). Visual short-term memory binding deficits in familial Alzheimer's disease. *Brain* 133, 2702–2713. doi: 10.1093/brain/awq148

Petrella, J. R., Sheldon, F. C., Prince, S. E., Calhoun, V. D., and Doraiswamy, P. M. (2011). Default mode network connectivity in stable vs progressive mild cognitive impairment. *Neurology* 76, 511–517. doi: 10.1212/wnl.0b013e31820af94e

Prestia, A., Caroli, A., van der Flier, W. M., Ossenkoppele, R., Van Berckel, B., and Barkhof, F. (2013). Prediction of dementia in MCI patients based on core diagnostic markers for Alzheimer disease. *Neurology* 80, 1048–1056. doi: 10.1212/wnl.0b013e3182872830

Rehmann-Sutter, Chr., and Müller, H. J. (2009). eds. *Disclosure dilemmas: ethics of genetic prognosis after the 'Right to Know/Not to Know' Debate.* Farnham: Ashgate.

Schicktanz, S., Schweda, M., and Wynne, B. (2012). The ethics of 'public understanding of ethics'—Why and how bioethics expertise should include public and patients' voices. *Med. Health Philos.* 15, 129–139. doi: 10.1007/s11019-011-9321-4

Shim, Y. S., and Morris, J. C. (2011). Biomarkers predicting Alzheimer's disease in cognitively normal aging. *J. Clin. Neurol.* 7, 60–68. doi: 10.3988/jcn.2011.7.2.60

Sperling, R. A., Aisen, P. S., Beckett, L. A., Bennett, D. A., Craft, S., Fagan, A. M., et al. (2011). Toward defining the preclinical stages of Alzheimer's disease: recommendation from the National Institute on Aging-Alzheimer's Association workgroups on diagnostic guidelines for Alzheimer's disease. *Alzheimers Dement.* 7, 280–292. doi: 10.1016/j.jalz.2011.03.003

Sperling, R. A., Karlawish, J., and Johnson, K. A. (2013). Preclinical Alzheimer disease—the challenges ahead. *Nat. Rev. Neurol.* 9, 54–58. doi: 10.1038/nrneurol.2012.241

Visser, P. J., Verhey, F., Knol, D. L., Scheltens, P., Wahlund, L. O., Freund-Levi, Y., et al. (2009). Prevalence and prognostic value of CSF marker of AD pathologies. *Lancet Neurol.* 8, 619–627. doi: 10.3410/f.1166395.627365

Waldemar, G., Dubois, B., Emre, M., Georges, J., McKeith, I. G., Rossor, M., et al. (2007). Recommendations for the diagnosis and management of Alzheimer's disease and other disorders associated with dementia: EFNS guideline. *Eur. J. Neurol.* 14, e1–e26. doi: 10.5772/55467

World Health Organization and Alzheimer's Disease International. (2012). *Dementia - A public health priority.* Geneva: WHO Press.

Wright, C. F., Hall, A., Matthews, F. E., and Brayne, C. (2009). Biomarkers, dementia and public health. *Ann. NY Acad. Sci.* 1180, 11–19. doi: 10.1111/j.1749-6632.2009.04942.x

3

Is integration and survival of newborn neurons the bottleneck for effective neural repair by endogenous neural precursor cells?

Ann M. Turnley*, Harleen S. Basrai and Kimberly J. Christie

Department of Anatomy and Neuroscience, The University of Melbourne, Parkville, VIC, Australia

Edited by:
Luca Bonfanti, University of Turin, Italy

Reviewed by:
Liliana Bernardino, University of Beira Interior, Portugal
Giorgia Quadrato, University of Tuebingen, Germany

****Correspondence:***
Ann M. Turnley, Department of Anatomy and Neuroscience, Melbourne Brain Centre, The University of Melbourne, 30 Royal Parade, Parkville, VIC 3010, Australia
e-mail: turnley@unimelb.edu.au

After two decades of research the existence of adult neural precursor cells and the phenomenon of adult neurogenesis is well established. However, there has been little or no effective harnessing of these endogenous cells to promote functional neuronal replacement following neural injury or disease. Neural precursor cells can respond to neural damage by proliferating, migrating to the site of injury, and differentiating into neuronal or glial lineages. However, after a month or so, very few or no newborn neurons can be detected, suggesting that even though neuroblasts are generated, they generally fail to survive as mature neurons and contribute to the local circuitry. Is this lack of survival and integration one of the major bottlenecks that inhibits effective neuronal replacement and subsequent repair of the nervous system following injury or disease? In this perspective article the possibility that this bottleneck can be targeted to enhance the integration and subsequent survival of newborn neurons will be explored and will suggest some possible mechanisms that may need to be modulated for this to occur.

Keywords: adult neurogenesis, neural stem cells, neural repair, SVZ, SGZ, hippocampus, olfactory bulb, neurite outgrowth

INTRODUCTION

Two decades of research has demonstrated that a surprisingly wide variety of factors can influence adult neural precursor cell biology (Christie and Turnley, 2012). This includes extrinsic factors, such as growth factors, cytokines, chemokines, neurotrophins, steroids and extracellular matrix molecules as well as cell intrinsic factors such as transcription factors and signal transduction pathway regulators (Christie and Turnley, 2012; Christie et al., 2013a). In general, endogenous adult neural precursor cells can be quite easily induced to proliferate and migrate, and depending on the context, differentiate into neuronal or glial cell types. However, fewer factors have been identified that induce newborn neurons to integrate into the local circuitry and survive more than a few weeks after their birth. Indeed at least 50% of newborn neurons fail to survive longer than a month or two after their generation (Petreanu and Alvarez-Buylla, 2002; Dayer et al., 2003). This makes sense under normal physiological conditions, where newborn neurons replenish local neurons lost due to normal turnover, to homeostatically maintain neuron numbers (Valley et al., 2009). Addition of newborn neurons to existing circuitry has specific functional outcomes. In the olfactory bulb, addition of new neurons is required for short-term olfactory memory, perceptual learning, and for innate olfactory responses (Breton-Provencher et al., 2009; Moreno et al., 2009; Sakamoto et al., 2011). In the hippocampus, adult neurogenesis plays roles in anxiety and affective behaviors, cognition and spatial memory (Ming and Song, 2011), and is proposed to be vital for forgetting of hippocampal-dependent short-term memories (Frankland et al., 2013). However, in instances of larger neuronal loss, such as following injury or disease, this failure of newborn neurons to increase their integration and survival in conjunction with increases in proliferation and redirected migration means that the full potential of adult neural progenitor cells (NPCs) to repair the damage may not be realized. This perspective article will explore some of the mechanisms and factors that may be targeted to enhance newborn neuron survival, summarized in **Table 1**.

SOURCE OF NEURAL STEM/PROGENITOR CELLS—SUBVENTRICULAR ZONE vs. HIPPOCAMPUS

There are two principle sources of neural progenitor cells in the adult brain: the subventricular zone (SVZ) lining the lateral walls of the lateral ventricles, which supplies new neurons to the olfactory bulb and the subgranular zone (SGZ) of the hippocampal dentate gyrus, which produces new hippocampal granule cell neurons. Under normal physiological conditions, both of these NPC populations primarily generate neurons, however there are differences in the neuroblasts and neurons they produce and their response to neural damage. SVZ-derived cells must migrate a long distance along the rostral migratory stream to reach the olfactory bulb, while hippocampal-derived cells only migrate a short distance from the SGZ into the granule cell layer directly adjacent. In response to neural damage, both populations increase their proliferation but apparently only SVZ-derived cells migrate to ectopic sites of damage (Ming and Song, 2011), while hippocampal cells remain within the granule cell layer. The differentiation fate of SVZ-derived cells is also more easily switched to a glial fate in response to damage and the subsequent production of

Table 1 | Factors that regulate or may be targeted to promote survival of adult newborn neurons.

Factor	Role	References
EXOGENOUS		
Neurotransmitters—GABA and glutamate	Activity induced survival and synaptic integration	Gascon et al., 2006; Ge et al., 2006; Platel et al., 2010; Kim et al., 2012; Chancey et al., 2013
Neurotrophins—BDNF	Enhances neurite outgrowth, dendritic arborization, and spine density	Miyamoto et al., 2006; Cheung et al., 2007; Chan et al., 2008; Gao and Chen, 2009; Gao et al., 2009; Bergami et al., 2013
ENDOGENOUS		
Rho GTPases	Cytoskeletal reorganization—dendrite/axon outgrowth, dendritic spine formation—regulation of plasticity induced survival	Nikolic, 2002; Keung et al., 2011; Christie et al., 2013b; Vadodaria et al., 2013
	NPC migration	Leong et al., 2011
	Extant neuron survival in stroke and Parkinson's disease models	Lemmens et al., 2013; Rodriguez-Perez et al., 2013
SOCS2	Regulation of growth factor signaling and neurite outgrowth	Goldshmit et al., 2004a,b; Basrai et al., 2013
TRANSCRIPTION FACTORS		
zif268/egr1, KLF9, NeuroD1, cAMP response element, ATF5, miR-132	Regulation of neuronal morphology and maturation	Giachino et al., 2005; Gao et al., 2009; Jagasia et al., 2009; Scobie et al., 2009; Pathania et al., 2012; Wang et al., 2012; Veyrac et al., 2013
p63	Anti-apoptotic	Cancino et al., 2013
NFATc4	Mediates BDNF-induced survival	Quadrato et al., 2012
OTHER POTENTIAL MODULATORS		
Ephs/ephrins	Regulation of axonal and dendritic sprouting, synaptic plasticity	Goldshmit et al., 2011; Overman et al., 2012; Spanevello et al., 2013
Peri-neuronal nets	Inhibits synaptic plasticity; degradation promotes plasticity	Kwok et al., 2011; Wang et al., 2011
Environmental enrichment/ Forced use	Enhances synaptic plasticity	Rochefort et al., 2002; Miwa and Storm, 2005; Yamaguchi and Mori, 2005; Alonso et al., 2006; Mandairon et al., 2006; Overman et al., 2012

chemokines and cytokines, while SGZ cell fate remains largely neuronal depending on type of damage (Christie and Turnley, 2012). However the end stage of neuronal integration and survival does not appear to differ greatly, with the majority of neurons failing to survive in both cases.

ADULT NEWBORN NEURONAL SURVIVAL UNDER NORMAL PHYSIOLOGICAL CONDITIONS

INTEGRATION OF NEWBORN NEURONS INTO EXISTING LOCAL CIRCUITRY

While there are homeostatic mechanisms in place to regulate the integration and subsequent survival of newborn neurons into local circuits under normal physiological conditions, this does not mean to imply that this process is always held at a constant level. Indeed, the numbers of newborn neurons that survive and integrate can be varied by altered levels of circuit activity/plasticity. In the olfactory bulb, alteration of local activity by complex odor environments or odor discrimination learning increases the survival of newborn neurons (Rochefort et al., 2002; Miwa and Storm, 2005; Alonso et al., 2006; Mandairon et al., 2006), while conversely at the critical time of neuronal integration, sensory deprivation and hence decreased circuit activity results in increased newborn neuron death (Yamaguchi and Mori, 2005). Similarly, numerous activity and environment-induced alterations in adult hippocampal neurogenesis have been described, including exercise, environmental enrichment and learning increasing newborn neuron numbers, with stress, steroids, and depression decreasing them. However, with some exceptions, these factors alter final mature newborn numbers by increasing or decreasing proliferation of neural precursor cells and hence production of new neurons, rather than acting primarily at the integration and survival stage. It seems that the newborn hippocampal neurons, during the critical few weeks after their generation, require activity in the form of effortful learning, to promote their survival (Shors et al., 2012).

So, how do newborn neurons integrate into the extant local circuitry? While the mechanisms are not yet well understood it seems that newly generated neurons compete for synaptic space, with only those that make successful connections surviving. The newborn neurons must compete not only with each other but also with older neurons to integrate into the circuitry. It should be noted that the regions into which newborn neurons integrate are actually open to the competition. In other words, they are very plastic regions of the CNS that unlike other CNS regions, are primed to allow new neurons to be added to the circuitry. This is highlighted in neural precursor cell transplantation studies, whereby new neurons were produced and survived if transplanted into neurogenic regions but not into non-neurogenic regions (Suhonen et al., 1996; Shihabuddin et al., 2000). While there are similarities in regulation of neuronal survival and integration of SVZ- and SGZ-derived neurons under normal physiological conditions, there are quite important differences following injury. This includes their ability to migrate to distant sites of damage and differences into which they integrate. The SVZ-derived cells will migrate to sites of damage in non-neurogenic regions, e.g., cortex or striatum and therefore need to try to integrate and survive in areas that are usually non-receptive to such processes. SGZ-derived cells remain in a neurogenic environment, although injury-induced plasticity may be increased (Perederiy et al., 2013). In the injured non-neurogenic CNS there is a variable degree of rewiring and plasticity occurring, which may change the normally non-neurogenic environment to a partially neurogenic environment in some instances and which may account for the various reports of newborn neurons at sites of injury or disease (Christie and Turnley, 2012). So, what can be taken from our knowledge of factors that regulate normal physiological adult newborn neuron integration and survival and be applied to the injured regions of the CNS?

FACTORS THAT ENHANCE NEWBORN NEURON INTEGRATION AND SURVIVAL UNDER NORMAL PHYSIOLOGICAL CONDITIONS

Compared to our knowledge of factors that promote adult neural precursor cell proliferation or differentiation, there is comparatively little known about factors that promote newborn neuron survival and integration *per se*. Broadly speaking, what information we do have centers on ways to alter plasticity—particularly at the synaptic or cell morphological level (dendrite and axon morphology). These may be categorized into factors that regulate circuit/neuronal activity (e.g., neurotransmitters) and factors that regulate cellular morphology (e.g., cytoskeletal regulators, neurotrophins), as well as less-defined but otherwise acknowledged general regulators of neural plasticity, such as environmental enrichment and use/activity induced plasticity.

These different signals converge on a range of transcription factors, the roles, and regulation of which are beginning to be elucidated (Christie et al., 2013a). These include transcription factors that regulate neurochemical and/or morphological maturation, such the inducible immediate early gene zif268/egr1 (Veyrac et al., 2013), KLF9 (Scobie et al., 2009), NeuroD1 (Gao et al., 2009), the cAMP response element (Giachino et al., 2005; Jagasia et al., 2009) and ATF5 (Wang et al., 2012), as well as the microRNA miR-132 (Pathania et al., 2012). The anti-apoptotic p63 (Cancino et al., 2013) and NFATc4, which mediates BDNF-dependent survival (Quadrato et al., 2012), also promote newborn neuron survival.

Neurotransmitters

Early in the life of a newborn neuron, before integration has taken place, the cells are responsive to non-synapse-mediated GABA stimulation. After further maturation, the cells become synoptically responsive to GABA with concomitant responsiveness to glutamate (Gascon et al., 2006; Ge et al., 2006; Kim et al., 2012; Chancey et al., 2013). It has been proposed that this responsiveness may allow synaptic integration into local circuitry to occur in a process whereby a highly motile filopodia of a newborn neuron contacts a pre-existing synapse, possibly in response to excess neurotransmitter release. This connection then matures, becomes stabilized and the filopodium develops into a mature dendritic spine. Astrocyte-released glutamatergic activation of neuroblast NMDA receptors has been shown to be required for synaptic integration (Platel et al., 2010), while the level of cell-intrinsic excitability also modulates survival (Lin et al., 2010). For such an interaction to be most effective, there likely needs to be a substantial degree of synaptic and dendritic remodeling occurring, as in the plastic neurogenic regions of the CNS, which requires substantial cytoskeletal rearrangement and regulation. Enhancing plasticity by enhancing cytoskeletal rearrangement provides another potential target for increasing the likelihood of integration and survival of newborn neurons.

Cytoskeletal rearrangement as a potential target for enhancing newborn neuron integration into local circuitry—modulating the RhoA family of small GTPases

While a multitude of factors have effects on cytoskeletal rearrangement, most of these converge on the family of small Rho GTPases, RhoA, Rac1, and cdc42. The Rho GTPases are regulators of neurite outgrowth, with RhoA activation inhibiting and Rac1 activation promoting neurite outgrowth and dendritic spine formation (Nikolic, 2002). Enhancement of a newborn neuron's ability to produce dendrites, axons, or dendritic spines may give it a competitive advantage, while increasing synaptic remodeling or turnover of existing local circuitry could also increase the chances of newborn neuron integration. A number of recent studies implicate these molecules in regulation of adult newborn hippocampal neuron maturation and survival, as recently reviewed (Vadodaria and Jessberger, 2013).

Conceptually, Rac1 may promote neuronal survival and integration while RhoA may oppose it, given the promotion and inhibition of neurite outgrowth and spine formation respectively. This indeed appears to be the case. Deletion or inhibition of Rac1 or cdc42 blocked dendrite and spine formation of adult hippocampal newborn neurons, although there were no effects on neuron survival (Vadodaria et al., 2013). Conversely, constitutive activation of RhoA decreased the percentage of newborn neurons (Keung et al., 2011), while inhibition of RhoA signaling specifically enhanced the survival of newborn hippocampal neurons, which correlated with enhanced spatial memory (Christie et al., 2013b). Rho kinase inhibition also promotes ectopic migration of SVZ-derived neural precursor cells and subsequent neuron survival (Leong et al., 2011). Therefore, activation of Rac1 or cdc42 or inhibition of RhoA signaling pathways may be of potential therapeutic effectiveness at promoting survival and integration of newborn neurons. Results are yet to be reported on effects on neurogenesis, however use of the Rho kinase inhibitor HA1077 (Fasudil) promotes extant neuron survival, regeneration and functional improvement, in Parkinson's disease and stroke models (Lemmens et al., 2013; Rodriguez-Perez et al., 2013).

FACTORS THAT REGULATE NEURONAL MORPHOLOGY AND SURVIVAL—OTHER POTENTIAL TARGETS TO ENHANCE SURVIVAL AND INTEGRATION OF NEWBORN ADULT NEURONS

While administration of Fasudil appeared to have few side effects, not many studies have been performed at present and so the possibility exists that problems may emerge. A number of other factors are known to regulate neuronal morphology and also play a role in neurogenesis and newborn neuron survival. These may, at least in part, signal via Rho GTPases to perform their function, but given the broad expression of Rho GTPases, in some instances it may be more prudent to target molecules that have a more limited expression profile, to avoid potential side effects. These have been recently reviewed (Vadodaria and Jessberger, 2013) so only a subset will be discussed briefly here.

SOCS2

An example of such a molecule is the intracellular regulator of cytokine and growth factor signaling, Suppressor of Cytokine Signaling-2 (SOCS2). Although best known as a negative feedback regulator of growth hormone signaling (Metcalf et al., 2000), it has a broader range of molecules it interacts with, including EGF and Epo (Basrai et al., 2013; Goldshmit et al., 2004a,b). Overexpression of SOCS2 enhances neurite length and branching, which may in part be due to activation of Rac1 and inhibition of Rho kinase (Goldshmit et al., 2004a,b). During development, SOCS2 is expressed widely throughout the developing brain and regulates developmental neurogenesis (Polizzotto et al., 2000; Turnley et al., 2002). In the adult its expression is primarily in the dentate gyrus and hippocampal CA3 region, suggesting it plays a role in adult neurogenesis. Overexpression of SOCS2 increased numbers of newborn adult hippocampal neurons without affecting their differentiation or proliferation of neural precursor cells (Ransome and Turnley, 2008). These results are in keeping with the idea that enhancing neurite outgrowth and complexity may enhance survival and integration of newborn neurons.

Neurotrophins

Although many growth factors have been shown to play a role in some aspect of adult neurogenesis, often promoting proliferation and survival of neural precursor cells (Christie and Turnley, 2012), few have been shown to play a role in the specific stage of neuronal maturation, integration and survival. The neurotrophin brain-derived neurotrophic factor, BDNF, is one such factor. BDNF has been shown to regulate neuronal morphology via activation of the Rho GTPases Rac1 and cdc42 (Miyamoto et al., 2006; Cheung et al., 2007). It is important for neurite outgrowth, dendritic arborization and spine density of adult hippocampal neurons, but not proliferation or cell fate specification (Chan et al., 2008; Gao and Chen, 2009; Gao et al., 2009; Bergami et al., 2013) and deletion of TrkB decreases survival and induces an anxiety-like phenotype (Bergami et al., 2008). Further, in the absence of hippocampal BDNF, there is increased death of adult newborn hippocampal neurons following traumatic brain injury (Gao and Chen, 2009).

OTHER MODULATORS OF NEURAL PLASTICITY THAT MAY BE HARNESSED TO PROMOTE SURVIVAL AND INTEGRATION

Normal physiological levels of neurogenesis, newborn neuron integration, and survival are enhanced by activity-induced plasticity. This can be applied to the therapeutic scenario, where environmental enrichment, exercise, or forced use can induce circuit sprouting and plasticity and lead to functional improvement. While this has been examined more in terms of axonal regeneration, such as by inhibition of repulsive axon guidance molecules, it is also applicable to enhancement of neuron integration into damaged circuitry. For example, blocking of members of the Eph/ephrin family promotes axonal and dendritic sprouting/regeneration and enhances functional recovery (Goldshmit et al., 2011; Overman et al., 2012; Spanevello et al., 2013). This sprouting/plasticity can be further enhanced with forced use of the affected limb (i.e., enhancing plasticity) in a stroke model (Overman et al., 2012). Altering the expression of different Ephs or ephrins has positive or negative effects on neurogenesis (Ricard et al., 2006; Chumley et al., 2007; Jiao et al., 2008; Hara et al., 2010; Murai et al., 2010; Ashton et al., 2012). It is likely that their neuronal progeny also express these molecules, suggesting that blocking them or modulating their signaling pathways (again, converging on Rho GTPases) may enhance newborn neuron survival and integration into damaged but sprouting local circuitry. Indeed, deletion of ephrinB3 leads to enhanced neurogenesis around the lesion site in a stroke model, however it also resulted in more severe ischemic damage (Doeppner et al., 2011). Targeting of other repulsive guidance molecules, such as Semaphorins, Slits, and DCC may also be advantageous (Christie and Turnley, 2012).

Another factor that inhibits neural regeneration and limits access to neuronal circuits is the peri-neuronal net (Kwok et al., 2011). This is made up of extracellular matrix, such as proteoglycans, surrounding neuronal cell bodies, and their processes. Degradation of the nets, for example using chondroitinases, enhances sprouting, plasticity, and functional improvement after injury (Wang et al., 2011). Given that breakdown of the peri-neuronal nets makes it easier for synaptic plasticity to occur, it may also allow easier access and integration of newborn neurons, although this has yet to be examined.

COMBINATION OF NEWBORN NEURON SURVIVAL PROMOTING AGENTS WITH NEUROPROTECTIVE, PROLIFERATIVE, OR PLASTICITY INDUCING AGENTS

While a number of factors have been described above that have the potential to enhance newborn neuron integration and survival in an injury or disease setting, we cannot forget that the damaged CNS environment is much different to the normal physiological neurogenic niches where neurogenesis normally takes place. On the plus side, the injured CNS undergoes a certain amount of sprouting and local circuit rearrangement, which may open up the opportunity for newborn neurons to compete for synaptic space along with sprouting extant neurons, unlike the comparatively non-plastic normal CNS parenchyma. On the minus side, the damaged CNS environment is quite an inhibitory environment, such that newborn neuroblasts may need to be protected so that they can differentiate and become mature neurons, rather than dying of other causes along the way. Neuroprotective or anti-inflammatory strategies probably also need to be included with therapy to improve newborn neuron maturation, integration, or plasticity. There are a number of promising molecules in this regard, such as erythropoietin (Epo) which is neuroprotective and enhances the numbers of neural precursor cells and neurons following neural injury (Shingo et al., 2001; Wang et al., 2004; Lu et al., 2005; Tsai et al., 2006; Byts and Siren, 2009; Zhang et al., 2012). It has shown promise in a large range of pre-clinical studies and is currently undergoing clinical trial for a range of conditions. Combinatorial studies now need to be performed, with for example Epo and inhibition of Rho kinase, to determine whether the outcome is further improved, and numbers of surviving and integrated newborn neurons is enhanced more than either factor alone.

CONCLUSIONS

There is a high rate of failure of newborn adult neurons to integrate into local circuitry and survive under physiological conditions and an even higher failure rate in injury or disease conditions. We propose that provision of factors that enhance the competitiveness of newborn neurons to integrate into circuitry, either by affecting the newborn neurons themselves or by affecting plasticity of the local circuitry, will improve this bottleneck of low newborn neuron survival, leading to improved functional outcome following neural damage. Further, it is likely that such treatments will be more effective if combined with treatments that will make the injured CNS a less toxic environment, by use of inflammatory modulators or neuroprotective agents. After two decades of research we know what needs to be done and we now have several avenues of approach to be tested that may actually allow the therapeutic promise of adult neural stem cells to be realized.

ACKNOWLEDGMENTS

This work is supported by an NHMRC of Australia grant (#1045125) and Fellowship (#628344) to Ann M. Turnley. We apologize to the authors of many papers we could not cite due to word limits.

REFERENCES

Alonso, M., Viollet, C., Gabellec, M. M., Meas-Yedid, V., Olivo-Marin, J. C., and Lledo, P. M. (2006). Olfactory discrimination learning increases the survival of adult-born neurons in the olfactory bulb. *J. Neurosci.* 26, 10508–10513. doi: 10.1523/JNEUROSCI.2633-06.2006

Ashton, R. S., Conway, A., Pangarkar, C., Bergen, J., Lim, K. I., Shah, P., et al. (2012). Astrocytes regulate adult hippocampal neurogenesis through ephrin-B signaling. *Nat. Neurosci.* 15, 1399–1406. doi: 10.1038/nn.3212

Basrai, H. S., Christie, K. J., and Turnley, A. M. (2013). "Regulation of basal and injury-induced fate decisions of adult neural precursor cells: focus on SOCS2 and related signalling pathways," in *Trends in Cell Signaling Pathways in Neuronal Fate Decision [Internet]. InTech Open.* Available online at: http://www.intechopen.com/books/trends-in-cell-signaling-pathways-in-neuronal-fate-decision/regulation-of-basal-and-injury-induced-fate-decisions-of-adult-neural-precursor-cells-focus-on-socs2

Bergami, M., Rimondini, R., Santi, S., Blum, R., Gotz, M., and Canossa, M. (2008). Deletion of TrkB in adult progenitors alters newborn neuron integration into hippocampal circuits and increases anxiety-like behavior. *Proc. Natl. Acad. Sci. U.S.A.* 105, 15570–15575. doi: 10.1073/pnas.0803702105

Bergami, M., Vignoli, B., Motori, E., Pifferi, S., Zuccaro, E., Menini, A., et al. (2013). TrkB signaling directs the incorporation of newly generated periglomerular cells in the adult olfactory bulb. *J. Neurosci.* 33, 11464–11478. doi: 10.1523/JNEUROSCI.4812-12.2013

Breton-Provencher, V., Lemasson, M., Peralta, M. R. 3rd., and Saghatelyan, A. (2009). Interneurons produced in adulthood are required for the normal functioning of the olfactory bulb network and for the execution of selected olfactory behaviors. *J. Neurosci.* 29, 15245–15257. doi: 10.1523/JNEUROSCI.3606-09.2009

Byts, N., and Siren, A. L. (2009). Erythropoietin: a multimodal neuroprotective agent. *Exp. Transl. Stroke Med.* 1, 4. doi: 10.1186/2040-7378-1-4

Cancino, G. I., Yiu, A. P., Fatt, M. P., Dugani, C. B., Flores, E. R., Frankland, P. W., et al. (2013). p63 Regulates adult neural precursor and newly born neuron survival to control hippocampal-dependent Behavior. *J. Neurosci.* 33, 12569–12585. doi: 10.1523/JNEUROSCI.1251-13.2013

Chan, J. P., Cordeira, J., Calderon, G. A., Iyer, L. K., and Rios, M. (2008). Depletion of central BDNF in mice impedes terminal differentiation of new granule neurons in the adult hippocampus. *Mol. Cell. Neurosci.* 39, 372–383. doi: 10.1016/j.mcn.2008.07.017

Chancey, J. H., Adlaf, E. W., Sapp, M. C., Pugh, P. C., Wadiche, J. I., and Overstreet-Wadiche, L. S. (2013). GABA depolarization is required for experience-dependent synapse unsilencing in adult-born neurons. *J. Neurosci.* 33, 6614–6622. doi: 10.1523/JNEUROSCI.0781-13.2013

Cheung, Z. H., Chin, W. H., Chen, Y., Ng, Y. P., and Ip, N. Y. (2007). Cdk5 is involved in BDNF-stimulated dendritic growth in hippocampal neurons. *PLoS Biol* 5:e63. doi: 10.1371/journal.pbio.0050063

Christie, K. J., Emery, B., Denham, M., Bujalka, H., Cate, H. S., and Turnley, A. M. (2013a). Transcriptional regulation and specification of neural stem cells. *Adv. Exp. Med. Biol.* 786, 129–155. doi: 10.1007/978-94-007-6621-1_8

Christie, K. J., Turbic, A., and Turnley, A. M. (2013b). Adult hippocampal neurogenesis, Rho kinase inhibition and enhancement of neuronal survival. *Neuroscience* 247, 75–83. doi: 10.1016/j.neuroscience.2013.05.019

Christie, K. J., and Turnley, A. M. (2012). Regulation of endogenous neural stem/progenitor cells for neural repair-factors that promote neurogenesis and gliogenesis in the normal and damaged brain. *Front. Cell. Neurosci.* 6:70. doi: 10.3389/fncel.2012.00070

Chumley, M. J., Catchpole, T., Silvany, R. E., Kernie, S. G., and Henkemeyer, M. (2007). EphB receptors regulate stem/progenitor cell proliferation, migration, and polarity during hippocampal neurogenesis. *J. Neurosci.* 27, 13481–13490. doi: 10.1523/JNEUROSCI.4158-07.2007

Dayer, A. G., Ford, A. A., Cleaver, K. M., Yassaee, M., and Cameron, H. A. (2003). Short-term and long-term survival of new neurons in the rat dentate gyrus. *J. Comp. Neurol.* 460, 563–572. doi: 10.1002/cne.10675

Doeppner, T. R., Bretschneider, E., Doehring, M., Segura, I., Senturk, A., Acker-Palmer, A., et al. (2011). Enhancement of endogenous neurogenesis in ephrin-B3 deficient mice after transient focal cerebral ischemia. *Acta Neuropathol.* 122, 429–442. doi: 10.1007/s00401-011-0856-5

Frankland, P. W., Kohler, S., and Josselyn, S. A. (2013). Hippocampal neurogenesis and forgetting. *Trends Neurosci.* 36, 497–503. doi: 10.1016/j.tins.2013.05.002

Gao, X., and Chen, J. (2009). Conditional knockout of brain-derived neurotrophic factor in the hippocampus increases death of adult-born immature neurons following traumatic brain injury. *J. Neurotrauma* 26, 1325–1335. doi: 10.1089/neu.2008-0744

Gao, X., Smith, G. M., and Chen, J. (2009). Impaired dendritic development and synaptic formation of postnatal-born dentate gyrus granular neurons in the absence of brain-derived neurotrophic factor signaling. *Exp. Neurol.* 215, 178–190. doi: 10.1016/j.expneurol.2008.10.009

Gao, Z., Ure, K., Ables, J. L., Lagace, D. C., Nave, K. A., Goebbels, S., et al. (2009). Neurod1 is essential for the survival and maturation of adult-born neurons. *Nat. Neurosci.* 12, 1090–1092. doi: 10.1038/nn.2385

Gascon, E., Dayer, A. G., Sauvain, M. O., Potter, G., Jenny, B., De Roo, M., et al. (2006). GABA regulates dendritic growth by stabilizing lamellipodia in newly generated interneurons of the olfactory bulb. *J. Neurosci.* 26, 12956–12966. doi: 10.1523/JNEUROSCI.4508-06.2006

Ge, S., Goh, E. L., Sailor, K. A., Kitabatake, Y., Ming, G. L., and Song, H. (2006). GABA regulates synaptic integration of newly generated neurons in the adult brain. *Nature* 439, 589–593. doi: 10.1038/nature04404

Giachino, C., De Marchis, S., Giampietro, C., Parlato, R., Perroteau, I., Schutz, G., et al. (2005). cAMP response element-binding protein regulates differentiation and survival of newborn neurons in the olfactory bulb. *J. Neurosci.* 25, 10105–10118. doi: 10.1523/JNEUROSCI.3512-05.2005

Goldshmit, Y., Greenhalgh, C. J., and Turnley, A. M. (2004a). Suppressor of cytokine signalling-2 and epidermal growth factor regulate neurite outgrowth of cortical neurons. *Eur. J. Neurosci.* 20, 2260–2266. doi: 10.1111/j.1460-9568.2004.03698.x

Goldshmit, Y., Walters, C. E., Scott, H. J., Greenhalgh, C. J., and Turnley, A. M. (2004b). SOCS2 induces neurite outgrowth by regulation of epidermal growth factor receptor activation. *J. Biol. Chem.* 279, 16349–16355. doi: 10.1074/jbc.M312873200

Goldshmit, Y., Spanevello, M. D., Tajouri, S., Li, L., Rogers, F., Pearse, M., et al. (2011). EphA4 blockers promote axonal regeneration and functional recovery following spinal cord injury in mice. *PLoS ONE* 6:e24636. doi: 10.1371/journal.pone.0024636

Hara, Y., Nomura, T., Yoshizaki, K., Frisen, J., and Osumi, N. (2010). Impaired hippocampal neurogenesis and vascular formation in ephrin-A5-deficient mice. *Stem Cells* 28, 974–983. doi: 10.1002/stem.427

Jagasia, R., Steib, K., Englberger, E., Herold, S., Faus-Kessler, T., Saxe, M., et al. (2009). GABA-cAMP response element-binding protein signaling regulates maturation and survival of newly generated neurons in the adult hippocampus. *J. Neurosci.* 29, 7966–7977. doi: 10.1523/JNEUROSCI.1054-09.2009

Jiao, J. W., Feldheim, D. A., and Chen, D. F. (2008). Ephrins as negative regulators of adult neurogenesis in diverse regions of the central nervous system. *Proc. Natl. Acad. Sci. U.S.A.* 105, 8778–8783. doi: 10.1073/pnas.0708861105

Keung, A. J., de Juan-Pardo, E. M., Schaffer, D. V., and Kumar, S. (2011). Rho GTPases mediate the mechanosensitive lineage commitment of neural stem cells. *Stem Cells* 29, 1886–1897. doi: 10.1002/stem.746

Kim, J. Y., Liu, C. Y., Zhang, F., Duan, X., Wen, Z., Song, J., et al. (2012). Interplay between DISC1 and GABA signaling regulates neurogenesis in mice and risk for schizophrenia. *Cell* 148, 1051–1064. doi: 10.1016/j.cell.2011.12.037

Kwok, J. C., Dick, G., Wang, D., and Fawcett, J. W. (2011). Extracellular matrix and perineuronal nets in CNS repair. *Dev. Neurobiol.* 71, 1073–1089. doi: 10.1002/dneu.20974

Lemmens, R., Jaspers, T., Robberecht, W., and Thijs, V. N. (2013). Modifying expression of EphA4 and its downstream targets improves functional recovery after stroke. *Hum. Mol. Genet.* 22, 2214–2220. doi: 10.1093/hmg/ddt073

Leong, S. Y., Faux, C. H., Turbic, A., Dixon, K. J., and Turnley, A. M. (2011). The Rho kinase pathway regulates mouse adult neural precursor cell migration. *Stem Cells* 29, 332–343. doi: 10.1002/stem.577

Lin, C. W., Sim, S., Ainsworth, A., Okada, M., Kelsch, W., and Lois, C. (2010). Genetically increased cell-intrinsic excitability enhances neuronal integration into adult brain circuits. *Neuron* 65, 32–39. doi: 10.1016/j.neuron.2009.12.001

Lu, D., Mahmood, A., Qu, C., Goussev, A., Schallert, T., and Chopp, M. (2005). Erythropoietin enhances neurogenesis and restores spatial memory in rats after traumatic brain injury. *J. Neurotrauma* 22, 1011–1017. doi: 10.1089/neu.2005.22.1011

Mandairon, N., Sacquet, J., Garcia, S., Ravel, N., Jourdan, F., and Didier, A. (2006). Neurogenic correlates of an olfactory discrimination task in the adult olfactory bulb. *Eur. J. Neurosci.* 24, 3578–3588. doi: 10.1111/j.1460-9568.2006.05235.x

Metcalf, D., Greenhalgh, C. J., Viney, E., Willson, T. A., Starr, R., Nicola, N. A., et al. (2000). Gigantism in mice lacking suppressor of cytokine signalling-2. *Nature* 405, 1069–1073. doi: 10.1038/35016611

Ming, G. L., and Song, H. (2011). Adult neurogenesis in the mammalian brain: significant answers and significant questions. *Neuron* 70, 687–702. doi: 10.1016/j.neuron.2011.05.001

Miwa, N., and Storm, D. R. (2005). Odorant-induced activation of extracellular signal-regulated kinase/mitogen-activated protein kinase in the olfactory bulb promotes survival of newly formed granule cells. *J. Neurosci.* 25, 5404–5412. doi: 10.1523/JNEUROSCI.1039-05.2005

Miyamoto, Y., Yamauchi, J., Tanoue, A., Wu, C., and Mobley, W. C. (2006). TrkB binds and tyrosine-phosphorylates Tiam1, leading to activation of Rac1 and induction of changes in cellular morphology. *Proc. Natl. Acad. Sci. U.S.A.* 103, 10444–1049. doi: 10.1073/pnas.0603914103

Moreno, M. M., Linster, C., Escanilla, O., Sacquet, J., Didier, A., and Mandairon, N. (2009). Olfactory perceptual learning requires adult neurogenesis. *Proc. Natl. Acad. Sci. U.S.A.* 106, 17980–17985. doi: 10.1073/pnas.0907063106

Murai, K., Qiu, R., Zhang, H., Wang, J., Wu, C., Neubig, R. R., et al. (2010). Galpha subunit coordinates with ephrin-B to balance self-renewal and differentiation in neural progenitor cells. *Stem Cells* 28, 1581–1589. doi: 10.1002/stem.474

Nikolic, M. (2002). The role of Rho GTPases and associated kinases in regulating neurite outgrowth. *Int. J. Biochem. Cell Biol.* 34, 731–745. doi: 10.1016/S1357-2725(01)00167-4

Overman, J. J., Clarkson, A. N., Wanner, I. B., Overman, W. T., Eckstein, I., Maguire, J. L., et al. (2012). A role for ephrin-A5 in axonal sprouting, recovery, and activity-dependent plasticity after stroke. *Proc. Natl. Acad. Sci. U.S.A.* 109, E2230–E2239. doi: 10.1073/pnas.1204386109

Pathania, M., Torres-Reveron, J., Yan, L., Kimura, T., Lin, T. V., Gordon, V., et al. (2012). miR-132 enhances dendritic morphogenesis, spine density, synaptic integration, and survival of newborn olfactory bulb neurons. *PLoS ONE* 7:e38174. doi: 10.1371/journal.pone.0038174

Perederiy, J. V., Luikart, B. W., Washburn, E. K., Schnell, E., and Westbrook, G. L. (2013). Neural injury alters proliferation and integration of adult-generated neurons in the dentate gyrus. *J. Neurosci.* 33, 4754–4767. doi: 10.1523/JNEUROSCI.4785-12.2013

Petreanu, L., and Alvarez-Buylla, A. (2002). Maturation and death of adult-born olfactory bulb granule neurons: role of olfaction. *J. Neurosci.* 22, 6106–6113.

Platel, J. C., Dave, K. A., Gordon, V., Lacar, B., Rubio, M. E., and Bordey, A. (2010). NMDA receptors activated by subventricular zone astrocytic glutamate are critical for neuroblast survival prior to entering a synaptic network. *Neuron* 65, 859–872. doi: 10.1016/j.neuron.2010.03.009

Polizzotto, M. N., Bartlett, P. F., and Turnley, A. M. (2000). Expression of "suppressor of cytokine signalling" (SOCS) genes in the developing and adult mouse nervous system. *J. Comp. Neurol.* 423, 348–358.

Quadrato, G., Benevento, M., Alber, S., Jacob, C., Floriddia, E. M., Nguyen, T., et al. (2012). Nuclear factor of activated T cells (NFATc4) is required for BDNF-dependent survival of adult-born neurons and spatial memory formation in the hippocampus. *Proc. Natl. Acad. Sci. U.S.A.* 109, E1499–E1508. doi: 10.1073/pnas.1202068109

Ransome, M. I., and Turnley, A. M. (2008). Growth hormone signaling and hippocampal neurogenesis: insights from genetic models. *Hippocampus* 18, 1034–1050. doi: 10.1002/hipo.20463

Ricard, J., Salinas, J., Garcia, L., and Liebl, D. J. (2006). EphrinB3 regulates cell proliferation and survival in adult neurogenesis. *Mol. Cell. Neurosci.* 31, 713–722. doi: 10.1016/j.mcn.2006.01.002

Rochefort, C., Gheusi, G., Vincent, J. D., and Lledo, P. M. (2002). Enriched odor exposure increases the number of newborn neurons in the adult olfactory bulb and improves odor memory. *J. Neurosci.* 22, 2679–2689.

Rodriguez-Perez, A. I., Dominguez-Meijide, A., Lanciego, J. L., Guerra, M. J., and Labandeira-Garcia, J. L. (2013). Inhibition of Rho kinase mediates the neuroprotective effects of estrogen in the MPTP model of Parkinson's disease. *Neurobiol. Dis.* 58, 209–219. doi: 10.1016/j.nbd.2013.06.004

Sakamoto, M., Imayoshi, I., Ohtsuka, T., Yamaguchi, M., Mori, K., and Kageyama, R. (2011). Continuous neurogenesis in the adult forebrain is required for innate olfactory responses. *Proc. Natl. Acad. Sci. U.S.A.* 108, 8479–8484. doi: 10.1073/pnas.1018782108

Scobie, K. N., Hall, B. J., Wilke, S. A., Klemenhagen, K. C., Fujii-Kuriyama, Y., Ghosh, A., et al. (2009). Kruppel-like factor 9 is necessary for late-phase neuronal maturation in the developing dentate gyrus and during adult hippocampal neurogenesis. *J. Neurosci.* 29, 9875–9887. doi: 10.1523/JNEUROSCI.2260-09.2009

Shihabuddin, L. S., Horner, P. J., Ray, J., and Gage, F. H. (2000). Adult spinal cord stem cells generate neurons after transplantation in the adult dentate gyrus. *J. Neurosci.* 20, 8727–8735.

Shingo, T., Sorokan, S. T., Shimazaki, T., and Weiss, S. (2001). Erythropoietin regulates the *in vitro* and *in vivo* production of neuronal progenitors by mammalian forebrain neural stem cells. *J. Neurosci.* 21, 9733–9743.

Shors, T. J., Anderson, M. L., Curlik, D. M. 2nd., and Nokia, M. S. (2012). Use it or lose it: how neurogenesis keeps the brain fit for learning. *Behav. Brain Res.* 227, 450–458. doi: 10.1016/j.bbr.2011.04.023

Spanevello, M. D., Tajouri, S. I., Mirciov, C., Kurniawan, N., Pearse, M. J., Fabri, L. J., et al. (2013). Acute delivery of EphA4-Fc improves functional recovery after contusive spinal cord injury in rats. *J Neurotrauma* 30, 1023–1034. doi: 10.1089/neu.2012.2729

Suhonen, J. O., Peterson, D. A., Ray, J., and Gage, F. H. (1996). Differentiation of adult hippocampus-derived progenitors into olfactory neurons *in vivo*. *Nature* 383, 624–627. doi: 10.1038/383624a0

Tsai, P. T., Ohab, J. J., Kertesz, N., Groszer, M., Matter, C., Gao, J., et al. (2006). A critical role of erythropoietin receptor in neurogenesis and post-stroke recovery. *J. Neurosci.* 26, 1269–1274. doi: 10.1523/JNEUROSCI.4480-05.2006

Turnley, A. M., Faux, C. H., Rietze, R. L., Coonan, J. R., and Bartlett, P. F. (2002). Suppressor of cytokine signaling 2 regulates neuronal differentiation by inhibiting growth hormone signaling. *Nat. Neurosci.* 5, 1155–1162. doi: 10.1038/nn954

Vadodaria, K. C., Brakebusch, C., Suter, U., and Jessberger, S. (2013). Stage-specific functions of the small Rho GTPases Cdc42 and Rac1 for adult hippocampal neurogenesis. *J. Neurosci.* 33, 1179–1189. doi: 10.1523/JNEUROSCI.2103-12.2013

Vadodaria, K. C., and Jessberger, S. (2013). Maturation and integration of adult born hippocampal neurons: signal convergence onto small Rho GTPases. *Front. Synaptic Neurosci.* 5:4. doi: 10.3389/fnsyn.2013.00004

Valley, M. T., Mullen, T. R., Schultz, L. C., Sagdullaev, B. T., and Firestein, S. (2009). Ablation of mouse adult neurogenesis alters olfactory bulb structure and olfactory fear conditioning. *Front. Neurosci.* 3:51. doi: 10.3389/neuro.22.003.2009

Veyrac, A., Gros, A., Bruel-Jungerman, E., Rochefort, C., Kleine Borgmann, F. B., Jessberger, S., et al. (2013). Zif268/egr1 gene controls the selection, maturation and functional integration of adult hippocampal newborn neurons by learning. *Proc. Natl. Acad. Sci. U.S.A.* 110, 7062–7067. doi: 10.1073/pnas.1220558110

Wang, D., Ichiyama, R. M., Zhao, R., Andrews, M. R., and Fawcett, J. W. (2011). Chondroitinase combined with rehabilitation promotes recovery of forelimb function in rats with chronic spinal cord injury. *J. Neurosci.* 31, 9332–9344. doi: 10.1523/JNEUROSCI.0983-11.2011

Wang, L., Zhang, Z., Wang, Y., Zhang, R., and Chopp, M. (2004). Treatment of stroke with erythropoietin enhances neurogenesis and angiogenesis and improves neurological function in rats. *Stroke* 35, 1732–1737. doi: 10.1161/01.STR.0000132196.49028.a4

Wang, S. Z., Ou, J., Zhu, L. J., and Green, M. R. (2012). Transcription factor ATF5 is required for terminal differentiation and survival of olfactory sensory neurons. *Proc. Natl. Acad. Sci. U.S.A.* 109, 18589–18594. doi: 10.1073/pnas.1210479109

Yamaguchi, M., and Mori, K. (2005). Critical period for sensory experience-dependent survival of newly generated granule cells in the adult mouse olfactory bulb. *Proc. Natl. Acad. Sci. U.S.A.* 102, 9697–9702. doi: 10.1073/pnas.0406082102

Zhang, Y., Chopp, M., Mahmood, A., Meng, Y., Qu, C., and Xiong, Y. (2012). Impact of inhibition of erythropoietin treatment-mediated neurogenesis in the dentate gyrus of the hippocampus on restoration of spatial learning after traumatic brain injury. *Exp. Neurol.* 235, 336–344. doi: 10.1016/j.expneurol.2012.02.015

4

Illuminating the role of cholinergic signaling in circuits of attention and emotionally salient behaviors

Antonio Luchicchi[1], Bernard Bloem[1,2], John Noel M. Viaña[1], Huibert D. Mansvelder[1]* and Lorna W. Role[3]*

[1] Department of Integrative Neurophysiology, Center for Neurogenomics and Cognitive Research, Neuroscience Campus Amsterdam, Vrije Universiteit, Amsterdam, Netherlands
[2] McGovern Institute for Brain Research, Massachusetts Institute of Technology, Cambridge, MA, USA
[3] Department of Neurobiology and Behavior, Stony Brook University, Stony Brook, NY, USA

Edited by:
Sukumar Vijayaraghavan, University of Colorado Health Science Center, USA

Reviewed by:
Dan McGehee, University of Chicago, USA
John A. Dani, Baylor College of Medicine, USA

***Correspondence:**
Huibert D. Mansvelder, Department of Integrative Neurophysiology, Center for Neurogenomics and Cognitive Research, Neuroscience Campus Amsterdam, Vrije Universiteit, de Boelelaan 1085, 1081 HV, Amsterdam, Netherlands
e-mail: h.d.mansvelder@vu.nl;
Lorna W. Role, Department of Neurobiology and Behavior, Stony Brook University, Stony Brook, NY 11794, USA
e-mail: lorna.role@stonybrook.edu

Acetylcholine (ACh) signaling underlies specific aspects of cognitive functions and behaviors, including attention, learning, memory and motivation. Alterations in ACh signaling are involved in the pathophysiology of multiple neuropsychiatric disorders. In the central nervous system, ACh transmission is mainly guaranteed by dense innervation of select cortical and subcortical regions from disperse groups of cholinergic neurons within the basal forebrain (BF; e.g., diagonal band, medial septal, nucleus basalis) and the pontine-mesencephalic nuclei, respectively. Despite the fundamental role of cholinergic signaling in the CNS and the long standing knowledge of the organization of cholinergic circuitry, remarkably little is known about precisely how ACh release modulates cortical and subcortical neural activity and the behaviors these circuits subserve. Growing interest in cholinergic signaling in the CNS focuses on the mechanism(s) of action by which endogenously released ACh regulates cognitive functions, acting as a neuromodulator and/or as a direct transmitter via nicotinic and muscarinic receptors. The development of optogenetic techniques has provided a valuable toolbox with which we can address these questions, as it allows the selective manipulation of the excitability of cholinergic inputs to the diverse array of cholinergic target fields within cortical and subcortical domains. Here, we review recent papers that use the light-sensitive opsins in the cholinergic system to elucidate the role of ACh in circuits related to attention and emotionally salient behaviors. In particular, we highlight recent optogenetic studies which have tried to disentangle the precise role of ACh in the modulation of cortical-, hippocampal- and striatal-dependent functions.

Keywords: acetylcholine, optogenetics, nicotinic receptors, limbic circuitries, attention

INTRODUCTION

Acetylcholine (ACh) is essential to normal CNS function, modulating cognitive, emotional and behavioral functions, including learning and memory (Kilgard and Merzenich, 1998; Hasselmo and Giocomo, 2006), reward (Leslie et al., 2013), wakefulness and attention (Klinkenberg et al., 2011; see Picciotto et al., 2012 for a recent review). Appropriate levels of ACh are required to process relevant sensory information and for encoding environmental cues that drive goal-directed behavior (Sarter et al., 2009). Disruptions of cholinergic transmission contribute to the pathophysiology of neuropsychiatric disorders, including Alzheimer's disease, schizophrenia and drug addiction (Court et al., 2001; Dani and Harris, 2005; Martin and Freedman, 2007). To support its prominent role in the brain, the cholinergic system sends dense projections from sparse cholinergic nuclei, that include the basal forebrain (BF), laterodorsal tegmental nucleus (LDTg), peduculopontine tegmentum (PPTg), and medial habenula (MHb; Woolf, 1991; Mesulam, 1995; Zaborszky et al., 1999; Ren et al., 2011). In addition, there is a small population of choline acetyltransferase (ChAT) positive interneurons in areas including the striatum and neocortex (Woolf, 1991; Mesulam, 1995; von Engelhardt et al., 2007). Cholinergic projections, from the BF, LDTg and PPTg nuclei extend throughout the main telencephalic and limbic structures delivering ACh to broad terminal fields. Released ACh activates via both ionotropic nicotinic and metabotropic muscarinic ACh receptors (nAChRs, and mAChRs, respectively) that vary in terms of cellular localization (pre- and/or postsynaptic), subunit composition, signaling mechanism(s) and affinity for ACh (for recent reviews see Wess, 2003; Gotti and Clementi, 2004; Changeux, 2010; Picciotto et al., 2012).

Although our understanding of the organization of the cholinergic system and its role in modulating certain behaviors is growing, many questions remain to be answered to understand the dynamics of ACh action and its involvement in (patho) physiology. The role of ACh in specific behaviors has been addressed using lesions of cholinergic projections or pharmacological interventions with ACh receptor activation. Such approaches, though informative, are confounded by issues of bioavailability, lack of complete reversibility and the fact that such interventions act on time scales of unknown relevance for cholinergic driven changes in excitability *in vivo*. Our understanding of how cholinergic projections innervate and modulate target circuitry remains rudimentary. In fact, it is not even clear whether ACh acts as a classic synaptic neurotransmitter—on the millisecond to tens of millisecond time scale—or whether it acts as a neuromodulator (at the hundreds of milliseconds to seconds time scale) or both (see Picciotto et al., 2012; Sarter et al., 2014). The latter hypothesis is supported by several investigations that emphasize the predominant role of ACh in modifying cell excitability and activity of entire networks of neurons (Wonnacott, 1997; Kawai et al., 2007). Moreover, a relatively modest specificity of the cholinergic system exists in terms of connectivity in crucial target regions such as the cortex (see Sarter et al., 2009, for a review). On the other hand, the presence of point-to-point sites of ACh release juxtaposed to cholinergic receptors suggests that the cholinergic system may also utilize fast synaptic signaling, typical of classic neurotransmitters (Smiley et al., 1997; Turrini et al., 2001). Indeed, the complexity of results obtained to date has led to the conclusion that ACh signaling may occur over a range of different time courses due, in part, to varied release mechanisms and proximity of release and receptive sites as well as to the involvement of distinct signaling cascades downstream of both nicotinic and muscarinic AChRs (e.g see Arroyo et al., 2014; Jiang et al., 2014). A lack of high-temporal resolution and accurate detection methods for ACh release has hampered our understanding of whether endogenous cholinergic signaling is mediated by rapid, transient release (millisecond time-scale) and/or by a more diffuse transmission (from second to minute time-scale).

With the exponential rise in the number and type of optogenetic tools developed over the last decade it is now possible to selectively stimulate or inhibit specific populations of CNS cholinergic neurons and/or their axonal terminal fields through the activation of light-sensitive opsins (for reviews see: Deisseroth, 2011; Yizhar et al., 2011; Poorthuis et al., 2014). Here, we review the recent studies that have used the expression of photo-sensitive opsins in the cholinergic system to elucidate the role of endogenous ACh signaling in different brain regions related to attention and emotionally salient/ limbic behaviors.

BASAL FOREBRAIN ACH AND NEOCORTICAL FUNCTION

The mechanisms by which ACh release in the neocortex influences cognitive functions and behaviors are still poorly understood. While early microdialysis studies in the medial prefrontal cortex (mPFC) reported a long-lasting ACh increase during attention-related performance tasks (Passetti et al., 2000), more recent works with faster, dynamic, electrochemical detection of choline, have shown that ACh can also be released briefly in concert with cue detection in a cued appetitive response task (Parikh et al., 2007; Parikh and Sarter, 2008). Thus, while the microdialysis assays are consistent with the idea that ACh release could promote a general state of cortical arousal, due to sustained levels of ACh over long time-scales, recent and more sensitive electrochemical assays highlight a faster, and more transient release of ACh. The latter observation modifies the prior view that ACh only acts through "volume transmission" (Sarter et al., 2009), and underscores the possibility of faster components of ACh action in the modulation of specific cholinergic functions. For example, the phasic release of ACh would support more rapid transitions of cortical states, consistent with cholinergic regulation of an animal's ability to incorporate the detection of a cue into new goal-directed behaviors (Sarter et al., 2014).

CHOLINERGIC FAST SYNAPTIC TRANSMISSION IN CORTEX

The application of optogenetic tools to the analysis of central cholinergic signaling using ChAT-Cre lines in either mice (Kalmbach et al., 2012; Huang and Zeng, 2013) or rats (Witten et al., 2011; see **Figure 1**) allows selective activation and silencing of cholinergic neurons and axonal projections, both *in vitro* and *in vivo*. Using this approach, several studies have now shown that ACh signaling occurs through direct, fast synaptic transmission—as well as over longer time scales consistent with more diffuse transmission—in the cortex (Letzkus et al., 2011; Arroyo et al., 2012, 2014; Bennett et al., 2012; Kimura et al., 2014). Activating channelrhodopsin (ChR2) in fibers from the BF elicited a barrage of inhibitory synaptic inputs to layer (L) 2/3 pyramidal cells, which depended on nAChR activation (Arroyo et al., 2012, 2014; Bennett et al., 2012; Kimura et al., 2014). Pyramidal neurons in L2/3 apparently do not express nAChRs themselves, but L2/3 interneurons do (Poorthuis et al., 2013). Activation of BF fibers produced cell type-specific responses in cortical interneurons. L1 and L2/3 LS neurons exhibited both a fast and a slow response, while L2/3 ChAT bipolar neurons exhibited only a slow response. Activation of L2/3 interneurons by ACh via both nicotinic and muscarinic receptors depressed pyramidal neuron firing thereby curtailing visual responses (Kimura et al., 2014). ACh-induced excitatory postsynaptic currents were generated by a mixed population of nAChRs (Arroyo et al., 2012). In addition to a slow dihydro-β-erythroidine (DHβE) sensitive non-α7*-mediated current, a fast component of excitatory postsynaptic potentials (EPSCs) was abolished by methyllycaconitine (MLA) in both L1 and 2/3 interneurons but not in ChAT+ cells. Comparing the reported time course of the inhibitory barrage received by L2/3 pyramidal neurons upon light-induced ACh release with the time course of the two different EPSC components, suggested that L2/3 pyramidal neuron inhibition is more likely dependent on the slow component, rather than the fast component of cholinergic activation. This was confirmed by bath application of DhβE, which prevented the inhibitory drive onto pyramidal cells. In a follow-up study, the same authors found a large trial-to trial variability of the fast component of the ACh-induced current components, indicative of direct synaptic transmission which they propose is mediated by synaptic α7*-containing (α7*) receptors. This was confirmed by lack of effect of AChE inhibitors on the amplitude or kinetics of this fast current component (Bennett et al., 2012; Arroyo et al., 2014). The slow component showed much less trial-to-trial variability and was sensitive to manipulation of AChE activity. From this, the authors conclude that the slow, non-α7* component involves diffusion of ACh over some distance, and arises from the effects of ACh on extra synaptic α4β2* nAChRs, while the faster nAChR EPSCs are mediated by direct transmission via synaptic or peri-synaptic α7* AChRs (Arroyo et al., 2012, 2014). These experiments demonstrate that in superficial layers of the somatosensory, visual and auditory cortex, L1 and L2/3 interneurons receive both direct and

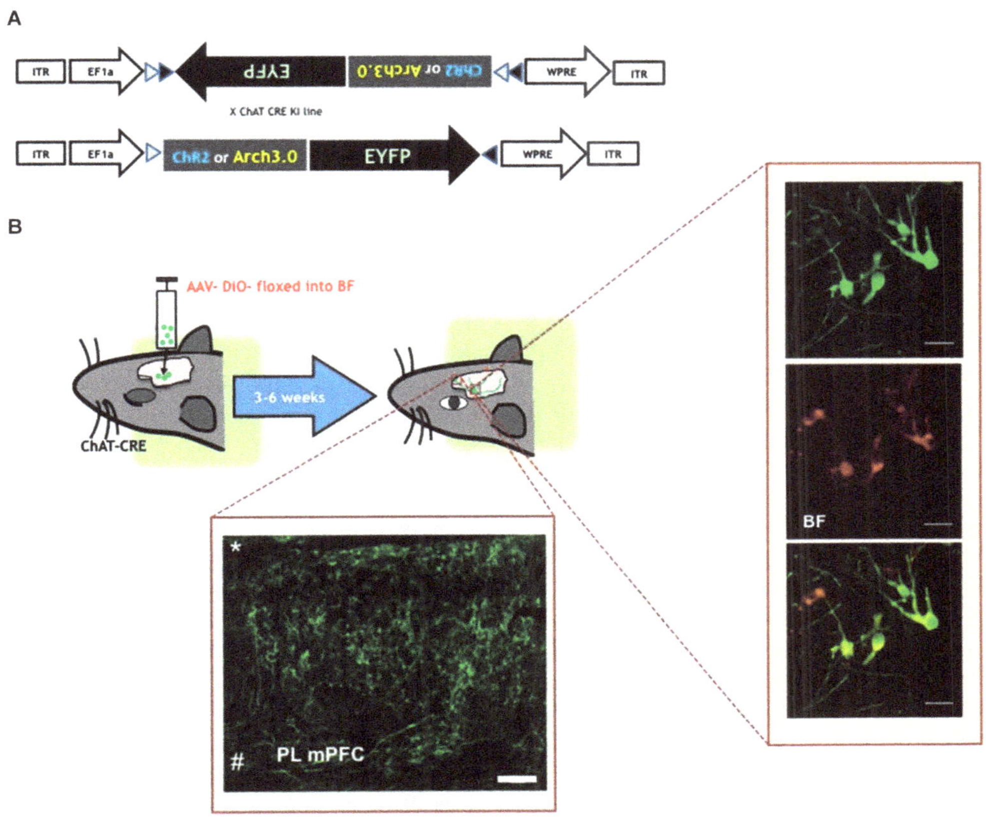

FIGURE 1 | Visualizing the cholinergic system in rodents. (A) Viral construct used to achieve selective expression of functional opsins (ChR2 or Arch3.0) in ChAT+ cells (Witten et al., 2011). Top panel shows the construct that is sterotactically injected in the basal forebrain region of ChAT-cre mice or rats. The portion of the construct encoding the opsin and fluorophore (Enhanced yellow fluorescent protein-EYFP) is inverted and flanked by double LoxP sites (black and white triangles). After virus delivery in the brain, and in presence of cre-recombinase, the coding fragment is oriented in the right direction, allowing the expression of functional light-sensitive opsins in the ChAT+ neurons. **(B)** Schematic representation of virus delivery and opsin expression in ChAT-cre mice/rats. Rodents undergo surgery to infuse the adeno-associated virus (AAV) construct with the coding information for opsins and/or fluorophores. After 3 to 6 weeks rodents have sustained expression of the flourophore and/or excitatory (ChR2, ChIEF etc.) or inhibitory (halorhodopsin or arch 3.0) in ChAT+ cell soma and fibers. Left inset is a confocal micrograph of the basal forebrain of a ChAT-cre rat. Green cells in the top panel express EYFP as result of the AAV-floxed EYFP injection. Middle panel is a confocal micrograph of ChAT+ neurons, confirmed by the presence of anti-ChAT antibody staining. Bottom panel is a confocal micrograph indicating that the EYFP probe is expressed only in ChAT+ cells. Scale bar is 40 μm (Luchicchi and Mansvelder, unpublished observations).Bottom inset confocal micrograph of EYFP+ labeled basal forebrain terminal fields within the mPFC (*pia; # white matter). Scale bar is 200 μm (Luchicchi and Mansvelder, unpublished observations). Figure is adapted from Jiang et al. (submitted).

diffuse cholinergic inputs, that enable the cholinergic system to manipulate neocortical processing on a millisecond time scale as well as on slower time scales (Arroyo et al., 2012, 2014; Kimura et al., 2014).

On a network level, BF stimulation in anesthetized animals results in a desynchronized state of field potentials (Goard and Dan, 2009; Kalmbach et al., 2012; reviewed in Bloem et al., 2014) and neuronal firing in the BF is correlated with a reduction in low frequency, and an increase of high frequency, oscillations in the cortex (Duque et al., 2000; Manns et al., 2000). Since the frequency band activity is related to the state of arousal and the extent of cortical activation (Uhlhaas et al., 2008; Wang, 2010; Deco and Thiele, 2011; Cachope et al., 2012), this supports the idea that ACh acts as a neuromodulator involved in setting the state of arousal. Mechanistically, it was shown that ACh activated mAChRs on cortical pyramidal neurons (Gulledge et al., 2009), thereby shifting firing modes from bursting to tonic and changing low frequency high amplitude oscillatory activity to high frequency low amplitude activity on a network level (Metherate et al., 1992).

Other studies have looked at the effect of ACh on the direction of the flow of information in the cortex. Again, these studies have been performed in sensory areas because in these regions, neuronal responses could be related to sensory stimulation. In this regard it is reasonably well established that ACh is directly involved in the enhancement of feed-forward thalamic input into the sensory cortical areas (see Bloem et al., 2014, for a review). In L4 of visual cortex, ACh increases the gain and reliability of neuronal responses (Goard and Dan, 2009; Soma et al., 2012, 2013), an effect that is mediated by heteromeric nAChRs (Roberts et al., 2005; Disney et al., 2007). A similar effect of ACh is observed in the barrel cortex (Oldford and Castro-Alamancos, 2003).

In L2/3, the picture is more complex. In general, cholinergic modulation reduces firing rate in these layers by increasing GABAergic inhibition through mAChRs and nAChRs (Disney et al., 2012; Alitto and Dan, 2013; Soma et al., 2013; Kimura et al., 2014). The ACh modulation in firing rates was associated with enhancement of the reliability of encoding and modulation by stimuli presented (Goard and Dan, 2009; Soma et al., 2013).

The cortical depression associated with whisker trimming is accompanied by an increase of heteromeric nAChRs on interneurons in L2/3 and blockade of these nAChRs can prevent the cortical depression. These observations support the contention that heteromeric nAChRs in L2/3 are required for regulating the input- dependent responsiveness of the somatosensory cortex (Brown et al., 2012a).

Intra-cortical projections that connect superficial layers between different cortical columns are also inhibited by ACh through activation of mAChRs (Kimura and Baughman, 1997). Based on this finding and the reduced activity in the superficial layers, it has been suggested that ACh reduces horizontal processing through cortico-cortical interactions (Hasselmo and Giocomo, 2006). Indeed it has been observed in slices, and *in vivo* animal experiments as well as in humans, that the spatial spread of excitation in response to stimuli is reduced in the presence of elevated levels of ACh (Kimura et al., 1999; Silver et al., 2008). Such a modulation of excitation could have a sharpening effect on tuning curves of receptive fields and on discrimination of sensory stimuli (Roberts et al., 2005; Thiele et al., 2012). The combined effects of ACh—e.g., reduction of lateral interactions and increased sensitivity to thalamic inputs, would be expected to increase network sensitivity to incoming information and enhance signal to noise. A similar selective gain-control effect of ACh is observed with enhanced attention (Briggs et al., 2013) and could be one of the core mechanisms through which ACh modulates selective attention (Hasselmo and Giocomo, 2006; Deco and Thiele, 2011; Hasselmo and Sarter, 2011).

The functional impact of ACh on the deeper L5 and 6 is less well understood. It is clear that deep layer pyramidal and interneurons are modulated by both nAChRs and mAChRs (Gulledge et al., 2007; Kassam et al., 2008; Poorthuis et al., 2013). ACh is associated with both response suppression and response facilitation, although the net effect of endogenous cholinergic signaling is not clear (Soma et al., 2013). In L1, most (if not all) interneurons contain α7* and /or non-α7* nAChRs (Christophe et al., 2002; Alitto and Dan, 2013). Since these neurons inhibit both L1-3 interneurons and L2/3 pyramidal cells, the effect of cholinergic L1 activation appears to be complex with both net inhibition as well as disinhibition of pyramidal cells in deeper layers, and it is likely dependent on the source and extent of ACh release in L1 (Letzkus et al., 2011; Bennett et al., 2012; Cruikshank et al., 2012; Jiang et al., 2013; Arroyo et al., 2014).

Thalamic inputs to L5 neurons are strongly regulated by nicotinic receptor activation (Lambe et al., 2003; Couey et al., 2007; Poorthuis et al., 2013). Whether these are targeted by direct cholinergic inputs is not known. However, within the thalamic reticular nucleus, neurons receive biphasic fast cholinergic inputs mediated by non-α7* nAChRs and mAChRs (Sun et al., 2013).

MANIPULATING THE CORTICAL CHOLINERGIC SYSTEM DURING BEHAVIOR

Despite new insights as to how rapidly ACh levels may rise and fall in prefrontal cortex during cue detection (Sarter et al., 2014), there is still no direct demonstration of the cellular and synaptic mechanisms by which ACh controls attentional behaviors. Hints emerge from the optogenetic data on the disinhibitory circuit mechanisms in superficial layers of sensory areas (Letzkus et al., 2011; Arroyo et al., 2014), but the architecture of the somatosensory cortex differs substantially from that of prefrontal cortical regions. Indeed, L4 is absent from rodent medial PFC (Uylings et al., 2003), and projections from the mediodorsal thalamus target all layers of mPFC, in contrast to the more discrete segregation of thalamo—cortical input seen in somatosensory areas (Douglas and Martin, 2004; Constantinople and Bruno, 2013). Few studies have appeared that manipulate the cholinergic system using optogenetics during cognitive tasks. In the primary visual cortex (V1) optogenetic stimulation of BF projections improved visual discrimination, a hallmark of visual attention, in a go-no-go task (Pinto et al., 2013). Inhibiting the BF cholinergic projections to the visual cortex with either halo-rhodopsin (NpHR) or archaerhodopsin (Arch) impaired mouse performance on the same tasks (Pinto et al., 2013; Arroyo et al., 2014 for review).

In a recent report of unpublished observations, Sarter et al. (2014) optogenetically manipulated the excitability of BF projections to the PFC in mice performing a sustained attention task (SAT). This would be the first report of optogenetic manipulation of ACh release in the PFC and modulation of attention performance. Using ChAT-Cre mice expressing ChR2 in the BF, the authors report that brief blue light stimulation during cue presentation increases detection of the cue. Optogenetic stimulation of BF fibers in the absence of a cue, which predict the presentation of reward, results in a higher number of false-positive responses in cue detection of ChR2 mice. Inhibition of ACh fibers with NpHR stimulation reduced cue detection (Sarter et al., 2014). Previous studies from the same group have identified transient release of ACh in the mPFC as a modulator of cue-directed attention. In particular, fast ACh release occurred when the cue trial was preceded by an actual or perceived non-cue trial (Howe et al., 2013). Therefore, cholinergic transients may be involved in state-shifting: i.e., in regulating the shift from generalized monitoring to one of cue-directed attention (Sarter et al., 2014). In this sense, the optogenetic increase in false-positive responses, where the animal responds incorrectly to a non-cue trial, might reveal the mechanism by which transient release of ACh in the mPFC determines the transition from cue detection to a behavioral response. Full appreciation of the data underlying these conclusions awaits publication of the primary data referred to in the Sarter review (Sarter et al., 2014).

OPTOGENETIC CONTROL OF CHOLINERGIC PROJECTIONS TO HIPPOCAMPUS AND AMYGDALA: SYNAPTIC PLASTICITY AND OSCILLATIONS

Hippocampal control over specific behaviors, such as learning and memory, is potently modulated by cholinergic signaling. Antagonists to both nicotinic and muscarinic AChRs impair performance in hippocampal-dependent memory tasks in rodents (Levin et al., 2002), as well as the ability to encode spatial information (Blokland et al., 1992). The majority of cholinergic inputs to the hippocampus (up to 90%) come from the medial septum and diagonal band via the fimbria/fornix, and enter the hippocampus through the stratum oriens (SO; Frotscher and Léránth, 1985; Dutar et al., 1995). In addition, sparse cholinergic interneurons have been reported in some regions of the hippocampus, where they usually impinge on GABAergic interneurons (Griguoli and Cherubini, 2012). Both nicotinic and muscarinic AChRs are involved in regulating hippocampal network activity, such as synchronization of neuronal activity and altering of synaptic weights, thereby influencing hippocampal support of cognitive function (Yakel, 2012). Exogenous application of nicotinic agonists in hippocampal slices affects synaptic plasticity in nearly all hippocampal areas (Tu et al., 2009; Yakel, 2012), and muscarinic agonists induce fast network oscillations (Mann et al., 2005). However, it is still not completely clear how cholinergic receptors regulate rhythmic and phasic oscillations and synaptic plasticity *in vivo*, during hippocampal-dependent cognitive functions.

By stimulating septal cholinergic projecting neurons to the SO using both electrical and optogenetic methods, Gu and Yakel disentangled the temporal requirements for ACh release in the cholinergic modulation of synaptic strength of Schaffer's collateral (SC) to CA1 synapses (Gu and Yakel, 2011). With precisely timed activation of septal cholinergic neurons in ChAT-cre mice expressing ChR2, Yakel et al. showed that when the light-evoked increase of ACh release in the SO preceded the SC stimulation by 100 ms, long-term potentiation (LTP) in the CA1 was triggered. This effect was dependent on the activation of α7* nAChRs in postsynaptic neurons. On the other hand, ChR2 activation of cholinergic terminals only 10 ms before the SC stimulation resulted in hippocampal short-term depression. In the latter case the effect was due to an α7* subunit-dependent inhibition of presynaptic glutamate release. Even more intriguing, the α7* component also altered synaptic plasticity when light pulses were delivered 10 ms *after* the SC activation. In fact, this latter protocol caused LTD in SO neurons by a mechanism which was attributed to mAChR activation, although whether the muscarinic component was pre- or postsynaptic is not clear (Gu and Yakel, 2011).

Muscarinic AChRs also modulate hippocampal activity by acting on interneurons (Bell et al., 2013). This is in line with the role of these receptors in orchestrating network oscillation within the hippocampus (Mann et al., 2005). Interestingly, interneuron network responses to light-evoked ACh release from the septum varied according to the level of cholinergic activity. In particular, low-intensity stimulation of cholinergic inputs was more likely to inhibit certain classes of interneurons via a mechanism dependent on the M4 type of mAChRs, whereas higher levels of ACh release triggered depolarization in other interneurons via broader muscarinic signaling. Cholinergic inputs from BF can also activate GABAergic interneurons through activation of α4β2* nAChRs in specific layers of the hippocampus (Bell et al., 2011).

Combining optogenetic stimulation of medial septum/diagonal band of Broca (MS/DBB) projections to the hippocampus with whole-cell patch clamp recordings and voltage sensitive dye (VSD) imaging it has been shown that inhibitory interneurons in the hippocampus receive cholinergic EPSPs in response to light stimulation of septal cholinergic fibers that are sensitive to DhβE, but not MLA (Bell et al., 2011). These light-evoked EPSPs have slow kinetics similar to the non-α7* component seen in interneurons in the somatosensory cortex (Arroyo et al., 2012). The interneurons that express α4β2* have their somata or dendrites in the SO or stratum lacunosum-moleculare (SLM) of the hippocampus. Finally, another recent optogenetic study implicates ACh release from the MS/DBB in the modulation of synaptic plasticity triggered by GABAergic interneurons of the stratum oriens lacunosum-maculare (OLM) in the SC-CA1 (Leão et al., 2012). Taken together, these data show that ACh inputs from the septum can influence hippocampal oscillations and plasticity in a highly specialized manner, resulting in a fine-tuning of hippocampal network activity in a layer specific manner and with millisecond timing. We still lack knowledge on the exact timing of activation of hippocampal cholinergic inputs during behavior. This will require both optogenetic manipulation of cholinergic projections, and concurrent visualization of activity of the BF projections in the hippocampus of awake-behaving animals.

Recently, optogenetic studies have been carried out to study the influence of other neuromodulatory systems interacting with cholinergic signaling to modulate hippocampal network activity. A set of studies conducted by Alger's group have very elegantly demonstrated that both the endocannabinoid (eCb) and endogenous opioid systems may participate in the generation of ACh-dependent modulation of hippocampal oscillatory activity (Nagode et al., 2011, 2014). With brief stimulation of the MS/DBB fibers in the CA1, Nagode et al. (2011) reported rhythmic inhibitory post-synaptic currents (IPSCs) in pyramidal neurons, accompanied by low frequency oscillation in hippocampal slices. Interestingly, the IPSCs, which were likely evoked by interneurons impinging on the pyramidal cells, were abolished by either GABA or mAChR antagonists. Moreover, the same events were also eCb-sensitive, supporting the presence of active cannabinoid receptor (CB-R1) in the presynaptic interneuron terminal. It is widely known that CB-Rs are expressed in the hippocampus, where they drive different forms of plasticity and mediate aspects of neuroprotection (Wilson and Nicoll, 2001). Only cholecystokinin (CCK) + interneurons in hippocampus have functional CB1-Rs; CB-Rs are not present on PV+ interneurons (Katona et al., 1999). For this reason, it is likely that the cholinergic modulation of low frequency oscillations observed in this study depends solely on CCK+ cell activity. Optogenetic inhibition of either PV+ interneurons or glutamic-acid decarboxylase-2 (GAD2)+ cells in the CA1 confirmed that the PV− population of GABAergic interneurons were required for ACh induction of low frequency oscillations. Surprisingly the ability of these PV− cells to trigger low frequency rhythms in the hippocampus was blocked by a mu-opioid receptor antagonist, and subsequent induction of IPSCs in pyramidal neurons by ACh release in ChAT-Cre mice was shown to be sensitive to both CB1 and mu-receptor blockade (Nagode et al., 2014). Overall, these studies provide new insights on the possible cross-communication between the eCb and cholinergic modulatory systems in the regulation of hippocampal network activity and perhaps, in memory functions.

The effects of cholinergic input in general, and of nAChRs in particular, in the basolateral amygdala is also under study with optogenetic labeling of the neurons and projections of the nucleus basalis (Role, 2014). These studies have revealed that cholinergic signaling potently modulates the plasticity of cortical synapses on basolateral amygdale (BLA) pyramidal neurons, decreasing the threshold for induction of LTP. Excitatory effects of nucleus basalis stimulation on BLA firing is confirmed in *in vivo* recording and, most striking, the rate of extinction of responses to a cue-associated fear conditioning paradigm is slowed by brief optogenetic activation of the cholinergic terminal fields in BLA during training (Role, 2014). These findings are consistent with the idea that cholinergic signaling reinforces amygdala-based memories, perhaps rendering them less susceptible to subsequent extinction (Role, 2014).

MODULATION OF STRIATAL CIRCUITS BY ACH

CHOLINERGIC INTERNEURONS MODULATE THE RELEASE OF MULTIPLE STRIATAL NEUROTRANSMITTERS

In addition to the robust modulatory activities of cholinergic signaling in cortex and hippocampus ACh is renowned for its strong regulatory role in subcortical brain regions within the midbrain and striatum. In particular, the core of the brain reward circuitry, comprising the ventral tegmental area (VTA) and the nucleus accumbens (NAc), is strongly modulated by ACh. The main source of ACh to the VTA neurons in the midbrain arises from the brainstem structures LDTg and PPTg, which play a role in acquisition of reward, and reward-related locomotor activity (Corrigall et al., 2002; Champtiaux et al., 2006). The main source of ACh for the NAc/ventral striatum, as well as for the dorsal striatum, is the cholinergic interneurons which comprise less than 2–5% of the total striatal neuron population (Descarries et al., 1997). Notwithstanding the paucity of striatal cholinergic interneurons, ACh signaling is directly involved in the modulation of (1) striatal dopamine (DA) release (Rice and Cragg, 2004; Exley and Cragg, 2008; Wang et al., 2014); (2) local network functionality (Galarraga et al., 1999; Koós and Tepper, 2002); and (3) striatal-dependent behaviors related to reward (Joshua et al., 2008).

The release of DA in striatum is crucial for functions such as motivation, reward and locomotor activity (see Cachope and Cheer, 2014, for a recent review) and cholinergic transmission can drive striatal DA release (Exley and Cragg, 2008). A recent study showed that selective optogenetic activation of accumbal cholinergic interneurons is sufficient to trigger DA release in the same region, and that this effect is independent of the suprathreshold activation of VTA DA neurons *per se* (Cachope et al., 2012; Threlfell et al., 2012; Wang et al., 2014). As such, the activity of cholinergic interneurons might boost the release of DA to encode aspects of reward-related events. This proposal is in line with studies in which photostimulation of cholinergic interneurons drove striatal DA release via activation of presynaptic nAChRs (Threlfell et al., 2012; Wang et al., 2014). On the other hand, Cachope et al. (2012) reported that the direct effect of cholinergic interneuron activation on DA release was only partially mediated by activation of AChRs. Combining optogenetic manipulation with *in vitro* pharmacology, revealed the collaboration of both nicotinic (β2*) and muscarinic receptors, together with the activation of α-amino-3-hydroxy-5-methyl-4-isoxazolepropionic acid (AMPA)-type glutamate receptors in the enhancement of striatal DA release. Thus, a synergy exists between ACh and glutamate in modulating the activity of the striatal network. The source of glutamate may be the striatal cholinergic interneurons themselves (Gras et al., 2008). Activating ChR2 in cholinergic striatal interneurons triggers postsynaptic responses onto medium spiny neurons (MSNs), the most abundant striatal cell type. Under the stimulation conditions used by Higley et al., the direct postsynaptic responses were blocked by glutamate receptor antagonists alone and were insensitive to AChR blockade (Higley et al., 2011). This suggests that at low levels of stimulation direct control of MSN firing by "cholinergic" interneurons may also rely on fast glutamatergic transmission.

A follow-up of this study was conducted looking at the connections between ACh interneurons and other local interneurons. including the PV+ interneurons, that also contact MSNs directly (Koós and Tepper, 1999; Gittis et al., 2010). Activating dorsal striatal ACh interneurons triggers the co-release of ACh and glutamate on PV+ interneurons, activating slow non-α7* nAChR currents, and both AMPA and N-methyl-D-aspartate (NMDA) receptors (Nelson et al., 2014). ACh and glutamate co-release was dependent on the presence of the vesicular glutamate transporter VGLUT3. This transporter is also involved in enhancing the vesicular loading of ACh and is important for di-synaptic inhibition of MSNs after PV+ excitation, a common feature in striatal information processing (Gras et al., 2008).

Activation of ChR2 in cholinergic interneurons in striatum also triggered GABA-A receptor-mediated postsynaptic currents in MSNs both *in vivo* and *in vitro* (Witten et al., 2010). Optogenetic stimulation of striatal cholinergic interneurons activated di-synaptic inhibitory responses in MSNs *in vitro* (Nelson et al., 2014). This effect was still present when PV+ neurons were ablated leading the authors to suggest that the di-synaptic inhibition of MSNs might be mediated by GABA release from DA terminals, that are studded with β2* nAChRs and targeted by cholinergic interneuronal projections. Thus, striatal network activity could be orchestrated by cholinergic interneurons through simultaneous regulation of DA and GABA release in the same striatal area.

OPTOGENETIC STUDIES OF ROLE OF CHOLINERGIC INTERNEURONS IN STRIATAL-DEPENDENT BEHAVIORS

Optogenetic studies have helped to define the role of striatal cholinergic interneurons in multiple aspects of motor control, associative learning and reward (see Jiang et al., 2014, for review; Exley and Cragg, 2008). During reward-related events, cholinergic interneurons initially increase their firing activity, and then pause, after which they start firing in a third phase of elevated activity (e.g., Morris et al., 2004). Most likely, these phasic activity periods support DA release from VTA projections, with the nAChR mediated component being *independent* of VTA action potential firing (e.g., see Wang et al., 2014). By combining pharmacological, optogenetic and electrophysiological techniques, Straub et al. (2014) recently suggested reward coding resides in the pause in striatal ACh interneuron activity that results from the direct effect of nigrostriatal DA projections via D2 dopamine receptors on cholinergic interneurons. The authors did not identify which neurotransmitter is involved in the rebound phase. Other studies have suggested that the pause of ACh interneuron firing may be caused by a GABA component. Activating VTA GABA neurons that project to the striatum with ChR2 and recording activity on ACh interneurons resulted in a pause of ACh interneuron firing (Van Bockstaele and Pickel, 1995; Tan et al., 2012; Van Zessen et al., 2012). Interestingly this effect was only observed in striatal ACh interneurons, sparing the other cell population and it was insensitive to DA receptor blockade. Behavioral studies have confirmed that GABA mediated inhibition of cholinergic interneurons is a requisite component of stimulus-outcome association under relevant learning conditions, pinpointing the pivotal role of ACh interneurons in goal directed behaviors (Brown et al., 2012b). In addition, Witten et al. (2010) have reported that cholinergic interneuron silencing by NpHR stimulation reduced cocaine preference in behaving mice.

Taken together, these findings support the idea that cholinergic interneurons play a crucial role in the modulation of striatal activity, and striatal-dependent behavior. Recent anatomical studies have also underscored the potential importance of direct projections from the brainstem (PPTg and LDTg) to striatal cells (Dautan et al., 2014). Hence, it will be interesting to learn how cooperation between these different elements of the cholinergic system modulates striatal activity.

SUMMARY AND CONCLUSIONS

The application of optogenetic tools has accelerated the acquisition of precise information about the varied modulatory and direct synaptic signaling by ACh in an array of brain regions and behaviors. Selective expression of optogenetic probes in ChAT+ neurons allows studies of the connectivity, functionality and anatomy of cholinergic neurons and circuits throughout the rodent brain (Atasoy et al., 2008; Witten et al., 2011; for reviews see: Arroyo et al., 2014; Jiang et al., 2014; Poorthuis et al., 2014). The application of these techniques has unveiled novel contributions of previously un-identified ChAT-positive neurons to activity-dependent proliferation and neurogenesis (Paez-Gonzalez et al., 2014) as well as implicating the co-storage—and perhaps co-release—of ACh and glutamate (e.g., see Higley et al., 2011). Many important challenges and new areas of exploration are now accessible to the cholinergic enthusiast. It will be particularly important to establish the precise mechanisms by which ACh modulates attention and contributes to top down executive control of directed behaviors. With the increasing number of research groups that have adopted the optogenetic toolbox, we can expect to learn more about these exciting topics in the not-so-distant future.

ACKNOWLEDGMENTS

Huibert D. Mansvelder received funding from the ERC StG “BrainSignals”, the Dutch Fund for Economic Structure Reinforcement (FES, 0908 “NeuroBasic PharmaPhenomics project”), EU 7th Framework Programme (HEALTH-F2-2009-242167 “SynSys”) and an NWO VICI grant. Lorna W. Role is the recipient of an NIH Directors Pioneer Award and was supported by NS22061. We thank Dr. Floris Wouterlood for help with immunostaining and confocal microscopy for images shown in the **Figure 1** and Dr. D. Talmage for critique of the manuscript.

REFERENCES

Alitto, H. J., and Dan, Y. (2013). Cell-type-specific modulation of neocortical activity by basal forebrain input. *Front. Syst. Neurosci.* 6:79. doi: 10.3389/fnsys.2012.00079

Arroyo, S., Bennett, C., Aziz, D., Brown, S. P., and Hestrin, S. (2012). Prolonged disynaptic inhibition in the cortex mediated by slow, non-α7 nicotinic excitation of a specific subset of cortical interneurons. *J. Neurosci.* 32, 3859–3864. doi: 10.1523/JNEUROSCI.0115-12.2012

Arroyo, S., Bennett, C., and Hestrin, S. (2014). Nicotinic modulation of cortical circuits. *Front. Neural Circuits* 8:30. doi: 10.3389/fncir.2014.00030

Atasoy, D., Aponte, Y., Su, H. H., and Sternson, S. M. (2008). A FLEX switch targets channelrhodopsin-2 to multiple cell types for imaging and long-range circuit mapping. *J. Neurosci.* 28, 7025–7030. doi: 10.1523/jneurosci.1954-08.2008

Bell, L. A., Bell, K. A., and McQuiston, A. R. (2013). Synaptic muscarinic response types in hippocampal CA1 interneurons depend on different levels of presynaptic activity and different muscarinic receptor subtypes. *Neuropharmacology* 73, 160–173. doi: 10.1016/j.neuropharm.2013.05.026

Bell, K. A., Shim, H., Chen, C. K., and McQuiston, A. R. (2011). Nicotinic excitatory postsynaptic potentials in hippocampal CA1 interneurons are predominantly mediated by nicotinic receptors that contain α4 and β2 subunits. *Neuropharmacology* 61, 1379–1388. doi: 10.1016/j.neuropharm.2011.08.024

Bennett, C., Arroyo, S., Berns, D., and Hestrin, S. (2012). Mechanisms generating dual-component nicotinic EPSCs in cortical interneurons. *J. Neurosci.* 32, 17287–17296. doi: 10.1523/jneurosci.3565-12.2012

Bloem, B., Poorthuis, R. B., and Mansvelder, H. D. (2014). Cholinergic modulation of the medial prefrontal cortex: the role of nicotinic receptors in attention and regulation of neuronal activity. *Front. Neural Circuits* 8:17. doi: 10.3389/fncir.2014.00017

Blokland, A., Honig, W., and Raaijmakers, W. G. M. (1992). Effects of intra-hippocampal scopolamine injections in a repeated spatial acquisition task in the rat. *Psychopharmacology (Berl)* 109, 373–376. doi: 10.1007/bf02245886

Briggs, F., Mangun, G. R., and Usrey, W. M. (2013). Attention enhances synaptic efficacy and the signal-to-noise ratio in neural circuits. *Nature* 499, 476–480. doi: 10.1038/nature12276

Brown, C. E., Sweetnam, D., Beange, M., Nahirney, P. C., and Nashmi, R. (2012a). $\alpha4^*$ nicotinic acetylcholine receptors modulate experience-based cortical depression in the adult mouse somatosensory cortex. *J. Neurosci.* 32, 1207–1219. doi: 10.1523/JNEUROSCI.4568-11.2012

Brown, M. T. C., Tan, K. R., O'Connor, E. C., Nikonenko, I., Muller, D., and Lüscher, C. (2012b). Ventral tegmental area GABA projections pause accumbal cholinergic interneurons to enhance associative learning. *Nature* 492, 452–456. doi: 10.1038/nature11657

Cachope, R., and Cheer, J. F. (2014). Local control of striatal dopamine release. *Front. Behav. Neurosci.* 8:188. doi: 10.3389/fnbeh.2014.00188

Cachope, R., Mateo, Y., Mathur, B. N., Irving, J., Wang, H. L., Morales, M., et al. (2012). Selective activation of cholinergic interneurons enhances accumbal phasic dopamine release: setting the tone for reward processing. *Cell Rep.* 2, 33–41. doi: 10.1016/j.celrep.2012.05.011

Champtiaux, N., Kalivas, P. W., and Bardo, M. T. (2006). Contribution of dihydro-beta-erythroidine sensitive nicotinic acetylcholine receptors in the ventral tegmental area to cocaine-induced behavioral sensitization in rats. *Behav. Brain Res.* 168, 120–126. doi: 10.1016/j.bbr.2005.10.017

Changeux, J.-P. (2010). Nicotine addiction and nicotinic receptors: lessons from genetically modified mice. *Nat. Rev. Neurosci.* 11, 389–401. doi: 10.1038/nrn2849

Christophe, E., Roebuck, A., Staiger, J. F., Lavery, D. J., Charpak, S., and Audinat, E. (2002). Two types of nicotinic receptors mediate an excitation of neocortical layer I interneurons. *J. Neurophysiol.* 88, 1318–1327. doi: 10.1152/jn.00199.2002

Constantinople, C. M., and Bruno, R. M. (2013). Deep cortical layers are activated directly by thalamus. *Science* 340, 1591–1594. doi: 10.1126/science.1236425

Corrigall, W. A., Coen, K. M., Zhang, J., and Adamson, L. K. (2002). Pharmacological manipulations of the pedunculopontine tegmental nucleus in the rat reduce self-administration of both nicotine and cocaine. *Psychopharmacology (Berl)* 160, 198–205. doi: 10.1007/s00213-001-0965-2

Couey, J. J., Meredith, R. M., Spijker, S., Poorthuis, R. B., Smit, A. B., Brussaard, A. B., et al. (2007). Distributed network actions by nicotine increase the threshold for spike-timing-dependent plasticity in prefrontal cortex. *Neuron* 54, 73–87. doi: 10.1016/j.neuron.2007.03.006

Court, J., Martin-Ruiz, C., Piggott, M., Spurden, D., Griffiths, M., and Perry, E. (2001). Nicotinic receptor abnormalities in Alzheimer's disease. *Biol. Psychiatry* 49, 175–184. doi: 10.1016/s0006-3223(00)01116-1

Cruikshank, S. J., Ahmed, O. J., Stevens, T. R., Patrick, S. L., Gonzalez, A. N., Elmaleh, M., et al. (2012). Thalamic control of layer 1 circuits in prefrontal cortex. *J. Neurosci.* 32, 17813–17823. doi: 10.1523/JNEUROSCI.3231-12.2012

Dani, J. A., and Harris, R. A. (2005). Nicotine addiction and comorbidity with alcohol abuse and mental illness. *Nat. Neurosci.* 8, 1465–1470. doi: 10.1038/nn1580

Dautan, D., Huerta-Ocampo, I., Witten, I. B., Deisseroth, K., Bolam, J. P., Gerdjikov, T., et al. (2014). A major external source of cholinergic innervation of the striatum and nucleus accumbens originates in the brainstem. *J. Neurosci.* 34, 4509–4518. doi: 10.1523/jneurosci.5071-13.2014

Deco, G., and Thiele, A. (2011). Cholinergic control of cortical network interactions enables feedback-mediated attentional modulation. *Eur. J. Neurosci.* 34, 146–157. doi: 10.1111/j.1460-9568.2011.07749.x

Deisseroth, K. (2011). Optogenetics. *Nat. Methods* 8, 26–29. doi: 10.1038/nmeth.f.324

Descarries, L., Gisiger, V., and Steriade, M. (1997). Diffuse transmission by acetylcholine in the CNS. *Prog. Neurobiol.* 53, 603–625. doi: 10.1016/s0301-0082(97)00050-6

Disney, A. A., Aoki, C., and Hawken, M. J. (2007). Gain modulation by nicotine in macaque V1. *Neuron* 56, 701–713. doi: 10.1016/j.neuron.2007.09.034

Disney, A. A., Aoki, C., and Hawken, M. J. (2012). Cholinergic suppression of visual responses in primate V1 is mediated by GABAergic inhibition. *J. Neurophysiol.* 108, 1907–1923. doi: 10.1152/jn.00188.2012

Douglas, R. J., and Martin, K. A. C. (2004). Neuronal circuits of the neocortex. *Annu. Rev. Neurosci.* 27, 419–451. doi: 10.1146/annurev.neuro.27.070203.144152

Duque, A., Balatoni, B., Detari, L., and Zaborszky, L. (2000). EEG correlation of the discharge properties of identified neurons in the basal forebrain. *J. Neurophysiol.* 84, 1627–1635.

Dutar, P., Bassant, M. H., Senut, M. C., and Lamour, Y. (1995). The septohippocampal pathway: structure and function of a central cholinergic system. *Physiol. Rev.* 75, 393–427.

Exley, R., and Cragg, S. J. (2008). Presynaptic nicotinic receptors: a dynamic and diverse cholinergic filter of striatal dopamine neurotransmission. *Br. J. Pharmacol.* 153(Suppl. 1), S283–S297. doi: 10.1038/sj.bjp.0707510

Frotscher, M., and Léránth, C. (1985). Cholinergic innervation of the rat hippocampus as revealed by choline acetyltransferase immunocytochemistry: a combined light and electron microscopic study. *J. Comp. Neurol.* 239, 237–246. doi: 10.1002/cne.902390210

Galarraga, E., Hernández-López, S., Reyes, A., Miranda, I., Bermudez-Rattoni, F., Vilchis, C., et al. (1999). Cholinergic modulation of neostriatal output: a functional antagonism between different types of muscarinic receptors. *J. Neurosci.* 19, 3629–3638.

Gittis, A. H., Nelson, A. B., Thwin, M. T., Palop, J. J., and Kreitzer, A. C. (2010). Distinct roles of GABAergic interneurons in the regulation of striatal output pathways. *J. Neurosci.* 30, 2223–2234. doi: 10.1523/jneurosci.4870-09.2010

Goard, M., and Dan, Y. (2009). Basal forebrain activation enhances cortical coding of natural scenes. *Nat. Neurosci.* 12, 1444–1449. doi: 10.1038/nn.2402

Gotti, C., and Clementi, F. (2004). Neuronal nicotinic receptors: from structure to pathology. *Prog. Neurobiol.* 74, 363–396. doi: 10.1016/j.pneurobio.2004.09.006

Gras, C., Amilhon, B., Lepicard, E. M., Poirel, O., Vinatier, J., Herbin, M., et al. (2008). The vesicular glutamate transporter VGLUT3 synergizes striatal acetylcholine tone. *Nat. Neurosci.* 11, 292–300. doi: 10.1038/nn2052

Griguoli, M., and Cherubini, E. (2012). Regulation of hippocampal inhibitory circuits by nicotinic acetylcholine receptors. *J. Physiol.* 590, 655–666. doi: 10.1113/jphysiol.2011.220095

Gu, Z., and Yakel, J. L. (2011). Timing-dependent septal cholinergic induction of dynamic hippocampal synaptic plasticity. *Neuron* 71, 155–165. doi: 10.1016/j.neuron.2011.04.026

Gulledge, A. T., Bucci, D. J., Zhang, S. S., Matsui, M., and Yeh, H. H. (2009). M1 receptors mediate cholinergic modulation of excitability in neocortical pyramidal neurons. *J. Neurosci.* 29, 9888–9902. doi: 10.1523/jneurosci.1366-09.2009

Gulledge, A. T., Park, S. B., Kawaguchi, Y., and Stuart, G. J. (2007). Heterogeneity of phasic cholinergic signaling in neocortical neurons. *J. Neurophysiol.* 97, 2215–2229. doi: 10.1152/jn.00493.2006

Hasselmo, M. E., and Giocomo, L. M. (2006). Cholinergic modulation of cortical function. *J. Mol. Neurosci.* 30, 133–136. doi: 10.1385/JMN:30:1:133

Hasselmo, M. E., and Sarter, M. (2011). Modes and models of forebrain cholinergic neuromodulation of cognition. *Neuropsychopharmacology* 36, 52–73. doi: 10.1038/npp.2010.104

Higley, M. J., Gittis, A. H., Oldenburg, I. A., Balthasar, N., Seal, R. P., Edwards, R. H., et al. (2011). Cholinergic interneurons mediate fast VGluT3-dependent glutamatergic transmission in the striatum. *PLoS One* 6:e19155. doi: 10.1371/journal.pone.0019155

Howe, W. M., Berry, A. S., Francois, J., Gilmour, G., Carp, J. M., Tricklebank, M., et al. (2013). Prefrontal cholinergic mechanisms instigating shifts from monitoring for cues to cue-guided performance: converging electrochemical and fMRI evidence from rats and humans. *J. Neurosci.* 33, 8742–8752. doi: 10.1523/jneurosci.5809-12.2013

Huang, Z. J., and Zeng, H. (2013). Genetic approaches to neural circuits in the mouse. *Annu. Rev. Neurosci.* 36, 183–215. doi: 10.1146/annurev-neuro-062012-170307

Jiang, L., López-Hernández, G. Y., Lederman, J., Talmage, D. A., and Role, W. L. (2014). Optogenetic studies of nicotinic contributions to cholinergic signaling in the central nervous system. *Rev. Neurosci.* doi: 10.1515/revneuro-2014-0032. [Epub ahead of print].

Jiang, X., Wang, G., Lee, A. J., Stornetta, R. L., and Zhu, J. J. (2013). The organization of two new cortical interneuronal circuits. *Nat. Neurosci.* 16, 210–218. doi: 10.1038/nn.3305

Joshua, M., Adler, A., Mitelman, R., Vaadia, E., and Bergman, H. (2008). Midbrain dopaminergic neurons and striatal cholinergic interneurons encode the difference between reward and aversive events at different epochs of probabilistic classical conditioning trials. *J. Neurosci.* 28, 11673–11684. doi: 10.1523/jneurosci.3839-08.2008

Kalmbach, A., Hedrick, T., and Waters, J. (2012). Selective optogenetic stimulation of cholinergic axons in neocortex. *J. Neurophysiol.* 107, 2008–2019. doi: 10.1152/jn.00870.2011

Kassam, S. M., Herman, P. M., Goodfellow, N. M., Alves, N. C., and Lambe, E. K. (2008). Developmental excitation of corticothalamic neurons by nicotinic acetylcholine receptors. *J. Neurosci.* 28, 8756–8764. doi: 10.1523/JNEUROSCI.2645-08.2008

Katona, I., Sperlágh, B., Sík, A., Käfalvi, A., Vizi, E. S., Mackie, K., et al. (1999). Presynaptically located CB1 cannabinoid receptors regulate GABA release from axon terminals of specific hippocampal interneurons. *J. Neurosci.* 19, 4544–4558.

Kawai, H., Lazar, R., and Metherate, R. (2007). Nicotinic control of axon excitability regulates thalamocortical transmission. *Nat. Neurosci.* 10, 1168–1175. doi: 10.1038/nn1956

Kilgard, M. P., and Merzenich, M. M. (1998). Cortical map reorganization enabled by nucleus basalis activity. *Science* 279, 1714–1718. doi: 10.1126/science.279.5357.1714

Kimura, F., and Baughman, R. W. (1997). Distinct muscarinic receptor subtypes suppress excitatory and inhibitory synaptic responses in cortical neurons. *J. Neurophysiol.* 77, 709–716.

Kimura, F., Fukuda, M., and Tsumoto, T. (1999). Acetylcholine suppresses the spread of excitation in the visual cortex revealed by optical recording: possible differential effect depending on the source of input. *Eur. J. Neurosci.* 11, 3597–3609. doi: 10.1046/j.1460-9568.1999.00779.x

Kimura, R., Safari, M.-S., Mirnajafi-Zadeh, J., Kimura, R., Ebina, T., Yanagawa, Y., et al. (2014). Curtailing effect of awakening on visual responses of cortical neurons by cholinergic activation of inhibitory circuits. *J. Neurosci.* 34, 10122–10133. doi: 10.1523/jneurosci.0863-14.2014

Klinkenberg, I., Sambeth, A., and Blokland, A. (2011). Acetylcholine and attention. *Behav. Brain Res.* 221, 430–442. doi: 10.1016/j.bbr.2010.11.033

Koós, T., and Tepper, J. M. (1999). Inhibitory control of neostriatal projection neurons by GABAergic interneurons. *Nat. Neurosci.* 2, 467–472. doi: 10.1038/8138

Koós, T., and Tepper, J. M. (2002). Dual cholinergic control of fast-spiking interneurons in the neostriatum. *J. Neurosci.* 22, 529–535.

Lambe, E. K., Picciotto, M. R., and Aghajanian, G. K. (2003). Nicotine induces glutamate release from thalamocortical terminals in prefrontal cortex. *Neuropsychopharmacology* 28, 216–225. doi: 10.1038/sj.npp.1300032

Leão, R. N., Mikulovic, S., Leão, K. E., Munguba, H., Gezelius, H., Enjin, A., et al. (2012). OLM interneurons differentially modulate CA3 and entorhinal inputs to hippocampal CA1 neurons. *Nat. Neurosci.* 15, 1524–1530. doi: 10.1038/nn.3235

Leslie, F. M., Mojica, C. Y., and Reynaga, D. D. (2013). Nicotinic receptors in addiction pathways. *Mol. Pharmacol.* 83, 753–758. doi: 10.1124/mol.112.083659

Letzkus, J. J., Wolff, S. B. E., Meyer, E. M. M., Tovote, P., Courtin, J., Herry, C., et al. (2011). A disinhibitory microcircuit for associative fear learning in the auditory cortex. *Nature* 480, 331–335. doi: 10.1038/nature10674

Levin, E. D., Bradley, A., Addy, N., and Sigurani, N. (2002). Hippocampal alpha 7 and alpha 4 beta 2 nicotinic receptors and working memory. *Neuroscience* 109, 757–765. doi: 10.1016/s0306-4522(01)00538-3

Mann, E. O., Suckling, J. M., Hajos, N., Greenfield, S. A., and Paulsen, O. (2005). Perisomatic feedback inhibition underlies cholinergically induced fast network oscillations in the rat hippocampus in vitro. *Neuron* 45, 105–117. doi: 10.1016/j.neuron.2004.12.016

Manns, I. D., Alonso, A., and Jones, B. E. (2000). Discharge profiles of juxtacellularly labeled and immunohistochemically identified GABAergic basal forebrain neurons recorded in association with the electroencephalogram in anesthetized rats. *J. Neurosci.* 20, 9252–9263.

Martin, L. F., and Freedman, R. (2007). Schizophrenia and the alpha7 nicotinic acetylcholine receptor. *Int. Rev. Neurobiol.* 78, 225–246. doi: 10.1016/S0074-7742(06)78008-4

Mesulam, M. M. (1995). Cholinergic pathways and the ascending reticular activating system of the human brain. *Ann. N Y Acad. Sci.* 757, 169–179. doi: 10.1111/j.1749-6632.1995.tb17472.x

Metherate, R., Cox, C. L., and Ashe, J. H. (1992). Cellular bases of neocortical activation: modulation of neural oscillations by the nucleus basalis and endogenous acetylcholine. *J. Neurosci.* 12, 4701–4711.

Morris, G., Arkadir, D., Nevet, A., Vaadia, E., and Bergman, H. (2004). Coincident but distinct messages of midbrain dopamine and striatal tonically active neurons. *Neuron* 43, 133–143. doi: 10.1016/j.neuron.2004.06.012

Nagode, D. A., Tang, A. H., Karson, M. A., Klugmann, M., and Alger, B. E. (2011). Optogenetic release of ACh induces rhythmic bursts of perisomatic IPSCs in hippocampus. *PLoS One* 6:e27691. doi: 10.1371/journal.pone.0027691

Nagode, D. A., Tang, A.-H., Yang, K., and Alger, B. E. (2014). Optogenetic identification of an intrinsic cholinergically driven inhibitory oscillator sensitive to cannabinoids and opioids in hippocampal CA1. *J. Physiol.* 592, 103–123. doi: 10.1113/jphysiol.2013.257428

Nelson, A. B., Hammack, N., Yang, C. F., Shah, N. M., Seal, R. P., and Kreitzer, A. C. (2014). Striatal cholinergic interneurons drive GABA release from dopamine terminals. *Neuron* 82, 63–70. doi: 10.1016/j.neuron.2014.01.023

Oldford, E., and Castro-Alamancos, M. A. (2003). Input-specific effects of acetylcholine on sensory and intracortical evoked responses in the "barrel cortex" in vivo. *Neuroscience* 117, 769–778. doi: 10.1016/s0306-4522(02)00663-2

Paez-Gonzalez, P., Asrican, B., Rodriguez, E., and Kuo, C. T. (2014). Identification of distinct ChAT(+) neurons and activity-dependent control of postnatal SVZ neurogenesis. *Nat. Neurosci.* 17, 934–942. doi: 10.1038/nn.3734

Parikh, V., Kozak, R., Martinez, V., and Sarter, M. (2007). Prefrontal acetylcholine release controls cue detection on multiple timescales. *Neuron* 56, 141–154. doi: 10.1016/j.neuron.2007.08.025

Parikh, V., and Sarter, M. (2008). Cholinergic mediation of attention. *Ann. N Y Acad. Sci.* 1129, 225–235. doi: 10.1196/annals.1417.021

Passetti, F., Dalley, J. W., O'Connell, M. T., Everitt, B. J., and Robbins, T. W. (2000). Increased acetylcholine release in the rat medial prefrontal cortex during performance of a visual attentional task. *Eur. J. Neurosci.* 12, 3051–3058. doi: 10.1046/j.1460-9568.2000.00183.x

Picciotto, M. R., Higley, M. J., and Mineur, Y. S. (2012). Acetylcholine as a neuromodulator: cholinergic signaling shapes nervous system function and behavior. *Neuron* 76, 116–129. doi: 10.1016/j.neuron.2012.08.036

Pinto, L., Goard, M. J., Estandian, D., Xu, M., Kwan, A. C., Lee, S.-H., et al. (2013). Fast modulation of visual perception by basal forebrain cholinergic neurons. *Nat. Neurosci.* 16, 1857–1863. doi: 10.1038/nn.3552

Poorthuis, R. B., Bloem, B., Schak, B., Wester, J., de Kock, C. P. J., and Mansvelder, H. D. (2013). Layer-specific modulation of the prefrontal cortex by nicotinic acetylcholine receptors. *Cereb. Cortex* 23, 148–161. doi: 10.1093/cercor/bhr390

Poorthuis, R. B., Enke, L., and Letzkus, J. J. (2014). Cholinergic circuit modulation through differential recruitment of neocortical interneuron types during behaviour. *J. Physiol.* 592, 4155–4164. doi: 10.1113/jphysiol.2014.273862

Ren, J., Qin, C., Hu, F., Tan, J., Qiu, L., Zhao, S., et al. (2011). Habenula "cholinergic" neurons corelease glutamate and acetylcholine and activate postsynaptic neurons via distinct transmission modes. *Neuron* 69, 445–452. doi: 10.1016/j.neuron.2010.12.038

Rice, M. E., and Cragg, S. J. (2004). Nicotine amplifies reward-related dopamine signals in striatum. *Nat. Neurosci.* 7, 583–584. doi: 10.1038/nn1244

Roberts, M. J., Zinke, W., Guo, K., Robertson, R., McDonald, J. S., and Thiele, A. (2005). Acetylcholine dynamically controls spatial integration in marmoset primary visual cortex. *J. Neurophysiol.* 93, 2062–2072. doi: 10.1152/jn.00911.2004

Role, L. W. (2014). "Cholinergic modulation of cortical-amygdala circuits and behavior. ABS S25," in *Nicotinic Acetylcholine Receptors, Wellcome Trust Scientific Conference*, eds I. Bermudez, N. Millar and S. Wonnacott.

Sarter, M., Lustig, C., Howe, W. M., Gritton, H., and Berry, A. S. (2014). Deterministic functions of cortical acetylcholine. *Eur. J. Neurosci.* 39, 1912–1920. doi: 10.1111/ejn.12515

Sarter, M., Parikh, V., and Howe, W. M. (2009). Phasic acetylcholine release and the volume transmission hypothesis: time to move on. *Nat. Rev. Neurosci.* 10, 383–390. doi: 10.1038/nrn2635

Silver, M. A., Shenhav, A., and D'Esposito, M. (2008). Cholinergic enhancement reduces spatial spread of visual responses in human early visual cortex. *Neuron* 60, 904–914. doi: 10.1016/j.neuron.2008.09.038

Smiley, J. F., Morrell, F., and Mesulam, M. M. (1997). Cholinergic synapses in human cerebral cortex: an ultrastructural study in serial sections. *Exp. Neurol.* 144, 361–368. doi: 10.1006/exnr.1997.6413

Soma, S., Shimegi, S., Osaki, H., and Sato, H. (2012). Cholinergic modulation of response gain in the primary visual cortex of the macaque. *J. Neurophysiol.* 107, 283–291. doi: 10.1152/jn.00330.2011

Soma, S., Shimegi, S., Suematsu, N., Tamura, H., and Sato, H. (2013). Modulation-specific and laminar-dependent effects of acetylcholine on visual responses in the rat primary visual cortex. *PLoS One* 8:e68430. doi: 10.1371/journal.pone.0068430

Straub, C., Tritsch, N. X., Hagan, N. A., Gu, C., and Sabatini, B. L. (2014). Multiphasic modulation of cholinergic interneurons by nigrostriatal afferents. *J. Neurosci.* 34, 8557–8569. doi: 10.1523/jneurosci.0589-14.2014

Sun, Y.-G., Pita-Almenar, J. D., Wu, C.-S., Renger, J. J., Uebele, V. N., Lu, H.-C., et al. (2013). Biphasic cholinergic synaptic transmission controls action potential activity in thalamic reticular nucleus neurons. *J. Neurosci.* 33, 2048–2059. doi: 10.1523/JNEUROSCI.3177-12.2013

Tan, K. R., Yvon, C., Turiault, M., Mirzabekov, J. J., Doehner, J., Labouèbe, G., et al. (2012). GABA neurons of the VTA drive conditioned place aversion. *Neuron* 73, 1173–1183. doi: 10.1016/j.neuron.2012.02.015

Thiele, A., Herrero, J. L., Distler, C., and Hoffmann, K.-P. (2012). Contribution of cholinergic and GABAergic mechanisms to direction tuning, discriminability, response reliability and neuronal rate correlations in macaque middle temporal area. *J. Neurosci.* 32, 16602–16615. doi: 10.1523/jneurosci.0554-12.2012

Threlfell, S., Lalic, T., Platt, N. J., Jennings, K. A., Deisseroth, K., and Cragg, S. J. (2012). Striatal dopamine release is triggered by synchronized activity in cholinergic interneurons. *Neuron* 75, 58–64. doi: 10.1016/j.neuron.2012.04.038

Tu, B., Gu, Z., Shen, J.-X., Lamb, P. W., and Yakel, J. L. (2009). Characterization of a nicotine-sensitive neuronal population in rat entorhinal cortex. *J. Neurosci.* 29, 10436–10448. doi: 10.1523/jneurosci.2580-09.2009

Turrini, P., Casu, M. A., Wong, T. P., De Koninck, Y., Ribeiro-da-Silva, A., and Cuello, A. C. (2001). Cholinergic nerve terminals establish classical synapses in the rat cerebral cortex: synaptic pattern and age-related atrophy. *Neuroscience* 105, 277–285. doi: 10.1016/s0306-4522(01)00172-5

Uhlhaas, P. J., Haenschel, C., Nikolić, D., and Singer, W. (2008). The role of oscillations and synchrony in cortical networks and their putative relevance for the pathophysiology of schizophrenia. *Schizophr. Bull.* 34, 927–943. doi: 10.1093/schbul/sbn062

Uylings, H. B. M., Groenewegen, H. J., and Kolb, B. (2003). Do rats have a prefrontal cortex? *Behav. Brain Res.* 146, 3–17. doi: 10.1016/j.bbr.2003.09.028

Van Bockstaele, E. J., and Pickel, V. M. (1995). GABA-containing neurons in the ventral tegmental area project to the nucleus accumbens in rat brain. *Brain Res.* 682, 215–221. doi: 10.1016/0006-8993(95)00334-m

Van Zessen, R., Phillips, J. L., Budygin, E. A., and Stuber, G. D. (2012). Activation of VTA GABA neurons disrupts reward consumption. *Neuron* 73, 1184–1194. doi: 10.1016/j.neuron.2012.02.016

von Engelhardt, J., Eliava, M., Meyer, A. H., Rozov, A., and Monyer, H. (2007). Functional characterization of intrinsic cholinergic interneurons in the cortex. *J. Neurosci.* 27, 5633–5642. doi: 10.1523/jneurosci.4647-06.2007

Wang, X.-J. (2010). Neurophysiological and computational principles of cortical rhythms in cognition. *Physiol. Rev.* 90, 1195–1268. doi: 10.1152/physrev.00035.2008

Wang, L., Shang, S., Kang, X., Teng, S., Zhu, F., Liu, B., et al. (2014). Modulation of dopamine release in the striatum by physiologically relevant levels of nicotine. *Nat. Commun.* 5:3925. doi: 10.1038/ncomms4925

Wess, J. (2003). Novel insights into muscarinic acetylcholine receptor function using gene targeting technology. *Trends Pharmacol. Sci.* 24, 414–420. doi: 10.1016/s0165-6147(03)00195-0

Wilson, R. I., and Nicoll, R. A. (2001). Endogenous cannabinoids mediate retrograde signalling at hippocampal synapses. *Nature* 410, 588–592. doi: 10.1038/35069076

Witten, I. B., Lin, S.-C., Brodsky, M., Prakash, R., Diester, I., Anikeeva, P., et al. (2010). Cholinergic interneurons control local circuit activity and cocaine conditioning. *Science* 330, 1677–1681. doi: 10.1126/science.1193771

Witten, I. B., Steinberg, E. E., Lee, S. Y., Davidson, T. J., Zalocusky, K. A., Brodsky, M., et al. (2011). Recombinase-driver rat lines: tools, techniques and optogenetic application to dopamine-mediated reinforcement. *Neuron* 72, 721–733. doi: 10.1016/j.neuron.2011.10.028

Wonnacott, S. (1997). Presynaptic nicotinic ACh receptors. *Trends Neurosci.* 20, 92–98. doi: 10.1016/s0166-2236(96)10073-4

Woolf, N. J. (1991). Cholinergic systems in mammalian brain and spinal cord. *Prog. Neurobiol.* 37, 475–524. doi: 10.1016/0301-0082(91)90006-m

Yakel, J. L. (2012). Nicotinic ACh receptors in the hippocampus: role in excitability and plasticity. *Nicotine Tob. Res.* 14, 1249–1257. doi: 10.1093/ntr/nts091

Yizhar, O., Fenno, L. E., Davidson, T. J., Mogri, M., and Deisseroth, K. (2011). Optogenetics in neural systems. *Neuron* 71, 9–34. doi: 10.1016/j.neuron.2011.06.004

Zaborszky, L., Pang, K., Somogyi, J., Nadasdy, Z., and Kallo, I. (1999). The basal forebrain corticopetal system revisited. *Ann. N Y Acad. Sci.* 877, 339–367. doi: 10.1111/j.1749-6632.1999.tb09276.x

5

Acetylcholine release and inhibitory interneuron activity in hippocampal CA1

A. Rory McQuiston *

Department of Anatomy and Neurobiology, Virginia Commonwealth University, Richmond, VA, USA

Edited by:
Sukumar Vijayaraghavan, University of Colorado Health Science Center, USA

Reviewed by:
Scott Thompson, University of Maryland School of Medicine, USA
Qian Sun, Columbia University, USA

***Correspondence:**
A. Rory McQuiston, Department of Anatomy and Neurobiology, Virginia Commonwealth University, Sanger Hall 9-060, 1101 E. Marshall St., Box 980709, Richmond, VA 23298, USA
e-mail: amcquiston@vcu.edu

Acetylcholine release in the central nervous system (CNS) has an important role in attention, recall, and memory formation. One region influenced by acetylcholine is the hippocampus, which receives inputs from the medial septum and diagonal band of Broca complex (MS/DBB). Release of acetylcholine from the MS/DBB can directly affect several elements of the hippocampus including glutamatergic and GABAergic neurons, presynaptic terminals, postsynaptic receptors, and astrocytes. A significant portion of acetylcholine's effect likely results from the modulation of GABAergic inhibitory interneurons, which have crucial roles in controlling excitatory inputs, synaptic integration, rhythmic coordination of principal neurons, and outputs in the hippocampus. Acetylcholine affects interneuron function in large part by altering their membrane potential via muscarinic and nicotinic receptor activation. This minireview describes recent data from mouse hippocampus that investigated changes in CA1 interneuron membrane potentials following acetylcholine release. The interneuron subtypes affected, the receptor subtypes activated, and the potential outcome on hippocampal CA1 network function is discussed.

Keywords: hippocampus, acetylcholine, muscarinic, nicotinic, inhibitory interneuron

INTRODUCTION

Acetylcholine is released throughout the mammalian central nervous system (CNS) where it impacts global brain function by affecting sleep-wake cycles, attention, and memory formation. One region of the brain heavily innervated by cholinergic afferents from the medial septum and diagonal band of Broca complex (MS/DBB) is the hippocampus (Dutar et al., 1995). Functionally, acetylcholine release in the hippocampus has been proposed to aid in the formation or retrieval of memories depending on the extracellular concentration of acetylcholine (Power et al., 2003; Hasselmo and Giocomo, 2006; Kenney and Gould, 2008; Deiana et al., 2011; Hasselmo and Sarter, 2011; Easton et al., 2012; Blake et al., 2014). The mechanism by which MS/DBB cholinergic terminals affect hippocampal network function is through the activation of both muscarinic and nicotinic receptors located on dendrites, cell bodies, and axon terminals of pyramidal neurons and inhibitory interneurons, as well as on astrocytes (Cobb and Davies, 2005; Teles-Grilo Ruivo and Mellor, 2013). Although acetylcholine affects multiple sites on several different cell types, a portion of its influence likely arises from its effects on interneuron function.

Inhibitory interneurons play a crucial role in information processing in the hippocampus. Interneurons are very diverse in anatomical structure and presumed function (Freund and Buzsaki, 1996; Klausberger and Somogyi, 2008). Depending on the interneuron subtype and where it innervates the pyramidal cell, an individual interneuron can completely block activity in a dendrite, change action potential firing phase at the soma, or completely prevent action potential firing at the pyramidal cell body (Miles et al., 1996; Larkum et al., 1999). At the network level, interneurons contribute to the generation of synchronous activity among populations of principal neurons at a variety of behaviorally relevant frequencies (Buzsaki, 2002; Buzsaki and Wang, 2012). Given the significant impact individual interneurons have on neuronal network function, it is probable that a considerable proportion of acetylcholine's influence on hippocampal activity arises through interneuron modulation. Although cholinergic receptors have been shown to affect inhibitory presynaptic terminals (Behrends and Ten Bruggencate, 1993; Tang et al., 2011) and interneuron excitability (McQuiston and Madison, 1999b; Griguoli et al., 2009; Cea-Del Rio et al., 2010, 2011), this minireview will limit its focus to recent studies that have investigated the effect of acetylcholine release on changes in interneuron membrane potential, specifically in hippocampal CA1.

MS/DBB CHOLINERGIC NEURON ACTIVITY AND ACETYLCHOLINE RELEASE IN HIPPOCAMPAL CA1

The impact that acetylcholine release has in hippocampal CA1 and the extent to which different interneuron subtypes are affected will depend on the specific location and density of cholinergic axon terminals as well as its inactivating enzyme, acetylcholinesterase. Notably, both cholinergic fibers and acetylcholinesterase have been shown to be differentially distributed across layers in hippocampal CA1. In mouse, cholinergic fibers were shown to be evenly distributed except for two bands of higher density in the stratum pyamidale (SP) and at the border between the stratum radiatum (SR) and stratum lacunosum-moleculare (SLM) (Aznavour et al., 2002). In rat, similar higher density bands were observed in the SP and at the border of SR and SLM. However, compared to the stratum oriens (SO), lower densities were seen in the SR and even lower densities in SLM (SO > SR > SLM) (Aznavour et al., 2002). The distribution of acetylcholinesterase in hippocampal CA1 complements that of cholinergic input, with higher densities observed between SP and SO as well as another peak in SLM near the border with SR (Storm-Mathisen, 1970). Consistent with these anatomical data, measurements of increased acetylcholine release during theta rhythms have shown that acetylcholine concentrations were highest near the stratum pyramidale (Zhang et al., 2010). This differential distribution of cholinergic fibers and extracellular acetylcholine levels is particularly important when considering that not all cholinergic terminals in the hippocampus appear to transmit acetylcholine synaptically. In both the hippocampus and neocortex, 85–93% of cholinergic axon terminals were estimated to have no postsynaptic specialization and thus the majority of cholinergic terminals were proposed to transmit acetylcholine by volume or non-synaptic transmission (Umbriaco et al., 1994, 1995). However, other groups have estimated that the majority of cholinergic terminals (66–67%) in the neocortex make classical synaptic connections (Smiley et al., 1997; Turrini et al., 2001). Regardless of this discrepancy, a significant portion of terminals appear to release acetylcholine into the extracellular space in a paracrine-like manner. This requires terminally released acetylcholine to diffuse significant distances past acetylcholinesterase to bind to receptors on postsynaptic elements. Thus, regions or layers with favorable densities of cholinergic terminals (higher) and/or acetylcholinesterase (lower) may result in larger extracellular concentrations of acetylcholine that may be more effective at transmitting acetylcholine through volume transmission. Furthermore, it is possible that there is a subset of terminals that are more active, have a higher probability of release, or may release more neurotransmitter. These terminals may be more effective at mediating volume transmission and influencing nearby inhibitory interneurons.

Acetylcholine release from cholinergic terminals will depend on the activity of the cholinergic neurons in the MS/DBB. However, the firing patterns of MS/DBB cholinergic neurons reported in the literature have shown some variability (Barrenechea et al., 1995; Brazhnik and Fox, 1997, 1999; Simon et al., 2006). A small number of anatomically identified MS/DBB cholinergic neurons recorded in awake restrained rodents have been reported to have low irregular firing rates (<2 Hz) (Simon et al., 2006). In contrast, anatomically unidentified neurons with action potential waveforms consistent with MS/DBB cholinergic neurons have been reported to fire at rates up to 30 Hz (Brazhnik and Fox, 1999). Thus, it remains unclear which rates best describe the firing patterns of cholinergic neurons in the MS/DBB or whether they fall along a wide continuum. Nevertheless, potential differences in the firing frequency or the duration of activity of cholinergic neurons could have variable effects on different interneuron subtypes through local differences in acetylcholine concentrations.

EFFECTS OF MUSCARINIC RECEPTOR ACTIVATION ON HIPPOCAMPAL CA1 INHIBITORY INTERNEURONS

Disruption of the MS/DBB cholinergic function by systemic blockade of muscarinic receptors or direct injection of muscarinic receptor antagonists into the hippocampus can impair memory and the encoding of spatial information (Blokland et al., 1992; Atri et al., 2004; Hasselmo, 2006). A potential role for inhibitory interneurons in muscarinic receptor modulation of hippocampal function was initially based on observations that the exogenous application of cholinergic agonists resulted in an increase in spontaneous inhibitory postsynaptic currents (sIPSCs) in CA1 pyramidal neurons (Pitler and Alger, 1992). These data indirectly suggested that a subset of inhibitory interneurons may be depolarized by muscarinic receptor activation and were subsequently confirmed by direct recordings (Parra et al., 1998; McQuiston and Madison, 1999a). However, not all interneurons responded to muscarinic receptor activation by depolarizing. Some interneurons were hyperpolarized or exhibited biphasic responses, and some failed to respond to the exogenous application of muscarinic agonist (Parra et al., 1998; McQuiston and Madison, 1999a). Moreover, each muscarinic response type could not be correlated with a morphological subtype of interneuron. These findings were further complicated by the observation that muscarinic receptors can inhibit the release of GABA from a subset of perisomatic inhibitory interneurons (Behrends and Ten Bruggencate, 1993; Fukudome et al., 2004; Szabo et al., 2010) and muscarinic receptor activation can increase interneuron excitability through the generation of after depolarizations (McQuiston and Madison, 1999b; Lawrence et al., 2006). Thus, the impact that acetylcholine release has on the interneuron population is complex and results in the recruitment of some interneurons while inhibiting others.

ACTIVATION OF MUSCARINIC RECEPTORS IN HIPPOCAMPAL CA1 INTERNEURONS FOLLOWING ACETYLCHOLINE RELEASE

Although cholinergic muscarinic synaptic responses were first measured in CA1 pyramidal neurons in 1983 (Cole and Nicoll, 1983), it was not until 2006 that muscarinic responses to electrically evoked acetylcholine release were measured in hippocampal CA1 inhibitory interneurons (Widmer et al., 2006). This study showed that terminally released acetylcholine had divergent effects on different interneuron subtypes. Interneurons could respond by depolarizing, hyperpolarizing, or with biphasic responses. Overall, the majority of responding interneurons produced depolarizations (64%) whereas hyperpolarizations were infrequently observed (13%) (Widmer et al., 2006). Moreover, like previous studies using exogenous application of muscarinic agonists (Parra et al., 1998; McQuiston and Madison, 1999a), the different electrically evoked muscarinic response types could not be correlated with specific interneuron anatomical subtypes (Widmer et al., 2006). These findings have been recently confirmed by optogenetic studies using evoked release in response to light-activation (Nagode et al., 2011; Bell et al., 2013). However, in one of these optogenetic studies, interneurons responding with biphasic (25%), hyperpolarizing (35%), and depolarizing (40%) muscarinic responses were more equally distributed among the different response types (Bell et al., 2013). Importantly, optogenetically released acetylcholine predominantly produced muscarinic responses (80%) vs. nicotinic responses (17%). The remaining 3% of responding interneurons had both muscarinic and nicotinic responses. Furthermore, the muscarinic hyperpolarizations were mediated by the activation of M_4 receptors whereas the depolarizations were likely produced by M_3 receptor activation (Bell et al., 2013). Similar to the electrical stimulation studies, muscarinic response type could not be correlated with anatomical interneuron subtypes. Importantly, both studies showed that perisomatically projecting interneurons (likely parvalbumin-expressing basket cells) could respond to acetylcholine release with any one of the three muscarinic response types (Widmer et al., 2006; Bell et al., 2013). In different optogenetic studies, CA1 interneuron membrane potential was indirectly assessed by measuring sIPSC frequency in CA1 pyramidal neurons (Nagode et al., 2011, 2014). Optogenetically released acetylcholine resulted in an increase in large amplitude sIPSCs with frequencies that fell within the theta bandwidth (4–12 Hz) (Nagode et al., 2011). Importantly, this increase in sIPSCs could be inhibited by endocannabinoids suggesting that they resulted from the activation of cholecystokinin positive interneurons (Nagode et al., 2011). Furthermore, the sIPSCs were not affected by optogenetic suppression of parvalbumin positive cells, suggesting they did not arise from the activation of parvalbumin basket cells, axo-axonic, bistratified or oriens-lacunosum-moleculare interneurons (Nagode et al., 2014). These findings are consistent with synaptic stimulation studies, which recorded from an interneuron with cholecystokinin basket cell morphology that produced a biphasic response to acetylcholine release (Widmer et al., 2006). Therefore, based on effects on the membrane potential alone, endogenously activated muscarinic receptors on hippocampal CA1 interneurons will have complex effects on network function (see **Table 1**).

Although different muscarinic response types were almost uniformly observed in CA1 interneurons, not all response types were as easily evoked by optogenetic stimulation (Bell et al., 2013). Consistent with some *in vivo* recordings (Brazhnik and Fox, 1999), acetylcholine released from MS/DBB cholinergic terminals by blue light flashes delivered at 20 Hz was capable of producing

Table 1 | Cholinergic responses vary in similar and different anatomical interneuron subtypes.

Interneuron axonal arborization	Muscarinic depol.	Muscarinic hyperpol.	Muscarinic biphasic	Nicotinic α7	Nicotinic α4β2	Nicotinic α2
Perisomatic SP	Agonist: Parra et al., 1998; McQuiston and Madison, 1999a	Agonist: McQuiston and Madison, 1999a	Agonist: McQuiston and Madison, 1999a	Agonist: McQuiston and Madison, 1999c; Buhler and Dunwiddie, 2001	Agonist: Not identified	Agonist: Not identified
	Synaptic: Widmer et al., 2006; Nagode et al., 2011, 2014; Bell et al., 2013	Synaptic: Widmer et al., 2006; Bell et al., 2013	Synaptic: Widmer et al., 2006; Bell et al., 2013	Synaptic: Not identified	Synaptic: Not identified	Synaptic: Not observed
Proximal dendritic SR or SO	Agonist: Parra et al., 1998; McQuiston and Madison, 1999a	Agonist: McQuiston and Madison, 1999a	Agonist: McQuiston and Madison, 1999a	Agonist: McQuiston and Madison, 1999c; Buhler and Dunwiddie, 2001	Agonist: Not identified	Agonist: Not identified
	Synaptic: Widmer et al., 2006; Bell et al., 2013	Synaptic: Widmer et al., 2006; Bell et al., 2013	Synaptic: Widmer et al., 2006; Bell et al., 2013	Synaptic: Not identified	Synaptic: Bell et al., 2011	Synaptic: Not observed
Distal dendritic SLM	Agonist: Parra et al., 1998; McQuiston and Madison, 1999a	Agonist: Parra et al., 1998; McQuiston and Madison, 1999a	Agonist: McQuiston and Madison, 1999a	Agonist: McQuiston and Madison, 1999c; Buhler and Dunwiddie, 2001; Griguoli et al., 2009	Agonist: Griguoli et al., 2009	Agonist: McQuiston and Madison, 1999c; Griguoli et al., 2009
	Synaptic: Widmer et al., 2006; Bell et al., 2013	Synaptic: Widmer et al., 2006; Bell et al., 2013	Synaptic: Bell et al., 2013	Synaptic: Not identified	Synaptic: Bell et al., 2011	Synaptic: Not observed

Cholinergic responsive interneurons are categorized based on the anatomical location of their axons (left column). References are reported for cholinergic response types observed in each class of interneuron. Agonist refers to responses elicited by exogenous agonist application. Stimulation refers to endogenous acetylcholine responses elicited electrically or optogenetically. Not identified—indicates that such a response type has not been observed in that class of interneuron. Not observed—indicates that no such response type has been observed in any interneuron class.

each response type in hippocampal CA1 interneurons (Bell et al., 2013). However, the number of flashes affected the probability of observing a particular response type. In hyperpolarizing interneurons, 10 flashes were sufficient (91% of hyperpolarizing interneurons) to observe a response. In contrast, 10 flashes were not sufficient to produce a response in the majority of depolarizing interneurons (58%). Similarly, the depolarizing phase could not be observed in the majority of biphasic interneurons (55%) when only 10 stimuli were delivered. Therefore, muscarinic hyperpolarizations may require less presynaptic MS/DBB cholinergic activity compared to depolarizing responses in hippocampal CA1 interneurons. It may be that suppression of interneuron excitability will be the predominant effect in response to low levels of MS/DBB cholinergic activity.

EFFECTS OF NICOTINIC RECEPTOR ACTIVATION ON HIPPOCAMPAL CA1 INTERNEURONS

Activation of nicotinic receptors in the hippocampus has a significant impact on physiological and pathophysiological memory formation (Levin, 2002; Levin et al., 2002, 2009; Buccafusco et al., 2005; Davis and Gould, 2006, 2009; Nott and Levin, 2006; Davis et al., 2007). Of the 11 different nicotinic receptor subunits found in the mammalian CNS, 9 have been reported to be expressed in hippocampal CA1 neurons (Sudweeks and Yakel, 2000). Using exogenous application of nicotinic agonists, functional nicotinic receptors that contain α7 (Alkondon et al., 1997; Jones and Yakel, 1997; Frazier et al., 1998b; McQuiston and Madison, 1999c), α4β2 (McQuiston and Madison, 1999c; Sudweeks and Yakel, 2000), or α2 subunits (McQuiston and Madison, 1999c; Sudweeks and Yakel, 2000; Jia et al., 2009) have been observed in hippocampal CA1 interneurons. Although hippocampal interneurons appeared to express a diverse collection nicotinic receptor subtypes, α7 containing receptors were more frequently observed and produced larger responses (McQuiston and Madison, 1999c; Sudweeks and Yakel, 2000). Indeed, α7 nicotinic receptors in the hippocampus have been associated with memory formation (Levin, 2002; Levin et al., 2002; Nott and Levin, 2006) and their dysfunction may play a role in some forms of schizophrenia (Freedman et al., 1994; Leonard et al., 1996; Adler et al., 1998). However, despite their lower expression levels, the α4β2 containing nicotinic receptors have been reported to play a significant role in memory formation (Davis and Gould, 2006; Davis et al., 2007) and in hippocampal-dependent nicotine addiction (Perry et al., 1999; Davis and Gould, 2009). α4β2 containing receptors have also been correlated with cognitive deficits associated with aging and Alzheimer's disease (Kellar et al., 1987; Wu et al., 2004; Gahring et al., 2005). To fully understand the role that different nicotinic subunits play in the hippocampus, the effect of endogenously released acetylcholine on individual hippocampal cells and the hippocampal network has begun to be investigated.

ACTIVATION OF NICOTINIC RECEPTORS IN HIPPOCAMPAL CA1 INTERNEURONS FOLLOWING ACETYLCHOLINE RELEASE

Acetylcholine release from MS/DBB cholinergic terminals in hippocampal CA1 has been demonstrated to activate nicotinic receptors on interneurons (Alkondon et al., 1998; Frazier et al., 1998a; Stone, 2007). Nicotinic excitatory postsynaptic currents (EPSCs) were first observed using electrical stimulation and whole cell patch clamping in acute rat brain slices. These nicotinic EPSCs had fast kinetics and were blocked by α7 nicotinic receptor antagonists (Alkondon et al., 1998; Frazier et al., 1998a), consistent with studies that applied nicotinic receptor agonists directly onto interneuron cell bodies (Alkondon et al., 1997; Jones and Yakel, 1997; Frazier et al., 1998b; McQuiston and Madison, 1999c). However, more recent optogenetic studies in mouse brain slices were not able to reproduce these earlier observations (Bell et al., 2011). Instead, optogenetically released acetylcholine primarily activated nicotinic receptors that contained α4β2 subunits. Furthermore, the α4β2 responses were mostly subthreshold and had very slow kinetics. These data were suggestive of acetylcholine diffusing a significant distance before binding to the α4β2 containing nicotinic receptors (McQuiston and Madison, 1999c; Bennett et al., 2012), consistent with volume or non-synaptic transmission (Vizi et al., 2010). Although these small nicotinic responses could temporally summate, their ability to excite interneurons was limited through muscarinic presynaptic inhibition. Because the nicotinic responses were mostly subthreshold, nicotinic transmission onto CA1 interneurons may be primarily modulatory in nature. The optogenetic studies also examined the nicotinic responses using voltage-sensitive dye (VSD) imaging. The nicotinic VSD signals were completely blocked by the α4β2 receptor antagonist DHβE and were found to be significantly larger in the distal dendritic region of CA1 pyramidal neurons, which overlaps with inputs from the entorhinal cortex and nucleus reuniens of the thalamus (Bell et al., 2011). Importantly, because the VSD stains all elements of the tissue, the VSD data suggest that α4β2 containing nicotinic receptors are the most prevalent receptor that mediates depolarizing nicotinic responses in mouse hippocampal CA1. Notably, nicotinic responses could be produced by a single flash of light (Bell et al., 2011) suggesting that acetylcholine release from MS/DBB cholinergic terminals may help recruit interneurons via nicotinic receptor activation before they are affected by muscarinic receptor activation.

EFFECTS OF ACETYLCHOLINE RELEASE ON HIPPOCAMPAL CA1 NETWORK FUNCTION FROM THE PERSPECTIVE OF THE INTERNEURON MEMBRANE POTENTIAL

Because CA1 inhibitory interneuron membrane potentials can be differentially modulated by both muscarinic and nicotinic receptor activation following acetylcholine release, the consequential effect on network function is undoubtedly complex. Muscarinic receptor activation can result in varying and opposing effects, even within the same interneuron (see **Table 1**). Unfortunately, our understanding of how each subtype of interneuron can be affected by muscarinic or nicotinic receptor activation remains incomplete. Nevertheless, the number of stimuli required to produce each type of response varied in a consistent manner. Nicotinic responses were most easily evoked requiring the fewest number of stimuli (Bell et al., 2011) whereas depolarizing muscarinic responses were the most difficult to produce requiring the largest number stimuli (Bell et al., 2013). Therefore, it can be hypothesized that low levels of MS/DBB cholinergic

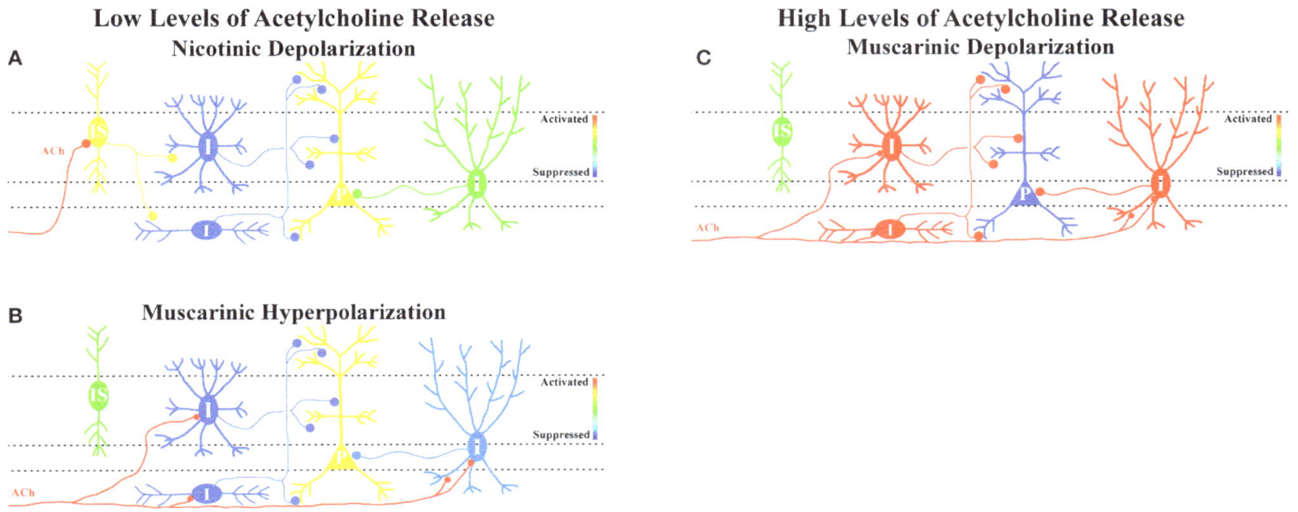

FIGURE 1 | Hypothesis that MS/DBB cholinergic inputs either suppress or activate interneuron networks in hippocampal CA1 depending on cholinergic neuron activity. (A) Low levels of MS/DBB cholinergic activity preferentially activate subsets of interneurons through the activation of nicotinic receptors. We postulate that nicotinic-driven interneurons are interneurons-selective interneurons (IS, yellow—activation) that specifically inhibit other interneurons (blue). Increasing their activity results in disinhibition of pyramidal neurons (P, yellow—activation, and increased output). **(B)** Low levels of MS/DBB cholinergic activity also hyperpolarize subsets of interneurons through the activation of muscarinic receptors (I, blue—suppression) resulting in disinhibition of pyramidal neurons (P, yellow—activation, and increased output). **(C)** Increasing cholinergic neuron activity causes subsets of interneurons to be depolarized by muscarinic receptor activation (I, red—activation, and increased synaptic inhibition) resulting in suppression of pyramidal neurons (P, blue—suppressed output).

neuron activity and lower concentrations of extracellular acetylcholine favor the activation nicotinic receptors or a muscarinic hyperpolarization in specific subsets of CA1 interneurons.

Because muscarinic hyperpolarization of CA1 interneurons requires less presynaptic cholinergic activity, disinhibition (indirect activation) of hippocampal CA1 pyramidal cells may be favored during low levels of MS/DBB cholinergic activity (**Figure 1B**). Furthermore, postulating that nicotinic responses preferentially affect interneurons that selectively inhibit other interneurons (interneuron-selective or IS), nicotinic receptor activation may also result in disinhibition of CA1 pyramidal neurons (**Figure 1A**). Together, low levels of MS/DBB cholinergic activity would favor a net disinhibition of hippocampal CA1 permitting higher probability of output from CA1 pyramidal neurons. Increased output from CA1 may result in the facilitation of recall and memory consolidation in other areas of the CNS as is thought to occur during slow wave sleep (Gais and Born, 2004; Hasselmo and McGaughy, 2004). In contrast, higher levels of MS/DBB cholinergic neuron activity coupled to higher extracellular concentrations of acetylcholine will subsequently recruit different subsets of interneurons that respond via muscarinic depolarizations. Some of these depolarizing interneurons may impose rhythmic inhibition of CA1 pyramidal neurons at theta frequencies (Nagode et al., 2011, 2014), a network rhythm observed during higher levels of acetylcholine release (Zhang et al., 2010). This would result in inhibition of hippocampal CA1 pyramidal neuron output (partly rhythmic) while facilitating synaptic integration within hippocampal CA1 pyramidal cell dendrites through cholinergic effects on glutamatergic receptors and dendritic function (**Figure 1C**) (Tsubokawa and Ross, 1997; Tsubokawa, 2000; Fernandez De Sevilla and Buno, 2010; Giessel and Sabatini, 2010). Indeed, such a dynamic role for acetylcholine concentrations in learning and memory formation has been previously proposed (Hasselmo, 2006; Hasselmo and Giocomo, 2006; Giocomo and Hasselmo, 2007; Hasselmo and Sarter, 2011). In this scheme, lower acetylcholine concentrations permit intrahippocampal (Schaffer collaterals) synaptic interactions to dominate thus increasing hippocampal CA1 output and memory retrieval, whereas higher acetylcholine concentrations favor processing of inputs from outside the hippocampus permitting the transient formation of memories in hippocampal CA1. Therefore, the combined effect of acetylcholine release on glutamatergic inputs and interneuron function may play important roles in tuning the hippocampal CA1 network for recall or to form new memories.

ACKNOWLEDGMENT

This work was supported by grants from the NIMH/NIH 5R01MH094626 and 1R21MH103695.

REFERENCES

Adler, L. E., Olincy, A., Waldo, M., Harris, J. G., Griffith, J., Stevens, K., et al. (1998). Schizophrenia, sensory gating, and nicotinic receptors. *Schizophr. Bull.* 24, 189–202. doi: 10.1093/oxfordjournals.schbul.a033320

Alkondon, M., Pereira, E. F., and Albuquerque, E. X. (1998). alpha-bungarotoxin- and methyllycaconitine-sensitive nicotinic receptors mediate fast synaptic transmission in interneurons of rat hippocampal slices. *Brain Res.* 810, 257–263. doi: 10.1016/S0006-8993(98)00880-4

Alkondon, M., Pereira, E. F., Barbosa, C. T., and Albuquerque, E. X. (1997). Neuronal nicotinic acetylcholine receptor activation modulates gamma-aminobutyric acid release from CA1 neurons of rat hippocampal slices. *J. Pharmacol. Exp. Ther.* 283, 1396–1411.

Atri, A., Sherman, S., Norman, K. A., Kirchhoff, B. A., Nicolas, M. M., Greicius, M. D., et al. (2004). Blockade of central cholinergic receptors impairs new learning and increases proactive interference in a word paired-associate memory task. *Behav. Neurosci.* 118, 223–236. doi: 10.1037/0735-7044.118.1.223

Aznavour, N., Mechawar, N., and Descarries, L. (2002). Comparative analysis of cholinergic innervation in the dorsal hippocampus of adult mouse and rat: a quantitative immunocytochemical study. *Hippocampus* 12, 206–217. doi: 10.1002/hipo.1108

Barrenechea, C., Pedemonte, M., Nunez, A., and Garcia-Austt, E. (1995). *In vivo* intracellular recordings of medial septal and diagonal band of Broca neurons: relationships with theta rhythm. *Exp. Brain Res.* 103, 31–40. doi: 10.1007/BF00241962

Behrends, J. C., and Ten Bruggencate, G. (1993). Cholinergic modulation of synaptic inhibition in the guinea pig hippocampus *in vitro*: excitation of GABAergic interneurons and inhibition of GABA-release. *J. Neurophysiol.* 69, 626–629.

Bell, K. A., Shim, H., Chen, C. K., and McQuiston, A. R. (2011). Nicotinic excitatory postsynaptic potentials in hippocampal CA1 interneurons are predominantly mediated by nicotinic receptors that contain alpha4 and beta2 subunits. *Neuropharmacology* 61, 1379–1388. doi: 10.1016/j.neuropharm.2011.08.024

Bell, L. A., Bell, K. A., and McQuiston, A. R. (2013). Synaptic muscarinic response types in hippocampal CA1 interneurons depend on different levels of presynaptic activity and different muscarinic receptor subtypes. *Neuropharmacology* 73, 160–173. doi: 10.1016/j.neuropharm.2013.05.026

Bennett, C., Arroyo, S., Berns, D., and Hestrin, S. (2012). Mechanisms generating dual-component nicotinic EPSCs in cortical interneurons. *J. Neurosci.* 32, 17287–17296. doi: 10.1523/JNEUROSCI.3565-12.2012

Blake, M. G., Krawczyk, M. C., Baratti, C. M., and Boccia, M. M. (2014). Neuropharmacology of memory consolidation and reconsolidation: insights on central cholinergic mechanisms. *J. Physiol. Paris.* doi: 10.1016/j.jphysparis.2014.04.005. [Epub ahead of print]

Blokland, A., Honig, W., and Raaijmakers, W. G. (1992). Effects of intra-hippocampal scopolamine injections in a repeated spatial acquisition task in the rat. *Psychopharmacology (Berl).* 109, 373–376. doi: 10.1007/BF02245886

Brazhnik, E. S., and Fox, S. E. (1997). Intracellular recordings from medial septal neurons during hippocampal theta rhythm. *Exp. Brain Res.* 114, 442–453. doi: 10.1007/PL00005653

Brazhnik, E. S., and Fox, S. E. (1999). Action potentials and relations to the theta rhythm of medial septal neurons *in vivo*. *Exp. Brain Res.* 127, 244–258. doi: 10.1007/s002210050794

Buccafusco, J. J., Letchworth, S. R., Bencherif, M., and Lippiello, P. M. (2005). Long-lasting cognitive improvement with nicotinic receptor agonists: mechanisms of pharmacokinetic-pharmacodynamic discordance. *Trends Pharmacol. Sci.* 26, 352–360. doi: 10.1016/j.tips.2005.05.007

Buhler, A. V., and Dunwiddie, T. V. (2001). Regulation of the activity of hippocampal stratum oriens interneurons by alpha7 nicotinic acetylcholine receptors. *Neuroscience* 106, 55–67. doi: 10.1016/S0306-4522(01)00257-3

Buzsaki, G. (2002). Theta oscillations in the hippocampus. *Neuron* 33, 325–340. doi: 10.1016/S0896-6273(02)00586-X

Buzsaki, G., and Wang, X. J. (2012). Mechanisms of gamma oscillations. *Annu. Rev. Neurosci.* 35, 203–225. doi: 10.1146/annurev-neuro-062111-150444

Cea-Del Rio, C. A., Lawrence, J. J., Erdelyi, F., Szabo, G., and McBain, C. J. (2011). Cholinergic modulation amplifies the intrinsic oscillatory properties of CA1 hippocampal cholecystokinin-positive interneurons. *J. Physiol.* 589, 609–627. doi: 10.1113/jphysiol.2010.199422

Cea-Del Rio, C. A., Lawrence, J. J., Tricoire, L., Erdelyi, F., Szabo, G., and McBain, C. J. (2010). M3 muscarinic acetylcholine receptor expression confers differential cholinergic modulation to neurochemically distinct hippocampal basket cell subtypes. *J. Neurosci.* 30, 6011–6024. doi: 10.1523/JNEUROSCI.5040-09.2010

Cobb, S. R., and Davies, C. H. (2005). Cholinergic modulation of hippocampal cells and circuits. *J. Physiol.* 562, 81–88. doi: 10.1113/jphysiol.2004.076539

Cole, A. E., and Nicoll, R. A. (1983). Acetylcholine mediates a slow synaptic potential in hippocampal pyramidal cells. *Science* 221, 1299–1301. doi: 10.1126/science.6612345

Davis, J. A., and Gould, T. J. (2006). The effects of DHBE and MLA on nicotine-induced enhancement of contextual fear conditioning in C57BL/6 mice. *Psychopharmacology (Berl).* 184, 345–352. doi: 10.1007/s00213-005-0047-y

Davis, J. A., and Gould, T. J. (2009). Hippocampal nAChRs mediate nicotine withdrawal-related learning deficits. *Eur. Neuropsychopharmacol.* 19, 551–561. doi: 10.1016/j.euroneuro.2009.02.003

Davis, J. A., Kenney, J. W., and Gould, T. J. (2007). Hippocampal alpha4beta2 nicotinic acetylcholine receptor involvement in the enhancing effect of acute nicotine on contextual fear conditioning. *J. Neurosci.* 27, 10870–10877. doi: 10.1523/JNEUROSCI.3242-07.2007

Deiana, S., Platt, B., and Riedel, G. (2011). The cholinergic system and spatial learning. *Behav. Brain Res.* 221, 389–411. doi: 10.1016/j.bbr.2010.11.036

Dutar, P., Bassant, M. H., Senut, M. C., and Lamour, Y. (1995). The septohippocampal pathway: structure and function of a central cholinergic system. *Physiol. Rev.* 75, 393–427.

Easton, A., Douchamps, V., Eacott, M., and Lever, C. (2012). A specific role for septohippocampal acetylcholine in memory? *Neuropsychologia* 50, 3156–3168. doi: 10.1016/j.neuropsychologia.2012.07.022

Fernandez De Sevilla, D., and Buno, W. (2010). The muscarinic long-term enhancement of NMDA and AMPA receptor-mediated transmission at Schaffer collateral synapses develop through different intracellular mechanisms. *J. Neurosci.* 30, 11032–11042. doi: 10.1523/JNEUROSCI.1848-10.2010

Frazier, C. J., Buhler, A. V., Weiner, J. L., and Dunwiddie, T. V. (1998a). Synaptic potentials mediated via alpha-bungarotoxin-sensitive nicotinic acetylcholine receptors in rat hippocampal interneurons. *J. Neurosci.* 18, 8228–8235.

Frazier, C. J., Rollins, Y. D., Breese, C. R., Leonard, S., Freedman, R., and Dunwiddie, T. V. (1998b). Acetylcholine activates an alpha-bungarotoxin-sensitive nicotinic current in rat hippocampal interneurons, but not pyramidal cells. *J. Neurosci.* 18, 1187–1195.

Freedman, R., Adler, L. E., Bickford, P., Byerley, W., Coon, H., Cullum, C. M., et al. (1994). Schizophrenia and nicotinic receptors. *Harv. Rev. Psychiatry* 2, 179–192. doi: 10.3109/10673229409017136

Freund, T. F., and Buzsaki, G. (1996). Interneurons of the hippocampus. *Hippocampus* 6, 347–470.

Fukudome, Y., Ohno-Shosaku, T., Matsui, M., Omori, Y., Fukaya, M., Tsubokawa, H., et al. (2004). Two distinct classes of muscarinic action on hippocampal inhibitory synapses: M2-mediated direct suppression and M1/M3-mediated indirect suppression through endocannabinoid signalling. *Eur. J. Neurosci.* 19, 2682–2692. doi: 10.1111/j.0953-816X.2004.03384.x

Gahring, L. C., Persiyanov, K., and Rogers, S. W. (2005). Mouse strain-specific changes in nicotinic receptor expression with age. *Neurobiol. Aging* 26, 973–980. doi: 10.1016/j.neurobiolaging.2004.07.005

Gais, S., and Born, J. (2004). Low acetylcholine during slow-wave sleep is critical for declarative memory consolidation. *Proc. Natl. Acad. Sci. U.S.A.* 101, 2140–2144. doi: 10.1073/pnas.0305404101

Giessel, A. J., and Sabatini, B. L. (2010). M1 muscarinic receptors boost synaptic potentials and calcium influx in dendritic spines by inhibiting postsynaptic SK channels. *Neuron* 68, 936–947. doi: 10.1016/j.neuron.2010.09.004

Giocomo, L. M., and Hasselmo, M. E. (2007). Neuromodulation by glutamate and acetylcholine can change circuit dynamics by regulating the relative influence of afferent input and excitatory feedback. *Mol. Neurobiol.* 36, 184–200. doi: 10.1007/s12035-007-0032-z

Griguoli, M., Scuri, R., Ragozzino, D., and Cherubini, E. (2009). Activation of nicotinic acetylcholine receptors enhances a slow calcium-dependent potassium conductance and reduces the firing of stratum oriens interneurons. *Eur. J. Neurosci.* 30, 1011–1022. doi: 10.1111/j.1460-9568.2009.06914.x

Hasselmo, M. E. (2006). The role of acetylcholine in learning and memory. *Curr. Opin. Neurobiol.* 16, 710–715. doi: 10.1016/j.conb.2006.09.002

Hasselmo, M. E., and Giocomo, L. M. (2006). Cholinergic modulation of cortical function. *J. Mol. Neurosci.* 30, 133–135. doi: 10.1385/JMN:30:1:133

Hasselmo, M. E., and McGaughy, J. (2004). High acetylcholine levels set circuit dynamics for attention and encoding and low acetylcholine levels set dynamics for consolidation. *Prog. Brain Res.* 145, 207–231. doi: 10.1016/S0079-6123(03)45015-2

Hasselmo, M. E., and Sarter, M. (2011). Modes and models of forebrain cholinergic neuromodulation of cognition. *Neuropsychopharmacology* 36, 52–73. doi: 10.1038/npp.2010.104

Jia, Y., Yamazaki, Y., Nakauchi, S., and Sumikawa, K. (2009). Alpha2 nicotine receptors function as a molecular switch to continuously excite a subset of interneurons in rat hippocampal circuits. *Eur. J. Neurosci.* 29, 1588–1603. doi: 10.1111/j.1460-9568.2009.06706.x

Jones, S., and Yakel, J. L. (1997). Functional nicotinic ACh receptors on interneurones in the rat hippocampus. *J. Physiol.* 504(Pt 3), 603–610. doi: 10.1111/j.1469-7793.1997.603bd.x

Kellar, K. J., Whitehouse, P. J., Martino-Barrows, A. M., Marcus, K., and Price, D. L. (1987). Muscarinic and nicotinic cholinergic binding sites in Alzheimer's disease cerebral cortex. *Brain Res.* 436, 62–68. doi: 10.1016/0006-8993(87)91556-3

Kenney, J. W., and Gould, T. J. (2008). Modulation of hippocampus-dependent learning and synaptic plasticity by nicotine. *Mol. Neurobiol.* 38, 101–121. doi: 10.1007/s12035-008-8037-9

Klausberger, T., and Somogyi, P. (2008). Neuronal diversity and temporal dynamics: the unity of hippocampal circuit operations. *Science* 321, 53–57. doi: 10.1126/science.1149381

Larkum, M. E., Zhu, J. J., and Sakmann, B. (1999). A new cellular mechanism for coupling inputs arriving at different cortical layers. *Nature* 398, 338–341. doi: 10.1038/18686

Lawrence, J. J., Statland, J. M., Grinspan, Z. M., and McBain, C. J. (2006). Cell type-specific dependence of muscarinic signalling in mouse hippocampal stratum oriens interneurones. *J. Physiol.* 570, 595–610. doi: 10.1113/jphysiol.2005.100875

Leonard, S., Adams, C., Breese, C. R., Adler, L. E., Bickford, P., Byerley, W., et al. (1996). Nicotinic receptor function in schizophrenia. *Schizophr. Bull.* 22, 431–445. doi: 10.1093/schbul/22.3.431

Levin, E. D. (2002). Nicotinic receptor subtypes and cognitive function. *J. Neurobiol.* 53, 633–640. doi: 10.1002/neu.10151

Levin, E. D., Bradley, A., Addy, N., and Sigurani, N. (2002). Hippocampal alpha 7 and alpha 4 beta 2 nicotinic receptors and working memory. *Neuroscience* 109, 757–765. doi: 10.1016/S0306-4522(01)00538-3

Levin, E. D., Petro, A., Rezvani, A. H., Pollard, N., Christopher, N. C., Strauss, M., et al. (2009). Nicotinic alpha7- or beta2-containing receptor knockout: effects on radial-arm maze learning and long-term nicotine consumption in mice. *Behav. Brain Res.* 196, 207–213. doi: 10.1016/j.bbr.2008.08.048

McQuiston, A. R., and Madison, D. V. (1999a). Muscarinic receptor activity has multiple effects on the resting membrane potentials of CA1 hippocampal interneurons. *J. Neurosci.* 19, 5693–5702.

McQuiston, A. R., and Madison, D. V. (1999b). Muscarinic receptor activity induces an afterdepolarization in a subpopulation of hippocampal CA1 interneurons. *J. Neurosci.* 19, 5703–5710.

McQuiston, A. R., and Madison, D. V. (1999c). Nicotinic receptor activation excites distinct subtypes of interneurons in the rat hippocampus. *J. Neurosci.* 19, 2887–2896.

Miles, R., Toth, K., Gulyas, A. I., Hajos, N., and Freund, T. F. (1996). Differences between somatic and dendritic inhibition in the hippocampus. *Neuron* 16, 815–823. doi: 10.1016/S0896-6273(00)80101-4

Nagode, D. A., Tang, A. H., Karson, M. A., Klugmann, M., and Alger, B. E. (2011). Optogenetic release of ACh induces rhythmic bursts of perisomatic IPSCs in hippocampus. *PLoS ONE* 6:e27691. doi: 10.1371/journal.pone.0027691

Nagode, D. A., Tang, A. H., Yang, K., and Alger, B. E. (2014). Optogenetic identification of an intrinsic cholinergically driven inhibitory oscillator sensitive to cannabinoids and opioids in hippocampal CA1. *J. Physiol.* 592, 103–123. doi: 10.1113/jphysiol.2013.257428

Nott, A., and Levin, E. D. (2006). Dorsal hippocampal alpha7 and alpha4beta2 nicotinic receptors and memory. *Brain Res.* 1081, 72–78. doi: 10.1016/j.brainres.2006.01.052

Parra, P., Gulyas, A. I., and Miles, R. (1998). How many subtypes of inhibitory cells in the hippocampus? *Neuron* 20, 983–993. doi: 10.1016/S0896-6273(00)80479-1

Perry, D. C., Davila-Garcia, M. I., Stockmeier, C. A., and Kellar, K. J. (1999). Increased nicotinic receptors in brains from smokers: membrane binding and autoradiography studies. *J. Pharmacol. Exp. Ther.* 289, 1545–1552.

Pitler, T. A., and Alger, B. E. (1992). Cholinergic excitation of GABAergic interneurons in the rat hippocampal slice. *J. Physiol.* 450, 127–142.

Power, A. E., Vazdarjanova, A., and McGaugh, J. L. (2003). Muscarinic cholinergic influences in memory consolidation. *Neurobiol. Learn. Mem.* 80, 178–193. doi: 10.1016/S1074-7427(03)00086-8

Simon, A. P., Poindessous-Jazat, F., Dutar, P., Epelbaum, J., and Bassant, M. H. (2006). Firing properties of anatomically identified neurons in the medial septum of anesthetized and unanesthetized restrained rats. *J. Neurosci.* 26, 9038–9046. doi: 10.1523/JNEUROSCI.1401-06.2006

Smiley, J. F., Morrell, F., and Mesulam, M. M. (1997). Cholinergic synapses in human cerebral cortex: an ultrastructural study in serial sections. *Exp. Neurol.* 144, 361–368. doi: 10.1006/exnr.1997.6413

Stone, T. W. (2007). Kynurenic acid blocks nicotinic synaptic transmission to hippocampal interneurons in young rats. *Eur. J. Neurosci.* 25, 2656–2665. doi: 10.1111/j.1460-9568.2007.05540.x

Storm-Mathisen, J. (1970). Quantitative histochemistry of acetylcholinesterase in rat hippocampal region correlated to histochemical staining. *J. Neurochem.* 17, 739–750. doi: 10.1111/j.1471-4159.1970.tb03344.x

Sudweeks, S. N., and Yakel, J. L. (2000). Functional and molecular characterization of neuronal nicotinic ACh receptors in rat CA1 hippocampal neurons. *J. Physiol.* 527(Pt 3), 515–528. doi: 10.1111/j.1469-7793.2000.00515.x

Szabo, G. G., Holderith, N., Gulyas, A. I., Freund, T. F., and Hajos, N. (2010). Distinct synaptic properties of perisomatic inhibitory cell types and their different modulation by cholinergic receptor activation in the CA3 region of the mouse hippocampus. *Eur. J. Neurosci.* 31, 2234–2246. doi: 10.1111/j.1460-9568.2010.07292.x

Tang, A. H., Karson, M. A., Nagode, D. A., McIntosh, J. M., Uebele, V. N., Renger, J. J., et al. (2011). Nerve terminal nicotinic acetylcholine receptors initiate quantal GABA release from perisomatic interneurons by activating axonal T-type (Cav3) Ca(2)(+) channels and Ca(2)(+) release from stores. *J. Neurosci.* 31, 13546–13561. doi: 10.1523/JNEUROSCI.2781-11.2011

Teles-Grilo Ruivo, L. M., and Mellor, J. R. (2013). Cholinergic modulation of hippocampal network function. *Front. Synaptic Neurosci.* 5:2. doi: 10.3389/fnsyn.2013.00002

Tsubokawa, H. (2000). Control of Na+ spike backpropagation by intracellular signaling in the pyramidal neuron dendrites. *Mol. Neurobiol.* 22, 129–141. doi: 10.1385/MN:22:1-3:129

Tsubokawa, H., and Ross, W. N. (1997). Muscarinic modulation of spike backpropagation in the apical dendrites of hippocampal CA1 pyramidal neurons. *J. Neurosci.* 17, 5782–5791.

Turrini, P., Casu, M. A., Wong, T. P., De, K. Y., Ribeiro-Da-Silva, A., and Cuello, A. C. (2001). Cholinergic nerve terminals establish classical synapses in the rat cerebral cortex: synaptic pattern and age-related atrophy. *Neuroscience* 105, 277–285. doi: 10.1016/S0306-4522(01)00172-5

Umbriaco, D., Garcia, S., Beaulieu, C., and Descarries, L. (1995). Relational features of acetylcholine, noradrenaline, serotonin and GABA axon terminals in the stratum radiatum of adult rat hippocampus (CA1). *Hippocampus* 5, 605–620. doi: 10.1002/hipo.450050611

Umbriaco, D., Watkins, K. C., Descarries, L., Cozzari, C., and Hartman, B. K. (1994). Ultrastructural and morphometric features of the acetylcholine innervation in adult rat parietal cortex: an electron microscopic study in serial sections. *J. Comp. Neurol.* 348, 351–373. doi: 10.1002/cne.903480304

Vizi, E. S., Fekete, A., Karoly, R., and Mike, A. (2010). Non-synaptic receptors and transporters involved in brain functions and targets of drug treatment. *Br. J. Pharmacol.* 160, 785–809. doi: 10.1111/j.1476-5381.2009.00624.x

Widmer, H., Ferrigan, L., Davies, C. H., and Cobb, S. R. (2006). Evoked slow muscarinic acetylcholinergic synaptic potentials in rat hippocampal interneurons. *Hippocampus* 16, 617–628. doi: 10.1002/hipo.20191

Wu, J., Kuo, Y. P., George, A. A., Xu, L., Hu, J., and Lukas, R. J. (2004). beta-Amyloid directly inhibits human alpha4beta2-nicotinic acetylcholine receptors heterologously expressed in human SH-EP1 cells. *J. Biol. Chem.* 279, 37842–37851. doi: 10.1074/jbc.M400335200

Zhang, H., Lin, S. C., and Nicolelis, M. A. (2010). Spatiotemporal coupling between hippocampal acetylcholine release and theta oscillations *in vivo*. *J. Neurosci.* 30, 13431–13440. doi: 10.1523/JNEUROSCI.1144-10.2010

6

How neurogenesis finds its place in a hardwired sensory system

Livio Oboti[1]* and Paolo Peretto[2]

[1] Children's National Health System, Center for Neuroscience Research, Washington, DC, USA
[2] Department of Life Sciences and Systems Biology, Neuroscience Institute Cavalieri Ottolenghi, University of Torino, Orbassano, Italy

Edited by:
Luca Bonfanti, University of Turin, Italy

Reviewed by:
Eric D. Laywell, The Florida State University College of Medicine, USA
José Luis Trejo, Institute Cajal - CSIC, Spain

***Correspondence:**
Livio Oboti, Children's National Health System, Center for Neuroscience Research, 111 Michigan Avenue, Washington, DC 20310, USA
e-mail: loboti@childrensnational.org

So far most studies on adult neurogenesis aimed to unravel mechanisms and molecules regulating the integration of newly generated neurons in the mature brain parenchyma. The exceedingly abundant amount of results that followed, rather than being beneficial in the perspective of brain repair, provided a clear evidence that adult neurogenesis constitutes a necessary feature to the correct functioning of the hosting brain regions. In particular, the rodent olfactory system represents a privileged model to study how neuronal plasticity and neurogenesis interact with sensory functions. Until recently, the vomeronasal system (VNS) has been commonly described as being specialized in the detection of innate chemosignals. Accordingly, its circuitry has been considered necessarily stable, if not hard-wired, in order to allow stereotyped behavioral responses. However, both first and second order projections of the rodent VNS continuously change their synaptic connectivity due to ongoing postnatal and adult neurogenesis. How the functional integrity of a neuronal circuit is maintained while newborn neurons are continuously added—or lost—is a fundamental question for both basic and applied neuroscience. The VNS is proposed as an alternative model to answer such question. Hereby the underlying motivations will be reviewed.

Keywords: accessory olfactory bulb, AOB, vomeronasal, VNO, neurogenesis, pheromones, plasticity, innate

INTRODUCTION

The idea of a mature brain as an organ with limited growth, cell renewal and rewiring has considerably changed since pioneer studies on adult neurogenesis (Altman and Das, 1966; Altman, 1969; Graziadei and Monti-Graziadei, 1979; Lledo and Gheusi, 2006; Kempermann, 2012). In the adult mammalian brain, neural progenitors are present in the subventricular zone (SVZ) of the lateral ventricles and the hippocampal subgranular zone (SGZ) where they give rise respectively to Dlx2/5/6-derived GABAergic olfactory bulb interneurons and glutamatergic granule cells of the dentate gyrus (DG) of the hippocampus (Doetsch et al., 1999; Seri et al., 2001; Kriegstein and Alvarez-Buylla, 2009). Admittedly, neurogenesis in other adult brain regions is generally believed to be very limited under physiological conditions (Nishiyama et al., 1996; Horner et al., 2000; Dawson et al., 2003; Luzzati et al., 2006, 2011; Bonfanti and Peretto, 2011), although it could be induced after injury (Ramaswamy et al., 2005; Gould, 2007; Yu et al., 2008; Kernie and Parent, 2010; Saha et al., 2013) or as a consequence of tissue inflammation and degeneration (Buffo et al., 2008; Ohira et al., 2010; Luzzati et al., 2011; Belarbi and Rosi, 2013). Nowadays several approaches have been developed to maintain and manipulate pluripotent stem cells *in-vitro* in the perspective of brain repair (Takahashi and Yamanaka, 2006; Yamanaka and Blau, 2010). Particularly the rodent olfactory bulb (OB) has been widely studied to clarify the logic of neuronal stem-cell biology in the SVZ opening new venues to brain-repair strategies, cell transplants techniques in disease models and other translational approaches (Gage and Temple, 2013).

However, the development of clinical translations cannot stand aside the basic research, focused in this case on the physiologic function of the neurogenic regions *in-vivo* (see for critical reviews on this point Lau et al., 2008; Lindvall and Kokaia, 2010).

In addition, studying OB neurogenesis may yield new insights in the biology of olfaction, being olfactory sensory activity and behaviors easy readouts of any experimental manipulation in rodents.

Understanding how the environment affects newborn neurons integration into mature networks, and consequently normal brain function, are certainly meaningful aims to define the boundaries between physiology and pathology in translational neuroscience. The restoration of brain connectivity after trauma or the comprehension of the etiology of major brain disorders may certainly move forward and undoubtedly more clinically oriented approaches would benefit from the unbiased attempts of basic research to address these issues (Fang and Casadevall, 2010;

Abbreviations: aAOB, anterior accessory olfactory bulb; AOB, accessory olfactory bulb; CR, calretinin; DCX, doublecortin; DG, dentate gyrus; ECL, external cellular layer; EGC, external granule cell; ET, external tufted; GAD, glutamic acid decarboxylase; GC, granule cell; Gl, glomerular layer; HMW, high molecular weight; ICL, internal cellular layer; IGC, internal granule cell; LMW, low molecular weight; LOT, lateral olfactory tract; MACs, main accessory cell; MOB, main olfactory bulb; MOE, main olfactory epithelium; MOS, main olfactory system; NSE, non-sensory epithelium; OB, olfactory bulb; OSNs, olfactory sensory neurons; pAOB, posterior accessory olfactory bulb; PC, principal cell; PG, periglomerular cell; PV, parvalbumin; SA, short axon cell; SGZ, subgranular zone; SVZ, subventricualr zone; TH, tyrosine hydroxylase; VNO, vomeronasal organ; VNS, vomeronasal system; VSNs, vomeronasal sensory neurons.

Enserink, 2013). In the present manuscript a special attention will be given to neurogenesis in a particular olfactory subsystem—namely the accessory/vomeronasal system (VNS)—due to the fact that, despite its behavioral relevance in rodent sociality, it received so far a minor deal of attention. The main point hereby stressed concerns the unclear relationship between form—plastic and changing—and function—presumably stable, innate—in the VNS. Due to its distinct peculiarities, compared to the rest of the olfactory system, the VNS offers an unparalleled opportunity to analyze how newborn neurons constantly integrate into mature circuits without interfering with the physiological behavioral and endocrine development. Recent findings on neurogenesis in the vomeronasal organ (VNO) and accessory olfactory bulb (AOB) will be listed and discussed with a particular emphasis on the AOB, since it represents the first central brain region of this olfactory pathway.

THE VOMERONASAL SYSTEM AS A MODEL TO STUDY ADULT NEUROGENESIS

Neurogenesis in the OB has been studied predominantly in the main olfactory pathway. The neurons constantly replaced in the main olfactory bulb (MOB) are GABAergic local interneurons (periglomerular, PGs, and granule cells, GCs) mainly derived from the Dlx2 subpallial domain in the SVZ (Puelles et al., 2000; Alvarez-Buylla and Garcia-Verdugo, 2002; Lledo and Gheusi, 2006; Whitman and Greer, 2009). These cells play a key role in regulating MOB input and output activity (Spors et al., 2012), and they have been proved to actively contribute to olfactory processing (Mandairon et al., 2011; Alonso et al., 2012) given their activity dependent survival and functional recruitment (Magavi et al., 2005; Mouret et al., 2008; Sultan et al., 2011a,b). In most of these reports the role of newborn neurons in the context of olfactory discrimination, short and long-term olfactory memory has been analyzed using synthetic odor compounds or artificial behavioral tasks. These paradigms are well suited to answer specific questions about the logic of sensory transduction (e.g., tuning, discrimination, detection threshold). However, framing the same analysis within the contexts of reproduction and sociality may be more informative to clarify whether neurogenesis itself is necessary or not to the mature brain. Indeed reproduction and sexual selection constitute a powerful evolutionary force and therefore the primary drive for any functional adaptation of a brain circuit. So far only few recent studies correlated MOB neurogenesis, with the regulation of social behavior in mice (see for example Larsen et al., 2008; Kageyama et al., 2012; Monteiro et al., 2013). The functional studies on the role of neurogenesis in the VNS are considerably fewer despite the major contribution of the VNS in rodent sociality (Tirindelli et al., 2009; Mucignat-Caretta, 2010; Chamero et al., 2012; Ibarra-Soria et al., 2013). Moreover the presence of neurogenesis in the AOB has been largely ignored, if not denied (Mak et al., 2007). However, neurogenesis occurs postnatally both at the VNS periphery, in the VNO, and more centrally, in the AOB (VNO: Barber and Raisman, 1978; Graziadei and Monti-Graziadei, 1979; Jia and Halpern, 1998; Giacobini et al., 2000; Martinez-Marcos et al., 2005; Weiler, 2005; Brann and Firestein, 2010; Enomoto et al., 2011; AOB: Bonfanti et al., 1997; Martínez-Marcos et al., 2001; Peretto et al., 2001; Huang and Bittman, 2002; Oboti et al., 2009, 2011; **Figure 1**). Interestingly cell survival in the AOB is higher after sensory stimulation around weaning and puberty onset (ca. 4 weeks in mice) when, after gonadal and endocrine maturation, social and reproductive behaviors become more clearly manifest (Oboti et al., 2011). Concurrently, despite the VNO seems to be already functional at birth (Coppola and O'Connell, 1989), the process of wiring and synaptogenesis of the VNO-AOB circuit has been shown to extend postnatally and to reach maturity only around the third postnatal week (Horowitz et al., 1999).

This seems to suggest the occurrence of a post-pubertal functional tuning of the VNS circuitry through neurogenesis, plasticity and constant rewiring, which goes beyond an early postnatal maturation of the system, similarly to the main olfactory system (**Figure 1**; Bonfanti and Peretto, 2011; Lepousez et al., 2013).

The reason why the VNS has been neglected by more recent studies on olfactory neurogenesis is possibly due to two main reasons. Firstly, the VNS is absent in humans, therefore limiting the interest in extending the study of olfactory neurogenesis to this system in rodents. Secondly, this sensory system has been traditionally associated to *pheromone* detection, innate signal processing and stereotyped endocrine responses, for which plasticity, neurogenesis, and rewiring are apparently not necessary. Nonetheless, regardless of any homologies in the mammalian olfactory systems, we undoubtedly share with rodents and other species the functions that this sensory pathway specifically regulates, when present (**Figure 2**). Therefore, one of the main reasons why neurogenesis in the rodent VNS deserves more attention is related to understanding the neural bases of mammalian neuroendocrine and behavioral development and how they are affected by environmental cues. Ultimately, the rodent VNS is a suitable and simple model to tackle wider issues related to other mammals in general, humans included.

The aim of the following paragraphs is to evaluate different aspects of VNS neurogenesis ranging from the phenotypes of newly generated neurons to their functional impact on specific circuits. The comparative description accompanying each of these points aims to open new questions for a wide range of approaches. These entailing the developmental, circuit, and system biology of olfaction. Aside, emerges the interesting—yet unanswered—question of how this olfactory subsystem acquires its function in the precise way it does, while its circuits are constantly changing. Rather than supporting the hardwired nature of this process, the evidences here reported suggest a necessary role for neurogenesis, neuronal plasticity, and environmental adaptation for its accomplishment.

NEUROGENESIS IN THE VOMERONASAL ORGAN

Olfactory sensory neurons (OSNs) are directly exposed to the environment to detect chemical stimuli through membrane bound receptors on their cilia (MOS) or microvilli (VNS). In the olfactory epithelia, ciliated and microvillus neurons, supporting cells and ensheating glial cells are constantly renewed during pre- and postnatal development (Murdoch and Roskams, 2008) by neural stem cells deriving from both neural crest and olfactory placode precursor lineages (Katoh et al., 2011; Heron et al., 2013; Suzuki et al., 2013). Due to this peripheral localization,

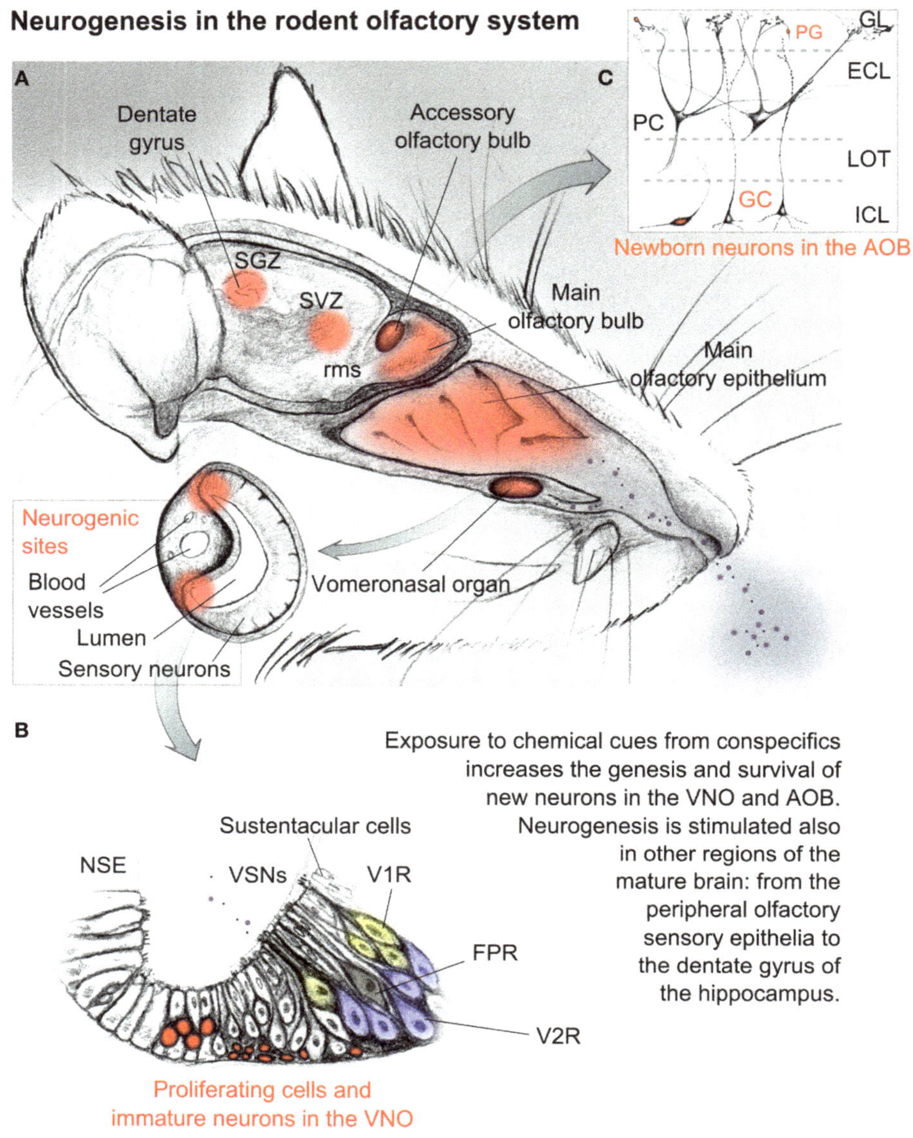

FIGURE 1 | Sketched representation of the mouse olfactory system. Central and peripheral neurogenic regions are evidenced in red. **(A)** Social odors and chemical cues are detected through the main olfactory epithelium and the vomeronasal organ, which is enclosed in a bony capsule opened rostrally toward the nasal cavity. A highly vascularized cavernous tissue flanking the organ allows tissue contraction and therefore the access of mucuous fluids transporting chemical cues toward the sensory epithelium. **(B)** Enlarged view of the vomeronasal sensory epithelium and its cell types. Proliferating cells are localized at the lateral and basal margins of the matured sensory epithelium. Sensory neurons here located send axonal projections to the accessory olfactory bulb. **(C)** Simplified anatomy of the accessory olfactory bulb cellular layers. Cells evidenced in red in **(B,C)** represent immature or regenerating neurons. Abbreviations: SGZ, subgranular zone; SVZ, subventricular zone; rms, rostral migratory stream; GL, glomerular layer; PG, periglomerular cell; ECL, external cellular layer; ICL, internal cellular layer; LOT, lateral olfactory tract; PC, principal cell; GC, granule cell; V1R, vomeronasal receptor neuron type1; V2R, vomeronasal receptor neuron type2; FPR, formyl peptide receptor neuron; VSNs, vomeronasal sensory neurons; NSE, non-sensory epithelium.

OSN renewal has been generally associated to tissue growth (during development), homeostasis and repair (during adulthood) as gene expression patterns are maintained very similar (Heron et al., 2013). In the VNO, as in the MOE, the proliferation of different subsets of neuronal progenitors gives rise to OMP-positive mature receptor neurons (Murdoch and Roskams, 2008; Enomoto et al., 2011) but begins slightly later. In the rat olfactory epithelium OMP starts to be expressed at E14, while in the VN epithelium it occurs only at P2 (Kulkarni-Narla et al., 1997). In the mouse OMP is expressed in vomeronasal sensory neurons (VSNs) a few days earlier, during the last week of gestation (Tarozzo et al., 1998). These data indicate that VSNs are not fully developed at birth as most of their maturation begins and occurs postnatally.

Mature VSNs can be divided in three main families, depending on the receptors expressed and the ligands they have been

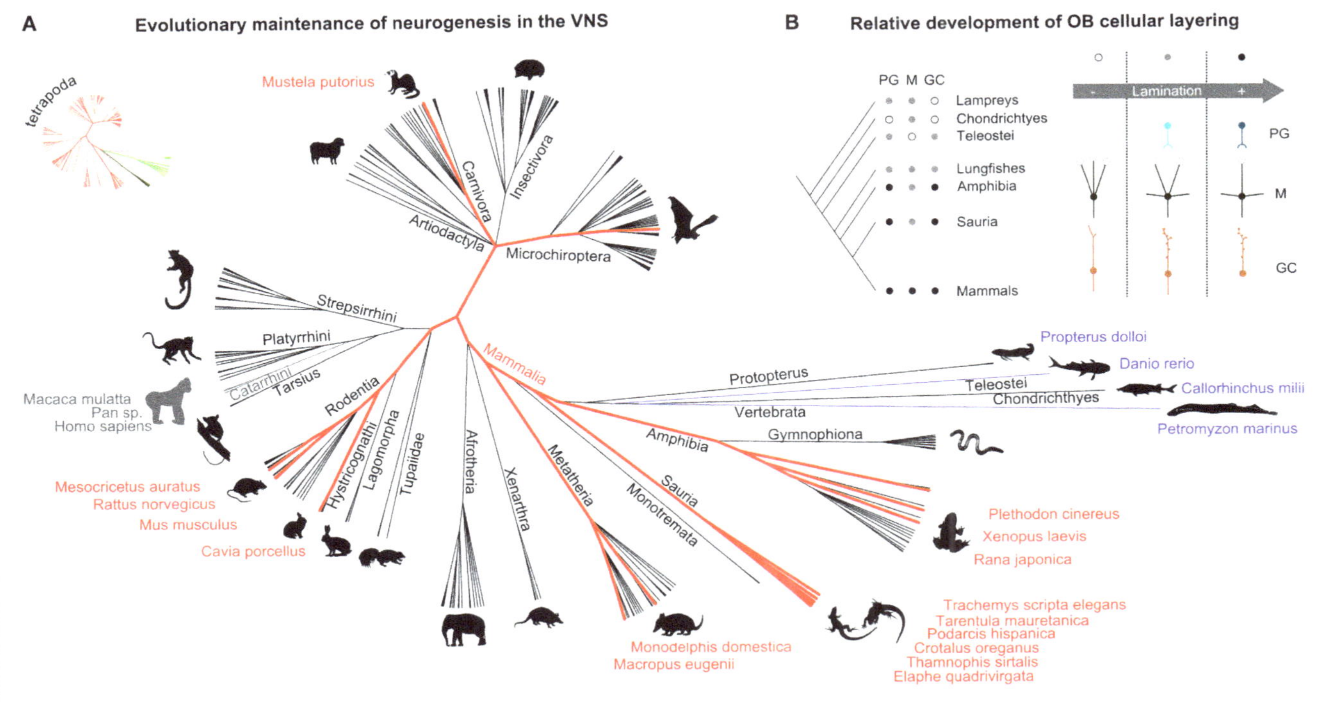

FIGURE 2 | Neuronal plasticity in the vomeronasal system is a conserved trait across several vertebrate species. The increased organizational complexity of the olfactory systems is plausibly related to their protracted development through postnatal neurogenesis. **(A)** Cladogram representing the main vertebrate taxa in which the presence of a vomeronasal system has been reported (black lines). Taxa indicated in blue possess the cellular and molecular elements of the VNS, without a defined structural organization. Old world monkeys are indicated in gray, as reference, although they generally do not possess a functional VNS. The species (and related taxa) in which neurogenesis in the VNS has been reported are highlighted in red. **(B)** Features of the vertebrate olfactory systems include: more defined cellular layering (white: low, gray: moderate, black: high lamination), presence of periglomerular cells, PG (white: absent, gray: ambiguous, black: present), development of mitral cell secondary dendrites, M (white: absent, only multiglomerular primary dendrites, gray: presence of both multiglomerular primary dendrites and secondary dendrites, black: monoglomerular primary dendrites and secondary dendrites), loss of granule cell axon, GC (white: smooth dendrites, axon, gray: spiny dendrites, axon, black: spiny dendrites, no axon). Sources: (Meisami and Bhatnagar, 1998; Eisthen, 2000; Halpern and Martinez-Marcos, 2003; Grus and Zhang, 2008; Eisthen and Polese, 2009; Mucignat-Caretta, 2010); NCBI.

reported to detect: V1Rs, activated preferentially by low molecular weight (LMW) hormone metabolites and other small molecules possibly contained in urine and bodily secretions; V2Rs, activated mainly by high molecular weight (HMW) peptidic compounds such as lipocalins, or smaller MHC peptides; formyl peptide receptors (FPRs), involved in the immune cell response to infections (Chamero et al., 2012; **Figure 1B**). V1R expressing neurons populate the apical portion of the sensory epithelium, V2Rs are located more basally while FPRs are more heterogeneously distributed (Rivière et al., 2009).

The earlier steps of VSNs differentiation are regulated by the proneural bHLH genes Mash1 and Neurogenin1, the former maintaining stem-cell progenitors, the second determining their multipotency (Cau et al., 2002), which is further regulated by the gene Ctip2 (Enomoto et al., 2011). Accordingly, loss of Ctip2 shifts the V1R/V2R differentiation ratio toward the V1R phenotype, suggesting a pivotal role in VSNs maturation and the possibility that the V2R-lineage entails both V1R and V2R committed neurons (Enomoto et al., 2011). The molecular mechanisms specifying the FPR lineage are not known.

VSNs proliferation is not homogeneous across the sensory epithelium but seems to be increasingly more localized at its margins, as development proceeds (Barber and Raisman, 1978; Giacobini et al., 2000; Martinez-Marcos et al., 2005; de la Rosa-Prieto et al., 2011). Although immature VSNs show limited migratory capabilities during adulthood (Martinez-Marcos et al., 2005; de la Rosa-Prieto et al., 2011), their proliferation increases until 2 months of age, in mice (Weiler, 2005; Brann and Firestein, 2010). Newborn VSNs are produced in clusters giving rise to patterned waves of migrating neurons (as observable by DCX immunohistochemistry). It would be interesting to clarify whether neurons expressing receptors of the same family are simultaneously generated at a given time. However, BrdU experiments suggested that both V1Rs and V2Rs are produced at the same pace in physiological conditions (de la Rosa-Prieto et al., 2010). Interestingly, postnatal development and growth seems to be present also in the non-sensory epithelium (NSE, **Figure 1B**) of the VNO (Garrosa et al., 1998; Elgayar et al., 2013).

Despite the vast number of MOE receptor genes (ca 1500 in the mouse) each OSN expresses only one of them. In the VNO this rule is not followed since each VSN may express more than one receptor gene (Martini et al., 2001; Silvotti et al., 2007; Ishii and Mombaerts, 2011). Interestingly, the phenotypic identity of newborn VSNs can be affected by histone modifications following application of urine ligands *in-vitro* (Xia et al., 2010). While application of HDAC inhibitors to cultured VSNs decreases the expression of immature neuronal marker Nestin, and increases the expression of markers of differentiation such as Map2, Neuro D1-D2, and V2R genes (Xia et al., 2010). It remains to be clarified whether these effects, represent a generalized adaptive response of the VNO epithelium to sensory stimulation or if it constitutes a mechanism to selectively specific subsets of newborn VSNs, as shown in the MOE (Watt et al., 2004; Dias and Ressler, 2013). Both simple parsimony and recent evidences suggest that this latter might be the case (Broad and Keverne, 2012). However, other factors such as odor exposure (Xia et al., 2006), hormonal changes (Kaba et al., 1988; Paternostro and Meisami, 1996) and sensory activity (Hovis et al., 2012) contribute to postnatal VNO neurogenesis and VNO-AOB rewiring indicating the persistence of constant adjustments in this circuit. Altogether these results strongly suggest that VNO neurogenesis do not serves mere tissue homeostasis and repair, but actively contributes to the functional tuning of the organ during postnatal development. A possibility still largely unexplored.

NEUROGENESIS IN THE ACCESSORY OLFACTORY BULB, A COMPARATIVE NOTE

Afferent axons from VSNs reach the brain at the level of the dorsal part of the OB. Here they form glomerular-like structures with the apical dendrites of a separate group of projection neurons which constitute the accessory olfactory bulb (AOB; **Figures 1A,C**). As for the MOB, their activity is regulated by inhibitory glomerular and granule cells (**Figure 1C**). Neurogenesis in the AOB involves mainly these two cell types (Oboti et al., 2009). Despite earlier doubts on its presence, several lines of evidence support the idea that adult neurogenesis represents a constitutive feature of the AOB. It can be found in adult mice of both genders (Oboti et al., 2009; Nunez-Parra et al., 2011), in adult rats (Peretto et al., 2001) and rabbits (personal observation). In addition, AOB neurogenesis has been reported not only in mammals (Altman and Das, 1966; Altman, 1969; Hinds, 1968a,b; Kaplan and Hinds, 1977; Bayer, 1983; Kaplan, 1985; Kishi, 1987), but also in other vertebrate species such as amphibians (Fritz et al., 1996), and reptiles (Garcia-Verdugo et al., 1989; Pérez-Cañellas and García-Verdugo, 1996; Pérez-Cañellas et al., 1997) indicating that it represents a conserved trait across different taxa (**Figure 2A**), rather than a parallel convergence. Neuronal plasticity in the olfactory system occurs independently of the presence of a discernible VNS, as in primates, fishes, cetaceans, and birds for example (García-Verdugo et al., 2002; Mucignat-Caretta, 2010); **Figure 2A**). In addition, taxa in which some of the typical cellular and molecular elements of the VNS are present, although with different levels of organization (as anurans, lungfishes, sea lampreys, teleosts, and cartilaginous fishes; Eisthen and Wyatt, 2006; **Figure 2A**), retain neuronal plasticity and neurogenesis in the primary olfactory structures during post-hatching and more mature stages. This indicates that a plastic VNS may not be an apomorphic (underived) trait of terrestrial vertebrates (**Figure 2A**; **Table 1**). In bat species, even though the VNS is not always developed, the presence of immature neurons typically expressing doublecortin (DCX) has been noted in the AOB (Amrein I., personal communication).

In mice, rats, rabbits and guinea pigs SVZ neuronal progenitors give rise to neuroblasts integrating in the AOB mainly as granule cells localized in the inner granule cell layer, below the lateral olfactory tract. The presence of newborn neurons in periglomerular layer is very limited, possibly reflecting a much slower turn-over rate of PGs (Martínez-Marcos et al., 2001; Peretto et al., 2001; Oboti et al., 2009; Nunez-Parra et al., 2011). A limited number of cells can be found in the plexiform layer between the GC and PG layers, where principal cells (PC) are located (Oboti et al., 2009; PCs are homologous to MOB mitral cells), possibly representing other cell types such as external granule cells and dwarf cells (Larriva-Sahd, 2008). The increasing importance of local interneurons for OB signal elaboration, reflected by the increased complexity in OB structural lamination (Eisthen and Polese, 2009; **Figure 2B**), implies a possible correlation with the maintenance of their turnover. Overall, OB neurogenesis may represent a necessary and conserved feature of the olfactory pathways, reminiscent of the higher neuronal plasticity showed by the paleocortex, to which it belongs (see **Table 1** for a list of representative studies explicitly focused on VNO or AOB postnatal development and neurogenesis). In the following paragraphs, attention will be given to the anatomy of the AOB, the phenotypes of AOB newborn cells and the possible role in its circuitry considering the present knowledge about its role in the VNS.

NEUROGENESIS IN THE TWO ACCESSORY OLFACTORY BULB SUBREGIONS

Both the glomerular and principal cell (PC) layer of the AOB look clearly partitioned by the segregated V1R/Gai2 and V2R/Gao afferent fibers. Axonal projections from these two neuronal populations establish synaptic contact with either the anterior (aAOB) or posterior (pAOB) AOB, respectively. This separation is visible in the PC layer neuropil (*linea alba*, Larriva-Sahd, 2008). In rodents the V1R and V2R pathways have been shown to selectively respond to low molecular weight organic molecules (Leinders-Zufall et al., 2000; Sugai et al., 2006) and high molecular weight compounds of peptidic nature, respectively (Leinders-Zufall et al., 2004, 2009; Kimoto et al., 2005). Accordingly to this functional dichotomy, differences in c-Fos expression patterns in the two AOB regions have been observed after exposure to gender related odors in male and female mice (Kumar et al., 1999; Halem et al., 2001). Interestingly, in mice and rats (Peretto et al., 2001; Oboti et al., 2009, but not in opossums Martínez-Marcos et al., 2001), newborn cells reaching the AOB in physiological conditions (no odor exposures) seem to be unequally distributed along the rostro-caudal axis. This may reflect a differential rate of development of the two AOB sub-regions or alternatively be related to the V1R/V2R functions being subjected to differential adaptive pressures in a given eco-ethological niche (Suárez et al., 2011a,b). Accordingly, recently a dual embryonic origin of the AOB has been proposed (Huilgol et al., 2013). In this study, Huilgol and coauthors showed that PCs in the pAOB derive from the thalamic eminences at the diencephalic/telencephalic boundary (DTB) from Lhx5 expressing neurons, as part of the amygdala,

Table 1 | List of representative studies explicitly focused on VNO and AOB neurogenesis.

Species	VNO	AOB
Mouse (*Mus musculus*)	Barber and Raisman, 1978 Monti-Graziadei, 1992 Cappello et al., 1999 Giacobini et al., 2000 Weiler, 2005 Martinez-Marcos et al., 2005 Murdoch and Roskams, 2008 Brann and Firestein, 2010 Enomoto et al., 2011	Hinds, 1968a,b Bonfanti et al., 1997 Oboti et al., 2009–2011 Veyrac and Bakker, 2011 Sakamoto et al., 2011 Nunez-Parra et al., 2011
Rat (*Rattus norvegicus*)	Monti-Graziadei, 1992 Weiler et al., 1999a–2005 Inamura et al., 2000 Martínez-Marcos et al., 2000 Matsuoka et al., 2002	Altman and Das, 1966 Altman, 1969 Kaplan and Hinds, 1977 Kishi, 1987 Bayer, 1983 Peretto et al., 2001 Corona et al., 2011 Portillo et al., 2012
Rabbit (*Oryctolagus cuniculus*)	Othman, 2011	Personal observation
Guinea pig (*Cavia porcellus*)		Personal observation
Hamster (*Mesocricetus auratus*)	Ichikawa et al., 1998 Taniguchi and Taniguchi, 2008	Huang and Bittman, 2002
Opossum (*Monodelphis domestica*)	Jia and Halpern, 1998	Shapiro et al., 1997
	Shapiro et al., 1997	Martínez-Marcos et al., 2001
Wallaby (*Macropus eugenii*)	Ashwell et al., 2008	Ashwell et al., 2008
Ferret (*Mustela putorius furo*)	Weiler et al., 1999b	
Bat (various spp.)		Amrein et al., 2007 (OB)
Garter snake (*Tamnophis sirtalis*)	Wang and Halpern, 1982	
Striped snake (*Elaphe quadrivirgata*)	Kondoh et al., 2012	
Wall lizard (Podarcis hispanica)		Garcia-Verdugo et al., 1989 Sampedro et al., 2008 Font et al., 2012
Red-eared slider (*Trachemys scripta elegans*)		Pérez-Cañellas et al., 1997
Gecko (*Tarentola mauritanica*)		Pérez-Cañellas and García-Verdugo, 1996
Clawed frog (*Xenopus laevis*)		
No	Hansen et al., 1998 Higgs and Burd, 2001	Fritz et al., 1996
Yes	Endo et al., 2011	
Salamander (*Plethodon cinereus*)	Dawley et al., 2000	
	Dawley and Crowder, 1995	
Japanese brown frog (*Rana japonica*)	Taniguchi et al., 1996	
Zebra fish (Danio rerio)		Byrd and Brunjes, 2001 *(OB)* Adolf et al., 2006 (OB)

Species in which neurogenesis in the VNS components of the olfactory system could be present are indicated italics.

BST and Cajal-Retzius neurons (Huilgol et al., 2013), while the aAOB PCs share common origin with MOB mitral cells, as indicated by Tbx21 expression in the OB primordium (Huilgol et al., 2013). The DTB is evolutionary conserved in amphibians and mammals indicating that the pAOB may be a residue of the earliest sensory systems originating from the thalamic eminences and controlling olfactory responses in amphibians (Krug et al., 1993; Huilgol et al., 2013). However, the apparent morphology of AOB granule cell layer does not reveal a similar dichotomy, as AOB granule cells connectivity may be more ambiguous (Larriva-Sahd, 2008). Despite the different origin of pAOB projection neurons, immature GABAergic interneurons of both the aAOB and pAOB may include cells derived from the same Dlx2/5/6, Emx1, and Meis2 lineages in the SVZ (Kohwi et al., 2007; Agoston et al., 2013). Overall this suggests the existence of different regulatory mechanisms locally specifying the phenotype of cells belonging to the same neuronal lineage but integrating in different circuits (aAOB vs. pAOB, but also AOB vs. MOB). Further understanding of the underlying mechanisms would extend our knowledge of the morphological and functional adaptations newborn neurons may be capable of. In addition, given the functional segregation of the VNS circuits (V1R-aAOB, V2R-pAOB), different levels of neuronal plasticity and neurogenesis may reflect a different degree of adaptability to the diversity of chemical stimuli each subsystem elaborates. However, despite the differences these features may have a similar functional relevance for their proper function.

PHENOTYPES OF NEWBORN NEURONS IN THE ACCESSORY OLFACTORY BULB

New neurons migrating from the SVZ through the rostral migratory stream, reach all AOB layers: glomerular (Gl), external (ECL), and internal (ICL) cellular layers (Larriva-Sahd, 2008). At present no detailed analysis has been made to identify these cell types. Moreover, the presence in the MOB of newly generated tbr2-derived glutamatergic cells (Brill et al., 2009) and GABAergic-serotonergic (Inta et al., 2008) interneurons has been recently proven, while in the AOB it remains to be verified.

In the MOB, the cell types forming the glomerulus (juxtaglomerular cells) are classified in periglomerular (PG), short axon (SA) and external tufted (ET) cells, based on their neurochemistry, morphology, and connectivity. Juxtaglomerular cells can be divided in two main GABAergic chemotypes based on the expression of different isoforms of the GABA synthesis enzyme—GAD-65, GAD-67—together with other markers such as dopamine (DA), or its synthesis enzyme tyrosine hydroxylase (TH), calbindin, calretinin, and others (Shipley et al., 2004). Virtually all dopaminergic neurons express GAD-67, while little if no overlap is present between the GAD-65 and the TH sub-populations (Kiyokage et al., 2010). As typical SA cells, TH-GAD-67 neurons innervate multiple glomeruli while GAD-65 neurons are mostly monoglomerular with only few secondary processes directed to other glomerular formations (Aungst et al., 2003; Kiyokage et al., 2010).

In the AOB glomerular layer scarce if not absent GAD-67 staining has been reported together with almost complete lack of TH expression (Mugnaini et al., 1984; Oboti et al., 2009). This possibly indicates a predominance in the AOB of the monoglomerular GAD-65 chemotype. However, newly generated cells with morphological features of both PG uniglomerular cells and SA multiglomerular cells have been identified in the AOB (Oboti et al., 2009) suggesting that the low levels of GAD-67 expression do not necessarily imply the absence of SA-like cells (Mugnaini et al., 1984; Larriva-Sahd, 2008).

In the MOB, dopaminergic PG cells are responsible of thresholding mitral cell firing in response to olfactory inputs (Pírez and Wachowiak, 2008). The lack of dopaminergic signaling in the AOB may imply a minor need for gain control of vomeronasal inputs on PCs being their firing threshold possibly determined by input coincidence from heterotypical glomerular afferents (Meeks et al., 2010).

Other inhibitory cells located more deeply in the AOB are external and internal granule cells, located above and below the lateral olfactory tract (LOT), respectively. Evidence showed the vast majority of newborn cells reaching the AOB is represented by internal granule cells (Oboti et al., 2009; Nunez-Parra et al., 2011). In the ICL main accessory cells are also present (MACs, Larriva-Sahd, 2008) and are distinguishable from granule cells by larger soma and nuclear size and by their sporadic presence in the LOT. Although newborn cells can be often found in the LOT, their nuclear size was always comparable to normal granule cells (external granule cells, in this case), thus limiting the likelihood for MACs to be regenerated during adulthood.

Recently, in the rat MOB the presence of newborn neurons in the external plexiform layer (EPL) has been proved (Yang, 2008). These neurons have been reported to be PV/CR expressing Van Gehuchten cells, multipolar cells and superficial SA cells (Yang, 2008). Since DCX- and BrdU-positive cells can be found in homologous locations in the AOB (ECL), the presence here of these cell types is possible but yet to be investigated.

It is not known whether SVZ-derived interneurons migrating to the AOB belong to the same lineage of those in the MOB. It is possible that genetically distinct populations of interneurons are heterogeneously distributed in the two OB sub-regions. Recently, viral fate-mapping experiments revealed the mosaic nature of the SVZ proliferative domains giving rise to different and heterogeneous pools of GABAergic interneurons (Merkle et al., 2007). However, upon inspection of the material used in this study, no apparent regionalization of either aAOB- or pAOB-committed progenitors was found (viral infected GFP+ cells were found in the AOB of mice injected at all SVZ levels, personal observation). Interestingly, although most of newborn AOB neurons labeled with BrdU coexpress NeuN at 4 weeks of age (80%) as in the MOB, the level of coexpression with other interneuronal markers is much lower (BrdU/GABA, BrDU/GAD-67, and BrdU/calretinin reach only about the 30%; Oboti et al., 2009) (MOB: BrdU/GAD67 is about 80% in the GrL and 30% in the GL; Parrish-Aungst et al., 2007). These results indicate that the phenotype of AOB newborn neurons is similar to the MOB but conserve some peculiarities specified either locally or in the SVZ. The different relative abundance of morpho- and chemo-types in this structure, renders the AOB an interesting circuit to study the differential role of a given cell type in different compartments of the bulbar circuitry. For example by studying PC (AOB mitral cell homolog) electrical responses to peripheral nerve stimulations it would be possible to clarify to which extent SA cells in the AOB may be dispensable—in case of their limited presence in this structure—for a certain olfactory coding task, or—by comparison—which specific function do they serve when present in other bulbar circuits.

SENSORY ACTIVITY-DEPENDENT SURVIVAL AND FUNCTION OF NEWBORN CELLS

As shown by olfactory enrichment or deprivation studies, the maturation and survival of newborn neurons in the MOB depends on sensory inputs (Cummings et al., 1997; Rochefort et al., 2002; Mandairon et al., 2006). Newborn neurons reach the MOB in massive waves but are gradually selected during integration into local circuits (Petreanu and Alvarez-Buylla, 2002) activated by sensory inputs (Magavi et al., 2005; Mouret et al., 2008; Sultan et al., 2011a,b). Importantly, loss or ablation of newborn neurons in the MOB can impair olfactory function (Breton-Provencher et al., 2009; Mandairon et al., 2011) since younger cells are preferentially involved in these circuits (Nissant et al., 2009; Alonso et al., 2012).

Although renewing at a slower rate (Oboti et al., 2009), newborn cells in the AOB are likely to similarly contribute to VNS function. As in the MOB, sensory activity increases the survival of newborn neurons in the AOB (Oboti et al., 2009, 2011; Nunez-Parra et al., 2011). This effect is mediated by chemical cues present in urine or bodily secretions (Nunez-Parra et al., 2011; Oboti et al., 2011), it is abolished after VNO genetic functional ablation in trpc2-ko mice (Oboti et al., 2011), it is persisting until 7 months of age (Nunez-Parra et al., 2011), and gives rise to neurons responding preferentially to experienced odor stimuli (Oboti et al., 2011).

The presence of gender related differences in AOB neurogenesis is controversial (no differences in CD1 mice Oboti et al., 2009, 2011; differences in B6 mice, Nunez-Parra et al., 2011). However, the effect of odor experience on AOB neurogenesis seems to be particularly evident in post-pubertal female mice after male odor stimulation (Oboti et al., 2009, 2011; Nunez-Parra et al., 2011). This seems particularly evident in the aAOB upon chronic exposure to low molecular weight (LMW) chemical cues present in male urine, which are mainly detected by the V1R neurons (Oboti et al., 2011). Larger protein compounds sensed through V2Rs are instead ineffective on neuronal survival in neither of the two AOB regions (Oboti et al., 2011). However, a lack of increase in surviving cells after sensory enrichment does not necessarily imply the absence of a sensory dependent functional recruitment of newborn elements, but only that the net amount of surviving cells remains stable. Considering that social odors are important primers on mice development and reproductive behavior, these findings suggest a possible role of AOB postnatal/adult neurogenesis in sensory processing in both genders. Accordingly, eliminating newborn cells in the whole bulb, AOB included, Sakamoto and colleagues showed for the first time an impairment in olfactory functions involving the VNS such as predator-odor avoidance, aggression and mounting in males (Sakamoto et al., 2011). A finding that has been extended to VNO-dependent mate recognition in females (Oboti et al., 2011). The effect of sensory inputs on AOB neurogenesis overall indicates that newborn neurons play an active and possibly relevant role on the vomeronasal circuitry during postnatal and adult life.

IMPACT OF NEWBORN NEURONS ON AOB CIRCUITS

A few comparative considerations with the MOB elementary functional unit—the olfactory column—can be insightful in defining the impact of newborn neurons on AOB network activity. The MOB olfactory column is considered equivalent to the cortical columns and barrels in the visual and somatosensory cortices (Shepherd, 2010). It comprises all OSNs projecting to a single glomerulus, all the mitral and tufted cells extending their dendrites to it and all the granule cells connected to these projection neurons. Granule cells can regulate mitral/tufted cell output providing self inhibition through dendrodendritic synapses on mitral cell lateral dendrites within the same column. In addition, they may exert lateral inhibition on adjacent columns by shunting the propagation of action potentials on distal lateral dendrites of extra-columnar mitral cells (Xiong and Chen, 2002). This implies a dual role of granule cells on mitral/tufted cell firing: through self-inhibition within the same column, granule cells may act synchronizing the firing rate of projection neurons belonging to different units while responding to the same sensory input (Dhawale et al., 2010); through lateral inhibition on extracolumnar mitral cells, granule cells may provide contrast enhancement between two different functional units (as other amacrine—axonless—cells in the retina for instance; Migliore and Shepherd, 2008). Both effects have been hypothesized to be relevant for olfactory discrimination (Migliore and Shepherd, 2008; Dhawale et al., 2010; see Lepousez et al., 2013 for a detailed review on this hypothesis). Given the apparent lack of columnar organization in the piriform cortex, this topological motif in the bulbar circuitry probably reflects its cortical like function and represents the modular unit encoding the diversity of olfactory inputs (Haberly, 2001; Migliore et al., 2007). Importantly, the constant re-adjustment of the synaptic inputs caused by renewal of both local interneurons and olfactory fibers has been associated with an optimization of this function (Alonso et al., 2006; Jones et al., 2008; Adam and Mizrahi, 2011).

The AOB appears structurally similar to the MOB, although it retains some peculiar features in both hodology and cell types. However, the occurrence of similar plastic events in both structures motivates the same reasoning done for the MOB. Olfactory glomeruli in the AOB are on average smaller than those in the MOB and appear to be clustered in pseudostratified formations. Contrarily to MOB glomeruli, they receive multiple inputs from different types of VSNs (Takami and Graziadei, 1991; Belluscio et al., 1999; Del Punta et al., 2002), with V1Rs projecting only to the aAOB and V2Rs to the pAOB. In addition, neurons expressing the same receptor/s in the VNO, may project to up to 20–30 different glomeruli (Belluscio et al., 1999), while same-receptor OSNs in the MOE project mainly to two symmetrical glomeruli in the MOB. This conserved pattern seems to underlie a higher degree of input convergence on MOB projection neurons and therefore functional specialization of each olfactory column in the MOB (Hildebrand and Shepherd, 1997; Su et al., 2009; Touhara and Vosshall, 2009) as mitral cells project to a single glomerulus, therefore receiving afferents from OSNs expressing the same receptor. Conversely, AOB PCs reach multiple glomeruli receiving inputs from different VSNs (a feature shared with the OB of fishes: Ngai et al., 1993; Speca et al., 1999). However, AOB projection neurons maintain V1R/V2R segregated apical dendritic arborizations depending on their location in the aAOB and pAOB

(Jia and Halpern, 1997). Nonetheless, a cross talk may exist between aAOB and pAOB principal cells via thinner lateral dendrites crossing the midline (Larriva-Sahd, 2008). As a result of their heterotypic connectivity, AOB PCs integrate inputs from different receptor types in the VNO and therefore different ligands. Slice recordings on *ex-vivo* VNO-AOB intact preparation showed that this is indeed the case (Meeks et al., 2010). Juxtaglomerular complexes in the AOB resemble the functional triads described in the MOB: PG and SA cells have inter- and intra-glomerular projections, external tufted cells contact a single glomerulus.

The limited extent by which AOB PGs are regenerated by SVZ-derived progenitors, together with the above mentioned lack of TH, could be explained by the lack of TH/GAD-67 cells in the AOB. Alternatively, since TH expression levels in PGs are traditionally used as a proxy for olfactory input (Nadi et al., 1981; Baker et al., 1983; Cho et al., 1996) and VNO activity is subordinated to initial odor detection by the MOE (Xu et al., 2005; Slotnick et al., 2010), the lack of TH and GAD-67 in the AOB could be just a consequence of the irregular nature of vomeronasal inputs. The expression patterns of other activity markers (such as cytochrome-c-oxydase or β-secretase-1) in the AOB glomerular layer resemble those in the MOB during sensory deprivation and therefore could support this hypothesis (Yan et al., 2007; He et al., 2014).

Conversely, granule cells in the AOB are the most represented cell type among newly generated neurons (Oboti et al., 2009; Nunez-Parra et al., 2011). They are typically located in the deep ICL (below the LOT) but also in the deeper portion of the ECL and in the LOT, just below PC somata. They project to PC dendrites belonging to the homologous region (aAOB or pAOB), but considering that PC axon collaterals cross repeatedly the two sub-regions, they could receive synaptic inputs from both. In addition their apical dendrites seem to reach the glomerular layer (Larriva-Sahd, 2008), although it is not clear whether they interact synaptically with the juxtaglomerular complex. Interestingly, while EGC dendritic processes appose on PC somata or proximal dendrites, those from IGC seem to localize preferentially on distal and apical processes, between glomeruli and PC somata (Larriva-Sahd, 2008), a feature confirmed by EM studies (Moriya-Ito et al., 2013). This distinction may imply a bias for AOB IGCs toward PC self-inhibition, instead of intercolumnar lateral inhibition. Eventually, since the vast majority of newly generated cells in the adult AOB are IGC, it is appealing to imagine neurogenesis in the AOB as a mechanism to shunt directly input signals from the VNO. Given the variable turnover rate of IGCs during postnatal development, this feature alone would be sufficient to justify changes in the response to vomeronasal sensory cues over time. In addition, given that both the survival and activation of newborn neurons is actively driven by vomeronasal sensory inputs, this selective shunting may contribute to encode stimulus familiarity. In general, a change in IGC turnover rate, together with other physiological changes, may set the timing for certain stimuli to be more or less effective as social signals or endocrine modulators (e.g., effect of male urine odors on female estrous varying depending on kinship or shared fostering). Ultimately, this could represent a possible answer to the question posed by the title of this manuscript.

Overall these observations suggest that newly generated GABAergic interneurons differently contribute to mature AOB circuits, if compared to the MOB. The different nature of GABAergic modulation of AOB output signals is further supported by the firing of AOB PCs, which appears to be longer sustained, if compared to MOB mitral cells (Meeks et al., 2010; Shpak et al., 2012). In addition, given PC heterogeneous glomerular connectivity and the convergence of their centripetal projections to more central targets (Salazar and Brennan, 2001), the information conveyed by their output signals is also different, and probably more complex. As a direct consequence and in the whole system perspective, the impact newborn IGCs have on PC output activity may definitely be higher than that of granule interneurons on MOB mitral cells.

CONCLUSIONS

Overall the considerations made in this manuscript are meant to underline that the VNS is not only constitutively plastic but also that this plasticity may constitute the basis for its peculiar function. Eventually the VNS circuitry cannot be considered hardwired but rather able to adjust its connectivity to environmental changes. If the function of the VNS described so far (see for critical views on this point Eisthen and Wyatt, 2006; Mucignat-Caretta et al., 2012) is the result of the interaction between plastic circuits and environmental stimuli, is definitely not known and certainly deserves further investigation. Plausibly neuronal plasticity and neurogenesis are indeed necessary to shape it and maintain it throughout postnatal life. Eventually different rates of neurogenesis can determine the extent by which VNS circuits adapt and tune to a given chemical environment, being it referred to social, reproductive, or aggressive/territorial behaviors. Even though the VNS is not simply the *pheromone-detector* in the nasal cavity of mammals or other vertebrates (Eisthen and Wyatt, 2006), it would be a challenge of future studies to test the impact of neuronal plasticity and neurogenesis on those functions, commonly associated to *pheromone* sensing. Indeed studying the molecular and genetic mechanisms underlying the neuroendocrine physiology of sociality may yield insights on the etiology of associated anomalies, even in those mammalian species, human included, in which this sensory pathway is not present. For this reason the rodent VNS may represent the unique opportunity to dissect this issue in an animal model in which these features strongly rely on its functional integrity and—plausibly—its capability of cell renewal through adult neurogenesis.

ACKNOWLEDGMENTS

We would like to thank Arturo Alvarez-Buylla for sending part of the tissues used for the viral fate-mapping analysis of the SVZ-OB and Carla Mucignat-Caretta, Jan Weiss, Martina Pyrski, and Roberto Tirindelli for their constructive comments on the manuscript.

REFERENCES

Adam, Y., and Mizrahi, A. (2011). Long-term imaging reveals dynamic changes in the neuronal composition of the glomerular layer. *J. Neurosci.* 31, 7967–7973. doi: 10.1523/JNEUROSCI.0782-11.2011

Adolf, B., Chapouton, P., Lam, C. S., Topp, S., Tannhäuser, B., Strähle, U., et al. (2006). Conserved and acquired features of adult neurogenesis in the zebrafish telencephalon. *Dev. biology*, 295, 278–293. doi: 10.1016/j.ydbio.2006.03.023

Agoston, Z., Heine, P., Brill, M. S., Grebbin, B. M., Hau, A.-C., Kallenborn-Gerhardt, W., et al. (2013). Meis2 is a Pax6 co-factor in neurogenesis and dopaminergic periglomerular fate specification in the adult olfactory bulb. *Development* 141, 28–38. doi: 10.1242/dev.097295

Alonso, M., Lepousez, G., Sebastien, W., Bardy, C., Gabellec, M.-M., Torquet, N., et al. (2012). Activation of adult-born neurons facilitates learning and memory. *Nat. Neurosci.* 15, 897–904. doi: 10.1038/nn.3108

Alonso, M., Viollet, C., Gabellec, M.-M., Meas-Yedid, V., Olivo-Marin, J.-C., and Lledo, P.-M. (2006). Olfactory discrimination learning increases the survival of adult-born neurons in the olfactory bulb. *J. Neurosci.* 26, 10508–10513. doi: 10.1523/JNEUROSCI.2633-06.2006

Altman, J. (1969). Autoradiographic and histological studies of postnatal neurogenesis. IV. Cell proliferation and migration in the anterior forebrain, with special reference to persisting neurogenesis in the olfactory bulb. *J. Comp. Neurol.* 137, 433–457. doi: 10.1002/cne.901370404

Altman, J., and Das, G. D. (1966). Autoradiographic and histological studies of postnatal neurogenesis. I. A longitudinal investigation of the kinetics, migration and transformation of cells incorporating tritiated thymidine in neonate rats, with special reference to postnatal neurogenesis. *J. Comp. Neurol.* 126, 337–389. doi: 10.1002/cne.901260302

Alvarez-Buylla, A., and Garcia-Verdugo, J. M. (2002). Neurogenesis in adult subventricular zone. *J. Neurosci.* 22, 629–634.

Amrein, I., Dechmann, D. K. N., Winter, Y., and Lipp, H.-P. (2007). Absent or low rate of adult neurogenesis in the hippocampus of bats (Chiroptera). *PLoS ONE*, 2:e455. doi: 10.1371/journal.pone.0000455

Ashwell, K. W. S., Marotte, L. R., and Cheng, G. (2008). Development of the olfactory system in a wallaby (*Macropus eugenii*). *Brain Behav. Evol.* 71, 216–230. doi: 10.1159/000119711

Aungst, J. L., Heyward, P. M., Puche, A. C., Karnup, S. V., Hayar, A., Szabo, G., et al. (2003). Centre-surround inhibition among olfactory bulb glomeruli. *Nature* 426, 623–629. doi: 10.1038/nature02185

Baker, H., Kawano, T., Margolis, F. L., and Joh, T. H. (1983). Transneuronal regulation of tyrosine hydroxylase expression in olfactory bulb of mouse and rat. *J. Neurosci.* 3, 69–78.

Barber, P. C., and Raisman, G. (1978). Cell division in the vomeronasal organ of the adult mouse. *Brain Res.* 141, 57–66. doi: 10.1016/0006-8993(78)90616-9

Bayer, S. A. (1983). 3H-thymidine-radiographic studies of neurogenesis in the rat olfactory bulb. *Exp. Brain Res.* 50, 329–340. doi: 10.1007/BF00239197

Belarbi, K., and Rosi, S. (2013). Modulation of adult-born neurons in the inflamed hippocampus. *Front. Cell. Neurosci.* 7:145. doi: 10.3389/fncel.2013.00145

Belluscio, L., Koentges, G., Axel, R., and Dulac, C. (1999). A map of pheromone receptor activation in the mammalian brain. *Cell* 97, 209–220. doi: 10.1016/S0092-8674(00)80731-X

Bonfanti, L., and Peretto, P. (2011). Adult neurogenesis in mammals–a theme with many variations. *Eur. J. Neurosci.* 34, 930–950. doi: 10.1111/j.1460-9568.2011.07832.x

Bonfanti, L., Peretto, P., Merighi, A., and Fasolo, A. (1997). Newly-generated cells from the rostral migratory stream in the accessory olfactory bulb of the adult rat. *Neuroscience* 81, 489–502. doi: 10.1016/S0306-4522(97)00090-0

Brann, J. H., and Firestein, S. (2010). Regeneration of new neurons is preserved in aged vomeronasal epithelia. *J. Neurosci.* 30, 15686–15694. doi: 10.1523/JNEUROSCI.4316-10.2010

Breton-Provencher, V., Lemasson, M., Peralta, M. R., and Saghatelyan, A. (2009). Interneurons produced in adulthood are required for the normal functioning of the olfactory bulb network and for the execution of selected olfactory behaviors. *J. Neurosci.* 29, 15245–15257. doi: 10.1523/JNEUROSCI.3606-09.2009

Brill, M. S., Ninkovic, J., Winpenny, E., Hodge, R. D., Ozen, I., Yang, R., et al. (2009). Adult generation of glutamatergic olfactory bulb interneurons. *Nat. Neurosci.* 12, 1524–1533. doi: 10.1038/nn.2416

Broad, K. D., and Keverne, E. B. (2012). The post-natal chemosensory environment induces epigenetic changes in vomeronasal receptor gene expression and a bias in olfactory preference. *Behav. Genet.* 42, 461–471. doi: 10.1007/s10519-011-9523-9

Buffo, A., Rite, I., Tripathi, P., Lepier, A., Colak, D., Horn, A.-P., et al. (2008). Origin and progeny of reactive gliosis: a source of multipotent cells in the injured brain. *Proc. Natl. Acad. Sci. U.S.A.* 105, 3581–3586. doi: 10.1073/pnas.0709002105

Byrd, C. A., and Brunjes, P. C. (2001). Neurogenesis in the olfactory bulb of adult zebrafish. *Neuroscience* 105, 793–801. doi: 10.1016/S0306-4522(01)00215-9

Cappello, P., Tarozzo, G., Benedetto, A., and Fasolo, A. (1999). Proliferation and apoptosis in the mouse vomeronasal organ during ontogeny. *Neurosci. Lett.* 266, 37–40. doi: 10.1016/S0304-3940(99)00262-1

Cau, E., Casarosa, S., and Guillemot, F. (2002). Mash1 and Ngn1 control distinct steps of determination and differentiation in the olfactory sensory neuron lineage. *Development* 129, 1871–1880.

Chamero, P., Leinders-Zufall, T., and Zufall, F. (2012). From genes to social communication: molecular sensing by the vomeronasal organ. *Trends Neurosci.* 35, 597–606. doi: 10.1016/j.tins.2012.04.011

Cho, J. Y., Min, N., Franzen, L., and Baker, H. (1996). Rapid down-regulation of tyrosine hydroxylase expression in the olfactory bulb of naris-occluded adult rats. *J. Comp. Neurol.* 369, 264–276. doi: 10.1002/(SICI)1096-9861(19960527)369:2<264::AID-CNE7>3.0.CO;2-1

Coppola, D. M., and O'Connell, R. J. (1989). Stimulus access to olfactory and vomeronasal receptors *in utero*. *Neurosci. Lett.* 106, 241–248. doi: 10.1016/0304-3940(89)90170-5

Corona, R., Larriva-Sahd, J., and Paredes, R. G. (2011). Paced-mating increases the number of adult new born cells in the internal cellular (granular) layer of the accessory olfactory bulb. *PLoS ONE* 6:e19380. doi: 10.1371/journal.pone.0019380

Cummings, D. M., Henning, H. E., and Brunjes, P. C. (1997). Olfactory bulb recovery after early sensory deprivation. *J. Neurosci.* 17, 7433–7440.

Dawley, E. M., and Crowder, J. (1995). Sexual and seasonal differences in the vomeronasal epithelium of the red-backed salamander (*Plethodon cinereus*). *J. Comp. Neurol.* 359, 382–390. doi: 10.1002/cne.903590303

Dawley, E. M., Fingerlin, A., Hwang, D., John, S. S., and Stankiewicz, C. A. (2000). Seasonal cell proliferation in the chemosensory epithelium and brain of red-backed salamanders, *Plethodon cinereus*. *Brain Behav. Evol.* 56, 1–13. doi: 10.1159/000006673

Dawson, M. R. L., Polito, A., Levine, J. M., and Reynolds, R. (2003). NG2-expressing glial progenitor cells: an abundant and widespread population of cycling cells in the adult rat CNS. *Mol. Cell. Neurosci.* 24, 476–488. doi: 10.1016/S1044-7431(03)00210-0

de la Rosa-Prieto, C., Saiz-Sanchez, D., Ubeda-Bañon, I., Argandoña-Palacios, L., Garcia-Muñozguren, S., and Martinez-Marcos, A. (2010). Neurogenesis in subclasses of vomeronasal sensory neurons in adult mice. *Dev. Neurobiol.* 70, 961–970. doi: 10.1002/dneu.20838

de la Rosa-Prieto, C., Saiz-Sánchez, D., Úbeda-Bañón, I., Mohedano-Moriano, A., and Martínez-Marcos, A. (2011). Maturation of newly born vomeronasal neurons in the adult mice. *Neuroreport* 22, 28–32. doi: 10.1097/WNR.0b013e328341fb66

Del Punta, K., Puche, A., Adams, N. C., Rodriguez, I., and Mombaerts, P. (2002). A divergent pattern of sensory axonal projections is rendered convergent by second-order neurons in the accessory olfactory bulb. *Neuron* 35, 1057–1066. doi: 10.1016/S0896-6273(02)00904-2

Dhawale, A. K., Hagiwara, A., Bhalla, U. S., Murthy, V. N., and Albeanu, D. F. (2010). Non-redundant odor coding by sister mitral cells revealed by light addressable glomeruli in the mouse. *Nat. Neurosci.* 13, 1404–1412. doi: 10.1038/nn.2673

Dias, B. G., and Ressler, K. J. (2013). Parental olfactory experience influences behavior and neural structure in subsequent generations. *Nat. Neurosci.* 17, 89–96. doi: 10.1038/nn.3594

Doetsch, F., García-Verdugo, J. M., and Alvarez-Buylla, A. (1999). Regeneration of a germinal layer in the adult mammalian brain. *Proc. Natl. Acad. Sci. U.S.A.* 96, 11619–11624. doi: 10.1073/pnas.96.20.11619

Eisthen, H. L. (2000). Presence of the vomeronasal system in acquatic salamanders. *Philos. Trans. R. Soc. Lond. B Biol. Sci.* 355, 1209–1213. doi: 10.1098/rstb.2000.0669

Eisthen, H. L., and Polese, G. (2009). "Evolution of the vertebrate olfactory subsystems," in *Evolutionary Neuroscience*, ed J. H. Kaas (Boston, MA: Academic Press), 447–492.

Eisthen, H. L., and Wyatt, T. D. (2006). The vomeronasal system and pheromones. *Curr. Biol.* 16, R73–R74. doi: 10.1016/j.cub.2006.01.038

Elgayar, S. A. M., Eltony, S. A., and Othman, M. A. (2013). Morphology of non-sensory epithelium during post-natal development of the rabbit vomeronasal organ. *Anat. Histol. Embryol.* doi: 10.1111/ahe.12073. [Epub ahead of print].

Endo, D., Yamamoto, Y., Nakamuta, N., and Taniguchi, K. (2011). Developmental changes in lectin-binding patterns of three nasal sensory epithelia in *Xenopus laevis*. *Anat. Rec.* 294, 839–846. doi: 10.1002/ar.21377

Enomoto, T., Ohmoto, M., Iwata, T., Uno, A., Saitou, M., Yamaguchi, T., et al. (2011). Bcl11b/Ctip2 controls the differentiation of vomeronasal sensory neurons in mice. *J. Neurosci.* 31, 10159–10173. doi: 10.1523/JNEUROSCI.1245-11.2011

Enserink, M. (2013). Europe. French mathematician tapped to head key funding agency. *Science* 342:545. doi: 10.1126/science.342.6158.545

Fang, F. C., and Casadevall, A. (2010). Lost in translation–basic science in the era of translational research. *Infect. Immun.* 78, 563–566. doi: 10.1128/IAI.01318-09

Font, E., Barbosa, D., Sampedro, C., and Carazo, P. (2012). Social behavior, chemical communication, and adult neurogenesis: studies of scent mark function in Podarcis wall lizards. *Gen. Comp. Endocrinol.* 177, 9–17. doi: 10.1016/j.ygcen.2012.02.015

Fritz, A., Gorlick, D. L., and Burd, G. D. (1996). Neurogenesis in the olfactory bulb of the frog *Xenopus laevis* shows unique patterns during embryonic development and metamorphosis. *Int. J. Dev. Neurosci.* 14, 931–943. doi: 10.1016/S0736-5748(96)00054-8

Gage, F. H., and Temple, S. (2013). Neural stem cells: generating and regenerating the brain. *Neuron* 80, 588–601. doi: 10.1016/j.neuron.2013.10.037

García-Verdugo, J. M., Ferrón, S., Flames, N., Collado, L., Desfilis, E., and Font, E. (2002). The proliferative ventricular zone in adult vertebrates: a comparative study using reptiles, birds, and mammals. *Brain Res. Bull.* 57, 765–775. doi: 10.1016/S0361-9230(01)00769-9

Garcia-Verdugo, J. M., Llahi, S., Ferrer, I., and Lopez-Garcia, C. (1989). Postnatal neurogenesis in the olfactory bulbs of a lizard. A tritiated thymidine autoradiographic study. *Neurosci. Lett.* 98, 247–252. doi: 10.1016/0304-3940(89)90408-4

Garrosa, M., Gayoso, M., and Esteban, F. (1998). Prenatal development of the mammalian vomeronasal organ. *Microsc. Res. Tech.* 41, 456–470. doi: 10.1002/(SICI)1097-0029(19980615)41:6<456::AID-JEMT2>3.0.CO;2-L

Giacobini, P., Benedetto, A., Tirindelli, R., and Fasolo, A. (2000). Proliferation and migration of receptor neurons in the vomeronasal organ of the adult mouse. *Brain Res. Dev. Brain Res.* 123, 33–40. doi: 10.1016/S0165-3806(00)00080-8

Gould, E. (2007). How widespread is adult neurogenesis in mammals? *Nat. Rev. Neurosci.* 8, 481–488. doi: 10.1038/nrn2147

Graziadei, P. P., and Monti-Graziadei, G. A. (1979). Neurogenesis and neuron regeneration in the olfactory system of mammals. I. Morphological aspects of differentiation and structural organization of the olfactory sensory neurons. *J. Neurocytol.* 8, 1–18. doi: 10.1007/BF01206454

Grus, W. E., and Zhang, J. (2008). Distinct evolutionary patterns between chemoreceptors of 2 vertebrate olfactory systems and the differential tuning hypothesis. *Mol. Biol. Evol.* 25, 1593–1601. doi: 10.1093/molbev/msn107

Haberly, L. B. (2001). Parallel-distributed processing in olfactory cortex: new insights from morphological and physiological analysis of neuronal circuitry. *Chem. Senses* 26, 551–576. doi: 10.1093/chemse/26.5.551

Halem, H. A., Baum, M. J., and Cherry, J. A. (2001). Sex difference and steroid modulation of pheromone-induced immediate early genes in the two zones of the mouse accessory olfactory system. *J. Neurosci.* 21, 2474–2480.

Halpern, M., and Martinez-Marcos, A. (2003). Structure and function of the vomeronasal system: an update. *Prog. Neurobiol.* 70, 245–318. doi: 10.1016/S0301-0082(03)00103-5

Hansen, A., Reiss, J. O., Gentry, C. L., and Burd, G. D. (1998). Ultrastructure of the olfactory organ in the clawed frog, *Xenopus laevis*, during larval development and metamorphosis. *J. Comp. Neurol.* 398, 273–288. doi: 10.1002/(SICI)1096-9861(19980824)398:2%3C273::AID-CNE8%3E3.0.CO;2-Y

He, X., Zhang, X.-M., Wu, J., Fu, J., Mou, L., Lu, D.-H., et al. (2014). Olfactory experience modulates immature neuron development in postnatal and adult guinea pig piriform cortex. *Neuroscience* 259, 101–112. doi: 10.1016/j.neuroscience.2013.11.056

Heron, P. M., Stromberg, A. J., Breheny, P., and McClintock, T. S. (2013). Molecular events in the cell types of the olfactory epithelium during adult neurogenesis. *Mol. Brain* 6:49. doi: 10.1186/1756-6606-6-49

Higgs, D. M., and Burd, G. D. (2001). Neuronal turnover in the *Xenopus laevis* olfactory epithelium during metamorphosis. *J. Comp. Neurol.* 433, 124–130. doi: 10.1002/cne.1130

Hildebrand, J. G., and Shepherd, G. M. (1997). Mechanisms of olfactory discrimination: converging evidence for common principles across phyla. *Annu. Rev. Neurosci.* 20, 595–631. doi: 10.1146/annurev.neuro.20.1.595

Hinds, J. W. (1968a). Autoradiographic study of histogenesis in the mouse olfactory bulb. I. Time of origin of neurons and neuroglia. *J. Comp. Neurol.* 134, 287–304. doi: 10.1002/cne.901340304

Hinds, J. W. (1968b). Autoradiographic study of histogenesis in the mouse olfactory bulb. II. Cell proliferation and migration. *J. Comp. Neurol.* 134, 305–322. doi: 10.1002/cne.901340305

Horner, P. J., Power, A. E., Kempermann, G., Kuhn, H. G., Palmer, T. D., Winkler, J., et al. (2000). Proliferation and differentiation of progenitor cells throughout the intact adult rat spinal cord. *J. Neurosci.* 20, 2218–2228.

Horowitz, L. F., Montmayeur, J. P., Echelard, Y., and Buck, L. B. (1999). A genetic approach to trace neural circuits. *Proc. Natl. Acad. Sci. U.S.A.* 96, 3194–3199. doi: 10.1073/pnas.96.6.3194

Hovis, K. R., Ramnath, R., Dahlen, J. E., Romanova, A. L., LaRocca, G., Bier, M. E., et al. (2012). Activity regulates functional connectivity from the vomeronasal organ to the accessory olfactory bulb. *J. Neurosci.* 32, 7907–7916. doi: 10.1523/JNEUROSCI.2399-11.2012

Huang, L., and Bittman, E. L. (2002). Olfactory bulb cells generated in adult male golden hamsters are specifically activated by exposure to estrous females. *Horm. Behav.* 41, 343–350. doi: 10.1006/hbeh.2002.1767

Huilgol, D., Udin, S., Shimogori, T., Saha, B., Roy, A., Aizawa, S., et al. (2013). Dual origins of the mammalian accessory olfactory bulb revealed by an evolutionarily conserved migratory stream. *Nat. Neurosci.* 16, 157–165. doi: 10.1038/nn.3297

Ibarra-Soria, X., Levitin, M. O., and Logan, D. W. (2013). The genomic basis of vomeronasal-mediated behaviour. *Mamm. Genome* 25, 75–86. doi: 10.1007/s00335-013-9463-1

Ichikawa, M., Osada, T., and Costanzo, R. M. (1998). Replacement of receptor cells in the hamster vomeronasal epithelium after nerve transection. *Chem. Senses* 23, 171–179. doi: 10.1093/chemse/23.2.171

Inamura, K., Sakamoto, H., Honda, N., and Kashiwayanagi, M. (2000). Cluster of proliferating cells in rat vomeronasal sensory epithelium. *Neuroreport* 11, 477–479. doi: 10.1097/00001756-200002280-00010

Inta, D., Alfonso, J., von Engelhardt, J., Kreuzberg, M. M., Meyer, A. H., van Hooft, J. A., et al. (2008). Neurogenesis and widespread forebrain migration of distinct GABAergic neurons from the postnatal subventricular zone. *Proc. Natl. Acad. Sci. U.S.A.* 105, 20994–20999. doi: 10.1073/pnas.0807059105

Ishii, T., and Mombaerts, P. (2011). Coordinated coexpression of two vomeronasal receptor V2R genes per neuron in the mouse. *Mol. Cell. Neurosci.* 46, 397–408. doi: 10.1016/j.mcn.2010.11.002

Jia, C., and Halpern, M. (1997). Segregated populations of mitral/tufted cells in the accessory olfactory bulb. *Neuroreport* 8, 1887–1890. doi: 10.1097/00001756-199705260-00019

Jia, C., and Halpern, M. (1998). Neurogenesis and migration of receptor neurons in the vomeronasal sensory epithelium in the opossum, *Monodelphis domestica*. *J. Comp. Neurol.* 400, 287–297. doi: 10.1002/(SICI)1096-9861(19981019)400:2%3C287::AID-CNE9%3E3.0.CO;2-5

Jones, S. V., Choi, D. C., Davis, M., and Ressler, K. J. (2008). Learning-dependent structural plasticity in the adult olfactory pathway. *J. Neurosci.* 28, 13106–13111. doi: 10.1523/JNEUROSCI.4465-08.2008

Kaba, H., Rosser, A. E., and Keverne, E. B. (1988). Hormonal enhancement of neurogenesis and its relationship to the duration of olfactory memory. *Neuroscience* 24, 93–98. doi: 10.1016/0306-4522(88)90314-4

Kageyama, R., Imayoshi, I., and Sakamoto, M. (2012). The role of neurogenesis in olfaction-dependent behaviors. *Behav. Brain Res.* 227, 459–463. doi: 10.1016/j.bbr.2011.04.038

Kaplan, M. S. (1985). Formation and turnover of neurons in young and senescent animals: an electronmicroscopic and morphometric analysis. *Ann. N. Y. Acad. Sci.* 457, 173–192. doi: 10.1111/j.1749-6632.1985.tb20805.x

Kaplan, M. S., and Hinds, J. W. (1977). Neurogenesis in the adult rat: electron microscopic analysis of light radioautographs. *Science* 197, 1092–1094. doi: 10.1126/science.887941

Katoh, H., Shibata, S., Fukuda, K., Sato, M., Satoh, E., Nagoshi, N., et al. (2011). The dual origin of the peripheral olfactory system: placode and neural crest. *Mol. Brain* 4:34. doi: 10.1186/1756-6606-4-34

Kempermann, G. (2012). New neurons for "survival of the fittest." *Nat. Rev. Neurosci.* 13, 727–736. doi: 10.1038/nrn3319

Kernie, S. G., and Parent, J. M. (2010). Forebrain neurogenesis after focal Ischemic and traumatic brain injury. *Neurobiol. Dis.* 37, 267–274. doi: 10.1016/j.nbd.2009.11.002

Kimoto, H., Haga, S., Sato, K., and Touhara, K. (2005). Sex-specific peptides from exocrine glands stimulate mouse vomeronasal sensory neurons. *Nature* 437, 898–901. doi: 10.1038/nature04033

Kishi, K. (1987). Golgi studies on the development of granule cells of the rat olfactory bulb with reference to migration in the subependymal layer. *J. Comp. Neurol.* 258, 112–124. doi: 10.1002/cne.902580109

Kiyokage, E., Pan, Y.-Z., Shao, Z., Kobayashi, K., Szabo, G., Yanagawa, Y., et al. (2010). Molecular identity of periglomerular and short axon cells. *J. Neurosci.* 30, 1185–1196. doi: 10.1523/JNEUROSCI.3497-09.2010

Kohwi, M., Petryniak, M. A., Long, J. E., Ekker, M., Obata, K., Yanagawa, Y., et al. (2007). A subpopulation of olfactory bulb GABAergic interneurons is derived from Emx1- and Dlx5/6-expressing progenitors. *J. Neurosci.* 27, 6878–6891. doi: 10.1523/JNEUROSCI.0254-07.2007

Kondoh, D., Yamamoto, Y., Nakamuta, N., and Taniguchi, K. (2012). Seasonal changes in the histochemical properties of the olfactory epithelium and vomeronasal organ in the Japanese striped snake, *Elaphe quadrivirgata. Anat. Histol. Embryol.* 41, 41–53. doi: 10.1111/j.1439-0264.2011.01101.x

Kriegstein, A., and Alvarez-Buylla, A. (2009). The glial nature of embryonic and adult neural stem cells. *Annu. Rev. Neurosci.* 32, 149–184. doi: 10.1146/annurev.neuro.051508.135600

Krug, L., Wicht, H., and Northcutt, R. G. (1993). Afferent and efferent connections of the thalamic eminence in the axolotl, Ambystoma mexicanum. *Neurosci. Lett.* 149, 145–148. doi: 10.1016/0304-3940(93)90757-C

Kulkarni-Narla, A., Getchell, T. V., and Getchell, M. L. (1997). Differential expression of manganese and copper-zinc superoxide dismutases in the olfactory and vomeronasal receptor neurons of rats during ontogeny. *J. Comp. Neurol.* 381, 31–40. doi: 10.1002/(SICI)1096-9861(19970428)381:1%3C31::AID-CNE3%3E3.0.CO;2-L

Kumar, A., Dudley, C. A., and Moss, R. L. (1999). Functional dichotomy within the vomeronasal system: distinct zones of neuronal activity in the accessory olfactory bulb correlate with sex-specific behaviors. *J. Neurosci.* 19, RC32.

Larriva-Sahd, J. (2008). The accessory olfactory bulb in the adult rat: a cytological study of its cell types, neuropil, neuronal modules, and interactions with the main olfactory system. *J. Comp. Neurol.* 510, 309–350. doi: 10.1002/cne.21790

Larsen, C. M., Kokay, I. C., and Grattan, D. R. (2008). Male pheromones initiate prolactin-induced neurogenesis and advance maternal behavior in female mice. *Horm. Behav.* 53, 509–517. doi: 10.1016/j.yhbeh.2007.11.020

Lau, D., Ogbogu, U., Taylor, B., Stafinski, T., Menon, D., and Caulfield, T. (2008). Stem cell clinics online: the direct-to-consumer portrayal of stem cell medicine. *Cell Stem Cell* 3, 591–594. doi: 10.1016/j.stem.2008.11.001

Leinders-Zufall, T., Brennan, P., Widmayer, P., S, P. C., Maul-Pavicic, A., Jäger, M., et al. (2004). MHC class I peptides as chemosensory signals in the vomeronasal organ. *Science* 306, 1033–1037. doi: 10.1126/science.1102818

Leinders-Zufall, T., Ishii, T., Mombaerts, P., Zufall, F., and Boehm, T. (2009). Structural requirements for the activation of vomeronasal sensory neurons by MHC peptides. *Nat. Neurosci.* 12, 1551–1558. doi: 10.1038/nn.2452

Leinders-Zufall, T., Lane, A. P., Puche, A. C., Ma, W., Novotny, M. V., Shipley, M. T., et al. (2000). Ultrasensitive pheromone detection by mammalian vomeronasal neurons. *Nature* 405, 792–796. doi: 10.1038/35015572

Lepousez, G., Valley, M. T., and Lledo, P.-M. (2013). The impact of adult neurogenesis on olfactory bulb circuits and computations. *Annu. Rev. Physiol.* 75, 339–363. doi: 10.1146/annurev-physiol-030212-183731

Lindvall, O., and Kokaia, Z. (2010). Stem cells in human neurodegenerative disorders–time for clinical translation? *J. Clin. Invest.* 120, 29–40. doi: 10.1172/JCI40543

Lledo, P.-M., and Gheusi, G. (2006). Adult neurogenesis: from basic research to clinical applications. *Bull. Acad. Natl. Méd.* 190, 385–402.

Luzzati, F., De Marchis, S., Fasolo, A., and Peretto, P. (2006). Neurogenesis in the caudate nucleus of the adult rabbit. *J. Neurosci.* 26, 609–621. doi: 10.1523/JNEUROSCI.4371-05.2006

Luzzati, F., De Marchis, S., Parlato, R., Gribaudo, S., Schütz, G., Fasolo, A., et al. (2011). New striatal neurons in a mouse model of progressive striatal degeneration are generated in both the subventricular zone and the striatal parenchyma. *PLoS ONE* 6:e25088. doi: 10.1371/journal.pone.0025088

Magavi, S. S. P., Mitchell, B. D., Szentirmai, O., Carter, B. S., and Macklis, J. D. (2005). Adult-born and preexisting olfactory granule neurons undergo distinct experience-dependent modifications of their olfactory responses *in vivo. J. Neurosci.* 25, 10729–10739. doi: 10.1523/JNEUROSCI.2250-05.2005

Mak, G. K., Enwere, E. K., Gregg, C., Pakarainen, T., Poutanen, M., Huhtaniemi, I., et al. (2007). Male pheromone-stimulated neurogenesis in the adult female brain: possible role in mating behavior. *Nat. Neurosci.* 10, 1003–1011. doi: 10.1038/nn1928

Mandairon, N., Sacquet, J., Jourdan, F., and Didier, A. (2006). Long-term fate and distribution of newborn cells in the adult mouse olfactory bulb: influences of olfactory deprivation. *Neuroscience* 141, 443–451. doi: 10.1016/j.neuroscience.2006.03.066

Mandairon, N., Sultan, S., Nouvian, M., Sacquet, J., and Didier, A. (2011). Involvement of newborn neurons in olfactory associative learning? The operant or non-operant component of the task makes all the difference. *J. Neurosci.* 31, 12455–12460. doi: 10.1523/JNEUROSCI.2919-11.2011

Martinez-Marcos, A., Jia, C., Quan, W., and Halpern, M. (2005). Neurogenesis, migration, and apoptosis in the vomeronasal epithelium of adult mice. *J. Neurobiol.* 63, 173–187. doi: 10.1002/neu.20128

Martínez-Marcos, A., Ubeda-Bañón, I., Deng, L., and Halpern, M. (2000). Neurogenesis in the vomeronasal epithelium of adult rats: evidence for different mechanisms for growth and neuronal turnover. *J. Neurobiol.* 44, 423–435. doi: 10.1002/1097-4695(20000915)44:4<423::AID-NEU5>3.0.CO;2-H

Martínez-Marcos, A., Ubeda-Bañón, I., and Halpern, M. (2001). Cell migration to the anterior and posterior divisions of the granule cell layer of the accessory olfactory bulb of adult opossums. *Brain Res. Dev. Brain Res.* 127, 95–98. doi: 10.1016/S0165-3806(01)00106-7

Martini, S., Silvotti, L., Shirazi, A., Ryba, N. J., and Tirindelli, R. (2001). Co-expression of putative pheromone receptors in the sensory neurons of the vomeronasal organ. *J. Neurosci.* 21, 843–848.

Matsuoka, M., Osada, T., Yoshida-Matsuoka, J., Ikai, A., Ichikawa, M., Norita, M., et al. (2002). A comparative immunocytochemical study of development and regeneration of chemosensory neurons in the rat vomeronasal system. *Brain. Res.* 946, 52–63. doi: 10.1016/S0006-8993(02)02823-8

Meeks, J. P., Arnson, H. A., and Holy, T. E. (2010). Representation and transformation of sensory information in the mouse accessory olfactory system. *Nat. Neurosci.* 13, 723–730. doi: 10.1038/nn.2546

Meisami, E., and Bhatnagar, K. P. (1998). Vomeronasal organ in bats and primates: extremes of structural variability and its phylogenetic implications. *Microsc. Res. Tech.* 43, 465–475. doi: 10.1002/(SICI)1097-0029(19981215)43:6<465::AID-JEMT1>3.0.CO;2-1

Merkle, F. T., Mirzadeh, Z., and varez-Buylla, A. (2007). Mosaic organization of neural stem cells in the adult brain. *Science* 317, 1095–9203. doi: 10.1126/science.1144914

Migliore, M., Inzirillo, C., and Shepherd, G. M. (2007). Learning mechanism for column formation in the olfactory bulb. *Front. Integr. Neurosci.* 1:12. doi: 10.3389/neuro.07.012.2007

Migliore, M., and Shepherd, G. M. (2008). Dendritic action potentials connect distributed dendrodendritic microcircuits. *J. Comput. Neurosci.* 24, 207–221. doi: 10.1007/s10827-007-0051-9

Monteiro, B. M. M., Moreira, F. A., Massensini, A. R., Moraes, M. F. D., and Pereira, G. S. (2013). Enriched environment increases neurogenesis and improves social memory persistence in socially isolated adult mice. *Hippocampus* 24, 239–248. doi: 10.1002/hipo.22218

Monti-Graziadei, A. G. (1992). Cell migration from the olfactory neuroepithelium of neonatal and adult rodents. *Brain Res. Dev. Brain Res.* 70, 65–74. doi: 10.1016/0165-3806(92)90104-5

Moriya-Ito, K., Endoh, K., Fujiwara-Tsukamoto, Y., and Ichikawa, M. (2013). Three-dimensional reconstruction of electron micrographs reveals intrabulbar circuit differences between accessory and main olfactory bulbs. *Front. Neuroanat.* 7:5. doi: 10.3389/fnana.2013.00005

Mouret, A., Gheusi, G., Gabellec, M.-M., de Chaumont, F., Olivo-Marin, J.-C., and Lledo, P.-M. (2008). Learning and survival of newly generated neurons: when time matters. *J. Neurosci.* 28, 11511–11516. doi: 10.1523/JNEUROSCI.2954-08.2008

Mucignat-Caretta, C. (2010). The rodent accessory olfactory system. *J. Comp. Phys.* 196, 767–777. doi: 10.1007/s00359-010-0555-z

Mucignat-Caretta, C., Redaelli, M., and Caretta, A. (2012). One nose, one brain: contribution of the main and accessory olfactory system to chemosensation. *Front. Neuroanat.* 6:46. doi: 10.3389/fnana.2012.00046

Mugnaini, E., Oertel, W. H., and Wouterlood, F. F. (1984). Immunocytochemical localization of GABA neurons and dopamine neurons in the rat main and accessory olfactory bulbs. *Neurosci. Lett.* 47, 221–226. doi: 10.1016/0304-3940(84)90517-2

Murdoch, B., and Roskams, A. J. (2008). A novel embryonic nestin-expressing radial glia-like progenitor gives rise to zonally restricted olfactory and vomeronasal neurons. *J. Neurosci.* 28, 4271–4282. doi: 10.1523/JNEUROSCI.5566-07.2008

Nadi, N. S., Head, R., Grillo, M., Hempstead, J., Grannot-Reisfeld, N., and Margolis, F. L. (1981). Chemical deafferentation of the olfactory bulb: plasticity of the levels of tyrosine hydroxylase, dopamine and norepinephrine. *Brain Res.* 213, 365–377. doi: 10.1016/0006-8993(81)90241-9

Ngai, J., Chess, A., Dowling, M. M., Necles, N., Macagno, E. R., and Axel, R. (1993). Coding of olfactory information: topography of odorant receptor expression in the catfish olfactory epithelium. *Cell* 72, 667–680. doi: 10.1016/0092-8674(93)90396-8

Nishiyama, A., Lin, X. H., Giese, N., Heldin, C. H., and Stallcup, W. B. (1996). Co-localization of NG2 proteoglycan and PDGF alpha-receptor on O2A progenitor cells in the developing rat brain. *J. Neurosci. Res.* 43, 299–314. doi: 10.1002/(SICI)1097-4547(19960201)43:3<299::AID-JNR5>3.0.CO;2-E

Nissant, A., Bardy, C., Katagiri, H., Murray, K., and Lledo, P.-M. (2009). Adult neurogenesis promotes synaptic plasticity in the olfactory bulb. *Nat. Neurosci.* 12, 728–730. doi: 10.1038/nn.2298

Nunez-Parra, A., Pugh, V., and Araneda, R. C. (2011). Regulation of adult neurogenesis by behavior and age in the accessory olfactory bulb. *Mol. Cell. Neurosci.* 47, 274–285. doi: 10.1016/j.mcn.2011.05.003

Oboti, L., Savalli, G., Giachino, C., De Marchis, S., Panzica, G. C., Fasolo, A., et al. (2009). Integration and sensory experience-dependent survival of newly-generated neurons in the accessory olfactory bulb of female mice. *Eur. J. Neurosci.* 29, 679–692. doi: 10.1111/j.1460-9568.2009.06614.x

Oboti, L., Schellino, R., Giachino, C., Chamero, P., Pyrski, M., Leinders-Zufall, T., et al. (2011). Newborn interneurons in the accessory olfactory bulb promote mate recognition in female mice. *Front. Neurosci.* 5:113. doi: 10.3389/fnins.2011.00113

Ohira, K., Furuta, T., Hioki, H., Nakamura, K. C., Kuramoto, E., Tanaka, Y., et al. (2010). Ischemia-induced neurogenesis of neocortical layer 1 progenitor cells. *Nat. Neurosci.* 13, 173–179. doi: 10.1038/nn.2473

Othman, M. A. (2011). Postnatal development of the female rabbit vomerosensory epithelium: a light and electron microscopy study. *Egypt. J. Histol.* 34, 69–79. doi: 10.1097/01.EHX.0000394886.69777.b0

Parrish-Aungst, S., Shipley, M. T., Erdelyi, F., Szabo, G., and Puche, A. C. (2007). Quantitative analysis of neuronal diversity in the mouse olfactory bulb. *J. Comp. Neurol.* 501, 825–836. doi: 10.1002/cne.21205

Paternostro, M. A., and Meisami, E. (1996). Essential role of thyroid hormones in maturation of olfactory receptor neurons: an immunocytochemical study of number and cytoarchitecture of OMP-positive cells in developing rats. *Int. J. Dev. Neurosci.* 14, 867–880. doi: 10.1016/S0736-5748(96)00064-0

Peretto, P., Giachino, C., Panzica, G. C., and Fasolo, A. (2001). Sexually dimorphic neurogenesis is topographically matched with the anterior accessory olfactory bulb of the adult rat. *Cell Tissue Res* 306, 385–389. doi: 10.1007/s00441-001-0471-1

Pérez-Cañellas, M. M., Font, E., and García-Verdugo, J. M. (1997). Postnatal neurogenesis in the telencephalon of turtles: evidence for nonradial migration of new neurons from distant proliferative ventricular zones to the olfactory bulbs. *Brain Res. Dev. Brain Res.* 101, 125–137.

Pérez-Cañellas, M. M., and García-Verdugo, J. M. (1996). Adult neurogenesis in the telencephalon of a lizard: a [3H]thymidine autoradiographic and bromodeoxyuridine immunocytochemical study. *Brain Res. Dev. Brain Res.* 93, 49–61.

Petreanu, L., and Alvarez-Buylla, A. (2002). Maturation and death of adult-born olfactory bulb granule neurons: role of olfaction. *J. Neurosci.* 22, 6106–6113. doi: 20026588

Pírez, N., and Wachowiak, M. (2008). *In vivo* modulation of sensory input to the olfactory bulb by tonic and activity-dependent presynaptic inhibition of receptor neurons. *J. Neurosci.* 28, 6360–6371. doi: 10.1523/JNEUROSCI.0793-08.2008

Portillo, W., Unda, N., Camacho, F. J., Sánchez, M., Corona, R., Arzate, D. M., et al. G. (2012). Sexual activity increases the number of newborn cells in the accessory olfactory bulb of male rats. *Front. Neuroanat.* 6:25. doi: 10.3389/fnana.2012.00025

Puelles, L., Kuwana, E., Puelles, E., Bulfone, A., Shimamura, K., Keleher, J., et al. (2000). Pallial and subpallial derivatives in the embryonic chick and mouse telencephalon, traced by the expression of the genes Dlx-2, Emx-1, Nkx-2.1, Pax-6, and Tbr-1. *J. Comp. Neurol.* 424, 409–438. doi: 10.1002/1096-9861(20000828)424:3%3C409::AID-CNE3%3E3.0.CO;2-7

Ramaswamy, S., Goings, G. E., Soderstrom, K. E., Szele, F. G., and Kozlowski, D. A. (2005). Cellular proliferation and migration following a controlled cortical impact in the mouse. *Brain Res.* 1053, 38–53. doi: 10.1016/j.brainres.2005.06.042

Rivière, S., Challet, L., Fluegge, D., Spehr, M., and Rodriguez, I. (2009). Formyl peptide receptor-like proteins are a novel family of vomeronasal chemosensors. *Nature* 459, 574–577. doi: 10.1038/nature08029

Rochefort, C., Gheusi, G., Vincent, J.-D., and Lledo, P.-M. (2002). Enriched odor exposure increases the number of newborn neurons in the adult olfactory bulb and improves odor memory. *J. Neurosci.* 22, 2679–2689. doi: 20026260

Saha, B., Peron, S., Murray, K., Jaber, M., and Gaillard, A. (2013). Cortical lesion stimulates adult subventricular zone neural progenitor cell proliferation and migration to the site of injury. *Stem Cell Res.* 11, 965–977. doi: 10.1016/j.scr.2013.06.006

Sakamoto, M., Imayoshi, I., Ohtsuka, T., Yamaguchi, M., Mori, K., and Kageyama, R. (2011). Continuous neurogenesis in the adult forebrain is required for innate olfactory responses. *Proc. Natl. Acad. Sci. U.S.A.* 108, 8479–8484. doi: 10.1073/pnas.1018782108

Salazar, I., and Brennan, P. A. (2001). Retrograde labelling of mitral/tufted cells in the mouse accessory olfactory bulb following local injections of the lipophilic tracer DiI into the vomeronasal amygdala. *Brain Res.* 896, 198–203. doi: 10.1016/S0006-8993(01)02225-9

Sampedro, C., Font, E., and Desfilis, E. (2008). Size variation and cell proliferation in chemosensory brain areas of a lizard (Podarcis hispanica): effects of sex and season. *Eur. J. Neurosci.* 28, 87–98. doi: 10.1111/j.1460-9568.2008.06287.x

Seri, B., García-Verdugo, J. M., McEwen, B. S., and Alvarez-Buylla, A. (2001). Astrocytes give rise to new neurons in the adult mammalian hippocampus. *J. Neurosci.* 21, 7153–7160.

Shapiro, L. S., Roland, R. M., and Halpern, M. (1997). Development of olfactory marker protein and N-CAM expression in chemosensory systems of the opossum, *Monodelphis domestica*. *J. Morphol.* 234, 109–129. doi: 10.1002/(SICI)1097-4687(199711)234:2<109::AID-JMOR1>3.0.CO;2-7

Shepherd, G. M. (2010), "New perspectives on olfactory processing and human smell," in *The Neurobiology of Olfaction*, Chapter 16, ed A. Menini (Boca Raton, FL: CRC Press), 395–403.

Shipley, M. T., Ennis, M., and Puche, A. C. (2004), "The olfactory system," in *The Rat Nervous System*, 3rd Edn, ed G. Paxinos (New York, NY: Elsevier), 921–962.

Shpak, G., Zylbertal, A., Yarom, Y., and Wagner, S. (2012). Calcium-activated sustained firing responses distinguish accessory from main olfactory bulb mitral cells. *J. Neurosci.* 32, 6251–6262. doi: 10.1523/JNEUROSCI.4397-11.2012

Silvotti, L., Moiani, A., Gatti, R., and Tirindelli, R. (2007). Combinatorial co-expression of pheromone receptors, V2Rs. *J. Neurochem.* 103, 1753–1763. doi: 10.1111/j.1471-4159.2007.04877.x

Slotnick, B., Restrepo, D., Schellinck, H., Archbold, G., Price, S., and Lin, W. (2010). Accessory olfactory bulb function is modulated by input from the main olfactory epithelium. *Eur. J. Neurosci.* 31, 1108–1116. doi: 10.1111/j.1460-9568.2010.07141.x

Speca, D. J., Lin, D. M., Sorensen, P. W., Isacoff, E. Y., Ngai, J., and Dittman, A. H. (1999). Functional identification of a goldfish odorant receptor. *Neuron* 23, 487–498. doi: 10.1016/S0896-6273(00)80802-8

Spors, H., Albeanu, D. F., Murthy, V. N., Rinberg, D., Uchida, N., Wachowiak, M., et al. (2012). Illuminating vertebrate olfactory processing. *J. Neurosci.* 32, 14102–14108. doi: 10.1523/JNEUROSCI.3328-12.2012

Su, C.-Y., Menuz, K., and Carlson, J. R. (2009). Olfactory perception: receptors, cells, and circuits. *Cell* 139, 45–59. doi: 10.1016/j.cell.2009.09.015

Suárez, R., Fernández-Aburto, P., Manger, P. R., and Mpodozis, J. (2011a). Deterioration of the Gαo vomeronasal pathway in sexually dimorphic mammals. *PLoS ONE* 6:e26436. doi: 10.1371/journal.pone.0026436

Suárez, R., Santibáñez, R., Parra, D., Coppi, A. A., Abrahão, L. M. B., Sasahara, T. H. C., et al. (2011b). Shared and differential traits in the accessory olfactory bulb of caviomorph rodents with particular reference to the semiaquatic capybara. *J. Anat.* 218, 558–565. doi: 10.1111/j.1469-7580.2011.01357.x

Sugai, T., Yoshimura, H., Kato, N., and Onoda, N. (2006). Component-dependent urine responses in the rat accessory olfactory bulb. *Neuroreport* 17, 1663–1667. doi: 10.1097/01.wnr.0000239950.14954.59

Sultan, S., Lefort, J. M., Sacquet, J., Mandairon, N., and Didier, A. (2011a). Acquisition of an olfactory associative task triggers a regionalized down-regulation of adult born neuron cell death. *Front. Neurosci.* 5:52. doi: 10.3389/fnins.2011.00052

Sultan, S., Rey, N., Sacquet, J., Mandairon, N., and Didier, A. (2011b). Newborn neurons in the olfactory bulb selected for long-term survival through olfactory learning are prematurely suppressed when the olfactory memory is erased. *J. Neurosci.* 31, 14893–14898. doi: 10.1523/JNEUROSCI.3677-11.2011

Suzuki, J., Yoshizaki, K., Kobayashi, T., and Osumi, N. (2013). Neural crest-derived horizontal basal cells as tissue stem cells in the adult olfactory epithelium. *Neurosci. Res.* 75, 112–120. doi: 10.1016/j.neures.2012.11.005

Takahashi, K., and Yamanaka, S. (2006). Induction of pluripotent stem cells from mouse embryonic and adult fibroblast cultures by defined factors. *Cell* 126, 663–676. doi: 10.1016/j.cell.2006.07.024

Takami, S., and Graziadei, P. P. (1991). Light microscopic Golgi study of mitral/tufted cells in the accessory olfactory bulb of the adult rat. *J. Comp. Neurol.* 311, 65–83. doi: 10.1002/cne.903110106

Taniguchi, K., and Taniguchi, K. (2008). Embryonic and postnatal differentiation of olfactory epithelium and vomeronasal organ in the Syrian hamster. *J. Vet. Med. Sci.* 70, 57–64. doi: 10.1292/jvms.70.57

Taniguchi, K., Toshima, Y., and Saito, T. R. (1996). Development of the olfactory epithelium and vomeronasal organ in the Japanese reddish frog, *Rana japonica*. *J. Vet. Med. Sci.* 58, 7–15. doi: 10.1292/jvms.58.7

Tarozzo, G., Cappello, P., De Andrea, M., Walters, E., Margolis, F. L., Oestreicher, B., et al. (1998). Prenatal differentiation of mouse vomeronasal neurones. *Eur. J. Neurosci.* 10, 392–396. doi: 10.1046/j.1460-9568.1998.00004.x

Tirindelli, R., Dibattista, M., Pifferi, S., and Menini, A. (2009). From pheromones to behavior. *Physiol. Rev.* 89, 921–956. doi: 10.1152/physrev.00037.2008

Touhara, K., and Vosshall, L. B. (2009). Sensing odorants and pheromones with chemosensory receptors. *Annu. Rev. Physiol.* 71, 307–332. doi: 10.1146/annurev.physiol.010908.163209

Veyrac, A., and Bakker, J. (2011). Postnatal and adult exposure to estradiol differentially influences adult neurogenesis in the main and accessory olfactory bulb of female mice. *FASEB J.* 25,1048–1057. doi: 10.1096/fj.10-172635

Wang, R. T., and Halpern, M. (1982). Neurogenesis in the vomeronasal epithelium of adult garter snakes. 1. Degeneration of bipolar neurons and proliferation of undifferentiated cells following experimental vomeronasal axotomy. *Brain Res.* 237, 23–39. doi: 10.1016/0006-8993(82)90555-8

Watt, W. C., Sakano, H., Lee, Z.-Y., Reusch, J. E., Trinh, K., and Storm, D. R. (2004). Odorant stimulation enhances survival of olfactory sensory neurons via MAPK and CREB. *Neuron* 41, 955–967. doi: 10.1016/S0896-6273(04)00075-3

Weiler, E. (2005). Postnatal development of the rat vomeronasal organ. *Chem. Senses* 27, 8 doi: 10.1093/chemse/bjh147

Weiler, E., Apfelbach, R., and Farbman, A. I. (1999b). The vomeronasal organ of the male ferret. *Chem. Senses* 24, 127–136. doi: 10.1093/chemse/24.2.127

Weiler, E., McCulloch, M. A., and Farbman, A. I. (1999a) Proliferation in the vomeronasal organ of the rat during postnatal development. *Eur. J. Neurosci.* 11, 700–711. doi: 10.1046/j.1460-9568.1999.00476.x

Whitman, M. C., and Greer, C. A. (2009). Adult neurogenesis and the olfactory system. *Prog. Neurobiol.* 89, 162–175. doi: 10.1016/j.pneurobio.2009.07.003

Xia, J., Broad, K. D., Emson, P. C., and Keverne, E. B. (2010). Epigenetic modification of vomeronasal (V2r) precursor neurons by histone deacetylation. *Neuroscience* 169, 1462–1472. doi: 10.1016/j.neuroscience.2010.05.071

Xia, J., Sellers, L. A., Oxley, D., Smith, T., Emson, P., and Keverne, E. B. (2006). Urinary pheromones promote ERK/Akt phosphorylation, regeneration and survival of vomeronasal (V2R) neurons. *E. J. Neurosci.* 24, 3333–3342. doi: 10.1111/j.1460-9568.2006.05244.x

Xiong, W., and Chen, W. R. (2002). Dynamic gating of spike propagation in the mitral cell lateral dendrites. *Neuron* 34, 115–126. doi: 10.1016/S0896-6273(02)00628-1

Xu, F., Schaefer, M., Kida, I., Schafer, J., Liu, N., Rothman, D. L., et al. (2005). Simultaneous activation of mouse main and accessory olfactory bulbs by odors or pheromones. *J. Comp. Neurol.* 489, 491–500. doi: 10.1002/cne.20652

Yamanaka, S., and Blau, H. M. (2010). Nuclear reprogramming to a pluripotent state by three approaches. *Nature* 465, 704–712. doi: 10.1038/nature09229

Yan, X.-X., Xiong, K., Luo, X.-G., Struble, R. G., and Clough, R. W. (2007). beta-Secretase expression in normal and functionally deprived rat olfactory bulbs: inverse correlation with oxidative metabolic activity. *J. Comp. Neurol.* 501, 52–69. doi: 10.1002/cne.21239

Yang, Z. (2008). Postnatal subventricular zone progenitors give rise not only to granular and periglomerular interneurons but also to interneurons in the external plexiform layer of the rat olfactory bulb. *J. Comp. Neurol.* 506, 347–358. doi: 10.1002/cne.21557

Yu, T.-S., Zhang, G., Liebl, D. J., and Kernie, S. G. (2008). Traumatic brain injury-induced hippocampal neurogenesis requires activation of early nestin-expressing progenitors. *J. Neurosci.* 28, 12901–12912. doi: 10.1523/JNEUROSCI.4629-08.2008

7

Striatal cholinergic interneuron regulation and circuit effects

Sean Austin O. Lim[1], Un Jung Kang[2] and Daniel S. McGehee[1,3]*

[1] Committee on Neurobiology, University of Chicago, Chicago, IL, USA
[2] Department of Neurology, Columbia University, New York, NY, USA
[3] Department of Anesthesia and Critical Care, University of Chicago, Chicago, IL, USA

Edited by:
Sukumar Vijayaraghavan, University of Colorado Health Science Center, USA

Reviewed by:
Maryka Quik, SRI International, USA
Teresa Morera-Herreras, University of the Basque Country, Spain

***Correspondence:**
Daniel S. McGehee, Department of Anesthesia and Critical Care, University of Chicago, 5841 S Maryland Ave., MC4028, Chicago, IL 60637, USA
e-mail: dmcgehee@uchicago.edu

The striatum plays a central role in motor control and motor learning. Appropriate responses to environmental stimuli, including pursuit of reward or avoidance of aversive experience all require functional striatal circuits. These pathways integrate synaptic inputs from limbic and cortical regions including sensory, motor and motivational information to ultimately connect intention to action. Although many neurotransmitters participate in striatal circuitry, one critically important player is acetylcholine (ACh). Relative to other brain areas, the striatum contains exceptionally high levels of ACh, the enzymes that catalyze its synthesis and breakdown, as well as both nicotinic and muscarinic receptor types that mediate its postsynaptic effects. The principal source of striatal ACh is the cholinergic interneuron (ChI), which comprises only about 1–2% of all striatal cells yet sends dense arbors of projections throughout the striatum. This review summarizes recent advances in our understanding of the factors affecting the excitability of these neurons through acute effects and long term changes in their synaptic inputs. In addition, we discuss the physiological effects of ACh in the striatum, and how changes in ACh levels may contribute to disease states during striatal dysfunction.

Keywords: acetylcholine, cholinergic interneuron, Parkinson's disease, plasticity, striatum

INTRODUCTION

The striatum is a subcortical brain region crucial for integrating motivation and action (Da Cunha et al., 2012). Convergence of inputs from motor cortex, thalamus and limbic areas create associations between actions and outcomes that ultimately contribute to survival. The essential nature of the striatum is evidenced by the presence of homologs structures throughout vertebrate evolution over hundreds of millions of years (Stephenson-Jones et al., 2011). Pathological changes in the striatum and associated basal ganglia structures are implicated in a wide variety of neurological and psychiatric disorders that involve the combination of motivation and action, including drug addiction (Koob, 1992), binge-eating (Norgren et al., 2006), obsessive-compulsive disorder (Aouizerate et al., 2004), attention deficit and hyperactivity disorder (Chudasama and Robbins, 2006), Huntington's disease (Cepeda et al., 2007), Parkinson's disease (Albin et al., 1989; Ellens and Leventhal, 2013), and L-DOPA induced dyskinesia (Barroso-Chinea and Bezard, 2010). Because so many human pathologies involve striatal dysfunction, a better understanding of neurotransmission in this brain structure will provide insight into the etiology of these conditions, potentially leading to the development of new pharmacotherapies. One neurotransmitter that is highly enriched in the striatum and vitally important for normal function is acetylcholine (ACh). This review will focus on the regulation of striatal ACh release as well as the functional consequences of cholinergic neurotransmission.

Unlike brain structures that show ordered laminar organization such as the hippocampus or cortex, the striatum is a heterogeneous mix of different cell types. The vast majority of striatal neurons (~95%) are the GABA-ergic medium spiny neurons (MSNs), also referred to as spiny projection neurons, which are the principal output cell type. The MSNs that express dopamine (DA) D1 receptors project to and inhibit cells in the internal capsule of the globus pallidus as well as the substantia nigra pars reticulata. These projections are referred to as the direct pathway, or the GO pathway, and activation of this class of cells leads to enhanced locomotion. Another MSN population expresses dopamine D2 receptors, and these projections inhibit cells in the external capsule of the globus pallidus. This is the indirect, or the NO-GO pathway, and activation of this pathway decreases locomotion. Both pathways eventually influence thalamic control of motor cortex to affect motor function. Approximately 6% of MSNs in the dorsal striatum express both D1 and D2 receptors. These cells produce both GABA and glutamate, allowing them to potentially modulate the basal ganglia network bidirectionally (Perreault et al., 2012). The MSN network of basal ganglia connectivity has provided a model for understanding striatal involvement in motor control (Albin et al., 1989; DeLong, 1990; Kravitz et al., 2010). In addition to the MSNs, approximately 4% of striatal neurons are GABA-ergic interneurons. These locally projecting inhibitory cells consist of three types: parvalbumin-expressing fast spiking interneurons (FSIs), NPY/SOM/NOS-expressing persistent depolarization low-threshold spiking interneurons, and the less understood calretinin-expressing low-threshold calcium spike interneurons (Kawaguchi, 1993). Each of these GABA-interneuron cell types possesses a unique gene expression profile and distinct electrophysiological properties (Tepper et al., 2010).

The remaining cells are the large, aspiny cholinergic interneurons (ChIs) originally described by the anatomist Kölliker in the late 1800's. Although recent tract tracing and electron microscopy studies report cholinergic projections from the rostral pedunculopontine nucleus into the striatum (Dautan et al., 2014), it is generally accepted that ChIs are the main source of striatal ACh (Woolf and Butcher, 1981). ChIs comprise ~1% of striatal cells, yet they ramify extensively and send projections widely throughout the striatum: each ChI is estimated to produce on average 500,000 axonal varicosities (Bolam et al., 1984; Contant et al., 1996). Anatomically, ChIs are easily distinguished from the other striatal cell types due to their large diameter somata (>15 microns). In addition, ChIs display unique electrophysiological characteristics, which include tonic action potential firing at a rate of 3–10 Hz (Wilson et al., 1990), depolarized resting membrane potential (~ −60 mV) (Lee et al., 1998), high input resistance (~ 200 MΩ) (Calabresi et al., 1997), prominent hyperpolarization-activated cation current (I_h) (Deng et al., 2007a), and broad action potential duration (Threlfell et al., 2012). The striatum has the highest levels of cholinergic markers in the brain, including ACh, choline acetyltransferase (ChAT), and acetylcholinesterase (AChE) (Macintosh, 1941; Hebb and Silver, 1961; Woolf et al., 1984). Such a high density of cholinergic markers underscores the importance of ACh neurotransmission in the striatum. Therefore, understanding striatal physiology requires careful consideration of the activity of ChIs and the consequences of changes in cholinergic signaling.

Classically, the striatum is subdivided according to synaptic connectivity. For example, the dorsal striatum receives DA-ergic input primarily from substantia nigra pars compacta (SNc) (Hattori et al., 1991) and sends projections to ventrolateral substantia nigra pars reticulata (SNr) and the globus pallidus. The ventral striatum receives the majority of DA from ventral tegmental area (VTA) projections, and in turn, sends inhibitory projections into the dorsomedial SNr (Maurin et al., 1999) and globus pallidus. In rodents, the dorsal and ventral striatum subserve different functions: The dorsal striatum is implicated in sensorimotor functions such as serial order learning (Yin, 2010), stimulus-response habit formation (Devan et al., 2011), and performance of learned instrumental tasks (Shiflett et al., 2010), whereas the ventral striatum is important for the reinforcement of appetitive behaviors including drugs of abuse (Robinson and Berridge, 2000) and healthy rewards, such as food intake (Kelley, 2004). Different functional roles are attributed to lateral vs. medial regions of the dorsal striatum. The dorsolateral region, or the "sensorimotor striatum," receives strong motor and premotor cortical inputs, and is therefore particularly important for habit formation (Künzle, 1975; Haber et al., 2000). The dorsomedial striatum, referred to as the "associative striatum," receives inputs from limbic regions as well as prefrontal cortex, and is involved in behavioral flexibility, reward-associated motor learning, and reaction time (Hauber and Schmidt, 1994; Ragozzino, 2003). Gradients of afferent connectivity most likely influence overall striatal output (Voorn et al., 2004), suggesting that these subdivisions are an oversimplification of striatal connectivity and function. Accepting that caveat, the distinctions in function of different striatal regions in the rodent brain provide a framework for ongoing investigations into the neural substrates of relevant behaviors, with an ultimate goal of understanding the functional role of analogous structures in the human brain.

ChIs are believed to be the analogs of tonically active neurons (TANs) identified by *in vivo* recordings in the putamen of primates. This correlation is based on similarities in ChAT immunoreactivity, electrophysiological, and morphological characteristics (Inokawa et al., 2010). Changes in TAN activity have been linked to motor and reinforcement learning. In classical sensorimotor Pavlovian conditioning, TANs pause activity within a second after presentation of the conditioned stimulus (CS), followed by a transient increase in activity before recovery to baseline firing. This stereotyped neural behavior was described as the "conditioned pause response" (Kimura et al., 1984; Aosaki et al., 1994). This CS-induced change in firing is not dependent on motor activity, as a similar firing profile was observed when the animal was trained to withhold movement after CS presentation in a NO-GO task (Apicella et al., 1991). TANs also pause in response to aversive-CS, but not to neutral stimuli (Ravel et al., 1999). The conditioned pause response is therefore believed to encode salience value to external stimuli. Thus, changes in TAN activity may contribute to associative learning, particularly the relationship between environmental cues and outcomes. The circuitry responsible for the pause response is debated. Some evidence implicates a dependence on SNc DA-ergic tone (Watanabe and Kimura, 1998; Reynolds et al., 2004; Straub et al., 2014), however others have observed a change in TAN firing even in response to aversive stimuli that do not increase DA-ergic firing (Mirenowicz and Schultz, 1996; Ravel et al., 1999). We know that ChIs respond to many neurotransmitters, and this stereotypical pause in activity could be mediated by a variety of inputs. Synchronous changes in afferent activity likely mediate the pause response among multiple ChIs, resulting in a coordinated change in striatal cholinergic tone. Understanding the connectivity and neurotransmission that influences these cells may thus provide insight into learning phenomena.

STRIATAL CHOLINERGIC DYSFUNCTION IN PARKINSON'S DISEASE AND TREATMENT

The necessity of proper striatal neurotransmission for normal motor function is dramatically and tragically evidenced by the deficits observed in Parkinson's disease (PD). The first medical characterization of PD was published in 1817 (Parkinson, 1817):

> The first symptoms perceived are, a slight sense of weakness, with a proneness to trembling in some particular part; sometimes in the head, but most commonly in one of the hands and arms... After a few more months the patient is found to be less strict than usual in preserving an upright posture: this being most observable whilst walking.

Although this is the first formal description of the disease in Western literature, descriptions of the disease appeared in Eastern texts as old as 600 BC (Manyam, 1990; Zhang et al., 2006; Raudino, 2012; Ovallath and Deepa, 2013). Some ancient cultures used treatments derived from herbal preparations that contain anticholinergic compounds with similar pharmacology to some therapies prescribed today (Manyam and Sánchez-Ramos, 1999).

Today, we know that the bradykinesia, resting tremor, rigidity, and difficulty in initiating movement observed in PD arise from deficits in basal ganglia DA transmission. However, it is important to consider the balance between the actions of striatal ACh and DA in the etiology of PD. Previous beliefs held that the two neurotransmitters had opposing actions, which was supported by the partial relief of PD symptoms with administration of anticholinergic compounds. These therapies may restore the balance between the two neurotransmitter systems. Drugs with similar pharmacological properties are still in use, particularly for younger PD patients whose primary symptom is tremor (Hristova and Koller, 2000), but cognitive and autonomic side effects preclude their widespread use. While anticholinergic drugs can improve some symptoms of PD (Whyte et al., 1971; Cantello et al., 1986; Baba et al., 2012), it has also been reported that elevation of ACh by treating patients with acetylcholinesterase inhibitors improves motor symptoms of PD (Chung et al., 2010). Although somewhat contradictory to the anticholinergic drug effects, inhibiting ACh degradation might enhance DA transmission through nicotinic acetylcholine receptors (nAChRs) on DA terminals. Alternatively, this treatment could promote cholinergic receptor desensitization to mimic anticholinergic drug effects. It is important to note that similar cholinesterase treatments have seen no effect on motor symptoms of PD (Poewe et al., 2006). Together, these observations highlight the importance of cholinergic transmission in striatal function under healthy and Parkinsonian conditions.

The physiology of ChIs is dramatically altered in PD. In humans, mutations in leucine-rich repeat kinase 2 (LRRK2) or the gene that encodes α-synuclein are both associated with a higher likelihood to develop PD (Simón-Sánchez et al., 2009). These genes are expressed in many basal ganglia cell types and the mechanisms that link these mutations to PD are the subject of ongoing studies (Gasser, 2009). ChIs in both rodents and humans express high levels of LRRK2 (Higashi et al., 2007; West et al., 2014), and abnormal kinase activity may contribute to pathological changes in ChI physiology. α-synuclein inclusions in the somata of ChIs are observed only in late PD but not early PD (Mori et al., 2008), suggesting that Lewy body-related interference of ChI physiology may be observed late in the disease.

In the 6-OHDA lesion model of PD, microdialysis studies have observed that striatal ACh levels are elevated in the DA depleted rat striatum (DeBoer et al., 1993), indicating a dysregulation of ChI excitability. Additionally, functional downregulation of M4—Cav2 coupling results in decreased sensitivity to autoinhibitory cholinergic transmission (Ding et al., 2006). Given the therapeutic effects of anticholinergic compounds in PD mentioned above, and the physiological changes in ChIs seen in animal models of the disease, it is evident that ACh is important in PD.

The development of DA replacement therapy to relieve the symptoms of PD in the 1960's revolutionized our understanding of neurotransmission in the dorsal striatum (Goetz, 2011). Currently, the biochemical precursor to DA, levodopa (L-DOPA) is the most effective clinical treatment for the motor symptoms of PD. L-DOPA crosses the blood brain barrier where it is then converted into DA by aromatic amino acid decarboxylase, thus increasing striatal levels of DA. Although L-DOPA effectively reverses PD locomotor disability, long-term treatment has its shortcomings, including shortening of the therapeutic window and psychiatric or mood disturbances such as impulse control disorders (Lesser et al., 1979; Voon et al., 2009; Santangelo et al., 2013a,b). Another debilitating side effect is the onset of levodopa-induced dyskinesia (LID), which is characterized by dystonia or choreic movements of the limbs, hands, or face. These side effects are potentially more debilitating than PD itself. This condition is highly prevalent, with LID development seen in approximately 40% of patients after 5 years of treatment, rising to nearly 90% after 10 years (Ahlskog and Muenter, 2001; Fabbrini et al., 2007). Interestingly, the age of onset of PD is a strong determinant for the development of LID, with earlier onset patients experiencing a more rapid expression of LID symptoms (Kostic et al., 1991; Kumar et al., 2005).

Pathological changes in striatal ACh signaling are related to the expression of LID. The anticholinergic benzatropine decreased dyskinesia in L-DOPA treated human PD patients (Pourcher et al., 1989), however, there are also reports of increased dyskinesia with anticholinergic treatment (Birket-Smith, 1974; Hauser and Olanow, 1993; Linazasoro, 1994). In a study of dyskinetic monkeys, the mAChR antagonist atropine changed the nature of dyskinesia from dystonia to chorea (Gomez-Mancilla and Bédard, 1993). Although these reports show mixed effects, they do suggest that cholinergic signaling influences the expression of LID. While examining a mouse model of LID, Ding et al. (2011b) observed enhanced levels of phosphorylated extracellular signal-regulated kinase (pERK) specifically in striatal ChIs. Electrophysiological recordings of ChIs revealed higher baseline and dopamine-induced firing rates in LID animals relative to vehicle-treated littermates. The increased ChI excitability and the expression of LID associated behaviors were both inhibited by blockers of MEK/ERK signaling (Ding et al., 2011b). Extending those studies, selective ablation of striatal ChIs decreases LID expression in a unilateral lesion model of PD (Won et al., 2014). Both nicotinic and muscarinic receptors are believed to contribute to LID. Treatment with either nAChR antagonists or nicotine improves abnormal involuntary movements (AIMs) in rodents and primates, which suggests that both drugs are decreasing nAChR function either through receptor blockade or desensitization (Quik et al., 2007; Bordia et al., 2010; Zhang et al., 2013). Although antimuscarinic drugs have mixed effects in human LID patients as mentioned above, there are reports of decreased LID expression (Pourcher et al., 1989), and a recent study of the Pitx3 mouse model of LID, a muscarinic receptor antagonist decreased behavioral expression of dyskinesia (Ding et al., 2011b). These findings support the conclusion that cholinergic transmission is important for mediating some aspects of LID and that pharmacological modulation of this system may help treat this debilitating condition.

Changes in striatal cholinergic signaling have been observed in patients with other movement disorders and psychiatric illnesses.

A partial list of these disorders and the nature of the changes in cholinergic activity can be found in **Table 1**. Considering the importance of striatal ChIs in both normal physiology and in disease, it is clear that this minority of cells plays a major role in the striatum. As such, understanding the nature of efferent and afferent synaptic connectivity of ChIs can provide important insights into striatal physiology.

AFFERENT CONNECTIONS TO ChIs

ChI excitability is affected by a remarkably large number of afferent input types and post-synaptic receptors. A simplified summary of this complex story is presented in **Table 2** and **Figures 1**, **2**. This section outlines the current state of our understanding of afferent control of ChIs.

GABA

ChIs receive a variety of GABA-ergic inputs, both local and extrastriatal in origin. GABA can inhibit cells by activating ionotropic $GABA_A$ receptors, which increases Cl- conductance. Of the $GABA_A$ receptor subunits, the α2, α4, β2/3 subunits are most highly expressed in the striatum (Persohn et al., 1992), and of potential interest, the α3 subunit is expressed only in choline acetyltransferase positive (ChAT+) cells (Rodríguez-Pallares et al., 2000). Local stimulation produces IPSCs in ChIs, and these events are blocked by bicuculline, indicating that ChIs express functional $GABA_A$ receptors (Sato et al., 2014). GABA also activates metabotropic $GABA_B$ receptors, G-protein coupled receptors (GPCRs) which decrease cell excitation by coupling to the $G_{i/o}$ protein and negatively regulating adenylyl cyclase (AC) (Bettler et al., 2004). Neither immunohistochemical examination of $GABA_B$ expression in ChIs nor the electrophysiological effects of selective $GABA_B$ activation on ChI excitability have been reported. *In vivo*, microdialysis experiments suggest that tonic activity at $GABA_A$ receptors regulates ChI excitability, whereas the $GABA_B$ receptors do not tonically inhibit ChI activity (DeBoer and Westerink, 1994).

Locally, GABA-ergic MSNs form synaptic connections with ChIs. Substance P-containing inputs are more prevalent than enkephalin-containing terminals, perhaps indicating that D1 MSNs have a more prominent influence over ChI activity compared to D2 MSNs (Martone et al., 1992). MSNs in the intact brain exist in one of two states of excitability, either an up or down state. In the up state, cells rest at a depolarized membrane potential, and are more likely to fire spontaneous action potentials compared to the relatively hyperpolarized down state (Wilson and Groves, 1981). The excitability state of MSNs will thus influence the inhibitory tone on ChIs. In the slice preparation MSNs are silent, and GABA released from these neurons will have minimal impact on ChIs. However, optogenetic activation of MSNs evoked a small amplitude IPSC in ~75% of ChIs, suggesting that the MSN-ChI connection is highly prevalent (Chuhma et al., 2011). Ultrastructural analysis of TAN connectivity in primates shows that approximately 24% of all synaptic contacts onto ChAT+ cells originate from MSN axon collaterals (Gonzales et al., 2013). In sum, GABA release from MSN onto ChIs is likely a major determinant of excitability of these cells *in vivo*.

ChIs also receive synaptic inputs from GABA-ergic interneurons. nAChR activation, presumably located on GABA-ergic interneurons, inhibits tonic firing of ChIs (De Rover et al., 2002; Sullivan et al., 2008). Not all GABA-ergic interneurons project to ChIs, however: PV positive FSIs project to MSNs and other interneurons, but do not inhibit ChIs (Szydlowski et al., 2013). Currently, NPY-expressing PLTS GABA-ergic interneurons are the best candidate for inhibition of ChIs, as ultrastructural analysis suggests synaptic connections with choline acetyltransferase-positive striatal neurons (Vuillet et al., 1992). However, there is no direct electrophysiological or functional evidence for this connection. It is unknown if calretinin positive interneurons form connections with ChIs.

Extrastriatal sources of GABA may also inhibit ChIs. Co-release of DA and GABA from nigrostriatal neurons onto MSNs occurs via a VMAT2-dependent vesicular mechanism (Tritsch et al., 2012). Cholinergic activation of nAChRs on those terminals was recently shown to enhance GABAergic inputs to MSNs (Nelson et al., 2014b). We know that DA projections form prominent synaptic contacts onto ChIs (Dimova et al., 1993; Li et al., 2002), and if some of these DA teminals co-release GABA, these inputs could profoundly affect tonic activity of ChIs *in vivo*. In addition, these projections may also have important implications in PD, as the loss of SNc projections could decrease this source of GABA-ergic tone onto ChIs, potentially contributing to increases in striatal ACh levels. Other non-dopaminergic projection neurons may contribute to GABA inhibition of ChIs. In addition to DA neurons, the VTA possesses GABA projection neurons that inhibit ventral striatum ChIs (Brown et al., 2012), but whether dorsal striatum ChIs receive GABA input from non-dopaminergic projection neurons in SNc or VTA is not known. Nigrostriatal non-dopaminergic projections have been observed (Gerfen et al., 1987; Rodríguez and González-Hernández, 1999), but the physiological effects of these presumed GABA projections on ChI activity have not been studied. These extrastriatal GABA projections may provide a means to inhibit ChIs that is independent of intrastriatal GABA sources.

GLUTAMATE – IONOTROPIC RECEPTORS

Glutamatergic innervation of ChIs is predominantly extrastriatal (Künzle, 1975). Glutamate induces rapid depolarization through activation of postsynaptically expressed AMPA, NMDA, or kainate receptors. About half of all ChIs are immunopositive for GluR1, GluR2, and GluR4 subunits (Bernard et al., 1997; Deng et al., 2007b), despite the presence of mRNA of all 4 GluR subunits (Richardson et al., 2000). AMPA receptors expressed on ChIs show rapid deactivation, desensitization, and a relatively high permeability to Ca^{2+}, and these properties differ from the AMPA receptors expressed by MSNs (Götz et al., 1997). mRNA for NR1 and NR2D are present at high levels in ChIs, while expression of NR2A mRNA is contested (Landwehrmeyer et al., 1995; Standaert et al., 1999; Richardson et al., 2000). 90% of ChIs are immunopositive for the kainate receptors GluR5/6/7 (Chen et al., 1996). In a slice preparation, bath application of an NMDAR positive allosteric modulator increases ChI firing rate (Feng et al., 2014), implying that glutamate tone in the slice preparation contributes to baseline ChI excitability. Considering the expression of these

Table 1 | Diseases associated with striatal cholinergic dysfunction.

Disorder	Nature of change	Species	Citations
Parkinson's disease (PD)	Smokers are less likely to develop PD	Human	Morens et al., 1995; Allam et al., 2004; Quik et al., 2012
	↓ symptoms with anticholinergic drugs	Human (drug trial)	Katzenschlager et al., 2003; Lanska, 2010; Fox et al., 2011; Fernandez, 2012
	↓ AChE activity	Human (PET Scan)	Gilman et al., 2010
	↓ nAChR binding	Human (postmortem)	Rinne et al., 1991; Aubert et al., 1992; Court et al., 2000; Hellström-Lindahl and Court, 2000; Bohr et al., 2005; Gotti et al., 2006a
		Monkey (MPTP lesion)	Kulak et al., 2002; Quik and McIntosh, 2006
	↓ M1 binding	Human (PM)	Sirviö et al., 1989; Lange et al., 1993; Piggott et al., 2003
	Changes in CHRNB3 gene	Human (genotyping)	Bar-Shira et al., 2014
Huntington's disease	↓ in symptoms with AChE inhibitor	Rat (3-NP lesion)	Kumar and Kumar, 2009
	↓ ChAT activity	Human	Bird and Iversen, 1974; Enna et al., 1976a; Suzuki et al., 2001a
	↓ ChAT mRNA	Mouse (R6/1 model)	Smith et al., 2006
	↓ mAChR binding	Human (postmortem)	Hiley and Bird, 1974; Enna et al., 1976a,b
Alzheimer's disease	↓ cognitive deficits with AChE	Rat (ketamine induced behavior)	Zugno et al., 2013
	↓ AChE levels (in NAc)	Human (PM)	Hammond and Brimijoin, 1988
	↓ nAChR binding sites in putamen, but not in caudate	Human (postmortem)	Shimohama et al., 1985
	No change in nAChR binding	Human (postmortem)	Aubert et al., 1992; Gotti et al., 2006a
	↓ cognitive deficits with α7 or α4β2 agonists	Human (drug trial)	Haydar and Dunlop, 2010
	↑ M1 binding	Human (postmortem)	Aubert et al., 1992
Schizophrenia	↑ likelihood to smoke	Human	Dalack et al., 1998; McEvoy and Allen, 2002
	↑ ChAT activity	Human (postmortem)	McGeer and McGeer, 1977
	↓ ChAT activity	Human (postmortem)	Bird et al., 1977
	↓ ChAT+ cells	Human (postmortem)	Holt et al., 1999
	↓ cognitive deficits with nicotine, α4β2 agonist	Human (drug trial)	Radek et al., 2010
	↑ nAChR binding	Human (postmortem)	Court et al., 2000
	↓ nAChR binding	Human (postmortem)	Durany et al., 2000
	↓ mAChR binding	Human (SPECT scan)	Raedler et al., 2003
	↓ M1 levels	Human (postmortem)	Dean et al., 1996
	Changes in CHNRA7 gene	Human (postmortem, genotyping)	Leonard et al., 2002
Bipolar disorder	↓ β2* nAChR binding	Human (PET scan)	Hannestad et al., 2013
	Changes in CHRNA7 gene	Human (genotyping)	Hong et al., 2004; Ancín et al., 2010
Tourette syndrome	↓ ChAT+ cells	Human (Postmortem)	Kataoka et al., 2010
	↓ tics with cholinesterase inhibitor	Mouse (DOI induced head tics)	Hayslett and Tizabi, 2003
		Human (drug trial)	Cubo et al., 2008
	↓ tics with nicotine	Mouse (DOI induced head tics)	Hayslett and Tizabi, 2003
		Human (drug trial)	Shytle et al., 1996; McEvoy and Allen, 2002
	↓ tics with nAChR antagonist	Mouse (DOI induced head tics)	Hayslett and Tizabi, 2003
		Human (drug trial)	Sanberg et al., 1998; Silver et al., 2000

(Continued)

Table 1 | Continued

Disorder	Nature of change	Species	Citations
	Alternative splicing in ACh related genes	Human (genotyping)	Tian et al., 2011
Attention Deficit Hyperactivity Disorder	No change in performance on attention tasks with nAChR agonist	Human (drug trial)	Jucaite et al., 2014
	↑ performance on attention tasks with nAChR agonist	Rat (MK801 induced attentional impairment)	Rezvani et al., 2012
		Human (drug trial)	Wilens and Decker, 2007; Bain et al., 2013; Potter et al., 2014
	Changes in choline transporter gene	Human (genotyping)	English et al., 2009
	Changes in CHRNA4 gene	Human (genotyping)	Todd et al., 2003; Lee et al., 2008; Guan et al., 2009; Wallis et al., 2009

glutamate receptors on ChIs, it is not surprising that application of AMPA, NMDA, or kainate excites ChIs (Calabresi et al., 1998b; Vorobjev et al., 2000; Cepeda et al., 2001). Collectively, the expression of the three functional classes of glutamate receptors support the idea that glutamate is an important determinant of ChI excitability.

Electron microscopy has revealed that glutamate synapses comprise 13% of total synaptic connections onto ChIs (Gonzales et al., 2013). In the dorsolateral striatum, glutamate is released from cells located in the sensorimotor cortex and the centromedian/parafascicular nucleus of the thalamus, with the vast majority of excitatory projections being thalamic in origin (Berendse and Groenewegen, 1990; Lapper and Bolam, 1992; Thomas et al., 2000; Ding et al., 2010). Glutamatergic inputs, predominantly thalamostriatal projections are likely responsible for synchronous activation of ChIs, which has been suggested to coordinate DA release through activation of nAChRs on DA terminals (Ding et al., 2010; Threlfell et al., 2012). Another source of glutamate, corelease from SNc dopamine terminals, is a topic of debate—Optogenetic activation of SNc dopaminergic axons can produce a small amplitude EPSC in dorsal striatum MSNs (Tritsch et al., 2012). However, using a similar optogenetic approach, others report that glutamate and DA are only coreleased in the ventral, but not dorsal striatum (Stuber et al., 2010). Both of these studies were performed while recording from MSNs, and the electrophysiological significance of SNc-derived glutamate on ChI excitability has not yet been reported. Due to the close proximity between MSNs and ChIs, one would also expect an influence of this source of glutamate on ChIs (Dimova et al., 1993; Li et al., 2002). In this case, the loss of SNc projections in PD may impact the degree to which glutamate modifies ChI activity.

Serotonergic (5-HT) projection neurons from the dorsal raphe nucleus also express glutamate-like immunoreactivity. In culture, 5-HT cells form glutamatergic autapses, indicating that 5-HT projections may functionally co-release glutamate (Nicholas et al., 1992; Johnson and Yee, 1995). The extent to which changes in 5-HT transmission are associated with altered striatal glutamatergic signaling is unknown, but this may contribute to striatal dysfunction in mood disorders. SSRI treatment of depression will prolong the action of synaptically released 5-HT, and may lead to presynaptic inhibition through autoreceptors. This may alter local excitation via co-released glutamate to decrease striatal excitation.

Striatal ChIs also co-release glutamate with ACh (Higley et al., 2011). One isoform of the vesicular glutamate transporter, VGLUT3, is highly expressed in ChIs, and evidence suggests co-expression of this transporter with the vesicular ACh transporter on the same synaptic vesicles. These transporters act synergistically to optimize vesicular loading of ACh and glutamate (Nelson et al., 2014a). Vglut3 knock-out mice have a hypocholinergic striatum, presumably due to a decrease in loading of both glutamate and ACh into vesicles, and also due to less excitatory drive onto synaptically connected ChIs (Gras et al., 2008). The functional consequences of these non-thalamic/non-cortical sources of glutamatergic drive onto ChIs have not been studied in depth.

GLUTAMATE – METABOTROPIC RECEPTORS

Glutamate also mediates long-term modulation of ChIs via metabotropic glutamate receptors (mGluRs). Excitatory group I mGluRs, which include mGluR1 and mGluR5, are highly expressed on ChIs (Tallaksen-Greene et al., 1998; Bell et al., 2002; Conn et al., 2005), and application of group I agonists induce excitation (Calabresi et al., 1999; Pisani et al., 2001; Berg et al., 2007). This excitation is mediated by a combination of cation currents through TrpC channels downstream of $G_{q\alpha}$, as well as inhibition of the chloride activated K^+ channel Slo2.1 (Berg et al., 2007). The group II mGluRs, which consist of mGluR2 and mGluR3, decrease excitability by inhibiting AC through activation of $G_{i/o\alpha}$ (Diraddo et al., 2014). mGluR2, mRNA expression on ChIs (Testa et al., 1994; Bell et al., 2002) indicate that agonists of these receptors would theoretically decrease cell excitability. However, group II mGluRs are more involved in the modulation of synaptic inputs onto ChIs, as activation of these receptors results in no change in membrane potential, but decreases the amplitude of both excitatory and inhibitory synaptic inputs onto ChIs (Pisani et al., 2002; Martella et al., 2009). Of the group III mGluRs, only mGluR7 is expressed on ChIs, at a prevalence of 38% with no expression of mGluR4, 6, or 8. As with group II mGluRs, group III mGluRs decrease presynaptic release probability by inhibition of the AC pathway (Bell et al., 2002). Although rapid ChI excitation and inhibition are mediated by ionotropic

Table 2 | Neurotransmitter systems and their effects on ChI activity.

Neurotransmitter	Source	Postsynaptic receptor targets	Effect on ChI
GABA	MSN PLTS interneurons SNc (?)	$GABA_A$	$GABA_A$: Inhibition DeBoer and Westerink, 1994
Glutamate	Intralaminar thalamic nuclei Sensorimotor cortex SNc Raphe nucleus ChI	GluR1, 2, 4 GluN1, 2D Kainate	AMPA, NMDA, Kainate: Excitation Calabresi et al., 1998b; Vorobjev et al., 2000; Cepeda et al., 2001 mGluR1,5: Excitation Calabresi et al., 1999; Pisani et al., 2001; Berg et al., 2007 mGluR2: Inhibition Martella et al., 2009 mGluR7: No direct effect Bell et al., 2002
Dopamine	SNc DA-ergic interneurons	D1 (low levels) D2 D5	Increased excitation Aosaki et al., 1998; Centonze et al., 2003; Ding et al., 2011b or Decreased excitation Deng et al., 2007a; Chuhma et al., 2014
5-HT	Raphe nucleus	5-HT2 5-HT6 5-HT7	Increased excitation Blomeley and Bracci, 2005 Excitation Bonsi et al., 2007 Excitation Bonsi et al., 2007 or No effect Blomeley and Bracci, 2005
Histamine	TMN Mast cells	H1 H2 H3	Depolarization and action potential firing Bell et al., 2000
Substance P	D1 MSNs	NK1	Depolarization, inward shift in holding current Aosaki and Kawaguchi, 1996 Increased ACh release Arenas et al., 1991; Preston et al., 2000
Enkephalin	D2 MSNs	DOR	Decreased excitation Mulder et al., 1984
		KOR	Decreased excitation Schoffelmeer et al., 1997 No effect on K+ induced ACh release Arenas et al., 1990; Jackisch et al., 1993
		MOR	Decreased excitation Ponterio et al., 2013
Dynorphin	D1 MSNs	KOR	Excitation at low concentrations of agonist Crain and Shen, 1996 Inhibition at higher concentrations of agonist Gross et al., 1990
Noradrenaline	Locus coeruleus	β1	Depolarization, increased action potential firing Pisani et al., 2003
Adenosine	Degradation of ATP	A_1 A_{2A}	Inhibition of ACh release Brown et al., 1990 Increased ACh release Kurokawa et al., 1994 No change in ACh release Jin and Fredholm, 1997
ATP	Synaptic release	P_2X P_2Y	No change in holding current Scheibler et al., 2004
Nitric oxide	NOS+ PLTS interneurons		Depolarization Centonze et al., 2001

Summary of the neurotransmitter systems and other neuromodulators involved in the regulation of ChI activity. "?" denotes potential yet untested source of neurotransmitter release.

receptors, it is important to consider that glutamate can have long term modulatory effects on ChI excitability via mGluR activation.

DOPAMINE

In addition to GABA and glutamate, there are a number of other neurotransmitter systems that affect ChI activity. Striatal dopamine levels are the highest of any region in the brain and it is a principal determinant of striatal function. The predominant source of dopaminergic innervation of the dorsal striatum is A9 neurons—neurons which have cell bodies in the SNc and project broadly into the striatum, forming hundreds of thousands of synaptic connections per neuron (Kubota et al., 1987; Chang, 1988; Arbuthnott and Wickens, 2007; Moss and Bolam, 2008; Matsuda et al., 2009; Threlfell and Cragg, 2011). Although synaptic connections to MSNs are well documented, some reports demonstrate dopamine cells synapse onto ChAT positive cells (Hattori et al., 1976) while others report that dopamine modulates ChIs through volume transmission (Lehmann and Langer,

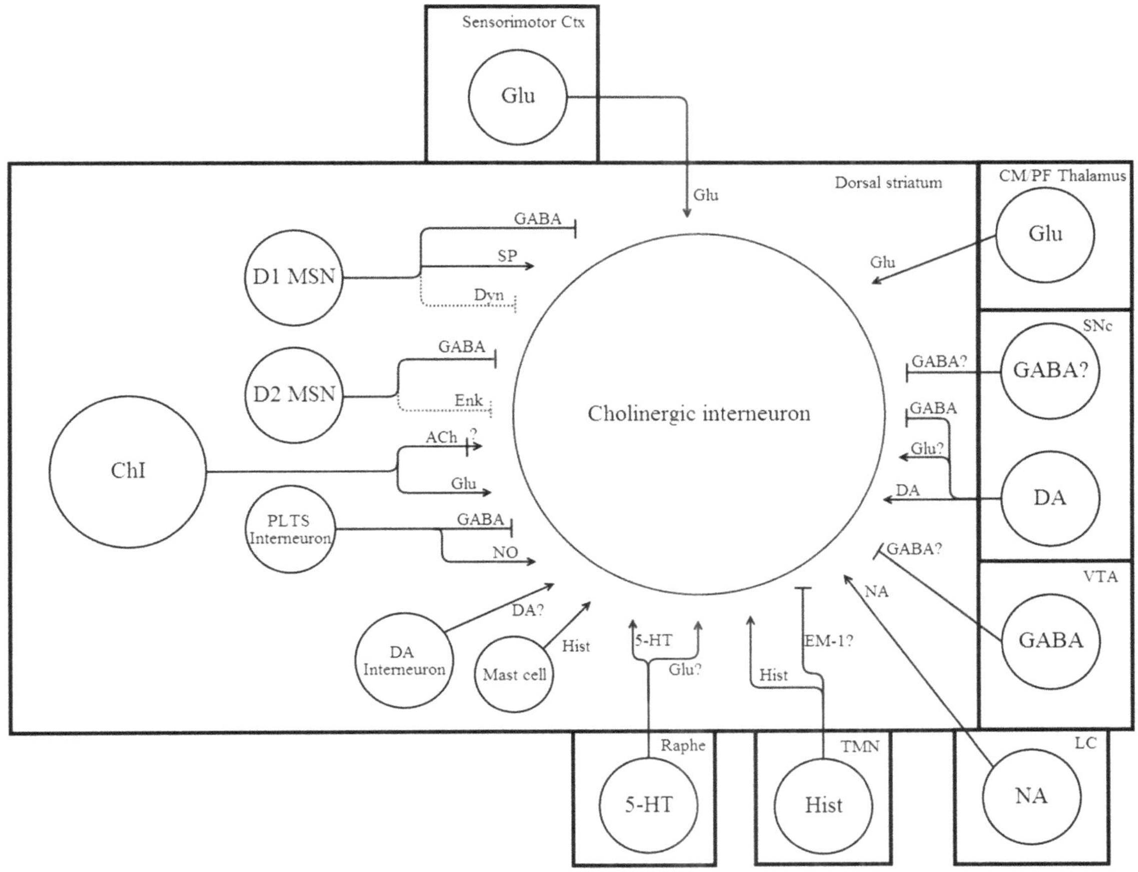

FIGURE 1 | Network connectivity of dorsal striatal cholinergic interneurons. Simplified schematic illustrating some of the afferent synaptic inputs onto ChIs. Arrow heads indicate excitation, while perpendicular lines indicate inhibition. Dotted lines indicate a weak synaptic input. "?" denotes uncertain or untested inputs that are expected by either anatomical or physiological results. References that support afferent connections to ChIs can be found in the text and **Table 2**.

1983). These nigral dopaminergic neurons may exist in 4 different activity states. The tonically active state is independent of excitatory drive, as the neurons will fire at a rate of around 3 Hz *in vivo* or *ex vivo* in a slice preparation (Grace and Bunney, 1984; Hyland et al., 2002; Zhou et al., 2006; Ding et al., 2011a; Henny et al., 2012; Guatteo et al., 2013). They also can transition to burst activity with excitatory inputs increasing activity to around 20 Hz (Grace and Bunney, 1984; Hyland et al., 2002). In addition to these two active states, the cells may exist in one of two silent states, either hyperpolarization below action potential threshold, or depolarization block. Activity of these neurons is crucially important to normal striatal function (Gasser, 2009).

Postsynaptically, the majority of ChIs express D2 and D5 receptors with only about 20% of the neurons expressing low levels of D1 receptors (Dawson et al., 1988; Bergson et al., 1995; Yan et al., 1997). D2 receptors generally decrease neuronal exitability through activation of $G_{i/o\alpha}$, which also inhibits AC activity to decrease cAMP levels. D5 receptors are members of the D1 family that activate AC through G_s and generally increase excitability (Beaulieu and Gainetdinov, 2011). In the slice preparation, bath application of DA can strongly excite ChIs (Aosaki et al., 1998; Centonze et al., 2003; Ding et al., 2011b), however others have reported that DA inhibits ChIs by prolonging slow afterhyperpolarization duration (Deng et al., 2007a), and that optogenetic activation of DA terminals induces a pause in ChI firing (Chuhma et al., 2014). It was also reported that amphetamine-induced increases in striatal DA rhas no effect on ACh efflux *in vivo* (Abercrombie and DeBoer, 1997), implying that, under those conditions, elevated DA does not significantly affect cholinergic tone. Clearly, DA can affect ChI excitability, and the conditions under which DA either excites or inhibits these neurons will require further study.

In addition to this important extrastriatal source of DA, there also exists a small population of striatal DA interneurons in both primates and rodents (Dubach et al., 1987; Cossette et al., 2005; Ibáñez-Sandoval et al., 2010). Interestingly, the number of striatal TH+ cells increases following acute experimental dopamine depletion in both rodents and primates (Tashiro et al., 1989; Betarbet et al., 1997; Smith and Kieval, 2000; Jollivet et al., 2004). This is potentially a compensatory mechanism designed to counteract the loss of DA-ergic innervation from SNc. Strangely, the number of striatal TH+ cells is decreased in humans with PD

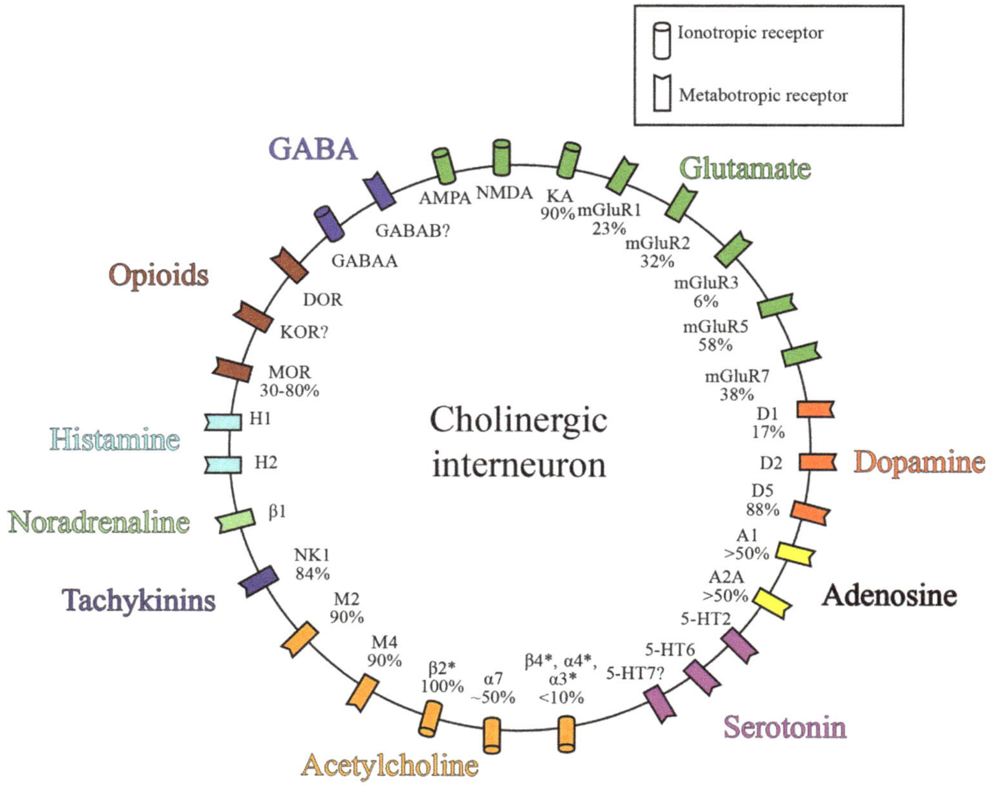

FIGURE 2 | Receptor expression on ChIs. Simplified diagram depicting a subset of known receptor classes expressed on ChIs grouped by neurotransmitter. Values represent percent of ChIs that express the given receptor. References for receptor expression by ChIs can be found in the text and **Table 2**.

(Huot et al., 2007), highlighting one difference between experimentally induced PD and the actual pathogenesis of the disease in humans. These DA interneurons form inhibitory GABA-ergic synapses with MSNs (Ibáñez-Sandoval et al., 2010). Whether or not these TH+ interneurons make DA-ergic and/or GABA-ergic synaptic contacts with ChIs is yet to be determined. Another interesting question to address would be whether or not these TH+ interneurons undergo changes in physiology that serve in a homeostatic role in the Parkinsonian striatum. Independent of changes in cell numbers outlined above, increased excitability following DA depletion may counteract low levels of striatal DA to help maintain striatal function. This small minority of striatal cells remains an interesting focus for future investigations.

ACETYLCHOLINE

ChIs receive synaptic inputs from other ChIs. Both nAChRs and mAChRs are expressed at various levels on ChIs. With respect to nAChR expression, *in situ* hybridization has shown that all ChIs express mRNA for β2 subunits, about half express α7 mRNA, while other subunit mRNAs are expressed at low levels (Azam et al., 2003). In support of the idea that ChIs express nAChRs, nicotine application to a slice preparation induces ACh release (Sandor et al., 1991). Interestingly, that effect was only seen in slices from animals that had undergone dopamine depletion with 6-OHDA treatment or in the presence of the D2 receptor antagonist sulpiride. These data suggest that resolving the nAChR-mediated ACh release requires elimination of D2 receptor mediated inhibition (Sandor et al., 1991).

The mAChR component of ACh modulation is through activation of the $G_{i/o}$ coupled M2 and M4 receptors (Weiner et al., 1990; Smiley et al., 1999; Ding et al., 2006), thus acting as an autoinhibitory clamp to prevent excessive ACh release. No co-expression of M1 and ChAT is observed in the striatum (Dawson et al., 1990; Alcantara et al., 2001).

Synchronized activity in ChIs is observed following presentation of behaviorally salient stimuli (Apicella et al., 1997; Ravel et al., 1999). Although this synchronous firing has been linked to coordinated thalamostriatal inputs (Ding et al., 2010), ChI projections to other ChIs may also contribute to this synchrony through positive feedback control to coordinate strong increases in ACh. Whether or not nAChR mediated transmission contributes to ChI-ChI signaling has yet to be reported.

SEROTONIN

Serotonin is a major determinant of ChI excitability. 5-HT-ergic projections originate from the raphe nucleus in the hind brain. These cells fire tonically at a rate of about 1–2 Hz (Innis and Aghajanian, 1987; Sprouse et al., 1989; Haj-Dahmane et al., 1991), releasing 5-HT into many brain areas including the striatum. 5-HT has an overall direct excitatory effect on ChIs, increasing action potential firing and membrane depolarization (Blomeley and Bracci, 2005; Bonsi et al., 2007). Activation of the G_q-coupled

5-HT2 receptors increases excitability due to a decrease in the amplitude of both the slow and medium afterhyperpolarization (AHP) (Blomeley and Bracci, 2005). It has not been examined if 5-HT receptor classes 1A, 3, or 4 are expressed on ChIs, however selective agonists of these receptor classes do not induce changes in ChI excitability (Blomeley and Bracci, 2005). 5-HT6 activation excites ChIs (Bonsi et al., 2007). The contribution of the 5-HT7 receptor to excitation is debated, as Blomeley and Bracci (2005) reported no effect, while Bonsi et al. (2007) observed depolarization.

HISTAMINE

Histamine (HA) is a neurotransmitter that was first identified as a peripheral vasodilator with an effect on respiratory patterns and muscle tone (Dale and Laidlaw, 1910). Originally described in the brain in 1984, HA immunoreactive fibers were found to project widely throughout the brain including the striatum (Haas et al., 2008). HA-ergic cell bodies reside only in a small region of the posterior hypothalamus, the tuberomamillary nucleus (Panula et al., 1984; Blandina et al., 2012). Histamine is also produced by mast cells (Schwartz et al., 1986).

HA can act on 4 different types of G-protein coupled receptors, H1 through H4 (Parsons and Ganellin, 2006). These receptors are widely expressed, but only H1, H2, and H3 are highly expressed in the striatum, with H1 and H2 expressed on ChIs, and the autoreceptor H3 being expressed presynaptically on HA-ergic terminals. H1 and H2 are excitatory, coupling to G_q and G_s respectively, while the inhibitory H3 receptor is coupled with G_i (Timmerman, 1989; Haas et al., 2008). HA application has the net result of depolarization of ChIs, presumably acting through by H1 receptors (Bell et al., 2000). In the ventral striatum, ACh overflow is increased following H1 activation, while blockade of H2 increases ACh overflow, presumably through activation of H2 on GABA interneurons (Prast et al., 1999b). The same group found an increase in ACh overflow with concurrent H3 activation, an effect mediated by presynaptically expressed GABA interneurons (Prast et al., 1999a).

OPIOIDS

ChIs are also sensitive to opioidergic modulation. δ, κ, and μ opioid receptors (DOR, KOR, and MOR, respectively) are the three major classes of opioid receptors in mammals. These receptors inhibit cell activity through coupling with $G_{i/o}$ proteins (Mansour et al., 1994; Tso and Wong, 2003), and are activated endogenously by a number of tightly regulated peptides. The endogenous opioid enkephalin activates DORs, and is produced by D2 expressing indirect pathway MSNs. mRNA for DORs is expressed in striatal ChIs (Le Moine et al., 1994), and activation of these receptors decreases ACh release (Mulder et al., 1984). The low number of synaptic connections between enkephalinergic cells and ChAT positive cells (Martone et al., 1992) suggests that enkephalin may only minimally inhibit ChI activity endogenously, but this does not preclude the possibility of volume transmission. Systematic investigation of endogenous DOR effects on ChI excitability has not been reported.

KOR is another major class of opioid receptors in the striatum. The endogenous opioid dynorphin is produced by D1 expressing direct pathway MSNs, and activates KORs. Like DORs, KORs are widely expressed in the striatum (Fallon and Leslie, 1986; Mansour et al., 1994). Compared to the DOR or MOR, the KOR receptor can be associated with $G_{i/o}$ as well as G_s. This bipolar effect of KOR activation is concentration dependent. At very low, subnanomolar concentrations of agonist, KOR preferably couples to G_s (Crain and Shen, 1996), but increasing the concentration results in the activation of signaling cascades downstream of $G_{i/o}$ (Gross et al., 1990; Claye et al., 1996). Thus, depending on the level of striatal dynorphin, ChIs may either increase or decrease their excitability. KOR activation decreases ACh release in the striatum (Mulder et al., 1991; Schoffelmeer et al., 1997), however, different studies showed no effect of KOR activation on ACh release (Arenas et al., 1990; Jackisch et al., 1993). These apparently contradictory findings could result from the biphasic dose-dependent intracellular coupling of the KOR. It is also possible that the KOR effects on ACh release occur through indirect modulation, as there has not been a direct demonstration of co-localization of KOR with ChAT expression in striatum, nor is there direct electrophysiological evidence of KOR expression on ChIs.

The MOR is also coexpressed on ChAT positive striatal cells, however with tremendous diurnal variation, fluctuating from 30% coexpression in the daytime to a peak of 80% coexpression in the afternoon (Jabourian et al., 2005). Activation of MOR by exogenous DAMGO decreases ChI firing (Ponterio et al., 2013). MOR-inhibition of ACh release lowers the DA release probability in striatum by limiting activation of presynaptic nAChRs (Britt and McGehee, 2008). Endomorphin-1 (EM-1), an endogenous agonist at the MOR, shows only weak immunoreactivity in the striatum. EM-1 may be co-released by histaminergic neurons, as the EM-1 immunoreactivity signal is very prominent in the posterior hypothalamus (Martin-Schild et al., 1999). In addition, some endogenous agonists have overlapping affinity for different opioid receptor classes, such as Leu-enkephalin, which activates both DORs, and MORs at physiological concentrations (Jabourian et al., 2005).

TACHYKININS

Tachykinins are another class of neuropeptides expressed in the striatum. In addition to producing GABA and dynorphin, D1-expressing MSNs also express the tachykinin Substance P. Terminals that contain Substance P. form synaptic connections with ChIs. Substance P. is a potent activator of NK1 receptors, which are expressed by ChIs (Bolam et al., 1986; Richardson et al., 2000). Activation of NK1 results in excitation (Aosaki and Kawaguchi, 1996) and increased ACh release (Arenas et al., 1991; Preston et al., 2000).

EFFERENT CONNECTIONS OF ChIs

Even though the ChIs make up a small fraction of cells in the striatum, they possess a large synaptic arbor and thus send ACh projections broadly throughout the striatum. As such, changes in ChI physiology influence a multitude of postsynaptic targets by activation of nicotinic and muscarinic ACh receptors. This section addresses the effects of ACh neurotransmission.

NICOTINIC ACETYLCHOLINE RECEPTORS

Nicotinic acetylcholine receptors (nAChRs) are ligand-gated, pentameric ion channels that are activated by endogenous ACh, exogenous nicotine, or other ligands. nAChRs can be expressed both pre and postsynaptically, where they induce depolarization and increase excitability. Presynaptic nAChRs enhance release of several different neurotransmitter types (MacDermott et al., 1999). The subunits that are assembled into neuronal nAChRs include α2-α10 and β2-β4 (Patrick et al., 1993; McGehee and Role, 1995; Dani, 2001). They can be composed of homomeric or heteromeric subunit combinations, which determine characteristic pharmacological and biophysical properties of the receptor (Fenster et al., 1997; Gotti et al., 2006b). In the striatum, the most common nAChR subunits are the α4, α6, α7, β2, and β3, although other subunits are present at lower levels (Quik et al., 2007). Generally, nAChR activation induces rapid depolarization, but Ca^{2+} entry, particularly through homomeric α7 nAChRs can lead to rapid changes in neurotransmitter release or long term changes in cellular function through activation of Ca^{2+} dependent intracellular cascades, such as altered transcription through pCREB activation (Mulle et al., 1992; Chang and Berg, 2001; Hu et al., 2002; Wu et al., 2009; Del Barrio et al., 2011).

MUSCARINIC ACETYLCHOLINE RECEPTORS

In comparison to the rapid, excitatory effect of nAChR activation, mAChR activation serves a more long-term modulatory role. Activation of mAChRs can either increase or decrease cell excitability. A total of 5 subtypes of mAChRs have been isolated and cloned, but they are generally divided into 2 classes based on differences in their intracellular signaling cascades. The excitatory mAChRs, consisting of M1, M3, and M5, couple to $G_{q/11}$ and induce activation of the phospholipase C pathway (Lin et al., 2004). The inhibitory receptors, M2, and M4, couple to $G_{i/o}$ proteins and decrease activity of adenylyl cyclase (Wess, 1996). All 5 mAChRs are expressed in the striatum (Yan et al., 2001), however M1 and M4 are more heavily expressed than other isoforms, with a small presence of M2 and very low levels of M3 and M5 expression (Yasuda et al., 1993). Muscarinic receptors are not limited to somatic expression, as terminal expression of mAChRs serves to modulate neurotransmitter release probability. Expression of M2 receptors on ChI terminals serves an autoinhibitory role (Hersch et al., 1994). Additionally, neurotransmitter release at incoming afferents can be sensitive to mAChR modulation, as these mAChRs can receive synaptic inputs from ChIs. Because mAChR activation can either increase or decrease cell excitability, the net effect of ACh release depends on the patterns of postsynaptic mAChR expression. For each major striatal postsynaptic target, both the nicotinic and muscarinic effects on neuronal excitability will be addressed.

MEDIUM SPINY NEURONS

GABA-ergic MSN projection neurons are the sole output of the striatum. Direct activation of AChRs on MSNs therefore represent a direct effect of ACh on striatal output. MSNs are generally believed to lack nAChRs (Matsubayashi et al., 2001; Luo et al., 2013), although Liu et al. (2007) reports that direct activation of nAChRs on MSNs by nicotine induces depolarization. This direct nAChR modulation of MSN activity has not been explored in depth, as the evidence that MSNs express nAChRs is quite limited. Interestingly, lesion studies indicate that only about 20% of α4β2 nAChRs are expressed on DA terminals (Quik and Wonnacott, 2011). Thus, the contribution of these receptors to striatal circuitry likey involves expression on GABAergic interneurons and presynaptic projections from a range of cell types. Resolving the complete physiological role of striatal α4β2 receptors is a topic of ongoing investigations.

The majority of studies of ACh-mediated modulation of MSNs focuses on mAChR activation. Bath application of the mAChR agonist carbachol increases MSN excitation in the absence of synaptic input, both in a slice preparation and in dissociated cell culture (Hsu et al., 1996; Galarraga et al., 1999). Two mechanisms have been proposed to explain this excitation. One involves an M1 mediated decrease in the inhibitory KCNQ potassium (Kv7) current (Shen et al., 2005), while the other an M1 mediated inhibition of Ca^{2+} entry through N and P/Q type channels, which in turn decreases the duration of the AHP (Pérez-Garci et al., 2003; Perez-Rosello et al., 2005). Neither of these studies differentiates between the direct and indirect pathway MSNs, and the mechanisms could differ between these cell types. Inhibitory M4 receptors are expressed on a subpopulation of MSNs (Bernard et al., 1992), and functional electrophysiological evidence suggests that M4 decreases Ca^{2+} influx to decrease excitability (Howe and Surmeier, 1995). Direct pathway MSNs express both M1 and M4, while indirect pathway MSNs express M1. Less than half of indirect pathway MSNs express M4 (Bernard et al., 1992; Yan et al., 2001). Both classes of MSNs would be excited with M1 activation, but the differential expression pattern of the inhibitory M4 could mean that ACh influences the two classes of MSNs in opposing directions.

GABA-ERGIC INTERNEURONS

In addition to directly acting on MSNs, ACh can also modify striatal output through receptors on GABA interneurons that project to MSNs. Optogenetic activation of cholinergic cells produced IPSCs and IPSPs in MSNs that were inhibited by nAChR blockade. This microcircuit is believed to be a disynaptic connection, consisting of nAChR-expressing GABA interneurons that are activated by ACh, which then release GABA onto MSNs (English et al., 2011). The GABA interneurons that contribute to this inhibition of MSNs are likely the parvalbumin-expressing FSIs (Chang and Kita, 1992) and/or the NPY-expressing PLTS interneurons (English et al., 2011). However, English and coworkers did not observe an involvement of FSIs in the ChI-MSN interaction. Consistent with nAChR activation leading to elevated striatal GABA, inhibition of α7 receptors resulted in a decrease in striatal GABA in awake behaving animals (Beggiato et al., 2013), while activation of α7 nAChRs increases GABA levels (Campos et al., 2010).

Muscarinic receptor activation of GABA interneurons that project to MSNs can influence striatal output. Subcellular localization of the M2 receptor has been demonstrated in the NPY+ PLTS interneurons (Bernard et al., 1998). Consistent with this result, ACh decreases striatal GABA release (Marchi et al., 1990). More specifically, this is mediated by an inhibitory mAChR, as muscarine decreases GABA release onto MSNs (Sugita et al., 1991). Thus far, there are no reports of M1 receptor expression on GABA interneurons, but it is possible that M1-mediated enhancement of GABA output from one of the other interneuron subtypes neurons could contribute to striatal circuitry.

GLUTAMATERGIC TERMINALS

Glutamatergic inputs into the dorsal striatum originate primarily from the intralaminar nuclei of the thalamus and from the sensorimotor cortex, with a small amount of glutamate co-released from other terminals as well (Higley et al., 2011). nAChR expression on glutamatergic terminals provides a mechanism for cholinergic enhancement of excitatory drive onto MSNs. Increased glutamate release through activation of presynaptic nAChRs has been observed in brain regions such as the hippocampus, medial habenula, olfactory bulb and human neocortex (McGehee et al., 1995; Gray et al., 1996; Fisher and Dani, 2000; Girod et al., 2000; Marchi et al., 2002). Glutamate release probability is also modulated by nAChRs in the striatum (Kaiser and Wonnacott, 2000). *In vivo* microdialysis studies demonstrate that α7 nAChR activation in striatum increases glutamate release (Campos et al., 2010). α7 nAChR antagonism decreases glutamate release (Carpenedo et al., 2001), indicating that baseline ACh levels contribute to glutamatergic tone. Because the homomeric α7 subtype is highly Ca^{2+} permeable compared to other nAChRs stoichiometries, Ca^{2+} entry through these receptors may lead directly to enhanced neurotransmitter release (Gray et al., 1996). Activation of the α4β2* subtype also increases glutamate release onto MSNs (Xiao et al., 2009). As glutamatergic inputs originate from various neuronal types and brain regions, differential expression of nAChR stoichiometries may allow ChIs to amplify glutamate inputs differentially.

In contrast, activation of mAChRs negatively modulates striatal glutamate release. In field potential recordings, a mAChR agonist suppressed corticostriatal glutamatergic transmission (Malenka and Kocsis, 1988). Increasing mAChR signaling either by increasing ChI firing rates, or exogenous agonist application decreases excitatory drive onto MSNs (Calabresi et al., 1998a; Pakhotin and Bracci, 2007; Pancani et al., 2014). Muscarinic modulation of glutamatergic terminals occurs through M2 or M4 receptor activation, as mRNA and protein levels for both mAChRs are observed at high levels in striatal somata as well as terminals (Levey et al., 1991; Hersch et al., 1994). M2 or, interestingly enough, M3 activation results in paired pulse facilitation, indicating that mAChR activation decreases glutamate release probability (Hernández-Echeagaray et al., 1998; Ding et al., 2010). The change in release probability is observed in both corticostriatal afferents and thalamostriatal afferents, and when recording from both direct and indirect MSNs, indicating that regardless of the origin of the terminal or the post-synaptic target, release probability at glutamatergic terminals is decreased with mAChR activation (Ding et al., 2010). In agreement with these observations, intrastriatal injections of an M2-selective antagonist increases glutamate overflow (Smolders et al., 1997), providing evidence that tonic levels of ACh contribute to striatal glutamate tone. Additionally, glutamate release is downregulated via mAChR activation (Dodt and Misgeld, 1986). ChIs are thus in a position to regulate excitatory inputs to MSN, both rapidly by acting on nAChRs, and more slowly and persistently via mAChR activation.

DOPAMINERGIC TERMINALS

ACh profoundly modulates DA release in the striatum. In a slice preparation, optogenetic activation of ChIs increases evoked DA release. The quantity of DA released is dependent on frequency of stimulation, and requires synchronous ChI cell activation as well as activation of β2-containing nAChRs expressed on dopaminergic terminals (Cachope et al., 2012; Threlfell et al., 2012). Although the physiological conditions that coordinate synchronous firing of large numbers of ChIs are unknown, cross-talk between ChIs may facilitate simultaneous firing of these neurons to enhance DA release.

Dopaminergic terminals express α4 and β2 subunits at high levels, along with α5, α6, α7, and β3 subunits at variable levels (Le Novère et al., 1996; Sharples et al., 2000; Jones et al., 2001; Klink et al., 2001; Quik et al., 2003; Grady et al., 2007; Keath et al., 2007). Nicotinic agonists increase the efflux of DA in striatal tissue, as measured by microdialysis (Puttfarcken et al., 2000; Campos et al., 2010), and as expected, nAChR antagonists decrease DA efflux by interfering with the effects of local ACh activation of presynaptic nAChRs on DA terminals (Wonnacott et al., 2000; Grady et al., 2007). There is evidence that enhancement of DA release by exogenous activation of nAChRs requires glutamatergic signaling (Garcia-Munoz et al., 1996; Wonnacott et al., 2000), but enhancement of DA release by coordinated ACh release from ChIs is not dependent upon glutamate transmission (Threlfell et al., 2012). Additionally, striatal dopaminergic terminals also corelease GABA. In a recent study, optogenetic activation of ChIs produces a GABAA receptor mediated synaptic response in MSNs. Pharmacological blockade of α4 nAChRs inhibits this GABA current, suggesting that striatal nAChRs regulate GABA levels via modulation of release probability from DA terminals (Nelson et al., 2014b).

The expression of nAChRs on DA terminals not only enhances DA transmission, chronic agonist exposure, such as that achieved in tobacco users can shift DA release probability to suppress release during low frequency activity, but maintain or enhance release during burst firing (Zhou et al., 2001; Rice and Cragg, 2004; Zhang and Sulzer, 2004). These observations were obtained using high resolution fast-scan cylclic voltammetry to assess extracellular DA levels, and they suggest that nicotine may enhance the impact of high frequency DA neuron activity to effectively increase the salience of environmental stimuli. Recent *in vivo* investigations suggest that a chronic nicotine exposure model, which mimics the daily pattern of nicotine exposure by smokers (2 weeks via drinking water), results in a downregulation of electrically stimulated DA release due to persistent desensitization of nAChRs on DA terminals (Koranda et al., 2014). This observation extends the results seen in other preparations including brain slices and non-human primates (Perez et al., 2012, 2013; Exley et al., 2013). Together, these findings have led to the intriguing speculation that the reported protective effects of smoking against PD may result from an adaptation in striatal circuitry to lower DA levels, thus delaying the onset of symptoms (Koranda et al., 2014).

Exogenous nicotine affects striatal dopamine in interesting and sometime counterintuitive ways, as the interplay between nAChR activation and desensitization can lead to contradictory effects. In contrast, endogenous ACh from ChIs is rapidly degraded by acetylcholinesterase, which is expressed at remarkably high levels in striatum. As alluded to above, synchronous ChI activation can have profound effects on DA release in striatum, through the coordinated activation of presynaptic nAChRs on DA terminals (Threlfell et al., 2012). This study from the Cragg laboratory used optogenetic stimulation to coordinate ChI activity selectively to demonstrate this phenomenon. This is relevant to endogenous activation of ChIs, as synchronous stimulation of these neurons has been reported through coordination of thalamostriatal inputs in response to salient environmental stimuli (Ding et al., 2010; Threlfell et al., 2012).

While mAChRs are also involved in modulation of DA release, the identity of mAChRs expressed by SNc DA cells is unclear, as some observe M2, M4, and M5 (Vilaró et al., 1990; Levey et al., 1991), while others report expression of only M5 receptors (Weiner et al., 1990). Agreement on M5 receptor expression suggests that dopaminergic terminals in the striatum express this mAChR subtype. Electrophysiological evidence supports this, as M5 KO mice show reduced oxotremorine enhancement of potassium-stimulated dopamine release (Zhang et al., 2002). M2 receptors are also involved in tonic DA release, as intrastriatal administration of an M2 antagonist dramatically increases DA levels in freely moving rats (Smolders et al., 1997). Non-selective activation of striatal mAChRs with oxotremorine increases DA release (Lehmann and Langer, 1982; Threlfell et al., 2010), suggesting that M5 activation plays a stronger role in the modulation of DA terminals.

PLASTICITY OF THE EXCITATORY INPUTS TO CHOLINERGIC INTERNEURONS

Activity-dependent modification of synaptic connections is believed to be an important cellular substrate for learning and memory. As the dorsal striatum is believed to be an important site of action for habit formation and motor learning, it is likely that synaptic plasticity contributes to that learning. Considerable effort has focused on understanding the plasticity of the excitatory inputs to MSNs (Calabresi et al., 1996; Mahon et al., 2004; Surmeier et al., 2007), however, LTP/LTD in ChIs has not been explored extensively. Recording in tissue slices from dorsal striatum, Suzuki et al. (2001b) demonstrated LTP in ChIs following a 1 s, 100 Hz train stimulation of the corpus callosum. This LTP was dependent on Ca^{2+} entry, as intrapipette BAPTA blocked LTP induction. The source of Ca^{2+} entry in these studies was not from NMDA receptors, as NMDA blockers had no effect on LTP induction. They also found this LTP to be D5 receptor dependent, as pharmacological blockade of D1/D5 receptors prevents the long term maintenance of enhanced synaptic strength, whereas D2 receptor blockade did not affect LTP induction (Suzuki et al., 2001b). Bonsi and co-workers observed a similar LTP (using three 1 s, 100 Hz trains), however they attribute LTP at these synapses to calcium entry via L-type HVA channels, and not to Ca^{2+} permeable AMPA receptors or NMDA receptors (Bonsi et al., 2004). Using the same HFS stimulation paradigm as Bonsi et al, Picconi and coworkers demonstrate that plasticity of ChIs is not observed in the R6/2 mouse model of Huntington's disease (Picconi et al., 2006). It is not clear why a Huntington's disease model should lack plasticity at these synapses, which highlights the need for better understanding of the underlying mechanisms and functional significance of synaptic plasticity of the inputs to striatal ChIs.

Spike-timing dependent plasticity (STDP) is another experimental paradigm used to induce plasticity. In accordance with Hebbian theory, changing the time between presynaptic activation and postsynaptic depolarization can elicit either a strengthening, weakening, or no change in synaptic strength. First discovered in the cortex, examples of STDP have been observed in other parts of the nervous system including the hippocampus, striatum neuromuscular junction, and cerebellum (Linden et al., 1991; Markram et al., 1997; Wan and Poo, 1999; Nishiyama et al., 2000; Plotkin et al., 2013). To date, only one group has reported STDP in ChIs. Fino and colleagues observed bidirectional plasticity in a majority of ChIs—Post-pre stimulation elicited an LTP in some cells and LTD in others, while pre-post stimulation results in only LTD. Using pharmacology, they found that both forms of plasticity depend upon mGluR activation (Fino et al., 2008). These findings contrast with the Suzuki study where HFS induced-LTP was insensitive to mGluR blockade (Suzuki et al., 2001b). Additionally, post-pre stimulation plasticity was inhibited by NMDA receptor blockade, suggesting that HFS induced-LTP occurs by another mechanism. Further exploration into LTP/LTD of the excitatory inputs to ChIs represents an exciting field of study, as changes in synaptic strength here may contribute to motor skill learning and habit formation.

SUMMARY

Even though ChIs only make up 1–2% of all striatal cells, they send dense projections throughout the striatum. ACh can affect the output of the striatum directly or indirectly, and a wide variety of neurotransmitter systems can influence the activity of these cells. Given that ChIs are in a position to integrate synaptic inputs and modulate the output of the striatum, understanding the physiology of these cells will contribute to our knowledge of striatal function.

ChIs receive afferent inputs from a wide variety of sources which can arise either locally from within the striatum, or from brain regions as distant as the brainstem. Some of these neurotransmitter systems alter cellular excitability rapidly through their actions on ionotropic receptors, producing rapid electrical signals on a millisecond time scale. These changes in membrane properties affect the firing activity of the ChIs, and given the hundreds of thousands of synaptic contacts formed by each ChI, several other cell types are influenced by changes ACh release. The inherent membrane properties of ChIs allows them to be easily modified in either direction during neurotransmitter release: their depolarized resting membrane potential allows excitatory neurotransmitters to easily enhance action potential firing rate, and considering their tonic activity, inhibitory neurotransmitters will inhibit firing, reducing total cholinergic tone. Thus, because these cells are resting at some intermediate state of activity, they are sensitive to incoming afferents. In addition to the ionotropic receptors on these cells, ChIs express a wide variety of GPCRs. Activation of GPCRs can have a multitude of cellular effects, including the opening of ion channels, changes in plasticity or protein transcription (Altier, 2012; Rojas and Dingledine, 2013). The long time course of the signaling cascades downstream of GPCR activation could indicate that a temporary increase in neurotransmitter activity may lead to long-lasting modifications in ChI physiology that increases or decreases the cellular response to other incoming afferents. Given the sensitivity of these cells to various synaptic inputs, understanding ChI connectivity provides insight into the striatal network.

ACh has a wide variety of effects following release, either by directly activating receptors on postsynaptic cells or indirectly via the modulation of neurotransmitter release at terminals. Changes in striatal cholinergic tone will thus result in a complex series of downstream effects which ultimately may affect the striatal output neurons. Considering the multiple ACh-sensitive neurotransmitter systems that are involved in the striatal network, changes in receptor function or expression on any class of cells may result in a shift in the balance of these systems, potentially resulting in dysfunction. Understanding the nature of synaptic connectivity and the location of receptor expression therefor has a direct connection with human pathology. Using this knowledge in conjunction with an understanding of the changes that occur in disease, we can work toward the development of novel therapies that are aimed at counteracting neurotransmitter dysregulation.

Often times, we oversimplify the nature of the neurotransmitters released at a given terminal, neglecting the co-release of other neurotransmitters whose post-synaptic effects can differ from the primary neurotransmitter. Although there is evidence that co-release occurs, very few have looked in detail at the functional consequences of multiple transmitter release, or whether or not these neurotransmitters are released in sufficient amounts to contribute to cell physiology.

New genetic techniques can improve our understanding of striatal neurotransmission in both the normal and abnormal brain. Optogenetic manipulation of excitability in specific neuronal subtypes is providing important insights into connectivity throughout the nervous system. This robust technology has advantages over other methods of exogenous neural control and certainly provides a means to explore ChI efferent and afferent connections, as well as the nature of the neurotransmitter phenotypes that influence the excitability of these neurons. Extending these methods to *in vivo* analyses can help provide causal links between synaptic information and behavior.

CLARITY is a potentially groundbreaking new technique that allows high resolution visualization of subcellular structures such as individual synapses in the whole brain (Chung and Deisseroth, 2013). Because the preparation for CLARITY removes brain lipids, antibodies can easily permeate the entirety of the brain, permitting the resolution of the striatal connectome in total. This anatomical information will precisely elucidate the synaptic connectivity between striatal cell types.

Ultimately, ongoing efforts to improve our understanding of striatal ChIs will provide valuable insights into the physiology of this important brain area and help identify new pharmacotherapies for striatal disorders.

ACKNOWLEDGMENTS

The authors thank Lisa Won for helpful comments on the manuscript. Supported by Michael J. Fox Foundation for Parkinson Research and NS 064439 (UJK).

REFERENCES

Abercrombie, E. D., and DeBoer, P. (1997). Substantia nigra D1 receptors and stimulation of striatal cholinergic interneurons by dopamine: a proposed circuit mechanism. *J. Neurosci.* 17, 8498–8505.

Ahlskog, J. E., and Muenter, M. D. (2001). Frequency of levodopa-related dyskinesias and motor fluctuations as estimated from the cumulative literature. *Mov. Disord. Off. J. Mov. Disord. Soc.* 16, 448–458. doi: 10.1002/mds.1090

Albin, R. L., Young, A. B., and Penney, J. B. (1989). The functional anatomy of basal ganglia disorders. *Trends Neurosci.* 12, 366–375. doi: 10.1016/0166-2236(89)90074-X

Alcantara, A. A., Mrzljak, L., Jakab, R. L., Levey, A. I., Hersch, S. M., and Goldman-Rakic, P. S. (2001). Muscarinic m1 and m2 receptor proteins in local circuit and projection neurons of the primate striatum: anatomical evidence for cholinergic modulation of glutamatergic prefronto-striatal pathways. *J. Comp. Neurol.* 434, 445–460. doi: 10.1002/cne.1186

Allam, M. F., Campbell, M. J., Del Castillo, A. S., and Fernández-Crehuet Navajas, R. (2004). Parkinson's disease protects against smoking? *Behav. Neurol.* 15, 65–71. doi: 10.1155/2004/516302

Altier, C. (2012). GPCR and voltage-gated calcium channels (VGCC) signaling complexes. *Subcell. Biochem.* 63, 241–262. doi: 10.1007/978-94-007-4765-4_13

Ancín, I., Barabash, A., Vázquez-Álvarez, B., Santos, J. L., Sánchez-Morla, E., Martínez, J. L., et al. (2010). Evidence for association of the non-duplicated region of CHRNA7 gene with bipolar disorder but not with Schizophrenia. *Psychiatr. Genet.* 20, 289–297. doi: 10.1097/YPG.0b013e32833a9b7a

Aosaki, T., and Kawaguchi, Y. (1996). Actions of substance P on rat neostriatal neurons *in vitro*. *J. Neurosci.* 16, 5141–5153.

Aosaki, T., Kiuchi, K., and Kawaguchi, Y. (1998). Dopamine D1-like receptor activation excites rat striatal large aspiny neurons *in vitro*. *J. Neurosci.* 18, 5180–5190.

Aosaki, T., Tsubokawa, H., Ishida, A., Watanabe, K., Graybiel, A. M., and Kimura, M. (1994). Responses of tonically active neurons in the primate's striatum undergo systematic changes during behavioral sensorimotor conditioning. *J. Neurosci.* 14, 3969–3984.

Aouizerate, B., Guehl, D., Cuny, E., Rougier, A., Bioulac, B., Tignol, J., et al. (2004). Pathophysiology of obsessive-compulsive disorder: a necessary link between phenomenology, neuropsychology, imagery and physiology. *Prog. Neurobiol.* 72, 195–221. doi: 10.1016/j.pneurobio.2004.02.004

Apicella, P., Legallet, E., and Trouche, E. (1997). Responses of tonically discharging neurons in the monkey striatum to primary rewards delivered during different behavioral states. *Exp. Brain Res.* 116, 456–466. doi: 10.1007/PL00005773

Apicella, P., Ljungberg, T., Scarnati, E., and Schultz, W. (1991). Responses to reward in monkey dorsal and ventral striatum. *Exp. Brain Res.* 85, 491–500. doi: 10.1007/BF00231732

Arbuthnott, G. W., and Wickens, J. (2007). Space, time and dopamine. *Trends Neurosci.* 30, 62–69. doi: 10.1016/j.tins.2006.12.003

Arenas, E., Alberch, J., Perez-Navarro, E., Solsona, C., and Marsal, J. (1991). Neurokinin receptors differentially mediate endogenous acetylcholine release evoked by tachykinins in the neostriatum. *J. Neurosci.* 11, 2332–2338.

Arenas, E., Alberch, J., Sanchez Arroyos, R., and Marsal, J. (1990). Effect of opioids on acetylcholine release evoked by K+ or glutamic acid from rat neostriatal slices. *Brain Res.* 523, 51–56. doi: 10.1016/0006-8993(90)91633-R

Aubert, I., Araujo, D. M., Cécyre, D., Robitaille, Y., Gauthier, S., and Quirion, R. (1992). Comparative alterations of nicotinic and muscarinic binding sites in Alzheimer's and Parkinson's diseases. *J. Neurochem.* 58, 529–541. doi: 10.1111/j.1471-4159.1992.tb09752.x

Azam, L., Winzer-Serhan, U., and Leslie, F. M. (2003). Co-expression of alpha7 and beta2 nicotinic acetylcholine receptor subunit mRNAs within rat brain cholinergic neurons. *Neuroscience* 119, 965–977. doi: 10.1016/S0306-4522(03)00220-3

Baba, Y., Higuchi, M.-A., Abe, H., Fukuyama, K., Onozawa, R., Uehara, Y., et al. (2012). Anti-cholinergics for axial symptoms in Parkinson's disease after subthalamic stimulation. *Clin. Neurol. Neurosurg.* 114, 1308–1311. doi: 10.1016/j.clineuro.2012.03.046

Bain, E. E., Robieson, W., Pritchett, Y., Garimella, T., Abi-Saab, W., Apostol, G., et al. (2013). A randomized, double-blind, placebo-controlled phase 2 study of α4β2 agonist ABT-894 in adults with ADHD. *Neuropsychopharmacol. Off. Publ. Am. Coll. Neuropsychopharmacol.* 38, 405–413. doi: 10.1038/npp.2012.194

Barroso-Chinea, P., and Bezard, E. (2010). Basal Ganglia circuits underlying the pathophysiology of levodopa-induced dyskinesia. *Front. Neuroanat.* 4:131. doi: 10.3389/fnana.2010.00131

Bar-Shira, A., Gana-Weisz, M., Gan-Or, Z., Giladi, E., Giladi, N., and Orr-Urtreger, A. (2014). CHRNB3 c.-57A>G functional promoter change affects Parkinson's disease and smoking. *Neurobiol. Aging* 35, 2179.e1–2179.e6. doi: 10.1016/j.neurobiolaging.2014.03.014

Beaulieu, J.-M., and Gainetdinov, R. R. (2011). The physiology, signaling, and pharmacology of dopamine receptors. *Pharmacol. Rev.* 63, 182–217. doi: 10.1124/pr.110.002642

Beggiato, S., Antonelli, T., Tomasini, M. C., Tanganelli, S., Fuxe, K., Schwarcz, R., et al. (2013). Kynurenic acid, by targeting α7 nicotinic acetylcholine receptors, modulates extracellular GABA levels in the rat striatum *in vivo*. *Eur. J. Neurosci.* 37, 1470–1477. doi: 10.1111/ejn.12160

Bell, M. I., Richardson, P. J., and Lee, K. (2000). Histamine depolarizes cholinergic interneurones in the rat striatum via a H(1)-receptor mediated action. *Br. J. Pharmacol.* 131, 1135–1142. doi: 10.1038/sj.bjp.0703692

Bell, M. I., Richardson, P. J., and Lee, K. (2002). Functional and molecular characterization of metabotropic glutamate receptors expressed in rat striatal cholinergic interneurones. *J. Neurochem.* 81, 142–149. doi: 10.1046/j.1471-4159.2002.00815.x

Berendse, H. W., and Groenewegen, H. J. (1990). Organization of the thalamostriatal projections in the rat, with special emphasis on the ventral striatum. *J. Comp. Neurol.* 299, 187–228. doi: 10.1002/cne.902990206

Berg, A. P., Sen, N., and Bayliss, D. A. (2007). TrpC3/C7 and Slo2.1 are molecular targets for metabotropic glutamate receptor signaling in rat striatal cholinergic interneurons. *J. Neurosci.* 27, 8845–8856. doi: 10.1523/JNEUROSCI.0551-07.2007

Bergson, C., Mrzljak, L., Smiley, J. F., Pappy, M., Levenson, R., and Goldman-Rakic, P. S. (1995). Regional, cellular, and subcellular variations in the distribution of D1 and D5 dopamine receptors in primate brain. *J. Neurosci.* 15, 7821–7836.

Bernard, V., Laribi, O., Levey, A. I., and Bloch, B. (1998). Subcellular redistribution of m2 muscarinic acetylcholine receptors in striatal interneurons *in vivo* after acute cholinergic stimulation. *J. Neurosci.* 18, 10207–10218.

Bernard, V., Normand, E., and Bloch, B. (1992). Phenotypical characterization of the rat striatal neurons expressing muscarinic receptor genes. *J. Neurosci.* 12, 3591–3600.

Bernard, V., Somogyi, P., and Bolam, J. P. (1997). Cellular, subcellular, and subsynaptic distribution of AMPA-type glutamate receptor subunits in the neostriatum of the rat. *J. Neurosci.* 17, 819–833.

Betarbet, R., Turner, R., Chockkan, V., DeLong, M. R., Allers, K. A., Walters, J., et al. (1997). Dopaminergic neurons intrinsic to the primate striatum. *J. Neurosci.* 17, 6761–6768.

Bettler, B., Kaupmann, K., Mosbacher, J., and Gassmann, M. (2004). Molecular structure and physiological functions of GABA(B) receptors. *Physiol. Rev.* 84, 835–867. doi: 10.1152/physrev.00036.2003

Bird, E. D., and Iversen, L. L. (1974). Huntington's chorea. Post-mortem measurement of glutamic acid decarboxylase, choline acetyltransferase and dopamine in basal ganglia. *Brain J. Neurol.* 97, 457–472. doi: 10.1093/brain/97.1.457

Bird, E. D., Spokes, E. G., Barnes, J., MacKay, A. V., Iversen, L. L., and Shepherd, M. (1977). Increased brain dopamine and reduced glutamic acid decarboxylase and choline acetyl transferase activity in schizophrenia and related psychoses. *Lancet* 2, 1157–1158. doi: 10.1016/S0140-6736(77)91542-2

Birket-Smith, E. (1974). Abnormal involuntary movements induced by anticholinergic therapy. *Acta Neurol. Scand.* 50, 801–811. doi: 10.1111/j.1600-0404.1974.tb02820.x

Blandina, P., Munari, L., Provensi, G., and Passani, M. B. (2012). Histamine neurons in the tuberomamillary nucleus: a whole center or distinct subpopulations? *Front. Syst. Neurosci.* 6:33. doi: 10.3389/fnsys.2012.00033

Blomeley, C., and Bracci, E. (2005). Excitatory effects of serotonin on rat striatal cholinergic interneurones. *J. Physiol.* 569, 715–721. doi: 10.1113/jphysiol.2005.098269

Bohr, I. J., Ray, M. A., McIntosh, J. M., Chalon, S., Guilloteau, D., McKeith, I. G., et al. (2005). Cholinergic nicotinic receptor involvement in movement disorders associated with Lewy body diseases. An autoradiography study using [(125)I]alpha-conotoxinMII in the striatum and thalamus. *Exp. Neurol.* 191, 292–300. doi: 10.1016/j.expneurol.2004.10.004

Bolam, J. P., Ingham, C. A., Izzo, P. N., Levey, A. I., Rye, D. B., Smith, A. D., et al. (1986). Substance P-containing terminals in synaptic contact with cholinergic neurons in the neostriatum and basal forebrain: a double immunocytochemical study in the rat. *Brain Res.* 397, 279–289. doi: 10.1016/0006-8993(86)90629-3

Bolam, J. P., Wainer, B. H., and Smith, A. D. (1984). Characterization of cholinergic neurons in the rat neostriatum. A combination of choline acetyltransferase immunocytochemistry, Golgi-impregnation and electron microscopy. *Neuroscience* 12, 711–718. doi: 10.1016/0306-4522(84)90165-9

Bonsi, P., Cuomo, D., Ding, J., Sciamanna, G., Ulrich, S., Tscherter, A., et al. (2007). Endogenous serotonin excites striatal cholinergic interneurons via the activation of 5-HT 2C, 5-HT6, and 5-HT7 serotonin receptors: implications for extrapyramidal side effects of serotonin reuptake inhibitors. *Neuropsychopharmacol. Off. Publ. Am. Coll. Neuropsychopharmacol.* 32, 1840–1854. doi: 10.1038/sj.npp.1301294

Bonsi, P., De Persis, C., Calabresi, P., Bernardi, G., and Pisani, A. (2004). Coordinate high-frequency pattern of stimulation and calcium levels control the induction of LTP in striatal cholinergic interneurons. *Learn. Mem.* 11, 755–760. doi: 10.1101/lm.82104

Bordia, T., Campos, C., McIntosh, J. M., and Quik, M. (2010). Nicotinic receptor-mediated reduction in L-DOPA-induced dyskinesias may occur via desensitization. *J. Pharmacol. Exp. Ther.* 333, 929–938. doi: 10.1124/jpet.109.162396

Britt, J. P., and McGehee, D. S. (2008). Presynaptic opioid and nicotinic receptor modulation of dopamine overflow in the nucleus accumbens. *J. Neurosci.* 28, 1672–1681. doi: 10.1523/JNEUROSCI.4275-07.2008

Brown, M. T. C., Tan, K. R., O'Connor, E. C., Nikonenko, I., Muller, D., and Lüscher, C. (2012). Ventral tegmental area GABA projections pause accumbal cholinergic interneurons to enhance associative learning. *Nature* 492, 452–456. doi: 10.1038/nature11657

Brown, S. J., James, S., Reddington, M., and Richardson, P. J. (1990). Both A1 and A2a purine receptors regulate striatal acetylcholine release. *J. Neurochem.* 55, 31–38. doi: 10.1111/j.1471-4159.1990.tb08817.x

Cachope, R., Mateo, Y., Mathur, B. N., Irving, J., Wang, H.-L., Morales, M., et al. (2012). Selective activation of cholinergic interneurons enhances accumbal phasic dopamine release: setting the tone for reward processing. *Cell Rep.* 2, 33–41. doi: 10.1016/j.celrep.2012.05.011

Calabresi, P., Ascone, C. M., Centonze, D., Pisani, A., Sancesario, G., D'Angelo, V., et al. (1997). Opposite membrane potential changes induced by glucose deprivation in striatal spiny neurons and in large aspiny interneurons. *J. Neurosci.* 17, 1940–1949.

Calabresi, P., Centonze, D., Gubellini, P., Pisani, A., and Bernardi, G. (1998a). Blockade of M2-like muscarinic receptors enhances long-term potentiation at corticostriatal synapses. *Eur. J. Neurosci.* 10, 3020–3023. doi: 10.1111/j.1460-9568.1998.00348.x

Calabresi, P., Centonze, D., Pisani, A., and Bernardi, G. (1999). Metabotropic glutamate receptors and cell-type-specific vulnerability in the striatum: implication for ischemia and Huntington's disease. *Exp. Neurol.* 158, 97–108. doi: 10.1006/exnr.1999.7092

Calabresi, P., Centonze, D., Pisani, A., Sancesario, G., Gubellini, P., Marfia, G. A., et al. (1998b). Striatal spiny neurons and cholinergic interneurons express differential ionotropic glutamatergic responses and vulnerability: implications for ischemia and Huntington's disease. *Ann. Neurol.* 43, 586–597. doi: 10.1002/ana.410430506

Calabresi, P., Siniscalchi, A., Pisani, A., Stefani, A., Mercuri, N. B., and Bernardi, G. (1996). A field potential analysis on the effects of lamotrigine, GP 47779, and felbamate in neocortical slices. *Neurology* 47, 557–562. doi: 10.1212/WNL.47.2.557

Campos, F., Alfonso, M., and Durán, R. (2010). *In vivo* modulation of alpha7 nicotinic receptors on striatal glutamate release induced by anatoxin-A. *Neurochem. Int.* 56, 850–855. doi: 10.1016/j.neuint.2010.03.010

Cantello, R., Riccio, A., Gilli, M., Delsedime, M., Scarzella, L., Aguggia, M., et al. (1986). Bornaprine vs placebo in Parkinson disease: double-blind controlled cross-over trial in 30 patients. *Ital. J. Neurol. Sci.* 7, 139–143. doi: 10.1007/BF02230432

Carpenedo, R., Pittaluga, A., Cozzi, A., Attucci, S., Galli, A., Raiteri, M., et al. (2001). Presynaptic kynurenate-sensitive receptors inhibit glutamate release. *Eur. J. Neurosci.* 13, 2141–2147. doi: 10.1046/j.0953-816x.2001.01592.x

Centonze, D., Grande, C., Usiello, A., Gubellini, P., Erbs, E., Martin, A. B., et al. (2003). Receptor subtypes involved in the presynaptic and postsynaptic actions of dopamine on striatal interneurons. *J. Neurosci.* 23, 6245–6254.

Centonze, D., Pisani, A., Bonsi, P., Giacomini, P., Bernardi, G., and Calabresi, P. (2001). Stimulation of nitric oxide-cGMP pathway excites striatal cholinergic interneurons via protein kinase G activation. *J. Neurosci.* 21, 1393–1400.

Cepeda, C., Itri, J. N., Flores-Hernández, J., Hurst, R. S., Calvert, C. R., and Levine, M. S. (2001). Differential sensitivity of medium- and large-sized striatal neurons to NMDA but not kainate receptor activation in the rat. *Eur. J. Neurosci.* 14, 1577–1589. doi: 10.1046/j.0953-816x.2001.01783.x

Cepeda, C., Wu, N., André, V. M., Cummings, D. M., and Levine, M. S. (2007). The corticostriatal pathway in Huntington's disease. *Prog. Neurobiol.* 81, 253–271. doi: 10.1016/j.pneurobio.2006.11.001

Chang, H. T. (1988). Dopamine-acetylcholine interaction in the rat striatum: a dual-labeling immunocytochemical study. *Brain Res. Bull.* 21, 295–304. doi: 10.1016/0361-9230(88)90244-4

Chang, H. T., and Kita, H. (1992). Interneurons in the rat striatum: relationships between parvalbumin neurons and cholinergic neurons. *Brain Res.* 574, 307–311. doi: 10.1016/0006-8993(92)90830-3

Chang, K. T., and Berg, D. K. (2001). Voltage-gated channels block nicotinic regulation of CREB phosphorylation and gene expression in neurons. *Neuron* 32, 855–865. doi: 10.1016/S0896-6273(01)00516-5

Chen, Q., Veenman, C. L., and Reiner, A. (1996). Cellular expression of ionotropic glutamate receptor subunits on specific striatal neuron types and its implication for striatal vulnerability in glutamate receptor-mediated excitotoxicity. *Neuroscience* 73, 715–731. doi: 10.1016/0306-4522(96)00011-5

Chudasama, Y., and Robbins, T. W. (2006). Functions of frontostriatal systems in cognition: comparative neuropsychopharmacological studies in rats, monkeys and humans. *Biol. Psychol.* 73, 19–38. doi: 10.1016/j.biopsycho.2006.01.005

Chuhma, N., Mingote, S., Moore, H., and Rayport, S. (2014). Dopamine neurons control striatal cholinergic neurons via regionally heterogeneous dopamine and glutamate signaling. *Neuron* 81, 901–912. doi: 10.1016/j.neuron.2013.12.027

Chuhma, N., Tanaka, K. F., Hen, R., and Rayport, S. (2011). Functional connectome of the striatal medium spiny neuron. *J. Neurosci.* 31, 1183–1192. doi: 10.1523/JNEUROSCI.3833-10.2011

Chung, K. A., Lobb, B. M., Nutt, J. G., and Horak, F. B. (2010). Effects of a central cholinesterase inhibitor on reducing falls in Parkinson disease. *Neurology* 75, 1263–1269. doi: 10.1212/WNL.0b013e3181f6128c

Chung, K., and Deisseroth, K. (2013). CLARITY for mapping the nervous system. *Nat. Methods* 10, 508–513. doi: 10.1038/nmeth.2481

Claye, L. H., Unterwald, E. M., Ho, A., and Kreek, M. J. (1996). Both dynorphin A(1-17) and [Des-Tyr1]dynorphin A(2-17) inhibit adenylyl cyclase activity in rat caudate putamen. *J. Pharmacol. Exp. Ther.* 277, 359–365.

Conn, P. J., Battaglia, G., Marino, M. J., and Nicoletti, F. (2005). Metabotropic glutamate receptors in the basal ganglia motor circuit. *Nat. Rev. Neurosci.* 6, 787–798. doi: 10.1038/nrn1763

Contant, C., Umbriaco, D., Garcia, S., Watkins, K. C., and Descarries, L. (1996). Ultrastructural characterization of the acetylcholine innervation in adult rat neostriatum. *Neuroscience* 71, 937–947. doi: 10.1016/0306-4522(95)00507-2

Cossette, M., Lecomte, F., and Parent, A. (2005). Morphology and distribution of dopaminergic neurons intrinsic to the human striatum. *J. Chem. Neuroanat.* 29, 1–11. doi: 10.1016/j.jchemneu.2004.08.007

Court, J. A., Piggott, M. A., Lloyd, S., Cookson, N., Ballard, C. G., McKeith, I. G., et al. (2000). Nicotine binding in human striatum: elevation in schizophrenia and reductions in dementia with Lewy bodies, Parkinson's disease and Alzheimer's disease and in relation to neuroleptic medication. *Neuroscience* 98, 79–87. doi: 10.1016/S0306-4522(00)00071-3

Crain, S. M., and Shen, K. F. (1996). Modulatory effects of Gs-coupled excitatory opioid receptor functions on opioid analgesia, tolerance, and dependence. *Neurochem. Res.* 21, 1347–1351. doi: 10.1007/BF02532375

Cubo, E., Fernández Jaén, A., Moreno, C., Anaya, B., González, M., and Kompoliti, K. (2008). Donepezil use in children and adolescents with tics and attention-deficit/hyperactivity disorder: an 18-week, single-center, dose-escalating, prospective, open-label study. *Clin. Ther.* 30, 182–189. doi: 10.1016/j.clinthera.2008.01.010

Da Cunha, C., Gomez, A.-A., and Blaha, C. D. (2012). The role of the basal ganglia in motivated behavior. *Rev. Neurosci.* 23, 747–767. doi: 10.1515/revneuro-2012-0063

Dalack, G. W., Healy, D. J., and Meador-Woodruff, J. H. (1998). Nicotine dependence in schizophrenia: clinical phenomena and laboratory findings. *Am. J. Psychiatry* 155, 1490–1501.

Dale, H. H., and Laidlaw, P. P. (1910). The physiological action of beta-iminazolylethylamine. *J. Physiol.* 41, 318–344.

Dani, J. A. (2001). Overview of nicotinic receptors and their roles in the central nervous system. *Biol. Psychiatry* 49, 166–174. doi: 10.1016/S0006-3223(00)01011-8

Dautan, D., Huerta-Ocampo, I., Witten, I. B., Deisseroth, K., Bolam, J. P., Gerdjikov, T., et al. (2014). A major external source of cholinergic innervation of the striatum and nucleus accumbens originates in the brainstem. *J. Neurosci.* 34, 4509–4518. doi: 10.1523/JNEUROSCI.5071-13.2014

Dawson, V. L., Dawson, T. M., Filloux, F. M., and Wamsley, J. K. (1988). Evidence for dopamine D-2 receptors on cholinergic interneurons in the rat caudate-putamen. *Life Sci.* 42, 1933–1939. doi: 10.1016/0024-3205(88)90492-4

Dawson, V. L., Dawson, T. M., and Wamsley, J. K. (1990). Muscarinic and dopaminergic receptor subtypes on striatal cholinergic interneurons. *Brain Res. Bull.* 25, 903–912. doi: 10.1016/0361-9230(90)90186-4

Dean, B., Crook, J. M., Opeskin, K., Hill, C., Keks, N., and Copolov, D. L. (1996). The density of muscarinic M1 receptors is decreased in the caudate-putamen of subjects with schizophrenia. *Mol. Psychiatry* 1, 54–58.

DeBoer, P., Abercrombie, E. D., Heeringa, M., and Westerink, B. H. (1993). Differential effect of systemic administration of bromocriptine and L-dopa on the release of acetylcholine from striatum of intact and 6-OHDA-treated rats. *Brain Res.* 608, 198–203. doi: 10.1016/0006-8993(93)91459-6

DeBoer, P., and Westerink, B. H. (1994). GABAergic modulation of striatal cholinergic interneurons: an *in vivo* microdialysis study. *J. Neurochem.* 62, 70–75. doi: 10.1046/j.1471-4159.1994.62010070.x

Del Barrio, L., Egea, J., León, R., Romero, A., Ruiz, A., Montero, M., et al. (2011). Calcium signalling mediated through α7 and non-α7 nAChR stimulation is differentially regulated in bovine chromaffin cells to induce catecholamine release. *Br. J. Pharmacol.* 162, 94–110. doi: 10.1111/j.1476-5381.2010.01034.x

DeLong, M. R. (1990). Primate models of movement disorders of basal ganglia origin. *Trends Neurosci.* 13, 281–285. doi: 10.1016/0166-2236(90)90110-V

Deng, P., Zhang, Y., and Xu, Z. C. (2007a). Involvement of I(h) in dopamine modulation of tonic firing in striatal cholinergic interneurons. *J. Neurosci.* 27, 3148–3156. doi: 10.1523/JNEUROSCI.5535-06.2007

Deng, Y. P., Xie, J. P., Wang, H. B., Lei, W. L., Chen, Q., and Reiner, A. (2007b). Differential localization of the GluR1 and GluR2 subunits of the AMPA-type glutamate receptor among striatal neuron types in rats. *J. Chem. Neuroanat.* 33, 167–192. doi: 10.1016/j.jchemneu.2007.02.008

De Rover, M., Lodder, J. C., Kits, K. S., Schoffelmeer, A. N. M., and Brussaard, A. B. (2002). Cholinergic modulation of nucleus accumbens medium spiny neurons. *Eur. J. Neurosci.* 16, 2279–2290. doi: 10.1046/j.1460-9568.2002.02289.x

Devan, B. D., Hong, N. S., and McDonald, R. J. (2011). Parallel associative processing in the dorsal striatum: segregation of stimulus-response and cognitive control subregions. *Neurobiol. Learn. Mem.* 96, 95–120. doi: 10.1016/j.nlm.2011.06.002

Dimova, R., Vuillet, J., Nieoullon, A., and Kerkerian-Le Goff, L. (1993). Ultrastructural features of the choline acetyltransferase-containing neurons and relationships with nigral dopaminergic and cortical afferent pathways in the rat striatum. *Neuroscience* 53, 1059–1071. doi: 10.1016/0306-4522(93)90489-3

Ding, J. B., Guzman, J. N., Peterson, J. D., Goldberg, J. A., and Surmeier, D. J. (2010). Thalamic gating of corticostriatal signaling by cholinergic interneurons. *Neuron* 67, 294–307. doi: 10.1016/j.neuron.2010.06.017

Ding, J., Guzman, J. N., Tkatch, T., Chen, S., Goldberg, J. A., Ebert, P. J., et al. (2006). RGS4-dependent attenuation of M4 autoreceptor function in striatal cholinergic interneurons following dopamine depletion. *Nat. Neurosci.* 9, 832–842. doi: 10.1038/nn1700

Ding, S., Wei, W., and Zhou, F.-M. (2011a). Molecular and functional differences in voltage-activated sodium currents between GABA projection neurons and dopamine neurons in the substantia nigra. *J. Neurophysiol.* 106, 3019–3034. doi: 10.1152/jn.00305.2011

Ding, Y., Won, L., Britt, J. P., Lim, S. A. O., McGehee, D. S., and Kang, U. J. (2011b). Enhanced striatal cholinergic neuronal activity mediates L-DOPA-induced dyskinesia in parkinsonian mice. *Proc. Natl. Acad. Sci. U.S.A.* 108, 840–845. doi: 10.1073/pnas.1006511108

Diraddo, J. O., Miller, E. J., Hathaway, H. A., Grajkowska, E., Wroblewska, B., Wolfe, B. B., et al. (2014). A real-time method for measuring cAMP production modulated by Gαi/o-coupled metabotropic glutamate receptors. *J. Pharmacol. Exp. Ther.* 349, 373–382. doi: 10.1124/jpet.113.211532

Dodt, H. U., and Misgeld, U. (1986). Muscarinic slow excitation and muscarinic inhibition of synaptic transmission in the rat neostriatum. *J. Physiol.* 380, 593–608.

Dubach, M., Schmidt, R., Kunkel, D., Bowden, D. M., Martin, R., and German, D. C. (1987). Primate neostriatal neurons containing tyrosine hydroxylase: immunohistochemical evidence. *Neurosci. Lett.* 75, 205–210. doi: 10.1016/0304-3940(87)90298-9

Durany, N., Zöchling, R., Boissl, K. W., Paulus, W., Ransmayr, G., Tatschner, T., et al. (2000). Human post-mortem striatal alpha4beta2 nicotinic acetylcholine receptor density in schizophrenia and Parkinson's syndrome. *Neurosci. Lett.* 287, 109–112. doi: 10.1016/S0304-3940(00)01144-7

Ellens, D. J., and Leventhal, D. K. (2013). Review: electrophysiology of basal ganglia and cortex in models of Parkinson disease. *J. Park. Dis.* 3, 241–254. doi: 10.3233/JPD-130204

English, B. A., Hahn, M. K., Gizer, I. R., Mazei-Robison, M., Steele, A., Kurnik, D. M., et al. (2009). Choline transporter gene variation is associated with attention-deficit hyperactivity disorder. *J. Neurodev. Disord.* 1, 252–263. doi: 10.1007/s11689-009-9033-8

English, D. F., Ibanez-Sandoval, O., Stark, E., Tecuapetla, F., Buzsaki, G., Deisseroth, K., et al. (2011). Novel GABAergic circuits mediate the reinforcement-related signals of striatal cholinergic interneurons. *Nat. Neurosci.* 15, 123–130. doi: 10.1038/nn.2984

Enna, S. J., Bennett, J. P. Jr., Bylund, D. B., Snyder, S. H., Bird, E. D., and Iversen, L. L. (1976a). Alterations of brain neurotransmitter receptor binding in Huntington's chorea. *Brain Res.* 116, 531–537. doi: 10.1016/0006-8993(76)90502-3

Enna, S. J., Bird, E. D., Bennett, J. P. Jr., Bylund, D. B., Yamamura, H. I., Iversen, L. L., et al. (1976b). Huntington's chorea. Changes in neurotransmitter receptors in the brain. *N. Engl. J. Med.* 294, 1305–1309. doi: 10.1056/NEJM197606102942402

Exley, R., Clements, M. A., Hartung, H., McIntosh, J. M., Franklin, M., Bermudez, I., et al. (2013). Striatal dopamine transmission is reduced after chronic nicotine with a decrease in α6-nicotinic receptor control in nucleus accumbens. *Eur. J. Neurosci.* 22, 1379–1389. doi: 10.1111/ejn.12298

Fabbrini, G., Brotchie, J. M., Grandas, F., Nomoto, M., and Goetz, C. G. (2007). Levodopa-induced dyskinesias. *Mov. Disord. Off. J. Mov. Disord. Soc.* 22, 1379–1389. doi: 10.1002/mds.21475

Fallon, J. H., and Leslie, F. M. (1986). Distribution of dynorphin and enkephalin peptides in the rat brain. *J. Comp. Neurol.* 249, 293–336. doi: 10.1002/cne.902490302

Feng, Z.-J., Zhang, X., and Chergui, K. (2014). Allosteric modulation of NMDA receptors alters neurotransmission in the striatum of a mouse model of Parkinson's disease. *Exp. Neurol.* 255, 154–160. doi: 10.1016/j.expneurol.2014.03.001

Fenster, C. P., Rains, M. F., Noerager, B., Quick, M. W., and Lester, R. A. (1997). Influence of subunit composition on desensitization of neuronal acetylcholine receptors at low concentrations of nicotine. *J. Neurosci.* 17, 5747–5759.

Fernandez, H. H. (2012). Updates in the medical management of Parkinson disease. *Cleve. Clin. J. Med.* 79, 28–35. doi: 10.3949/ccjm.78gr.11005

Fino, E., Deniau, J.-M., and Venance, L. (2008). Cell-specific spike-timing-dependent plasticity in GABAergic and cholinergic interneurons in corticostriatal rat brain slices. *J. Physiol.* 586, 265–282. doi: 10.1113/jphysiol.2007.144501

Fisher, J. L., and Dani, J. A. (2000). Nicotinic receptors on hippocampal cultures can increase synaptic glutamate currents while decreasing the NMDA-receptor component. *Neuropharmacology* 39, 2756–2769. doi: 10.1016/S0028-3908(00)00102-7

Fox, S. H., Katzenschlager, R., Lim, S.-Y., Ravina, B., Seppi, K., Coelho, M., et al. (2011). The movement disorder society evidence-based medicine review update: treatments for the motor symptoms of Parkinson's disease. *Mov. Disord. Off. J. Mov. Disord. Soc.* 26(Suppl. 3), S2–S41. doi: 10.1002/mds.23829

Galarraga, E., Hernández-López, S., Reyes, A., Miranda, I., Bermudez-Rattoni, F., Vilchis, C., et al. (1999). Cholinergic modulation of neostriatal output: a functional antagonism between different types of muscarinic receptors. *J. Neurosci.* 19, 3629–3638.

Garcia-Munoz, M., Patino, P., Young, S. J., and Groves, P. M. (1996). Effects of nicotine on dopaminergic nigrostriatal axons requires stimulation of presynaptic glutamatergic receptors. *J. Pharmacol. Exp. Ther.* 277, 1685–1693.

Gasser, T. (2009). Molecular pathogenesis of Parkinson disease: insights from genetic studies. *Expert Rev. Mol. Med.* 11, e22. doi: 10.1017/S1462399409001148

Gerfen, C. R., Herkenham, M., and Thibault, J. (1987). The neostriatal mosaic: II. Patch- and matrix-directed mesostriatal dopaminergic and non-dopaminergic systems. *J. Neurosci.* 7, 3915–3934.

Gilman, S., Koeppe, R. A., Nan, B., Wang, C.-N., Wang, X., Junck, L., et al. (2010). Cerebral cortical and subcortical cholinergic deficits in parkinsonian syndromes. *Neurology* 74, 1416–1423. doi: 10.1212/WNL.0b013e3181dc1a55

Girod, R., Barazangi, N., McGehee, D., and Role, L. W. (2000). Facilitation of glutamatergic neurotransmission by presynaptic nicotinic acetylcholine receptors. *Neuropharmacology* 39, 2715–2725. doi: 10.1016/S0028-3908(00)00145-3

Goetz, C. G. (2011). The history of Parkinson's disease: early clinical descriptions and neurological therapies. *Cold Spring Harb. Perspect. Med.* 1:a008862. doi: 10.1101/cshperspect.a008862

Gomez-Mancilla, B., and Bédard, P. J. (1993). Effect of nondopaminergic drugs on L-dopa-induced dyskinesias in MPTP-treated monkeys. *Clin. Neuropharmacol.* 16, 418–427. doi: 10.1097/00002826-199310000-00004

Gonzales, K. K., Pare, J.-F., Wichmann, T., and Smith, Y. (2013). GABAergic inputs from direct and indirect striatal projection neurons onto cholinergic interneurons in the primate putamen. *J. Comp. Neurol.* 521, 2502–2522. doi: 10.1002/cne.23295

Gotti, C., Moretti, M., Bohr, I., Ziabreva, I., Vailati, S., Longhi, R., et al. (2006a). Selective nicotinic acetylcholine receptor subunit deficits identified in Alzheimer's disease, Parkinson's disease and dementia with Lewy bodies by immunoprecipitation. *Neurobiol. Dis.* 23, 481–489. doi: 10.1016/j.nbd.2006.04.005

Gotti, C., Zoli, M., and Clementi, F. (2006b). Brain nicotinic acetylcholine receptors: native subtypes and their relevance. *Trends Pharmacol. Sci.* 27, 482–491. doi: 10.1016/j.tips.2006.07.004

Götz, T., Kraushaar, U., Geiger, J., Lübke, J., Berger, T., and Jonas, P. (1997). Functional properties of AMPA and NMDA receptors expressed in identified types of basal ganglia neurons. *J. Neurosci.* 17, 204–215.

Grace, A. A., and Bunney, B. S. (1984). The control of firing pattern in nigral dopamine neurons: single spike firing. *J. Neurosci.* 4, 2866–2876.

Grady, S. R., Salminen, O., Laverty, D. C., Whiteaker, P., McIntosh, J. M., Collins, A. C., et al. (2007). The subtypes of nicotinic acetylcholine receptors on dopaminergic terminals of mouse striatum. *Biochem. Pharmacol.* 74, 1235–1246. doi: 10.1016/j.bcp.2007.07.032

Gras, C., Amilhon, B., Lepicard, E. M., Poirel, O., Vinatier, J., Herbin, M., et al. (2008). The vesicular glutamate transporter VGLUT3 synergizes striatal acetylcholine tone. *Nat. Neurosci.* 11, 292–300. doi: 10.1038/nn2052

Gray, R., Rajan, A. S., Radcliffe, K. A., Yakehiro, M., and Dani, J. A. (1996). Hippocampal synaptic transmission enhanced by low concentrations of nicotine. *Nature* 383, 713–716. doi: 10.1038/383713a0

Gross, R. A., Moises, H. C., Uhler, M. D., and Macdonald, R. L. (1990). Dynorphin A and cAMP-dependent protein kinase independently regulate neuronal calcium currents. *Proc. Natl. Acad. Sci. U.S.A.* 87, 7025–7029. doi: 10.1073/pnas.87.18.7025

Guan, L., Wang, B., Chen, Y., Yang, L., Li, J., Qian, Q., et al. (2009). A high-density single-nucleotide polymorphism screen of 23 candidate genes in attention deficit hyperactivity disorder: suggesting multiple susceptibility genes among Chinese Han population. *Mol. Psychiatry* 14, 546–554. doi: 10.1038/sj.mp.4002139

Guatteo, E., Yee, A., McKearney, J., Cucchiaroni, M. L., Armogida, M., Berretta, N., et al. (2013). Dual effects of L-DOPA on nigral dopaminergic neurons. *Exp. Neurol.* 247, 582–594. doi: 10.1016/j.expneurol.2013.02.009

Haas, H. L., Sergeeva, O. A., and Selbach, O. (2008). Histamine in the nervous system. *Physiol. Rev.* 88, 1183–1241. doi: 10.1152/physrev.00043.2007

Haber, S. N., Fudge, J. L., and McFarland, N. R. (2000). Striatonigrostriatal pathways in primates form an ascending spiral from the shell to the dorsolateral striatum. *J. Neurosci.* 20, 2369–2382. doi: 10.0270-6474/00/202369-14

Haj-Dahmane, S., Hamon, M., and Lanfumey, L. (1991). K+ channel and 5-hydroxytryptamine1A autoreceptor interactions in the rat dorsal raphe nucleus: an *in vitro* electrophysiological study. *Neuroscience* 41, 495–505. doi: 10.1016/0306-4522(91)90344-N

Hammond, P., and Brimijoin, S. (1988). Acetylcholinesterase in Huntington's and Alzheimer's diseases: simultaneous enzyme assay and immunoassay of multiple brain regions. *J. Neurochem.* 50, 1111–1116. doi: 10.1111/j.1471-4159.1988.tb10580.x

Hannestad, J. O., Cosgrove, K. P., DellaGioia, N. F., Perkins, E., Bois, F., Bhagwagar, Z., et al. (2013). Changes in the cholinergic system between bipolar depression and euthymia as measured with [123I]5IA single photon emission computed tomography. *Biol. Psychiatry* 74, 768–776. doi: 10.1016/j.biopsych.2013.04.004

Hattori, T., Singh, V. K., McGeer, E. G., and McGeer, P. L. (1976). Immunohistochemical localization of choline acetyltransferase containing neostriatal neurons and their relationship with dopaminergic synapses. *Brain Res.* 102, 164–173. doi: 10.1016/0006-8993(76)90583-7

Hattori, T., Takada, M., Moriizumi, T., and Van der Kooy, D. (1991). Single dopaminergic nigrostriatal neurons form two chemically distinct synaptic types: possible transmitter segregation within neurons. *J. Comp. Neurol.* 309, 391–401. doi: 10.1002/cne.903090308

Hauber, W., and Schmidt, W. J. (1994). Differential effects of lesions of the dorsomedial and dorsolateral caudate-putamen on reaction time performance in rats. *Behav. Brain Res.* 60, 211–215. doi: 10.1016/0166-4328(94)90149-X

Hauser, R. A., and Olanow, C. W. (1993). Orobuccal dyskinesia associated with trihexyphenidyl therapy in a patient with Parkinson's disease. *Mov. Disord. Off. J. Mov. Disord. Soc.* 8, 512–514. doi: 10.1002/mds.870080417

Haydar, S. N., and Dunlop, J. (2010). Neuronal nicotinic acetylcholine receptors - targets for the development of drugs to treat cognitive impairment associated with schizophrenia and Alzheimer's disease. *Curr. Top. Med. Chem.* 10, 144–152. doi: 10.2174/156802610790410983

Hayslett, R. L., and Tizabi, Y. (2003). Effects of donepezil on DOI-induced head twitch response in mice: implications for Tourette syndrome. *Pharmacol. Biochem. Behav.* 76, 409–415. doi: 10.1016/j.pbb.2003.08.015

Hebb, C. O., and Silver, A. (1961). Gradient of choline acetylase activity. *Nature* 189, 123–125. doi: 10.1038/189123a0

Hellström-Lindahl, E., and Court, J. A. (2000). Nicotinic acetylcholine receptors during prenatal development and brain pathology in human aging. *Behav. Brain Res.* 113, 159–168. doi: 10.1016/S0166-4328(00)00210-2

Henny, P., Brown, M. T. C., Northrop, A., Faunes, M., Ungless, M. A., Magill, P. J., et al. (2012). Structural correlates of heterogeneous *in vivo* activity of midbrain dopaminergic neurons. *Nat. Neurosci.* 15, 613–619. doi: 10.1038/nn.3048

Hernández-Echeagaray, E., Galarraga, E., and Bargas, J. (1998). 3-Alpha-chloro-imperialine, a potent blocker of cholinergic presynaptic modulation of glutamatergic afferents in the rat neostriatum. *Neuropharmacology* 37, 1493–1502. doi: 10.1016/S0028-3908(98)00131-2

Hersch, S. M., Gutekunst, C. A., Rees, H. D., Heilman, C. J., and Levey, A. I. (1994). Distribution of m1-m4 muscarinic receptor proteins in the rat striatum: light and electron microscopic immunocytochemistry using subtype-specific antibodies. *J. Neurosci.* 14, 3351–3363.

Higashi, S., Biskup, S., West, A. B., Trinkaus, D., Dawson, V. L., Faull, R. L. M., et al. (2007). Localization of Parkinson's disease-associated LRRK2 in normal and pathological human brain. *Brain Res.* 1155, 208–219. doi: 10.1016/j.brainres.2007.04.034

Higley, M. J., Gittis, A. H., Oldenburg, I. A., Balthasar, N., Seal, R. P., Edwards, R. H., et al. (2011). Cholinergic interneurons mediate fast VGluT3-dependent glutamatergic transmission in the striatum. *PLoS ONE* 6:e19155. doi: 10.1371/journal.pone.0019155

Hiley, C. R., and Bird, E. D. (1974). Decreased muscarinic receptor concentration in post-mortem brain in Huntington's chorea. *Brain Res.* 80, 355–358. doi: 10.1016/0006-8993(74)90700-8

Holt, D. J., Herman, M. M., Hyde, T. M., Kleinman, J. E., Sinton, C. M., German, D. C., et al. (1999). Evidence for a deficit in cholinergic interneurons in the striatum in schizophrenia. *Neuroscience* 94, 21–31. doi: 10.1016/S0306-4522(99)00279-1

Hong, C.-J., Lai, I.-C., Liou, L.-L., and Tsai, S.-J. (2004). Association study of the human partially duplicated alpha7 nicotinic acetylcholine receptor genetic variant with bipolar disorder. *Neurosci. Lett.* 355, 69–72. doi: 10.1016/j.neulet.2003.10.043

Howe, A. R., and Surmeier, D. J. (1995). Muscarinic receptors modulate N-, P-, and L-type Ca2+ currents in rat striatal neurons through parallel pathways. *J. Neurosci.* 15, 458–469.

Hristova, A. H., and Koller, W. C. (2000). Early Parkinson's disease: what is the best approach to treatment. *Drugs Aging* 17, 165–181. doi: 10.2165/00002512-200017030-00002

Hsu, K. S., Yang, C. H., Huang, C. C., and Gean, P. W. (1996). Carbachol induces inward current in neostriatal neurons through M1-like muscarinic receptors. *Neuroscience* 73, 751–760. doi: 10.1016/0306-4522(96)00066-8

Hu, M., Liu, Q., Chang, K. T., and Berg, D. K. (2002). Nicotinic regulation of CREB activation in hippocampal neurons by glutamatergic and nonglutamatergic pathways. *Mol. Cell. Neurosci.* 21, 616–625. doi: 10.1006/mcne.2002.1202

Huot, P., Lévesque, M., and Parent, A. (2007). The fate of striatal dopaminergic neurons in Parkinson's disease and Huntington's chorea. *Brain J. Neurol.* 130, 222–232. doi: 10.1093/brain/awl332

Hyland, B. I., Reynolds, J. N. J., Hay, J., Perk, C. G., and Miller, R. (2002). Firing modes of midbrain dopamine cells in the freely moving rat. *Neuroscience* 114, 475–492. doi: 10.1016/S0306-4522(02)00267-1

Ibáñez-Sandoval, O., Tecuapetla, F., Unal, B., Shah, F., Koós, T., and Tepper, J. M. (2010). Electrophysiological and morphological characteristics and synaptic connectivity of tyrosine hydroxylase-expressing neurons in adult mouse striatum. *J. Neurosci.* 30, 6999–7016. doi: 10.1523/JNEUROSCI.5996-09.2010

Innis, R. B., and Aghajanian, G. K. (1987). Pertussis toxin blocks 5-HT1A and GABAB receptor-mediated inhibition of serotonergic neurons. *Eur. J. Pharmacol.* 143, 195–204. doi: 10.1016/0014-2999(87)90533-4

Inokawa, H., Yamada, H., Matsumoto, N., Muranishi, M., and Kimura, M. (2010). Juxtacellular labeling of tonically active neurons and phasically active neurons in the rat striatum. *Neuroscience* 168, 395–404. doi: 10.1016/j.neuroscience.2010.03.062

Jabourian, M., Venance, L., Bourgoin, S., Ozon, S., Pérez, S., Godeheu, G., et al. (2005). Functional mu opioid receptors are expressed in cholinergic interneurons of the rat dorsal striatum: territorial specificity and diurnal variation. *Eur. J. Neurosci.* 21, 3301–3309. doi: 10.1111/j.1460-9568.2005.04154.x

Jackisch, R., Hotz, H., and Hertting, G. (1993). No evidence for presynaptic opioid receptors on cholinergic, but presence of kappa-receptors on dopaminergic neurons in the rabbit caudate nucleus: involvement of endogenous opioids. *Naunyn. Schmiedebergs Arch. Pharmacol.* 348, 234–241. doi: 10.1007/BF00169150

Jin, S., and Fredholm, B. B. (1997). Adenosine A2A receptor stimulation increases release of acetylcholine from rat hippocampus but not striatum, and does not affect catecholamine release. *Naunyn. Schmiedebergs Arch. Pharmacol.* 355, 48–56. doi: 10.1007/PL00004917

Johnson, M. D., and Yee, A. G. (1995). Ultrastructure of electrophysiologically-characterized synapses formed by serotonergic raphe neurons in culture. *Neuroscience* 67, 609–623. doi: 10.1016/0306-4522(95)00010-G

Jollivet, C., Montero-Menei, C. N., Venier-Julienne, M.-C., Sapin, A., Benoit, J.-P., and Menei, P. (2004). Striatal tyrosine hydroxylase immunoreactive neurons are induced by L-dihydroxyphenylalanine and nerve growth factor treatment in 6-hydroxydopamine lesioned rats. *Neurosci. Lett.* 362, 79–82. doi: 10.1016/j.neulet.2004.02.068

Jones, I. W., Bolam, J. P., and Wonnacott, S. (2001). Presynaptic localisation of the nicotinic acetylcholine receptor beta2 subunit immunoreactivity in rat nigrostriatal dopaminergic neurones. *J. Comp. Neurol.* 439, 235–247. doi: 10.1002/cne.1345

Jucaite, A., Öhd, J., Potter, A. S., Jaeger, J., Karlsson, P., Hannesdottir, K., et al. (2014). A randomized, double-blind, placebo-controlled crossover study of α4β 2* nicotinic acetylcholine receptor agonist AZD1446 (TC-6683) in adults with attention-deficit/hyperactivity disorder. *Psychopharmacology (Berl.)* 231, 1251–1265. doi: 10.1007/s00213-013-3116-7

Kaiser, S., and Wonnacott, S. (2000). Alpha-bungarotoxin-sensitive nicotinic receptors indirectly modulate [(3)H]dopamine release in rat striatal slices via glutamate release. *Mol. Pharmacol.* 58, 312–318. doi: 10.1124/mol.58.2.312

Kataoka, Y., Kalanithi, P. S. A., Grantz, H., Schwartz, M. L., Saper, C., Leckman, J. F., et al. (2010). Decreased number of parvalbumin and cholinergic interneurons in the striatum of individuals with Tourette syndrome. *J. Comp. Neurol.* 518, 277–291. doi: 10.1002/cne.22206

Katzenschlager, R., Sampaio, C., Costa, J., and Lees, A. (2003). Anticholinergics for symptomatic management of Parkinson's disease. *Cochrane Database Syst. Rev.* CD003735. doi: 10.1002/14651858.CD003735

Kawaguchi, Y. (1993). Physiological, morphological, and histochemical characterization of three classes of interneurons in rat neostriatum. *J. Neurosci.* 13, 4908–4923.

Keath, J. R., Iacoviello, M. P., Barrett, L. E., Mansvelder, H. D., and McGehee, D. S. (2007). Differential modulation by nicotine of substantia nigra versus ventral tegmental area dopamine neurons. *J. Neurophysiol.* 98, 3388–3396. doi: 10.1152/jn.00760.2007

Kelley, A. E. (2004). Ventral striatal control of appetitive motivation: role in ingestive behavior and reward-related learning. *Neurosci. Biobehav. Rev.* 27, 765–776. doi: 10.1016/j.neubiorev.2003.11.015

Kimura, M., Rajkowski, J., and Evarts, E. (1984). Tonically discharging putamen neurons exhibit set-dependent responses. *Proc. Natl. Acad. Sci. U.S.A.* 81, 4998–5001. doi: 10.1073/pnas.81.15.4998

Klink, R., de Kerchove d'Exaerde, A., Zoli, M., and Changeux, J. P. (2001). Molecular and physiological diversity of nicotinic acetylcholine receptors in the midbrain dopaminergic nuclei. *J. Neurosci.* 21, 1452–1463.

Koob, G. F. (1992). Neural mechanisms of drug reinforcement. *Ann. N.Y. Acad. Sci.* 654, 171–191. doi: 10.1111/j.1749-6632.1992.tb25966.x

Koranda, J. L., Cone, J. J., McGehee, D. S., Roitman, M. F., Beeler, J. A., and Zhuang, X. (2014). Nicotinic receptors regulate the dynamic range of dopamine release *in vivo*. *J. Neurophysiol.* 111, 103–111. doi: 10.1152/jn.00269.2013

Kostic, V., Przedborski, S., Flaster, E., and Sternic, N. (1991). Early development of levodopa-induced dyskinesias and response fluctuations in young-onset Parkinson's disease. *Neurology* 41, 202–205. doi: 10.1212/WNL.41.2_Part_1.202

Kravitz, A. V., Freeze, B. S., Parker, P. R. L., Kay, K., Thwin, M. T., Deisseroth, K., et al. (2010). Regulation of parkinsonian motor behaviours by optogenetic control of basal ganglia circuitry. *Nature* 466, 622–626. doi: 10.1038/nature09159

Kubota, Y., Inagaki, S., Shimada, S., Kito, S., Eckenstein, F., and Tohyama, M. (1987). Neostriatal cholinergic neurons receive direct synaptic inputs from dopaminergic axons. *Brain Res.* 413, 179–184. doi: 10.1016/0006-8993(87)90167-3

Kulak, J. M., Musachio, J. L., McIntosh, J. M., and Quik, M. (2002). Declines in different beta2* nicotinic receptor populations in monkey striatum after nigrostriatal damage. *J. Pharmacol. Exp. Ther.* 303, 633–639. doi: 10.1124/jpet.102.039347

Kumar, N., Van Gerpen, J. A., Bower, J. H., and Ahlskog, J. E. (2005). Levodopa-dyskinesia incidence by age of Parkinson's disease onset. *Mov. Disord. Off. J. Mov. Disord. Soc.* 20, 342–344. doi: 10.1002/mds.20360

Kumar, P., and Kumar, A. (2009). Protective effect of rivastigmine against 3-nitropropionic acid-induced Huntington's disease like symptoms: possible behavioural, biochemical and cellular alterations. *Eur. J. Pharmacol.* 615, 91–101. doi: 10.1016/j.ejphar.2009.04.058

Künzle, H. (1975). Bilateral projections from precentral motor cortex to the putamen and other parts of the basal ganglia. An autoradiographic study in *Macaca fascicularis*. *Brain Res.* 88, 195–209. doi: 10.1016/0006-8993(75)90384-4

Kurokawa, M., Kirk, I. P., Kirkpatrick, K. A., Kase, H., and Richardson, P. J. (1994). Inhibition by KF17837 of adenosine A2A receptor-mediated modulation of striatal GABA and ACh release. *Br. J. Pharmacol.* 113, 43–48. doi: 10.1111/j.1476-5381.1994.tb16171.x

Landwehrmeyer, G. B., Standaert, D. G., Testa, C. M., Penney, J. B. Jr., and Young, A. B. (1995). NMDA receptor subunit mRNA expression by projection neurons and interneurons in rat striatum. *J. Neurosci.* 15, 5297–5307.

Lange, K. W., Wells, F. R., Jenner, P., and Marsden, C. D. (1993). Altered muscarinic and nicotinic receptor densities in cortical and subcortical brain regions in Parkinson's disease. *J. Neurochem.* 60, 197–203. doi: 10.1111/j.1471-4159.1993.tb05838.x

Lanska, D. J. (2010). Chapter 33: the history of movement disorders. *Handb. Clin. Neurol.* 95, 501–546. doi: 10.1016/S0072-9752(08)02133-7

Lapper, S. R., and Bolam, J. P. (1992). Input from the frontal cortex and the parafascicular nucleus to cholinergic interneurons in the dorsal striatum of the rat. *Neuroscience* 51, 533–545. doi: 10.1016/0306-4522(92)90293-B

Lee, J., Laurin, N., Crosbie, J., Ickowicz, A., Pathare, T., Malone, M., et al. (2008). Association study of the nicotinic acetylcholine receptor alpha4 subunit gene, CHRNA4, in attention-deficit hyperactivity disorder. *Genes Brain Behav.* 7, 53–60. doi: 10.1111/j.1601-183X.2007.00325.x

Lee, K., Dixon, A. K., Freeman, T. C., and Richardson, P. J. (1998). Identification of an ATP-sensitive potassium channel current in rat striatal cholinergic interneurones. *J. Physiol.* 510(Pt 2), 441–453. doi: 10.1111/j.1469-7793.1998.441bk.x

Lehmann, J., and Langer, S. Z. (1982). Muscarinic receptors on dopamine terminals in the cat caudate nucleus: neuromodulation of [3H]dopamine release *in vitro* by endogenous acetylcholine. *Brain Res.* 248, 61–69. doi: 10.1016/0006-8993(82)91147-7

Lehmann, J., and Langer, S. Z. (1983). The striatal cholinergic interneuron: synaptic target of dopaminergic terminals? *Neuroscience* 10, 1105–1120. doi: 10.1016/0306-4522(83)90102-1

Le Moine, C., Kieffer, B., Gaveriaux-Ruff, C., Befort, K., and Bloch, B. (1994). Delta-opioid receptor gene expression in the mouse forebrain: localization in cholinergic neurons of the striatum. *Neuroscience* 62, 635–640. doi: 10.1016/0306-4522(94)90464-2

Le Novère, N., Zoli, M., and Changeux, J. P. (1996). Neuronal nicotinic receptor alpha 6 subunit mRNA is selectively concentrated in catecholaminergic nuclei of the rat brain. *Eur. J. Neurosci.* 8, 2428–2439. doi: 10.1111/j.1460-9568.1996.tb01206.x

Leonard, S., Gault, J., Hopkins, J., Logel, J., Vianzon, R., Short, M., et al. (2002). Association of promoter variants in the alpha7 nicotinic acetylcholine receptor subunit gene with an inhibitory deficit found in schizophrenia. *Arch. Gen. Psychiatry* 59, 1085–1096. doi: 10.1001/archpsyc.59.12.1085

Lesser, R. P., Fahn, S., Snider, S. R., Cote, L. J., Isgreen, W. P., and Barrett, R. E. (1979). Analysis of the clinical problems in parkinsonism and the complications of long-term levodopa therapy. *Neurology* 29, 1253–1260. doi: 10.1212/WNL.29.9_Part_1.1253

Levey, A. I., Kitt, C. A., Simonds, W. F., Price, D. L., and Brann, M. R. (1991). Identification and localization of muscarinic acetylcholine receptor proteins in brain with subtype-specific antibodies. *J. Neurosci.* 11, 3218–3226.

Li, J.-L., Kaneko, T., and Mizuno, N. (2002). Synaptic association of dopaminergic axon terminals and neurokinin-1 receptor-expressing intrinsic neurons in the striatum of the rat. *Neurosci. Lett.* 324, 9–12. doi: 10.1016/S0304-3940(02)00138-6

Lin, J. Y., Chung, K. K. H., de Castro, D., Funk, G. D., and Lipski, J. (2004). Effects of muscarinic acetylcholine receptor activation on membrane currents and intracellular messengers in medium spiny neurones of the rat striatum. *Eur. J. Neurosci.* 20, 1219–1230. doi: 10.1111/j.1460-9568.2004.03576.x

Linazasoro, G. (1994). Anticholinergics and dyskinesia. *Mov. Disord. Off. J. Mov. Disord. Soc.* 9, 689. doi: 10.1002/mds.870090618

Linden, D. J., Dickinson, M. H., Smeyne, M., and Connor, J. A. (1991). A long-term depression of AMPA currents in cultured cerebellar Purkinje neurons. *Neuron* 7, 81–89. doi: 10.1016/0896-6273(91)90076-C

Liu, Z., Otsu, Y., Vasuta, C., Nawa, H., and Murphy, T. H. (2007). Action-potential-independent GABAergic tone mediated by nicotinic stimulation of immature striatal miniature synaptic transmission. *J. Neurophysiol.* 98, 581–593. doi: 10.1152/jn.00768.2006

Luo, R., Janssen, M. J., Partridge, J. G., and Vicini, S. (2013). Direct and GABA-mediated indirect effects of nicotinic ACh receptor agonists on striatal neurones. *J. Physiol.* 591, 203–217. doi: 10.1113/jphysiol.2012.241786

MacDermott, A. B., Role, L. W., and Siegelbaum, S. A. (1999). Presynaptic ionotropic receptors and the control of transmitter release. *Annu. Rev. Neurosci.* 22, 443–485. doi: 10.1146/annurev.neuro.22.1.443

Macintosh, F. C. (1941). The distribution of acetylcholine in the peripheral and the central nervous system. *J. Physiol.* 99, 436–442.

Mahon, S., Deniau, J.-M., and Charpier, S. (2004). Corticostriatal plasticity: life after the depression. *Trends Neurosci.* 27, 460–467. doi: 10.1016/j.tins.2004.06.010

Malenka, R. C., and Kocsis, J. D. (1988). Presynaptic actions of carbachol and adenosine on corticostriatal synaptic transmission studied *in vitro*. *J. Neurosci.* 8, 3750–3756.

Mansour, A., Fox, C. A., Burke, S., Meng, F., Thompson, R. C., Akil, H., et al. (1994). Mu, delta, and kappa opioid receptor mRNA expression in the rat CNS: an *in situ* hybridization study. *J. Comp. Neurol.* 350, 412–438. doi: 10.1002/cne.903500307

Manyam, B. V. (1990). Paralysis agitans and levodopa in "Ayurveda": ancient Indian medical treatise. *Mov. Disord. Off. J. Mov. Disord. Soc.* 5, 47–48. doi: 10.1002/mds.870050112

Manyam, B. V., and Sánchez-Ramos, J. R. (1999). Traditional and complementary therapies in Parkinson's disease. *Adv. Neurol.* 80, 565–574.

Marchi, M., Risso, F., Viola, C., Cavazzani, P., and Raiteri, M. (2002). Direct evidence that release-stimulating alpha7* nicotinic cholinergic receptors are localized on human and rat brain glutamatergic axon terminals. *J. Neurochem.* 80, 1071–1078. doi: 10.1046/j.0022-3042.2002.00805.x

Marchi, M., Sanguineti, P., and Raiteri, M. (1990). Muscarinic receptors mediate direct inhibition of GABA release from rat striatal nerve terminals. *Neurosci. Lett.* 116, 347–351. doi: 10.1016/0304-3940(90)90099-U

Markram, H., Lübke, J., Frotscher, M., and Sakmann, B. (1997). Regulation of synaptic efficacy by coincidence of postsynaptic APs and EPSPs. *Science* 275, 213–215. doi: 10.1126/science.275.5297.213

Martella, G., Platania, P., Vita, D., Sciamanna, G., Cuomo, D., Tassone, A., et al. (2009). Enhanced sensitivity to group II mGlu receptor activation at corticostriatal synapses in mice lacking the familial parkinsonism-linked genes PINK1 or Parkin. *Exp. Neurol.* 215, 388–396. doi: 10.1016/j.expneurol.2008.11.001

Martin-Schild, S., Gerall, A. A., Kastin, A. J., and Zadina, J. E. (1999). Differential distribution of endomorphin 1- and endomorphin 2-like immunoreactivities in the CNS of the rodent. *J. Comp. Neurol.* 405, 450–471.

Martone, M. E., Armstrong, D. M., Young, S. J., and Groves, P. M. (1992). Ultrastructural examination of enkephalin and substance P input to cholinergic neurons within the rat neostriatum. *Brain Res.* 594, 253–262. doi: 10.1016/0006-8993(92)91132-X

Matsubayashi, H., Amano, T., Amano, H., and Sasa, M. (2001). Excitation of rat striatal large neurons by dopamine and/or glutamate released from nerve terminals via presynaptic nicotinic receptor (A4beta2 type) stimulation. *Jpn. J. Pharmacol.* 86, 429–436. doi: 10.1254/jjp.86.429

Matsuda, W., Furuta, T., Nakamura, K. C., Hioki, H., Fujiyama, F., Arai, R., et al. (2009). Single nigrostriatal dopaminergic neurons form widely spread and highly dense axonal arborizations in the neostriatum. *J. Neurosci.* 29, 444–453. doi: 10.1523/JNEUROSCI.4029-08.2009

Maurin, Y., Banrezes, B., Menetrey, A., Mailly, P., and Deniau, J. M. (1999). Three-dimensional distribution of nigrostriatal neurons in the rat: relation to the topography of striatonigral projections. *Neuroscience* 91, 891–909. doi: 10.1016/S0306-4522(98)00681-2

McEvoy, J. P., and Allen, T. B. (2002). The importance of nicotinic acetylcholine receptors in schizophrenia, bipolar disorder and Tourette's syndrome. *Curr. Drug Targets CNS Neurol. Disord.* 1, 433–442. doi: 10.2174/1568007023339210

McGeer, P. L., and McGeer, E. G. (1977). Possible changes in striatal and limbic cholinergic systems in schizophrenia. *Arch. Gen. Psychiatry* 34, 1319–1323. doi: 10.1001/archpsyc.1977.01770230061003

McGehee, D. S., Heath, M. J., Gelber, S., Devay, P., and Role, L. W. (1995). Nicotine enhancement of fast excitatory synaptic transmission in CNS by presynaptic receptors. *Science* 269, 1692–1696. doi: 10.1126/science.7569895

McGehee, D. S., and Role, L. W. (1995). Physiological diversity of nicotinic acetylcholine receptors expressed by vertebrate neurons. *Annu. Rev. Physiol.* 57, 521–546. doi: 10.1146/annurev.ph.57.030195.002513

Mirenowicz, J., and Schultz, W. (1996). Preferential activation of midbrain dopamine neurons by appetitive rather than aversive stimuli. *Nature* 379, 449–451. doi: 10.1038/379449a0

Morens, D. M., Grandinetti, A., Reed, D., White, L. R., and Ross, G. W. (1995). Cigarette smoking and protection from Parkinson's disease: false association or etiologic clue? *Neurology* 45, 1041–1051. doi: 10.1212/WNL.45.6.1041

Mori, F., Tanji, K., Zhang, H., Kakita, A., Takahashi, H., and Wakabayashi, K. (2008). alpha-Synuclein pathology in the neostriatum in Parkinson's disease. *Acta Neuropathol. (Berl.)* 115, 453–459. doi: 10.1007/s00401-007-0316-4

Moss, J., and Bolam, J. P. (2008). A dopaminergic axon lattice in the striatum and its relationship with cortical and thalamic terminals. *J. Neurosci.* 28, 11221–11230. doi: 10.1523/JNEUROSCI.2780-08.2008

Mulder, A. H., Burger, D. M., Wardeh, G., Hogenboom, F., and Frankhuyzen, A. L. (1991). Pharmacological profile of various kappa-agonists at kappa-, mu- and delta-opioid receptors mediating presynaptic inhibition of neurotransmitter release in the rat brain. *Br. J. Pharmacol.* 102, 518–522. doi: 10.1111/j.1476-5381.1991.tb12203.x

Mulder, A. H., Wardeh, G., Hogenboom, F., and Frankhuyzen, A. L. (1984). Kappa- and delta-opioid receptor agonists differentially inhibit striatal dopamine and acetylcholine release. *Nature* 308, 278–280. doi: 10.1038/308278a0

Mulle, C., Choquet, D., Korn, H., and Changeux, J. P. (1992). Calcium influx through nicotinic receptor in rat central neurons: its relevance to cellular regulation. *Neuron* 8, 135–143. doi: 10.1016/0896-6273(92)90115-T

Nelson, A. B., Bussert, T. G., Kreitzer, A. C., and Seal, R. P. (2014a). Striatal cholinergic neurotransmission requires VGLUT3. *J. Neurosci.* 34, 8772–8777. doi: 10.1523/JNEUROSCI.0901-14.2014

Nelson, A. B., Hammack, N., Yang, C. F., Shah, N. M., Seal, R. P., and Kreitzer, A. C. (2014b). Striatal cholinergic interneurons drive GABA release from dopamine terminals. *Neuron* 82, 63–70. doi: 10.1016/j.neuron.2014.01.023

Nicholas, A. P., Pieribone, V. A., Arvidsson, U., and Hökfelt, T. (1992). Serotonin-, substance P- and glutamate/aspartate-like immunoreactivities in medullo-spinal pathways of rat and primate. *Neuroscience* 48, 545–559. doi: 10.1016/0306-4522(92)90401-M

Nishiyama, M., Hong, K., Mikoshiba, K., Poo, M. M., and Kato, K. (2000). Calcium stores regulate the polarity and input specificity of synaptic modification. *Nature* 408, 584–588. doi: 10.1038/35046067

Norgren, R., Hajnal, A., and Mungarndee, S. S. (2006). Gustatory reward and the nucleus accumbens. *Physiol. Behav.* 89, 531–535. doi: 10.1016/j.physbeh.2006.05.024

Ovallath, S., and Deepa, P. (2013). The history of parkinsonism: descriptions in ancient Indian medical literature. *Mov. Disord. Off. J. Mov. Disord. Soc.* 28, 566–568. doi: 10.1002/mds.25420

Pakhotin, P., and Bracci, E. (2007). Cholinergic interneurons control the excitatory input to the striatum. *J. Neurosci.* 27, 391–400. doi: 10.1523/JNEUROSCI.3709-06.2007

Pancani, T., Bolarinwa, C., Smith, Y., Lindsley, C. W., Conn, P. J., and Xiang, Z. (2014). M4 mAChR-mediated modulation of glutamatergic transmission at corticostriatal synapses. *ACS Chem. Neurosci.* 5, 318–324. doi: 10.1021/cn500003z

Panula, P., Yang, H. Y., and Costa, E. (1984). Histamine-containing neurons in the rat hypothalamus. *Proc. Natl. Acad. Sci. U.S.A.* 81, 2572–2576. doi: 10.1073/pnas.81.8.2572

Parkinson, J. (1817). *An Essay on the Shaking Palsy.* London: Whittingham and Rowland for Sherwood, Needly and Jones.

Parsons, M. E., and Ganellin, C. R. (2006). Histamine and its receptors. *Br. J. Pharmacol.* 147(Suppl. 1), S127–S135. doi: 10.1038/sj.bjp.0706440

Patrick, J., Séquéla, P., Vernino, S., Amador, M., Luetje, C., and Dani, J. A. (1993). Functional diversity of neuronal nicotinic acetylcholine receptors. *Prog. Brain Res.* 98, 113–120. doi: 10.1016/S0079-6123(08)62387-0

Pérez-Garci, E., Bargas, J., and Galarraga, E. (2003). The role of Ca2+ channels in the repetitive firing of striatal projection neurons. *Neuroreport* 14, 1253–1256. doi: 10.1097/01.wnr.0000081861.45938.71

Perez-Rosello, T., Figueroa, A., Salgado, H., Vilchis, C., Tecuapetla, F., Guzman, J. N., et al. (2005). Cholinergic control of firing pattern and neurotransmission in rat neostriatal projection neurons: role of CaV2.1 and CaV2.2 Ca2+ channels. *J. Neurophysiol.* 93, 2507–2519. doi: 10.1152/jn.00853.2004

Perez, X. A., Ly, J., McIntosh, J. M., and Quik, M. (2012). Long-term nicotine exposure depresses dopamine release in nonhuman primate nucleus accumbens. *J. Pharmacol. Exp. Ther.* 342, 335–344. doi: 10.1124/jpet.112.194084

Perez, X. A., McIntosh, J. M., and Quik, M. (2013). Long-term nicotine treatment down-regulates α6β2* nicotinic receptor expression and function in nucleus accumbens. *J. Neurochem.* 127, 762–771. doi: 10.1111/jnc.12442

Perreault, M. L., Fan, T., Alijaniaram, M., O'Dowd, B. F., and George, S. R. (2012). Dopamine D1-D2 receptor heteromer in dual phenotype GABA/glutamate-coexpressing striatal medium spiny neurons: regulation of BDNF, GAD67 and VGLUT1/2. *PLoS ONE* 7:e33348. doi: 10.1371/journal.pone.0033348

Persohn, E., Malherbe, P., and Richards, J. G. (1992). Comparative molecular neuroanatomy of cloned GABAA receptor subunits in the rat CNS. *J. Comp. Neurol.* 326, 193–216. doi: 10.1002/cne.903260204

Picconi, B., Passino, E., Sgobio, C., Bonsi, P., Barone, I., Ghiglieri, V., et al. (2006). Plastic and behavioral abnormalities in experimental Huntington's disease: a crucial role for cholinergic interneurons. *Neurobiol. Dis.* 22, 143–152. doi: 10.1016/j.nbd.2005.10.009

Piggott, M. A., Owens, J., O'Brien, J., Colloby, S., Fenwick, J., Wyper, D., et al. (2003). Muscarinic receptors in basal ganglia in dementia with Lewy bodies, Parkinson's disease and Alzheimer's disease. *J. Chem. Neuroanat.* 25, 161–173. doi: 10.1016/S0891-0618(03)00002-4

Pisani, A., Bonsi, P., Catania, M. V., Giuffrida, R., Morari, M., Marti, M., et al. (2002). Metabotropic glutamate 2 receptors modulate synaptic inputs and calcium signals in striatal cholinergic interneurons. *J. Neurosci.* 22, 6176–6185.

Pisani, A., Bonsi, P., Centonze, D., Bernardi, G., and Calabresi, P. (2001). Functional coexpression of excitatory mGluR1 and mGluR5 on striatal cholinergic interneurons. *Neuropharmacology* 40, 460–463. doi: 10.1016/S0028-3908(00)00184-2

Pisani, A., Bonsi, P., Centonze, D., Martorana, A., Fusco, F., Sancesario, G., et al. (2003). Activation of beta1-adrenoceptors excites striatal cholinergic interneurons through a cAMP-dependent, protein kinase-independent pathway. *J. Neurosci.* 23, 5272–5282.

Plotkin, J. L., Shen, W., Rafalovich, I., Sebel, L. E., Day, M., Chan, C. S., et al. (2013). Regulation of dendritic calcium release in striatal spiny projection neurons. *J. Neurophysiol.* 110, 2325–2336. doi: 10.1152/jn.00422.2013

Poewe, W., Wolters, E., Emre, M., Onofrj, M., Hsu, C., Tekin, S., et al. (2006). Long-term benefits of rivastigmine in dementia associated with Parkinson's disease: an active treatment extension study. *Mov. Disord. Off. J. Mov. Disord. Soc.* 21, 456–461. doi: 10.1002/mds.20700

Ponterio, G., Tassone, A., Sciamanna, G., Riahi, E., Vanni, V., Bonsi, P., et al. (2013). Powerful inhibitory action of mu opioid receptors (MOR) on cholinergic interneuron excitability in the dorsal striatum. *Neuropharmacology* 75, 78–85. doi: 10.1016/j.neuropharm.2013.07.006

Potter, A. S., Dunbar, G., Mazzulla, E., Hosford, D., and Newhouse, P. A. (2014). AZD3480, a novel nicotinic receptor agonist, for the treatment of attention-deficit/hyperactivity disorder in adults. *Biol. Psychiatry* 75, 207–214. doi: 10.1016/j.biopsych.2013.06.002

Pourcher, E., Bonnet, A. M., Kefalos, J., Dubois, B., and Agid, Y. (1989). Effects of etybenzatropine and diazepam on levodopa-induced diphasic dyskinesias in Parkinson's disease. *Mov. Disord. Off. J. Mov. Disord. Soc.* 4, 195–201. doi: 10.1002/mds.870040301

Prast, H., Tran, M. H., Fischer, H., Kraus, M., Lamberti, C., Grass, K., et al. (1999a). Histaminergic neurons modulate acetylcholine release in the ventral striatum: role of H3 histamine receptors. *Naunyn. Schmiedebergs Arch. Pharmacol.* 360, 558–564. doi: 10.1007/s002109900097

Prast, H., Tran, M. H., Lamberti, C., Fischer, H., Kraus, M., Grass, K., et al. (1999b). Histaminergic neurons modulate acetylcholine release in the ventral striatum: role of H1 and H2 histamine receptors. *Naunyn. Schmiedebergs Arch. Pharmacol.* 360, 552–557. doi: 10.1007/s002109900098

Preston, Z., Lee, K., Widdowson, L., Richardson, P. J., and Pinnock, R. D. (2000). Tachykinins increase [3H]acetylcholine release in mouse striatum through multiple receptor subtypes. *Neuroscience* 95, 367–376. doi: 10.1016/S0306-4522(99)00440-6

Puttfarcken, P. S., Jacobs, I., and Faltynek, C. R. (2000). Characterization of nicotinic acetylcholine receptor-mediated [(3)H]-dopamine release from rat cortex and striatum. *Neuropharmacology* 39, 2673–2680. doi: 10.1016/S0028-3908(00)00131-3

Quik, M., Bordia, T., and O'Leary, K. (2007). Nicotinic receptors as CNS targets for Parkinson's disease. *Biochem. Pharmacol.* 74, 1224–1234. doi: 10.1016/j.bcp.2007.06.015

Quik, M., and McIntosh, J. M. (2006). Striatal alpha6* nicotinic acetylcholine receptors: potential targets for Parkinson's disease therapy. *J. Pharmacol. Exp. Ther.* 316, 481–489. doi: 10.1124/jpet.105.094375

Quik, M., Perez, X. A., and Bordia, T. (2012). Nicotine as a potential neuroprotective agent for Parkinson's disease. *Mov. Disord. Off. J. Mov. Disord. Soc.* 27, 947–957. doi: 10.1002/mds.25028

Quik, M., Sum, J. D., Whiteaker, P., McCallum, S. E., Marks, M. J., Musachio, J., et al. (2003). Differential declines in striatal nicotinic receptor subtype function after nigrostriatal damage in mice. *Mol. Pharmacol.* 63, 1169–1179. doi: 10.1124/mol.63.5.1169

Quik, M., and Wonnacott, S. (2011). α6β2* and α4β2* nicotinic acetylcholine receptors as drug targets for Parkinson's disease. *Pharmacol. Rev.* 63, 938–966. doi: 10.1124/pr.110.003269

Radek, R. J., Kohlhaas, K. L., Rueter, L. E., and Mohler, E. G. (2010). Treating the cognitive deficits of schizophrenia with alpha4beta2 neuronal nicotinic receptor agonists. *Curr. Pharm. Des.* 16, 309–322. doi: 10.2174/138161210790170166

Raedler, T. J., Knable, M. B., Jones, D. W., Urbina, R. A., Gorey, J. G., Lee, K. S., et al. (2003). *In vivo* determination of muscarinic acetylcholine receptor availability in schizophrenia. *Am. J. Psychiatry* 160, 118–127. doi: 10.1176/appi.ajp.160.1.118

Ragozzino, M. E. (2003). Acetylcholine actions in the dorsomedial striatum support the flexible shifting of response patterns. *Neurobiol. Learn. Mem.* 80, 257–267. doi: 10.1016/S1074-7427(03)00077-7

Raudino, F. (2012). The parkinson disease before james parkinson. *Neurol. Sci. Off. J. Ital. Neurol. Soc. Ital. Soc. Clin. Neurophysiol.* 33, 945–948. doi: 10.1007/s10072-011-0816-9

Ravel, S., Legallet, E., and Apicella, P. (1999). Tonically active neurons in the monkey striatum do not preferentially respond to appetitive stimuli. *Exp. Brain Res.* 128, 531–534. doi: 10.1007/s002210050876

Reynolds, J. N. J., Hyland, B. I., and Wickens, J. R. (2004). Modulation of an afterhyperpolarization by the substantia nigra induces pauses in the tonic firing of striatal cholinergic interneurons. *J. Neurosci.* 24, 9870–9877. doi: 10.1523/JNEUROSCI.3225-04.2004

Rezvani, A. H., Cauley, M. C., Johnson, E. C., Gatto, G. J., and Levin, E. D. (2012). Effects of AZD3480, a neuronal nicotinic acetylcholine receptor agonist, and donepezil on dizocilpine-induced attentional impairment in rats. *Psychopharmacology (Berl.)* 223, 251–258. doi: 10.1007/s00213-012-2712-2

Rice, M. E., and Cragg, S. J. (2004). Nicotine amplifies reward-related dopamine signals in striatum. *Nat. Neurosci.* 7, 583–584. doi: 10.1038/nn1244

Richardson, P. J., Dixon, A. K., Lee, K., Bell, M. I., Cox, P. J., Williams, R., et al. (2000). Correlating physiology with gene expression in striatal cholinergic neurones. *J. Neurochem.* 74, 839–846. doi: 10.1046/j.1471-4159.2000.740839.x

Rinne, J. O., Laihinen, A., Lönnberg, P., Marjamäki, P., and Rinne, U. K. (1991). A post-mortem study on striatal dopamine receptors in Parkinson's disease. *Brain Res.* 556, 117–122. doi: 10.1016/0006-8993(91)90554-9

Robinson, T. E., and Berridge, K. C. (2000). The psychology and neurobiology of addiction: an incentive-sensitization view. *Addict. Abingdon Engl.* 95(Suppl. 2), S91–S117. doi: 10.1080/09652140050111681

Rodríguez, M., and González-Hernández, T. (1999). Electrophysiological and morphological evidence for a GABAergic nigrostriatal pathway. *J. Neurosci.* 19, 4682–4694.

Rodríguez-Pallares, J., Labandeira-García, J. L., Muñoz, A., and Caruncho, H. J. (2000). Morphology and neurochemistry of two striatal neuronal subtypes expressing the GABA(A) receptor alpha3-subunit in the rat. *Brain Res.* 876, 124–130. doi: 10.1016/S0006-8993(00)02636-6

Rojas, A., and Dingledine, R. (2013). Ionotropic glutamate receptors: regulation by G-protein-coupled receptors. *Mol. Pharmacol.* 83, 746–752. doi: 10.1124/mol.112.083352

Sanberg, P. R., Shytle, R. D., and Silver, A. A. (1998). Treatment of Tourette's syndrome with mecamylamine. *Lancet* 352, 705–706. doi: 10.1016/S0140-6736(05)60822-7

Sandor, N. T., Zelles, T., Kiss, J., Sershen, H., Torocsik, A., Lajtha, A., et al. (1991). Effect of nicotine on dopaminergic-cholinergic interaction in the striatum. *Brain Res.* 567, 313–316. doi: 10.1016/0006-8993(91)90810-I

Santangelo, G., Barone, P., Trojano, L., and Vitale, C. (2013a). Pathological gambling in Parkinson's disease. A comprehensive review. *Parkinsonism Relat. Disord.* 19, 645–653. doi: 10.1016/j.parkreldis.2013.02.007

Santangelo, G., Trojano, L., Barone, P., Errico, D., Grossi, D., and Vitale, C. (2013b). Apathy in Parkinson's disease: diagnosis, neuropsychological correlates, pathophysiology and treatment. *Behav. Neurol.* 27, 501–513. doi: 10.3233/BEN-129025

Sato, A., Sasaoka, T., Nishijo, T., and Momiyama, T. (2014). GABAergic synaptic transmission onto striatal cholinergic interneurons in dopamine D2 receptor knock-out mice. *Neuroscience* 263, 138–147. doi: 10.1016/j.neuroscience.2014.01.010

Scheibler, P., Pesic, M., Franke, H., Reinhardt, R., Wirkner, K., Illes, P., et al. (2004). P2X2 and P2Y1 immunofluorescence in rat neostriatal medium-spiny projection neurones and cholinergic interneurones is not linked to respective purinergic receptor function. *Br. J. Pharmacol.* 143, 119–131. doi: 10.1038/sj.bjp.0705916

Schoffelmeer, A. N., Hogenboom, F., and Mulder, A. H. (1997). Kappa1- and kappa2-opioid receptors mediating presynaptic inhibition of dopamine and acetylcholine release in rat neostriatum. *Br. J. Pharmacol.* 122, 520–524. doi: 10.1038/sj.bjp.0701394

Schwartz, J. C., Arrang, J. M., Garbarg, M., and Korner, M. (1986). Properties and roles of the three subclasses of histamine receptors in brain. *J. Exp. Biol.* 124, 203–224.

Sharples, C. G., Kaiser, S., Soliakov, L., Marks, M. J., Collins, A. C., Washburn, M., et al. (2000). UB-165: a novel nicotinic agonist with subtype selectivity implicates the alpha4beta2* subtype in the modulation of dopamine release from rat striatal synaptosomes. *J. Neurosci.* 20, 2783–2791.

Shen, W., Hamilton, S. E., Nathanson, N. M., and Surmeier, D. J. (2005). Cholinergic suppression of KCNQ channel currents enhances excitability of striatal medium spiny neurons. *J. Neurosci.* 25, 7449–7458. doi: 10.1523/JNEUROSCI.1381-05.2005

Shiflett, M. W., Brown, R. A., and Balleine, B. W. (2010). Acquisition and performance of goal-directed instrumental actions depends on ERK signaling in distinct regions of dorsal striatum in rats. *J. Neurosci.* 30, 2951–2959. doi: 10.1523/JNEUROSCI.1778-09.2010

Shimohama, S., Taniguchi, T., Fujiwara, M., and Kameyama, M. (1985). Biochemical characterization of the nicotinic cholinergic receptors in human brain: binding of (-)-[3H]nicotine. *J. Neurochem.* 45, 604–610. doi: 10.1111/j.1471-4159.1985.tb04029.x

Shytle, R. D., Silver, A. A., Philipp, M. K., McConville, B. J., and Sanberg, P. R. (1996). Transdermal nicotine for Tourette's syndrome. *Drug Dev. Res.* 38, 290–298. doi: 10.1002/(SICI)1098-2299(199607/08)38:3/4<290::AID-DDR18>3.0.CO;2-2

Silver, A. A., Shytle, R. D., and Sanberg, P. R. (2000). Mecamylamine in Tourette's syndrome: a two-year retrospective case study. *J. Child Adolesc. Psychopharmacol.* 10, 59–68. doi: 10.1089/cap.2000.10.59

Simón-Sánchez, J., Schulte, C., Bras, J. M., Sharma, M., Gibbs, J. R., Berg, D., et al. (2009). Genome-wide association study reveals genetic risk underlying Parkinson's disease. *Nat. Genet.* 41, 1308–1312. doi: 10.1038/ng.487

Sirviö, J., Rinne, J. O., Valjakka, A., Rinne, U. K., Riekkinen, P. J., and Paljärvi, L. (1989). Different forms of brain acetylcholinesterase and muscarinic binding in Parkinson's disease. *J. Neurol. Sci.* 90, 23–32. doi: 10.1016/0022-510X(89)90042-7

Smiley, J. F., Levey, A. I., and Mesulam, M. M. (1999). m2 muscarinic receptor immunolocalization in cholinergic cells of the monkey basal forebrain and striatum. *Neuroscience* 90, 803–814. doi: 10.1016/S0306-4522(98)00527-2

Smith, R., Chung, H., Rundquist, S., Maat-Schieman, M. L. C., Colgan, L., Englund, E., et al. (2006). Cholinergic neuronal defect without cell loss in Huntington's disease. *Hum. Mol. Genet.* 15, 3119–3131. doi: 10.1093/hmg/ddl252

Smith, Y., and Kieval, J. Z. (2000). Anatomy of the dopamine system in the basal ganglia. *Trends Neurosci.* 23, S28–S33. doi: 10.1016/S1471-1931(00)00023-9

Smolders, I., Bogaert, L., Ebinger, G., and Michotte, Y. (1997). Muscarinic modulation of striatal dopamine, glutamate, and GABA release, as measured with *in vivo* microdialysis. *J. Neurochem.* 68, 1942–1948. doi: 10.1046/j.1471-4159.1997.68051942.x

Sprouse, J. S., Bradberry, C. W., Roth, R. H., and Aghajanian, G. K. (1989). MDMA (3,4-methylenedioxymethamphetamine) inhibits the firing of dorsal raphe neurons in brain slices via release of serotonin. *Eur. J. Pharmacol.* 167, 375–383. doi: 10.1016/0014-2999(89)90446-9

Standaert, D. G., Friberg, I. K., Landwehrmeyer, G. B., Young, A. B., and Penney, J. B. Jr. (1999). Expression of NMDA glutamate receptor subunit mRNAs in neurochemically identified projection and interneurons in the striatum of the rat. *Brain Res. Mol. Brain Res.* 64, 11–23. doi: 10.1016/S0169-328X(98)00293-9

Stephenson-Jones, M., Samuelsson, E., Ericsson, J., Robertson, B., and Grillner, S. (2011). Evolutionary conservation of the basal ganglia as a common vertebrate mechanism for action selection. *Curr. Biol.* 21, 1081–1091. doi: 10.1016/j.cub.2011.05.001

Straub, C., Tritsch, N. X., Hagan, N. A., Gu, C., and Sabatini, B. L. (2014). Multiphasic modulation of cholinergic interneurons by nigrostriatal afferents. *J. Neurosci.* 34, 8557–8569. doi: 10.1523/JNEUROSCI.0589-14.2014

Stuber, G. D., Hnasko, T. S., Britt, J. P., Edwards, R. H., and Bonci, A. (2010). Dopaminergic terminals in the nucleus accumbens but not the dorsal striatum corelease glutamate. *J. Neurosci.* 30, 8229–8233. doi: 10.1523/JNEUROSCI.1754-10.2010

Sugita, S., Uchimura, N., Jiang, Z. G., and North, R. A. (1991). Distinct muscarinic receptors inhibit release of gamma-aminobutyric acid and excitatory amino acids in mammalian brain. *Proc. Natl. Acad. Sci. U.S.A.* 88, 2608–2611. doi: 10.1073/pnas.88.6.2608

Sullivan, M. A., Chen, H., and Morikawa, H. (2008). Recurrent inhibitory network among striatal cholinergic interneurons. *J. Neurosci.* 28, 8682–8690. doi: 10.1523/JNEUROSCI.2411-08.2008

Surmeier, D. J., Ding, J., Day, M., Wang, Z., and Shen, W. (2007). D1 and D2 dopamine-receptor modulation of striatal glutamatergic signaling in striatal medium spiny neurons. *Trends Neurosci.* 30, 228–235. doi: 10.1016/j.tins.2007.03.008

Suzuki, M., Desmond, T. J., Albin, R. L., and Frey, K. A. (2001a). Vesicular neurotransmitter transporters in Huntington's disease: initial observations and comparison with traditional synaptic markers. *Synapse* 41, 329–336. doi: 10.1002/syn.1089

Suzuki, T., Miura, M., Nishimura, K., and Aosaki, T. (2001b). Dopamine-dependent synaptic plasticity in the striatal cholinergic interneurons. *J. Neurosci.* 21, 6492–6501.

Szydlowski, S. N., Pollak Dorocic, I., Planert, H., Carlén, M., Meletis, K., and Silberberg, G. (2013). Target selectivity of feedforward inhibition by striatal fast-spiking interneurons. *J. Neurosci.* 33, 1678–1683. doi: 10.1523/JNEUROSCI.3572-12.2013

Tallaksen-Greene, S. J., Kaatz, K. W., Romano, C., and Albin, R. L. (1998). Localization of mGluR1a-like immunoreactivity and mGluR5-like immunoreactivity in identified populations of striatal neurons. *Brain Res.* 780, 210–217. doi: 10.1016/S0006-8993(97)01141-4

Tashiro, Y., Sugimoto, T., Hattori, T., Uemura, Y., Nagatsu, I., Kikuchi, H., et al. (1989). Tyrosine hydroxylase-like immunoreactive neurons in the striatum of the rat. *Neurosci. Lett.* 97, 6–10. doi: 10.1016/0304-3940(89)90130-4

Tepper, J. M., Tecuapetla, F., Koós, T., and Ibáñez-Sandoval, O. (2010). Heterogeneity and diversity of striatal GABAergic interneurons. *Front. Neuroanat.* 4:150. doi: 10.3389/fnana.2010.00150

Testa, C. M., Standaert, D. G., Young, A. B., and Penney, J. B. Jr. (1994). Metabotropic glutamate receptor mRNA expression in the basal ganglia of the rat. *J. Neurosci.* 14, 3005–3018.

Thomas, T. M., Smith, Y., Levey, A. I., and Hersch, S. M. (2000). Cortical inputs to m2-immunoreactive striatal interneurons in rat and monkey. *Synapse* 37, 252–261. doi: 10.1002/1098-2396(20000915)37:4<252::AID-SYN2>3.0.CO;2-A

Threlfell, S., Clements, M. A., Khodai, T., Pienaar, I. S., Exley, R., Wess, J., et al. (2010). Striatal muscarinic receptors promote activity dependence of dopamine transmission via distinct receptor subtypes on cholinergic interneurons in ventral versus dorsal striatum. *J. Neurosci.* 30, 3398–3408. doi: 10.1523/JNEUROSCI.5620-09.2010

Threlfell, S., and Cragg, S. J. (2011). Dopamine signaling in dorsal versus ventral striatum: the dynamic role of cholinergic interneurons. *Front. Syst. Neurosci.* 5:11. doi: 10.3389/fnsys.2011.00011

Threlfell, S., Lalic, T., Platt, N. J., Jennings, K. A., Deisseroth, K., and Cragg, S. J. (2012). Striatal dopamine release is triggered by synchronized activity in cholinergic interneurons. *Neuron* 75, 58–64. doi: 10.1016/j.neuron.2012.04.038

Tian, Y., Gunther, J. R., Liao, I. H., Liu, D., Ander, B. P., Stamova, B. S., et al. (2011). GABA- and acetylcholine-related gene expression in blood correlate with tic severity and microarray evidence for alternative splicing in Tourette syndrome: a pilot study. *Brain Res.* 1381, 228–236. doi: 10.1016/j.brainres.2011.01.026

Timmerman, H. (1989). Histamine receptors in the central nervous system. *Pharm. Weekbl. Sci.* 11, 146–150. doi: 10.1007/BF01959461

Todd, R. D., Lobos, E. A., Sun, L.-W., and Neuman, R. J. (2003). Mutational analysis of the nicotinic acetylcholine receptor alpha 4 subunit gene in attention deficit/hyperactivity disorder: evidence for association of an intronic polymorphism with attention problems. *Mol. Psychiatry* 8, 103–108. doi: 10.1038/sj.mp.4001257

Tritsch, N. X., Ding, J. B., and Sabatini, B. L. (2012). Dopaminergic neurons inhibit striatal output through non-canonical release of GABA. *Nature* 490, 262–266. doi: 10.1038/nature11466

Tso, P. H., and Wong, Y. H. (2003). Molecular basis of opioid dependence: role of signal regulation by G-proteins. *Clin. Exp. Pharmacol. Physiol.* 30, 307–316. doi: 10.1046/j.1440-1681.2003.03835.x

Vilaró, M. T., Palacios, J. M., and Mengod, G. (1990). Localization of m5 muscarinic receptor mRNA in rat brain examined by *in situ* hybridization histochemistry. *Neurosci. Lett.* 114, 154–159. doi: 10.1016/0304-3940(90)90064-G

Voon, V., Fernagut, P.-O., Wickens, J., Baunez, C., Rodriguez, M., Pavon, N., et al. (2009). Chronic dopaminergic stimulation in Parkinson's disease: from dyskinesias to impulse control disorders. *Lancet Neurol.* 8, 1140–1149. doi: 10.1016/S1474-4422(09)70287-X

Voorn, P., Vanderschuren, L. J. M. J., Groenewegen, H. J., Robbins, T. W., and Pennartz, C. M. A. (2004). Putting a spin on the dorsal-ventral divide of the striatum. *Trends Neurosci.* 27, 468–474. doi: 10.1016/j.tins.2004.06.006

Vorobjev, V. S., Sharonova, I. N., Haas, H. L., and Sergeeva, O. A. (2000). Differential modulation of AMPA receptors by cyclothiazide in two types of striatal neurons. *Eur. J. Neurosci.* 12, 2871–2880. doi: 10.1046/j.1460-9568.2000.00175.x

Vuillet, J., Dimova, R., Nieoullon, A., and Kerkerian-Le Goff, L. (1992). Ultrastructural relationships between choline acetyltransferase- and neuropeptide y-containing neurons in the rat striatum. *Neuroscience* 46, 351–360. doi: 10.1016/0306-4522(92)90057-9

Wallis, D., Arcos-Burgos, M., Jain, M., Castellanos, F. X., Palacio, J. D., Pineda, D., et al. (2009). Polymorphisms in the neural nicotinic acetylcholine receptor α4 subunit (CHRNA4) are associated with ADHD in a genetic isolate. *Atten. Deficit Hyperact. Disord.* 1, 19–24. doi: 10.1007/s12402-009-0003-5

Wan, J., and Poo, M. (1999). Activity-induced potentiation of developing neuromuscular synapses. *Science* 285, 1725–1728. doi: 10.1126/science.285.5434.1725

Watanabe, K., and Kimura, M. (1998). Dopamine receptor-mediated mechanisms involved in the expression of learned activity of primate striatal neurons. *J. Neurophysiol.* 79, 2568–2580.

Weiner, D. M., Levey, A. I., and Brann, M. R. (1990). Expression of muscarinic acetylcholine and dopamine receptor mRNAs in rat basal ganglia. *Proc. Natl. Acad. Sci. U.S.A.* 87, 7050–7054. doi: 10.1073/pnas.87.18.7050

Wess, J. (1996). Molecular biology of muscarinic acetylcholine receptors. *Crit. Rev. Neurobiol.* 10, 69–99. doi: 10.1615/CritRevNeurobiol.v10.i1.40

West, A. B., Cowell, R. M., Daher, J. P. L., Moehle, M. S., Hinkle, K. M., Melrose, H. L., et al. (2014). Differential LRRK2 expression in the cortex, striatum, and substantia nigra in transgenic and nontransgenic rodents. *J. Comp. Neurol.* 522, 2465–2480. doi: 10.1002/cne.23583

Whyte, R. K., Hunter, K. R., Laurence, D. R., Stern, G. M., and Armitage, P. (1971). Levodopa and orphenadrine hydrochloride in Parkinsonism. *Eur. J. Clin. Pharmacol.* 4, 18–21. doi: 10.1007/BF00568893

Wilens, T. E., and Decker, M. W. (2007). Neuronal nicotinic receptor agonists for the treatment of attention-deficit/hyperactivity disorder: focus on cognition. *Biochem. Pharmacol.* 74, 1212–1223. doi: 10.1016/j.bcp.2007.07.002

Wilson, C. J., Chang, H. T., and Kitai, S. T. (1990). Firing patterns and synaptic potentials of identified giant aspiny interneurons in the rat neostriatum. *J. Neurosci.* 10, 508–519.

Wilson, C. J., and Groves, P. M. (1981). Spontaneous firing patterns of identified spiny neurons in the rat neostriatum. *Brain Res.* 220, 67–80. doi: 10.1016/0006-8993(81)90211-0

Won, L., Ding, Y., Singh, P., and Kang, U. J. (2014). Striatal cholinergic cell ablation attenuates L-DOPA induced dyskinesia in Parkinsonian mice. *J. Neurosci.* 34, 3090–3094. doi: 10.1523/JNEUROSCI.2888-13.2014

Wonnacott, S., Kaiser, S., Mogg, A., Soliakov, L., and Jones, I. W. (2000). Presynaptic nicotinic receptors modulating dopamine release in the rat striatum. *Eur. J. Pharmacol.* 393, 51–58. doi: 10.1016/S0014-2999(00)00005-4

Woolf, N. J., and Butcher, L. L. (1981). Cholinergic neurons in the caudate-putamen complex proper are intrinsically organized: a combined Evans blue and acetylcholinesterase analysis. *Brain Res. Bull.* 7, 487–507. doi: 10.1016/0361-9230(81)90004-6

Woolf, N. J., Eckenstein, F., and Butcher, L. L. (1984). Cholinergic systems in the rat brain: I. projections to the limbic telencephalon. *Brain Res. Bull.* 13, 751–784. doi: 10.1016/0361-9230(84)90236-3

Wu, J. C. F., Chruscinski, A., De Jesus Perez, V. A., Singh, H., Pitsiouni, M., Rabinovitch, M., et al. (2009). Cholinergic modulation of angiogenesis: role of the 7 nicotinic acetylcholine receptor. *J. Cell. Biochem.* 108, 433–446. doi: 10.1002/jcb.22270

Xiao, C., Nashmi, R., McKinney, S., Cai, H., McIntosh, J. M., and Lester, H. A. (2009). Chronic nicotine selectively enhances alpha4beta2* nicotinic acetylcholine receptors in the nigrostriatal dopamine pathway. *J. Neurosci.* 29, 12428–12439. doi: 10.1523/JNEUROSCI.2939-09.2009

Yan, Z., Flores-Hernandez, J., and Surmeier, D. J. (2001). Coordinated expression of muscarinic receptor messenger RNAs in striatal medium spiny neurons. *Neuroscience* 103, 1017–1024. doi: 10.1016/S0306-4522(01)00039-2

Yan, Z., Song, W. J., and Surmeier, J. (1997). D2 dopamine receptors reduce N-type Ca2+ currents in rat neostriatal cholinergic interneurons through a membrane-delimited, protein-kinase-C-insensitive pathway. *J. Neurophysiol.* 77, 1003–1015.

Yasuda, R. P., Ciesla, W., Flores, L. R., Wall, S. J., Li, M., Satkus, S. A., et al. (1993). Development of antisera selective for m4 and m5 muscarinic cholinergic receptors: distribution of m4 and m5 receptors in rat brain. *Mol. Pharmacol.* 43, 149–157.

Yin, H. H. (2010). The sensorimotor striatum is necessary for serial order learning. *J. Neurosci.* 30, 14719–14723. doi: 10.1523/JNEUROSCI.3989-10.2010

Zhang, D., Mallela, A., Sohn, D., Carroll, F. I., Bencherif, M., Letchworth, S., et al. (2013). Nicotinic receptor agonists reduce L-DOPA-induced dyskinesias in a monkey model of Parkinson's disease. *J. Pharmacol. Exp. Ther.* 347, 225–234. doi: 10.1124/jpet.113.207639

Zhang, H., and Sulzer, D. (2004). Frequency-dependent modulation of dopamine release by nicotine. *Nat. Neurosci.* 7, 581–582. doi: 10.1038/nn1243

Zhang, W., Yamada, M., Gomeza, J., Basile, A. S., and Wess, J. (2002). Multiple muscarinic acetylcholine receptor subtypes modulate striatal dopamine release, as studied with M1-M5 muscarinic receptor knock-out mice. *J. Neurosci.* 22, 6347–6352.

Zhang, Z.-X., Dong, Z.-H., and Román, G. C. (2006). Early descriptions of Parkinson disease in ancient China. *Arch. Neurol.* 63, 782–784. doi: 10.1001/archneur.63.5.782

Zhou, F. M., Liang, Y., and Dani, J. A. (2001). Endogenous nicotinic cholinergic activity regulates dopamine release in the striatum. *Nat. Neurosci.* 4, 1224–1229. doi: 10.1038/nn769

Zhou, F.-W., Xu, J.-J., Zhao, Y., LeDoux, M. S., and Zhou, F.-M. (2006). Opposite functions of histamine H1 and H2 receptors and H3 receptor in substantia nigra pars reticulata. *J. Neurophysiol.* 96, 1581–1591. doi: 10.1152/jn.00148.2006

Zugno, A. I., Julião, R. F., Budni, J., Volpato, A. M., Fraga, D. B., Pacheco, F. D., et al. (2013). Rivastigmine reverses cognitive deficit and acetylcholinesterase activity induced by ketamine in an animal model of schizophrenia. *Metab. Brain Dis.* 28, 501–508. doi: 10.1007/s11011-013-9417-z

8

Notching up neural stem cell homogeneity in homeostasis and disease

Claudio Giachino and Verdon Taylor*

Department of Biomedicine, University of Basel, Basel, Switzerland

Edited by:
Paolo Peretto, Università Degli Studi di Torino, Italy

Reviewed by:
Armen Saghatelyan, Université Laval, Canada
Harold Cremer, Centre National de la Recherche Scientifique, France

*Correspondence:
Verdon Taylor, Department of Biomedicine, University of Basel, Mattenstrasse 28, 4058 Basel, Switzerland
e-mail: verdon.taylor@unibas.ch

Adult neural stem cells (NSCs) are perceived as a homogeneous population of cells that divide infrequently and are capable of multi-lineage differentiation. However, recent data revealed that independent stem cell lineages act in parallel to maintain neurogenesis and provide a cellular source for tissue repair. In addition, even within the same lineage, the stem and progenitor cells are strikingly heterogeneous including NSCs that are dormant or mitotically active. We will discuss these different NSC populations and activity states with relation to their role in neurogenesis and regeneration but also how these different stem cells respond to aging. NSCs depend on Notch signaling for their maintenance. While Notch-dependence is a common feature among NSC populations, we will discuss how differences in Notch signaling might contribute to adult NSC heterogeneity. Understanding the fate of multiple NSC populations with distinct functions has implications for the mechanisms of aging and regeneration.

Keywords: Notch signaling, subventricular zone, hippocampal dentate gyrus, neurogenesis, aging

INTRODUCTION

Neural stem cells (NSCs) remain neurogenic during postnatal life within two regions of the mammalian brain, the subgranular zone (SGZ) of the hippocampal dentate gyrus (DG) and the subventricular zone (SVZ) of the wall of the lateral ventricles. The discovery of adult neurogenesis in mammals opened new avenues for research in regenerative medicine, with a goal of manipulating endogenous NSCs for brain repair (Gage and Temple, 2013). Over the last twenty years we have made considerable progress in our understanding of adult neurogenesis in homeostasis and disease (Ming and Song, 2011). However, several gaps remain in our knowledge that have to be filled before the potential of adult NSCs for regeneration can be fully exploited.

One such gap, and a field of active research, relates to the presence of heterogeneous subpopulations of NSCs within the same neurogenic niche (Alvarez-Buylla et al., 2008; Bonaguidi et al., 2012). The properties, functions, and lineage relationships between these subpopulations are still ill defined. Notch signaling is one molecular pathway involved in the regulation of NSC maintenance, proliferation, quiescence, and cell fate decisions. We propose that Notch signaling strength and diversity of downstream targets might, in concert with other molecular pathways, niche signals, and intrinsic factors, contribute to establishing adult NSC heterogeneity.

THE ADULT NEUROGENIC LINEAGE IN SHORT

Work from the 90's and early 2000's discovered the sequential developmental stages that cells undergo during lineage progression within the adult neurogenic niches (Alvarez-Buylla et al., 2001; Kempermann et al., 2004). Adult NSCs share ultrastructural and antigenic features with astrocytes (Kriegstein and Alvarez-Buylla, 2009). Most adult NSCs are quiescent or intermittently dividing, which explains their resistance to antimitotic drug and high dose tritiated-thymidine treatment (Morshead et al., 1994; Doetsch et al., 1999; Seri et al., 2001). In the SVZ, NSCs that proliferate likely undergo asymmetric cell divisions to self-renew and generate committed intermediate progenitors (IPs). These mitotically active IPs generate neuroblasts that migrate to the olfactory bulb (OB) where they mature into multiple types of neurons (Alvarez-Buylla et al., 2008). In the SGZ, NSCs also generate IPs that pass through a series of maturation stages before they differentiate into neuroblasts and subsequently granule neurons of the DG. This early work already implied some degree of heterogeneity in adult NSC and IP populations (Kempermann et al., 2004), suggesting that progression through the neurogenic lineage may be a more complex process than the simple NSC to IP to neuroblast transition. Later work added new insights into this emerging complexity and even proposed the coexistence of independent stem cell lineages acting in parallel.

ADULT NEURAL STEM AND PROGENITOR CELL HETEROGENEITY WITHIN THE SAME LINEAGE

The ability of adult NSCs to survive antimitotic drug treatment and regenerate the neurogenic lineage suggested that they rarely divide (Doetsch et al., 1999; Seri et al., 2001). This relative quiescence of NSCs is potentially linked to their potential for long-term maintenance over the lifespan of an organism (Kippin et al., 2005; Porlan et al., 2013). Indeed, quiescence of adult NSCs is actively promoted through several mechanisms including BMP and Notch signaling (Imayoshi et al., 2010; Mira et al., 2010), neurotransmitters (Berg et al., 2013), cell adhesion molecules (Kokovay et al., 2012), cell-cycle inhibitors (Kippin et al., 2005), and intrinsic factors (Martynoga et al., 2013). However, quiescence is not a prerequisite for somatic stem cell identity, and proliferating stem cell exist alongside more quiescent stem cell pools in several organs (Li and Clevers, 2010). A similar situation of dual stem cell populations may also exist in the neurogenic niches of the adult mammalian brain. A small but detectable fraction of adult NSCs proliferate quite rapidly in both the SVZ and SGZ (Encinas et al., 2011; Ponti et al., 2013). Even though NSCs can shuttle between active and quiescent states (Lugert et al., 2010; Bonaguidi et al., 2011), not all NSCs that proliferate re-enter a quiescent state, but some divide repeatedly (Lugert et al., 2010; Encinas et al., 2011; Ponti et al., 2013). Similarly, although quiescent NSCs enter cell-cycle to generate active NSCs (Bonaguidi et al., 2011; Encinas et al., 2011) and their exit from the quiescent state is augmented in response to neurogenic stimuli and during regeneration (Morshead et al., 1994; Doetsch et al., 1999; Lugert et al., 2010; Lopez-Juarez et al., 2013), it remains unclear what proportion of NSCs can be activated during homeostatic neurogenesis. Thus, it is possible that active and quiescent NSCs represent distinct pools where transition between the two is limited and tightly controlled, at least in the absence of injury, rather than all adult NSCs being equal in their ability to switch from quiescence to activity and back.

Discrimination of quiescent from activated NSC populations and niche astrocytes has proven difficult, but progress has been made toward this end in recent years (Pastrana et al., 2009; Beckervordersandforth et al., 2010; Mira et al., 2010; Ferron et al., 2011). Active NSCs within the SVZ express the epidermal growth factor receptor, respond to EGF with increased proliferation, and are eliminated by antimitotic drug treatment, similar to IPs, but retain expression of astrocytic and radial glia markers (Pastrana et al., 2009; Giachino et al., 2014). In the adult DG, a non-radial morphology correlates with the active state (Suh et al., 2007; Lugert et al., 2010), but molecular markers that demarcate quiescent and active NSC populations have still to be defined. Interestingly, genetic lineage tracing using promoters that potentially over-represent either quiescent or active cells suggest differences in the contribution of these populations to long-term neurogenesis (DeCarolis et al., 2013). Identifying markers that discriminate between NSCs with distinct proliferative activities is needed to develop genetic tools for independent and simultaneous lineage tracing of active and quiescent NSC pools, and determine their respective lifespan and inter-conversion *in vivo*. Lineage tracing approaches with inducible-cre/flp technologies and intersectional analyses combining promoters of cell-cycle marker genes with NSC marker genes may be useful to this end.

Heterogeneity in the adult neurogenic lineage is not restricted to NSCs. In the SVZ, a proportion of Ascl1+ IPs expresses radial glia markers whereas others do not (Pastrana et al., 2009; Giachino et al., 2014). In the SGZ, a combination of Nestin, Ascl1, Tbr2, and Doublecortin expression defines at least three stages of committed progenitors (Kempermann et al., 2004; Hodge et al., 2008). It is still unclear if marker heterogeneity of IPs reflects differences in their self-renewal abilities, but it is interesting that differences in cell-cycle dynamics of IP populations in the SVZ have been recently reported (Ponti et al., 2013). Moreover, late IPs and neuroblasts make up a large fraction of proliferating cells in both neurogenic niches (Hodge et al., 2008; Lugert et al., 2012; Ponti et al., 2013), proposing that substantial lineage amplification occurs right before cell-cycle exit and terminal differentiation.

HETEROGENEOUS NSC LINEAGES ACTING IN PARALLEL

Adult NSCs are capable of multi-lineage differentiation and able to clonally generate multiple neural lineages under appropriate conditions *in vitro* (Suh et al., 2007; Pastrana et al., 2011). Moreover, they show some degree of lineage plasticity upon heterotopic or heterochronic transplantation into neurogenic niches distinct to their origin (Suhonen et al., 1996; Sequerra et al., 2010). Indeed, elegant lineage tracing experiments demonstrated that DG NSCs are bi-potent at the single cell level and self-renew *in vivo* (Suh et al., 2007; Bonaguidi et al., 2011). SVZ NSCs are able to generate neurons, astrocytes and oligodendrocytes at the population level *in vivo* (Alvarez-Buylla et al., 2001; Menn et al., 2006; Benner et al., 2013). However, and apparently in contrast to these findings, other fate-mapping and transplantation studies demonstrated that SVZ NSCs are heterogeneous and their spatial distribution correlates with cell fate (Kelsch et al., 2007; Merkle et al., 2007). NSCs show a preference toward the production of distinct types of neurons depending on their dorsal-ventral position within the adult SVZ, and this differentiation bias seems to be intrinsic as it is maintained after *in vitro* passage and heterotopic transplantation (Merkle et al., 2007). In the same line, NSCs cultured in the absence of growth factors are able to generate either neurons or oligodendrocytes, in addition to astrocytes, but not both neurons and oligodendrocytes within the same lineage tree (Ortega et al., 2013). NSCs with oligodendrocytic potential are enriched in the dorsal and anterior SVZ (Gritti et al., 2002; Ortega et al., 2013). Genetic fate mapping indicates that these heterogeneous NSC populations in the adult SVZ are remnants of distinct germinative niches of the embryonic forebrain and derive from Emx1, Dbx1, Gsh2, Nkx2.1 or Nkx6.2 expressing lineages (Kohwi et al., 2007; Ventura and Goldman, 2007; Young et al., 2007; Lopez-Juarez et al., 2013; Merkle et al., 2014). These data suggest that the SVZ is arranged as a mosaic that is established during embryogenesis and the location within the niche can predict the type of progeny that NSCs give rise to. Whether this heterogeneity of lineages is intrinsically determined or regulated by extrinsic cues at distinct locations within the niche, or a combination of both, is still a matter of debate (Sequerra et al., 2013). The fact that manipulation of morphogen signals skews NSC differentiation potential *in vivo* suggest that the local environment plays a role in regional specification of adult NSCs (Ihrie et al., 2011). Moreover, pathological conditions stimulate NSCs to produce progenies that are different from the ones generated during homeostasis and these can migrate toward non-canonical locations, suggesting that cell fate is not fixed (Kernie and Parent, 2010; Ohira, 2011). Defining the degree of lineage plasticity of adult NSCs and the signals that can override their intrinsic programming has important implications for developing cell replacement strategies based on the mobilization of endogenous cells.

CONTRIBUTION OF NOTCH SIGNALING TO HETEROGENEITY OF THE ADULT NSC POOL

Notch signaling is a key mediator of NSC maintenance in the developing and adult brains (Ables et al., 2011; Pierfelice et al., 2011). Notchs are transmembrane receptors and undergo a series of proteolytic cleavages that liberate the Notch intracellular domain (NICD) upon binding to their ligands. The canonical

Notch signal links the NICD to the nuclear CSL (RBP-J in mice) transcriptional complex (Mumm and Kopan, 2000). The activity of Notch target genes of the *Hes/Hey* family is fundamental for maintaining NSCs in an undifferentiated state, suppressing the expression of proneural genes including Ascl1 (Louvi and Artavanis-Tsakonas, 2006). Inhibition of Notch or RBP-J in adult NSCs results in NSC loss and impaired neurogenesis (Breunig et al., 2007; Andreu-Agullo et al., 2009; Ables et al., 2010; Aguirre et al., 2010; Chapouton et al., 2010; Ehm et al., 2010; Imayoshi et al., 2010; Lugert et al., 2010; Imayoshi and Kageyama, 2011). Canonical Notch signaling activity and *Hes5* expression in particular distinguish NSCs from IPs in the developing and adult brain (Basak and Taylor, 2007; Mizutani et al., 2007; Andreu-Agullo et al., 2009; Imayoshi et al., 2010; Lugert et al., 2010; Giachino et al., 2014). It is unclear if Notch signaling contributes to adult NSC heterogeneity, but studies revealing that impairing distinct Notch pathway components affects distinct stages of the neurogenic lineage suggest that this might be the case. Notch1 promotes adult NSC proliferation whilst maintaining the undifferentiated state, proposing a role of the pathway in the maintenance of the active NSC subpopulation (Nyfeler et al., 2005; Androutsellis-Theotokis et al., 2006; Breunig et al., 2007; Ables et al., 2010; Aguirre et al., 2010; Basak et al., 2012). In contrast, activation of the RBP-J mediated canonical Notch pathway, potentially promoted by Dll1 ligand expressed by proliferating NSCs and IPs, preserves the quiescent NSC pool (Carlen et al., 2009; Ehm et al., 2010; Imayoshi et al., 2010; Basak et al., 2012; Kawaguchi et al., 2013). These data suggest that Notch can differentially regulate active and quiescent NSC populations in a context-dependent manner. Given that *Hes5* is expressed in both dividing and dormant adult NSCs, Notch is unlikely to be the only key to NSC heterogeneity (Lugert et al., 2010; Giachino et al., 2014). However, differences in the strength, dynamics, and targets of the pathway may contribute to heterogeneity and explain the discrepancies observed in mouse mutant phenotypes. Low levels of Notch activation (NICD) for instance promote proliferation of embryonic neural progenitors, whereas high levels lead to growth arrest *in vitro* (Guentchev and McKay, 2006). Therefore, one possibility is that the differential actions of Notch on proliferation vs. quiescence of adult NSCs are a function of dose. Another possibility is that oscillatory vs. sustained expression of Notch targets differentiate active and quiescent NSC pools. In mouse embryonic NSCs and progenitors, levels of Hes1/Hes5 oscillate in anti-phase with their repressed target Ascl1, and this oscillatory expression promotes proliferation (Imayoshi et al., 2013). In contrast, sustained Hes1 expression inhibits NSC proliferation and neurogenesis in the developing central nervous system (Baek et al., 2006). It is currently not known if the expression of *Hes* genes is sustained or oscillatory in adult NSCs, and the available tools are not adequate to address this issue *in vivo*. However, oscillatory expression of Notch targets together with low refractory expression of Ascl1 in adult NSCs that are in the cell-cycle would be compatible with data showing that the *Ascl1::CreER* locus can be used to lineage trace a subpopulation of neurogenic NSCs *in vivo* (Kim et al., 2011). Conversely, quiescent adult NSCs express high levels of Id proteins (Nam and Benezra, 2009), which can interfere with the negative autoregulation of *Hes1* and therefore modulate its oscillatory expression (Bai et al., 2007). These findings prompt to speculate that *Hes* genes are persistently expressed at high levels in quiescent NSCs.

Another possible scenario to explain the multifaceted functions of Notch in adult NSCs would be that distinct pathway components are differentially engaged in Notch signaling activity in different cell subpopulations. It has been proposed that Notch1 is required to maintain the active adult NSC pool but is dispensable during quiescence (Ables et al., 2010; Basak et al., 2012). This suggests that other members of the Notch family could provide a maintenance signal for quiescent NSCs and compensate for the absence of Notch1 in this population (Basak et al., 2012). Heterogeneity of Notch activity is related to cellular diversity in the neurogenic niches of the adult zebrafish brain, where Notch3 gates NSC activation whereas Notch1b maintains activated progenitors (Alunni et al., 2013). Interestingly, Notch3 restricts stem cell activation in muscle and mammary, while Notch1 is associated with proliferation (Carlson et al., 2008; Kitamoto and Hanaoka, 2010; Bjornson et al., 2012; Mourikis et al., 2012; Lafkas et al., 2013). It is tempting to speculate that distinct Notch receptors differentially regulate quiescent and active stem cell subpopulations in the adult mammalian brain. In addition to NSC heterogeneity within the same lineage, independent NSC lineages are fated to generate distinct OB neurons in the SVZ. Lineage tracing experiments with *Hes5::CreER* transgenic mice demonstrated that NSCs with active canonical Notch signaling generate multiple neuron subtypes in the OB (Giachino et al., 2014) implying that all adult NSC lineages require Notch for maintenance. However, this does not exclude that different receptors or receptor combinations mediate Notch activity within the NSCs of each lineage. Interestingly, genetic fate mapping of cells expressing individual Notchs revealed multiple lineages in bone marrow and mammary gland (Lafkas et al., 2013; Oh et al., 2013; Sale et al., 2013).

Not only the activity of Notch paralogues, but also combinations of different Notch target genes in NSC subpopulations may be a source of heterogeneity. NSCs in the developing neural tube of the mouse are heterogeneous based on their expression of *Hes* family genes, with cohorts of radial glia cells expressing either *Hes1* or *Hes5*, or both (Basak and Taylor, 2007; Nelson et al., 2013). Brain lipid binding protein (BLBP), a direct target of Notch signaling (Anthony et al., 2005), is also expressed heterogeneously by radial glia (Hartfuss et al., 2001). Recently, it was shown that different combinations of *Her/Hes* family genes correlate with the proliferation rate of NSCs and progenitors in the adult zebrafish (Chapouton et al., 2011). In the same line, BLBP expression positively correlates with proliferation of *Hes5*-expressing NSCs in the adult mouse SVZ, whereas most quiescent NSCs express *Hes5* but not BLBP (Giachino et al., 2014). How combinatorial or selective expression of Notch targets regulates the fate and activity of adult NSC subpopulations deserves closer scrutiny in the future.

IMPLICATIONS OF ADULT NSC HETEROGENEITY FOR AGING AND REGENERATION

The adult mammalian neurogenic niches show a remarkable capacity for self-repair and remodeling in response to lesion (Doetsch et al., 1999; Seri et al., 2001; Kuo et al., 2006; Nomura et al., 2010). However, neurogenesis declines with age in both the SVZ and SGZ (Lazarov et al., 2010) and most neuron subtypes produced in the OB are equally affected (Shook et al., 2012). Understanding the basis of this overall age-related decline in neurogenesis, and the mechanisms controlling self-renewal over the life on an individual, is fundamental to exploit the regenerative potential of adult NSCs.

One cause of reduced neurogenesis during aging is the impairment of the NSC compartment. An open question is whether this impairment reflects depletion or increased quiescence of NSCs (Hattiangady and Shetty, 2008; Lugert et al., 2010; Encinas et al., 2011; Shook et al., 2012; Giachino et al., 2014). This issue remains debated as most studies did not take into account the differential effects that aging may have on NSC subpopulations. One possibility is that active NSCs are more susceptible to imbalances between maintenance and differentiation signals that may occur during aging. These imbalances affect self-renewal, and therefore active NSCs are preferentially lost compared to quiescent populations (Lugert et al., 2010; Encinas et al., 2011; Giachino et al., 2014). Furthermore, some quiescent NSCs may activate to replenish an exhausted active NSC pool and thereby also be lost during aging. This is supported by findings that quiescent NSCs are reduced with time following depletion of the active NSC pool either by genetic means (Basak et al., 2012), or chronic treatment with antimitotic drugs (Doetsch et al., 1999). However, a variable but substantial proportion of NSCs is preserved in both the SGZ and SVZ of old mice, but these are dormant rather than senescent and can be reactivated (Jin et al., 2003; Hattiangady and Shetty, 2008; Lugert et al., 2010; Giachino et al., 2014). It will be important to genetically trace the progeny of distinct NSC populations during aging to assess differences in their lifespan, lineage plasticity and regenerative potential. Understanding the mechanisms responsible for NSC dormancy in the mouse neurogenic niches could help to understand why most NSCs in the human brain stop generating neurons after birth (Sanai et al., 2011).

REFERENCES

Ables, J. L., Breunig, J. J., Eisch, A. J., and Rakic, P. (2011). Not(ch) just development: notch signalling in the adult brain. *Nat. Rev. Neurosci.* 12, 269–283. doi: 10.1038/nrn3024

Ables, J. L., Decarolis, N. A., Johnson, M. A., Rivera, P. D., Gao, Z., Cooper, D. C., et al. (2010). Notch1 is required for maintenance of the reservoir of adult hippocampal stem cells. *J. Neurosci.* 30, 10484–10492. doi: 10.1523/JNEUROSCI.4721-09.2010

Aguirre, A., Rubio, M. E., and Gallo, V. (2010). Notch and EGFR pathway interaction regulates neural stem cell number and self-renewal. *Nature* 467, 323–327. doi: 10.1038/nature09347

Alunni, A., Krecsmarik, M., Bosco, A., Galant, S., Pan, L., Moens, C. B., et al. (2013). Notch3 signaling gates cell cycle entry and limits neural stem cell amplification in the adult pallium. *Development* 140, 3335–3347. doi: 10.1242/dev.095018

Alvarez-Buylla, A., Garcia-Verdugo, J. M., and Tramontin, A. D. (2001). A unified hypothesis on the lineage of neural stem cells. *Nat. Rev. Neurosci.* 2, 287–293. doi: 10.1038/35067582

Alvarez-Buylla, A., Kohwi, M., Nguyen, T. M., and Merkle, F. T. (2008). The heterogeneity of adult neural stem cells and the emerging complexity of their niche. *Cold Spring Harb. Symp. Quant. Biol.* 73, 357–365. doi: 10.1101/sqb.2008.73.019

Andreu-Agullo, C., Morante-Redolat, J. M., Delgado, A. C., and Farinas, I. (2009). Vascular niche factor PEDF modulates Notch-dependent stemness in the adult subependymal zone. *Nat. Neurosci.* 12, 1514–1523. doi: 10.1038/nn.2437

Androutsellis-Theotokis, A., Leker, R. R., Soldner, F., Hoeppner, D. J., Ravin, R., Poser, S. W., et al. (2006). Notch signalling regulates stem cell numbers *in vitro* and *in vivo*. *Nature* 442, 823–826. doi: 10.1038/nature04940

Anthony, T. E., Mason, H. A., Gridley, T., Fishell, G., and Heintz, N. (2005). Brain lipid-binding protein is a direct target of Notch signaling in radial glial cells. *Genes Dev.* 19, 1028–1033. doi: 10.1101/gad.1302105

Baek, J. H., Hatakeyama, J., Sakamoto, S., Ohtsuka, T., and Kageyama, R. (2006). Persistent and high levels of Hes1 expression regulate boundary formation in the developing central nervous system. *Development* 133, 2467–2476. doi: 10.1242/dev.02403

Bai, G., Sheng, N., Xie, Z., Bian, W., Yokota, Y., Benezra, R., et al. (2007). Id sustains Hes1 expression to inhibit precocious neurogenesis by releasing negative autoregulation of Hes1. *Dev. Cell* 13, 283–297. doi: 10.1016/j.devcel.2007.05.014

Basak, O., Giachino, C., Fiorini, E., Macdonald, H. R., and Taylor, V. (2012). Neurogenic subventricular zone stem/progenitor cells are Notch1-dependent in their active but not quiescent state. *J. Neurosci.* 32, 5654–5666. doi: 10.1523/JNEUROSCI.0455-12.2012

Basak, O., and Taylor, V. (2007). Identification of self-replicating multipotent progenitors in the embryonic nervous system by high Notch activity and Hes5 expression. *Eur. J. Neurosci.* 25, 1006–1022. doi: 10.1111/j.1460-9568.2007.05370.x

Beckervordersandforth, R., Tripathi, P., Ninkovic, J., Bayam, E., Lepier, A., Stempfhuber, B., et al. (2010). *In vivo* fate mapping and expression analysis reveals molecular hallmarks of prospectively isolated adult neural stem cells. *Cell Stem Cell* 7, 744–758. doi: 10.1016/j.stem.2010.11.017

Benner, E. J., Luciano, D., Jo, R., Abdi, K., Paez-Gonzalez, P., Sheng, H., et al. (2013). Protective astrogenesis from the SVZ niche after injury is controlled by Notch modulator Thbs4. *Nature* 497, 369–373. doi: 10.1038/nature12069

Berg, D. A., Belnoue, L., Song, H., and Simon, A. (2013). Neurotransmitter-mediated control of neurogenesis in the adult vertebrate brain. *Development* 140, 2548–2561. doi: 10.1242/dev.088005

Bjornson, C. R., Cheung, T. H., Liu, L., Tripathi, P. V., Steeper, K. M., and Rando, T. A. (2012). Notch signaling is necessary to maintain quiescence in adult muscle stem cells. *Stem Cells* 30, 232–242. doi: 10.1002/stem.773

Bonaguidi, M. A., Song, J., Ming, G. L., and Song, H. (2012). A unifying hypothesis on mammalian neural stem cell properties in the adult hippocampus. *Curr. Opin. Neurobiol.* 22, 754–761. doi: 10.1016/j.conb.2012.03.013

Bonaguidi, M. A., Wheeler, M. A., Shapiro, J. S., Stadel, R. P., Sun, G. J., Ming, G. L., et al. (2011). *In vivo* clonal analysis reveals self-renewing and multipotent adult neural stem cell characteristics. *Cell* 145, 1142–1155. doi: 10.1016/j.cell.2011.05.024

Breunig, J. J., Silbereis, J., Vaccarino, F. M., Sestan, N., and Rakic, P. (2007). Notch regulates cell fate and dendrite morphology of newborn neurons in the postnatal dentate gyrus. *Proc. Natl. Acad. Sci. U.S.A.* 104, 20558–20563. doi: 10.1073/pnas.0710156104

Carlen, M., Meletis, K., Goritz, C., Darsalia, V., Evergren, E., Tanigaki, K., et al. (2009). Forebrain ependymal cells are Notch-dependent and generate neuroblasts and astrocytes after stroke. *Nat. Neurosci.* 12, 259–267. doi: 10.1038/nn.2268

Carlson, M. E., Hsu, M., and Conboy, I. M. (2008). Imbalance between pSmad3 and Notch induces CDK inhibitors in old muscle stem cells. *Nature* 454, 528–532. doi: 10.1038/nature07034

Chapouton, P., Skupien, P., Hesl, B., Coolen, M., Moore, J. C., Madelaine, R., et al. (2010). Notch activity levels control the balance between quiescence and recruitment of adult neural stem cells. *J. Neurosci.* 30, 7961–7974. doi: 10.1523/JNEUROSCI.6170-09.2010

Chapouton, P., Webb, K. J., Stigloher, C., Alunni, A., Adolf, B., Hesl, B., et al. (2011). Expression of hairy/enhancer of split genes in neural progenitors and neurogenesis domains of the adult zebrafish brain. *J. Comp. Neurol.* 519, 1748–1769. doi: 10.1002/cne.22599

DeCarolis, N. A., Mechanic, M., Petrik, D., Carlton, A., Ables, J. L., Malhotra, S., et al. (2013). *In vivo* contribution of nestin- and GLAST-lineage cells to adult hippocampal neurogenesis. *Hippocampus* 23, 708–719. doi: 10.1002/hipo.22130

Doetsch, F., Garcia-Verdugo, J. M., and Alvarez-Buylla, A. (1999). Regeneration of a germinal layer in the adult mammalian brain. *Proc. Natl. Acad. Sci. U.S.A.* 96, 11619–11624. doi: 10.1073/pnas.96.20.11619

Ehm, O., Goritz, C., Covic, M., Schaffner, I., Schwarz, T. J., Karaca, E., et al. (2010). RBPJkappa-dependent signaling is essential for long-term maintenance of neural stem cells in the adult hippocampus. *J. Neurosci.* 30, 13794–13807. doi: 10.1523/JNEUROSCI.1567-10.2010

Encinas, J. M., Michurina, T. V., Peunova, N., Park, J. H., Tordo, J., Peterson, D. A., et al. (2011). Division-coupled astrocytic differentiation and age-related depletion of neural stem cells in the adult hippocampus. *Cell Stem Cell* 8, 566–579. doi: 10.1016/j.stem.2011.03.010

Ferron, S. R., Charalambous, M., Radford, E., McEwen, K., Wildner, H., Hind, E., et al. (2011). Postnatal loss of Dlk1 imprinting in stem cells and niche astrocytes regulates neurogenesis. *Nature* 475, 381–385. doi: 10.1038/nature10229

Gage, F. H., and Temple, S. (2013). Neural stem cells: generating and regenerating the brain. *Neuron* 80, 588–601. doi: 10.1016/j.neuron.2013.10.037

Giachino, C., Basak, O., Lugert, S., Knuckles, P., Obernier, K., Fiorelli, R., et al. (2014). Molecular diversity subdivides the adult forebrain neural stem cell population. *Stem Cells* 32, 70–84. doi: 10.1002/stem.1520

Gritti, A., Bonfanti, L., Doetsch, F., Caille, I., Alvarez-Buylla, A., Lim, D. A., et al. (2002). Multipotent neural stem cells reside into the rostral extension and olfactory bulb of adult rodents. *J. Neurosci.* 22, 437–445.

Guentchev, M., and McKay, R. D. (2006). Notch controls proliferation and differentiation of stem cells in a dose-dependent manner. *Eur. J. Neurosci.* 23, 2289–2296. doi: 10.1111/j.1460-9568.2006.04766.x

Hartfuss, E., Galli, R., Heins, N., and Gotz, M. (2001). Characterization of CNS precursor subtypes and radial glia. *Dev. Biol.* 229, 15–30. doi: 10.1006/dbio.2000.9962

Hattiangady, B., and Shetty, A. K. (2008). Aging does not alter the number or phenotype of putative stem/progenitor cells in the neurogenic region of the hippocampus. *Neurobiol. Aging* 29, 129–147. doi: 10.1016/j.neurobiolaging.2006.09.015

Hodge, R. D., Kowalczyk, T. D., Wolf, S. A., Encinas, J. M., Rippey, C., Enikolopov, G., et al. (2008). Intermediate progenitors in adult hippocampal neurogenesis: Tbr2 expression and coordinate regulation of neuronal output. *J. Neurosci.* 28, 3707–3717. doi: 10.1523/JNEUROSCI.4280-07.2008

Ihrie, R. A., Shah, J. K., Harwell, C. C., Levine, J. H., Guinto, C. D., Lezameta, M., et al. (2011). Persistent sonic hedgehog signaling in adult brain determines neural stem cell positional identity. *Neuron* 71, 250–262. doi: 10.1016/j.neuron.2011.05.018

Imayoshi, I., Isomura, A., Harima, Y., Kawaguchi, K., Kori, H., Miyachi, H., et al. (2013). Oscillatory control of factors determining multipotency and fate in mouse neural progenitors. *Science* 342, 1203–1208. doi: 10.1126/science.1242366

Imayoshi, I., and Kageyama, R. (2011). The role of Notch signaling in adult neurogenesis. *Mol. Neurobiol.* 44, 7–12. doi: 10.1007/s12035-011-8186-0

Imayoshi, I., Sakamoto, M., Yamaguchi, M., Mori, K., and Kageyama, R. (2010). Essential roles of Notch signaling in maintenance of neural stem cells in developing and adult brains. *J. Neurosci.* 30, 3489–3498. doi: 10.1523/JNEUROSCI.4987-09.2010

Jin, K., Sun, Y., Xie, L., Batteur, S., Mao, X. O., Smelick, C., et al. (2003). Neurogenesis and aging: FGF-2 and HB-EGF restore neurogenesis in hippocampus and subventricular zone of aged mice. *Aging Cell* 2, 175–183. doi: 10.1046/j.1474-9728.2003.00046.x

Kawaguchi, D., Furutachi, S., Kawai, H., Hozumi, K., and Gotoh, Y. (2013). Dll1 maintains quiescence of adult neural stem cells and segregates asymmetrically during mitosis. *Nat. Commun.* 4, 1880. doi: 10.1038/ncomms2895

Kelsch, W., Mosley, C. P., Lin, C. W., and Lois, C. (2007). Distinct mammalian precursors are committed to generate neurons with defined dendritic projection patterns. *PLoS Biol.* 5:e300. doi: 10.1371/journal.pbio.0050300

Kempermann, G., Jessberger, S., Steiner, B., and Kronenberg, G. (2004). Milestones of neuronal development in the adult hippocampus. *Trends Neurosci.* 27, 447–452. doi: 10.1016/j.tins.2004.05.013

Kernie, S. G., and Parent, J. M. (2010). Forebrain neurogenesis after focal Ischemic and traumatic brain injury. *Neurobiol. Dis.* 37, 267–274. doi: 10.1016/j.nbd.2009.11.002

Kim, E. J., Ables, J. L., Dickel, L. K., Eisch, A. J., and Johnson, J. E. (2011). Ascl1 (Mash1) defines cells with long-term neurogenic potential in subgranular and subventricular zones in adult mouse brain. *PLoS ONE* 6:e18472. doi: 10.1371/journal.pone.0018472

Kippin, T. E., Martens, D. J., and van der Kooy, D. (2005). p21 loss compromises the relative quiescence of forebrain stem cell proliferation leading to exhaustion of their proliferation capacity. *Genes Dev.* 19, 756–767. doi: 10.1101/gad.1272305

Kitamoto, T., and Hanaoka, K. (2010). Notch3 null mutation in mice causes muscle hyperplasia by repetitive muscle regeneration. *Stem Cells* 28, 2205–2216. doi: 10.1002/stem.547

Kohwi, M., Petryniak, M. A., Long, J. E., Ekker, M., Obata, K., Yanagawa, Y., et al. (2007). A subpopulation of olfactory bulb GABAergic interneurons is derived from Emx1- and Dlx5/6-expressing progenitors. *J. Neurosci.* 27, 6878–6891. doi: 10.1523/JNEUROSCI.0254-07.2007

Kokovay, E., Wang, Y., Kusek, G., Wurster, R., Lederman, P., Lowry, N., et al. (2012). VCAM1 is essential to maintain the structure of the SVZ niche and acts as an environmental sensor to regulate SVZ lineage progression. *Cell Stem Cell* 11, 220–230. doi: 10.1016/j.stem.2012.06.016

Kriegstein, A., and Alvarez-Buylla, A. (2009). The glial nature of embryonic and adult neural stem cells. *Annu. Rev. Neurosci.* 32, 149–184. doi: 10.1146/annurev.neuro.051508.135600

Kuo, C. T., Mirzadeh, Z., Soriano-Navarro, M., Rasin, M., Wang, D., Shen, J., et al. (2006). Postnatal deletion of Numb/Numblike reveals repair and remodeling capacity in the subventricular neurogenic niche. *Cell* 127, 1253–1264. doi: 10.1016/j.cell.2006.10.041

Lafkas, D., Rodilla, V., Huyghe, M., Mourao, L., Kiaris, H., and Fre, S. (2013). Notch3 marks clonogenic mammary luminal progenitor cells *in vivo*. *J. Cell Biol.* 203, 47–56. doi: 10.1083/jcb.201307046

Lazarov, O., Mattson, M. P., Peterson, D. A., Pimplikar, S. W., and van Praag, H. (2010). When neurogenesis encounters aging and disease. *Trends Neurosci.* 33, 569–579. doi: 10.1016/j.tins.2010.09.003

Li, L., and Clevers, H. (2010). Coexistence of quiescent and active adult stem cells in mammals. *Science* 327, 542–545. doi: 10.1126/science.1180794

Lopez-Juarez, A., Howard, J., Ullom, K., Howard, L., Grande, A., Pardo, A., et al. (2013). Gsx2 controls region-specific activation of neural stem cells and injury-induced neurogenesis in the adult subventricular zone. *Genes Dev.* 27, 1272–1287. doi: 10.1101/gad.217539.113

Louvi, A., and Artavanis-Tsakonas, S. (2006). Notch signalling in vertebrate neural development. *Nat. Rev. Neurosci.* 7, 93–102. doi: 10.1038/nrn1847

Lugert, S., Basak, O., Knuckles, P., Haussler, U., Fabel, K., Gotz, M., et al. (2010). Quiescent and active hippocampal neural stem cells with distinct morphologies respond selectively to physiological and pathological stimuli and aging. *Cell Stem Cell* 6, 445–456. doi: 10.1016/j.stem.2010.03.017

Lugert, S., Vogt, M., Tchorz, J. S., Muller, M., Giachino, C., and Taylor, V. (2012). Homeostatic neurogenesis in the adult hippocampus does not involve amplification of Ascl1(high) intermediate progenitors. *Nat. Commun.* 3, 670. doi: 10.1038/ncomms1670

Martynoga, B., Mateo, J. L., Zhou, B., Andersen, J., Achimastou, A., Urban, N., et al. (2013). Epigenomic enhancer annotation reveals a key role for NFIX in neural stem cell quiescence. *Genes Dev.* 27, 1769–1786. doi: 10.1101/gad.216804.113

Menn, B., Garcia-Verdugo, J. M., Yaschine, C., Gonzalez-Perez, O., Rowitch, D., and Alvarez-Buylla, A. (2006). Origin of oligodendrocytes in the subventricular zone of the adult brain. *J. Neurosci.* 26, 7907–7918. doi: 10.1523/JNEUROSCI.1299-06.2006

Merkle, F. T., Fuentealba, L. C., Sanders, T. A., Magno, L., Kessaris, N., and Alvarez-Buylla, A. (2014). Adult neural stem cells in distinct microdomains generate previously unknown interneuron types. *Nat. Neurosci.* 17, 207–214. doi: 10.1038/nn.3610

Merkle, F. T., Mirzadeh, Z., and Alvarez-Buylla, A. (2007). Mosaic organization of neural stem cells in the adult brain. *Science* 317, 381–384. doi: 10.1126/science.1144914

Ming, G. L., and Song, H. (2011). Adult neurogenesis in the mammalian brain: significant answers and significant questions. *Neuron* 70, 687–702. doi: 10.1016/j.neuron.2011.05.001

Mira, H., Andreu, Z., Suh, H., Lie, D. C., Jessberger, S., Consiglio, A., et al. (2010). Signaling through BMPR-IA regulates quiescence and long-term activity of neural stem cells in the adult hippocampus. *Cell Stem Cell* 7, 78–89. doi: 10.1016/j.stem.2010.04.016

Mizutani, K., Yoon, K., Dang, L., Tokunaga, A., and Gaiano, N. (2007). Differential Notch signalling distinguishes neural stem cells from intermediate progenitors. *Nature* 449, 351–355. doi: 10.1038/nature06090

Morshead, C. M., Reynolds, B. A., Craig, C. G., McBurney, M. W., Staines, W. A., Morassutti, D., et al. (1994). Neural stem cells in the adult mammalian forebrain: a relatively quiescent subpopulation of subependymal cells. *Neuron* 13, 1071–1082. doi: 10.1016/0896-6273(94)90046-9

Mourikis, P., Sambasivan, R., Castel, D., Rocheteau, P., Bizzarro, V., and Tajbakhsh, S. (2012). A critical requirement for notch signaling in maintenance of the quiescent skeletal muscle stem cell state. *Stem Cells* 30, 243–252. doi: 10.1002/stem.775

Mumm, J. S., and Kopan, R. (2000). Notch signaling: from the outside in. *Dev. Biol.* 228, 151–165. doi: 10.1006/dbio.2000.9960

Nam, H. S., and Benezra, R. (2009). High levels of Id1 expression define B1 type adult neural stem cells. *Cell Stem Cell* 5, 515–526. doi: 10.1016/j.stem.2009.08.017

Nelson, B. R., Hodge, R. D., Bedogni, F., and Hevner, R. F. (2013). Dynamic interactions between intermediate neurogenic progenitors and radial glia in embryonic mouse neocortex: potential role in Dll1-Notch signaling. *J. Neurosci.* 33, 9122–9139. doi: 10.1523/JNEUROSCI.0791-13.2013

Nomura, T., Goritz, C., Catchpole, T., Henkemeyer, M., and Frisen, J. (2010). EphB signaling controls lineage plasticity of adult neural stem cell niche cells. *Cell Stem Cell* 7, 730–743. doi: 10.1016/j.stem.2010.11.009

Nyfeler, Y., Kirch, R. D., Mantei, N., Leone, D. P., Radtke, F., Suter, U., et al. (2005). Jagged1 signals in the postnatal subventricular zone are required for neural stem cell self-renewal. *EMBO J.* 24, 3504–3515. doi: 10.1038/sj.emboj.7600816

Oh, P., Lobry, C., Gao, J., Tikhonova, A., Loizou, E., Manent, J., et al. (2013). *In vivo* mapping of notch pathway activity in normal and stress hematopoiesis. *Cell Stem Cell* 13, 190–204. doi: 10.1016/j.stem.2013.05.015

Ohira, K. (2011). Injury-induced neurogenesis in the mammalian forebrain. *Cell. Mol. Life Sci.* 68, 1645–1656. doi: 10.1007/s00018-010-0552-y

Ortega, F., Gascon, S., Masserdotti, G., Deshpande, A., Simon, C., Fischer, J., et al. (2013). Oligodendrogliogenic and neurogenic adult subependymal zone neural stem cells constitute distinct lineages and exhibit differential responsiveness to Wnt signalling. *Nat. Cell Biol.* 15, 602–613. doi: 10.1038/ncb2736

Pastrana, E., Cheng, L. C., and Doetsch, F. (2009). Simultaneous prospective purification of adult subventricular zone neural stem cells and their progeny. *Proc. Natl. Acad. Sci. U.S.A.* 106, 6387–6392. doi: 10.1073/pnas.0810407106

Pastrana, E., Silva-Vargas, V., and Doetsch, F. (2011). Eyes wide open: a critical review of sphere-formation as an assay for stem cells. *Cell Stem Cell* 8, 486–498. doi: 10.1016/j.stem.2011.04.007

Pierfelice, T., Alberi, L., and Gaiano, N. (2011). Notch in the vertebrate nervous system: an old dog with new tricks. *Neuron* 69, 840–855. doi: 10.1016/j.neuron.2011.02.031

Ponti, G., Obernier, K., Guinto, C., Jose, L., Bonfanti, L., and Alvarez-Buylla, A. (2013). Cell cycle and lineage progression of neural progenitors in the ventricular-subventricular zones of adult mice. *Proc. Natl. Acad. Sci. U.S.A.* 110, E1045–E1054. doi: 10.1073/pnas.1219563110

Porlan, E., Morante-Redolat, J. M., Marques-Torrejon, M. A., Andreu-Agullo, C., Carneiro, C., Gomez-Ibarlucea, E., et al. (2013). Transcriptional repression of Bmp2 by p21(Waf1/Cip1) links quiescence to neural stem cell maintenance. *Nat. Neurosci.* 16, 1567–1575. doi: 10.1038/nn.3545

Sale, S., Lafkas, D., and Artavanis-Tsakonas, S. (2013). Notch2 genetic fate mapping reveals two previously unrecognized mammary epithelial lineages. *Nat. Cell Biol.* 15, 451–460. doi: 10.1038/ncb2725

Sanai, N., Nguyen, T., Ihrie, R. A., Mirzadeh, Z., Tsai, H. H., Wong, M., et al. (2011). Corridors of migrating neurons in the human brain and their decline during infancy. *Nature* 478, 382–386. doi: 10.1038/nature10487

Sequerra, E. B., Costa, M. R., Menezes, J. R., and Hedin-Pereira, C. (2013). Adult neural stem cells: plastic or restricted neuronal fates? *Development* 140, 3303–3309. doi: 10.1242/dev.093096

Sequerra, E. B., Miyakoshi, L. M., Froes, M. M., Menezes, J. R., and Hedin-Pereira, C. (2010). Generation of glutamatergic neurons from postnatal and adult subventricular zone with pyramidal-like morphology. *Cereb. Cortex* 20, 2583–2591. doi: 10.1093/cercor/bhq006

Seri, B., Garcia-Verdugo, J. M., McEwen, B. S., and Alvarez-Buylla, A. (2001). Astrocytes give rise to new neurons in the adult mammalian hippocampus. *J. Neurosci.* 21, 7153–7160.

Shook, B. A., Manz, D. H., Peters, J. J., Kang, S., and Conover, J. C. (2012). Spatiotemporal changes to the subventricular zone stem cell pool through aging. *J. Neurosci.* 32, 6947–6956. doi: 10.1523/JNEUROSCI.5987-11.2012

Suh, H., Consiglio, A., Ray, J., Sawai, T., D'Amour, K. A., and Gage, F. H. (2007). *In vivo* fate analysis reveals the multipotent and self-renewal capacities of Sox2+ neural stem cells in the adult hippocampus. *Cell Stem Cell* 1, 515–528. doi: 10.1016/j.stem.2007.09.002

Suhonen, J. O., Peterson, D. A., Ray, J., and Gage, F. H. (1996). Differentiation of adult hippocampus-derived progenitors into olfactory neurons *in vivo*. *Nature* 383, 624–627. doi: 10.1038/383624a0

Ventura, R. E., and Goldman, J. E. (2007). Dorsal radial glia generate olfactory bulb interneurons in the postnatal murine brain. *J. Neurosci.* 27, 4297–4302. doi: 10.1523/JNEUROSCI.0399-07.2007

Young, K. M., Fogarty, M., Kessaris, N., and Richardson, W. D. (2007). Subventricular zone stem cells are heterogeneous with respect to their embryonic origins and neurogenic fates in the adult olfactory bulb. *J. Neurosci.* 27, 8286–8296. doi: 10.1523/JNEUROSCI.0476-07.2007

9

Interhemispheric synchrony in the neonatal EEG revisited: activation synchrony index as a promising classifier

Ninah Koolen[1,2*†], Anneleen Dereymaeker[3†], Okko Räsänen[4], Katrien Jansen[3], Jan Vervisch[3], Vladimir Matic[1,2], Maarten De Vos[5,6], Sabine Van Huffel[1,2], Gunnar Naulaers[3] and Sampsa Vanhatalo[7]

[1] Division STADIUS, Department of Electrical Engineering (ESAT), University of Leuven, Leuven, Belgium
[2] iMinds-KU Leuven Medical IT Department, Leuven, Belgium
[3] Department of Development and Regeneration, University of Leuven, Leuven, Belgium
[4] Department of Signal Processing and Acoustics, Aalto University, Espoo, Finland
[5] Department of Psychology, University of Oldenburg, Oldenburg, Germany
[6] Department of Engineering Science, Institute of Biomedical Engineering, University of Oxford, Oxford, UK
[7] Department of Children's Clinical Neurophysiology, HUS Medical Imaging Center and Children's Hospital, Helsinki University Central Hospital and University of Helsinki, Helsinki, Finland

Edited by:
Silvia Comani, Università degli Studi "G. d'Annunzio," Italy

Reviewed by:
Simon Farmer, National Hospital for Neurology and Neurosurgery and University College London, UK
Andrea Guzzetta, University of Pisa, Italy

***Correspondence:**
Ninah Koolen, Division STADIUS-BIOMED, Department of Electrical Engineering, University of Leuven, Kasteelpark Arenberg 10 - Bus 2446, 3000 Leuven, Belgium
e-mail: ninah.koolen@esat.kuleuven.be

† These authors are joint first authors.

A key feature of normal neonatal EEG at term age is interhemispheric synchrony (IHS), which refers to the temporal co-incidence of bursting across hemispheres during trace alternant EEG activity. The assessment of IHS in both clinical and scientific work relies on visual, qualitative EEG assessment without clearly quantifiable definitions. A quantitative measure, activation synchrony index (ASI), was recently shown to perform well as compared to visual assessments. The present study was set out to test whether IHS is stable enough for clinical use, and whether it could be an objective feature of EEG normality. We analyzed 31 neonatal EEG recordings that had been clinically classified as normal ($n = 14$) or abnormal ($n = 17$) using holistic, conventional visual criteria including amplitude, focal differences, qualitative synchrony, and focal abnormalities. We selected 20-min epochs of discontinuous background pattern. ASI values were computed separately for different channel pair combinations and window lengths to define them for the optimal ASI intraindividual stability. Finally, ROC curves were computed to find trade-offs related to compromised data lengths, a common challenge in neonatal EEG studies. Using the average of four consecutive 2.5-min epochs in the centro-occipital bipolar derivations gave ASI estimates that very accurately distinguished babies clinically classified as normal vs. abnormal. It was even possible to draw a cut-off limit (ASI~3.6) which correctly classified the EEGs in 97% of all cases. Finally, we showed that compromising the length of EEG segments from 20 to 5 min leads to increased variability in ASI-based classification. Our findings support the prior literature that IHS is an important feature of normal neonatal brain function. We show that ASI may provide diagnostic value even at individual level, which strongly supports its use in prospective clinical studies on neonatal EEG as well as in the feature set of upcoming EEG classifiers.

Keywords: interhemispheric synchrony, biomarker, preterm infant, brain monitoring, neonatal EEG

INTRODUCTION

Recent progress in basic neuroscience, neuroimaging, and neonatal care has raised interest in the understanding of physiological and pathological processes in the preterm and neonatal brain. Electroencephalography (EEG) is a non-invasive and sensitive tool for evaluating brain function in the neonatal period. A key component in early brain functional development is the emergence of functional networks, the long range connectivity between and within brain hemispheres, which lay the basis for the development of neurocognitive capabilities (Uhlhaas et al., 2010; Lubsen et al., 2011; Omidvarnia et al., 2014). In this context, it is intriguing that synchrony between hemispheres has been considered as an important feature of normal neonatal brain function since the seminal studies in the late 1970s (Lombroso, 1979).

Clinical classification of spontaneous neonatal EEG is traditionally based on visual assessment of multiple features: continuity, quality of sleep wake organization, interhemispheric synchrony (IHS), symmetry and amplitude. However, visual EEG interpretation requires expertise, and there are no objective standards for classification schemes, nor any other established method to yield appropriate diagnostic accuracy to support modern neuroscience or evidence based medicine. This has greatly compromised comparisons of results between different studies. A quantitative analysis of EEG activity, including automated analysis of selected features of cortical function, could create an objective and appropriate classification scheme for neonatal EEG. Moreover, it could also support and accelerate visual EEG analyses in medical centers without access to highly skilled EEG interpretation.

Visual estimation of IHS is based on observation of co-incidence of bursts in spontaneous background EEG activity during tracé alternant/discontinue (Holmes and Lombroso, 1993). IHS is interpreted as a sign of connectivity or functional interaction between hemispheres and is hence considered an important feature of normal brain function, resulting from the development of callosal connections (Kostovic and Jovanov-Milosevic, 2006; Dudink et al., 2008).

Despite the long and widespread clinical use of IHS, there is no physiologically plausible definition of IHS for visual EEG reading (for more details, please see Räsänen et al., 2013). A quantitative measure for IHS, the activation synchrony index (ASI), was recently developed by Räsänen et al. (2013). The ASI is based on statistically measuring the temporal delay between two signal energies, and was shown to correlate with visually rated IHS grades. It was also shown to clearly outperform other methods proposed for the same purpose in the recent literature (Räsänen et al., 2013).

Our ultimate aim is to use ASI more widely as a clinical biomarker or as a feature in EEG classifiers, which poses special requirements for individual stability. In addition, the analysis settings such as the epoch lengths need to be practical with respect to clinical reality, where obtaining longer high quality epochs is often challenging due to intermittent, trivial artifacts. The aim of this study was to test the ability of the ASI to distinguish normal and abnormal neonatal EEG recordings. Therefore, we first defined the optimal ASI parameters to maximize its intraindividual and technical stability, and then tested ASI as an input for a classifier to identify abnormal EEG activity.

MATERIALS AND METHODS

The present study consisted of two discrete phases (see **Figure 1**). First, we optimized the intraindividual stability of ASI. The earlier development of ASI had aimed to optimize parameter settings for maximal distinction between asynchrony grades as well as robustness against artifacts. Our present study continued ASI optimization by searching for EEG epoch lengths and channel derivations that would strike a balance between technical reliability and clinical practice. For clinical practice, an important consideration is that the algorithm should work equally well on EEG samples either with longer continuous epochs or with multiple shorter epochs. In addition, we tested our optimized ASI protocol on a new EEG dataset that had been classified using conventional clinical criteria, with the aim of seeing how well ASI alone is able to distinguish normal and abnormal EEG recordings. This latter aim is also a rigorous test of the conventional, albeit quantitatively untested assumption, that interhemispheric asynchrony would be an essential property in the abnormal EEG near term age.

SUBJECTS AND EEG RECORDINGS

A total of 31 neonatal EEG traces [postmenstrual age (PMA) 36–42 weeks], were retrospectively selected by an expert (A.D.) to assess the spontaneous background EEG activity. These EEG recordings were collected from a larger EEG dataset, recorded for clinical purposes. All EEG data were recorded at 256 Hz with a video-synchronized EEG device (BRAIN RT, OSG equipment, Mechelen, Belgium). After skin preparation (Nuprep Gel), 10–17 Ag/AgCl cup electrodes were placed according to the international 10–20 standard locations. The reference electrode was Cz. Electrode impedance was below 10 kΩ at the start, and the signal quality was monitored visually throughout the recording. The minimum recording time was 4 h to record multiple vigilance states. The protocol was reviewed and approved by the relevant Ethics Committee of the University Hospitals of Leuven, Belgium.

The EEG records were reviewed for clinical purposes by two independent raters (A.D. and K.J.) who were not aware of the later use of the EEG for this study. Hence, they were fully blinded to both the overall design as well as the numerical ASI results. The clinical assessment is based on holistic, conventional visual criteria (see Table 1 in Supplementary Material). If there was any difference in the interpretation of an EEG, a consensus was reached after re-evaluation (2 patients, Table 1 in Supplementary Material). The following parameters were assessed on the whole measurement, according to standard developmental features in preterm and term EEG (Scher et al., 2005; André et al., 2010; Shellhaas et al., 2011; Hayashi-Kurahashi et al., 2012): (1) brain activity cycling as being normal or abnormal for the age; (2) grade of continuity; (3) age-specific landmarks: amplitude, disorganization, and dysmaturation patterns; and (4) qualitative synchrony in quiet sleep. The overall clinical classification of the EEG recording as normal ($n = 14$) vs. abnormal ($n = 17$) was based on observing at least two features that were not appropriate for age.

ACTIVATION SYNCHRONY INDEX

The ASI algorithm implemented in Matlab is described in full detail in the original publication (Räsänen et al., 2013). It takes two EEG-signals (e.g., bipolar derivations in left and right hemispheres, respectively) as inputs to be processed through four main stages (**Figure 1C**): (1) preprocessing; (2) computation of signal amplitude envelope; (3) quantization of the amplitude envelope; and (4) calculation of the ASI value, a single scalar value, from the temporal relationship of the two quantized signals. Technical details of the algorithm can be found in the Supplementary Material. For as long as the peaks in energy envelopes are temporally co-incident (clinically perceived as "synchronized"), their dependency is highest at zero lag and diminishes with increasing relative lag between the two channels, thereby leading to a high ASI value. On the other hand, lack of temporal co-incidence, the signature of low-synchrony, will result in low ASI (for example signals, see **Figure 1B** or Räsänen et al., 2013).

PARAMETER OPTIMIZATION

The prior work on ASI development defined the main parameter settings, the most important of which appeared to be the definition of the frequency band, and the weighting of higher frequencies (a.k.a. "pre-emphasis"). These yielded an ASI that can discriminate between different visually rated IHS grades, and which clearly outperforms the other methods proposed earlier in

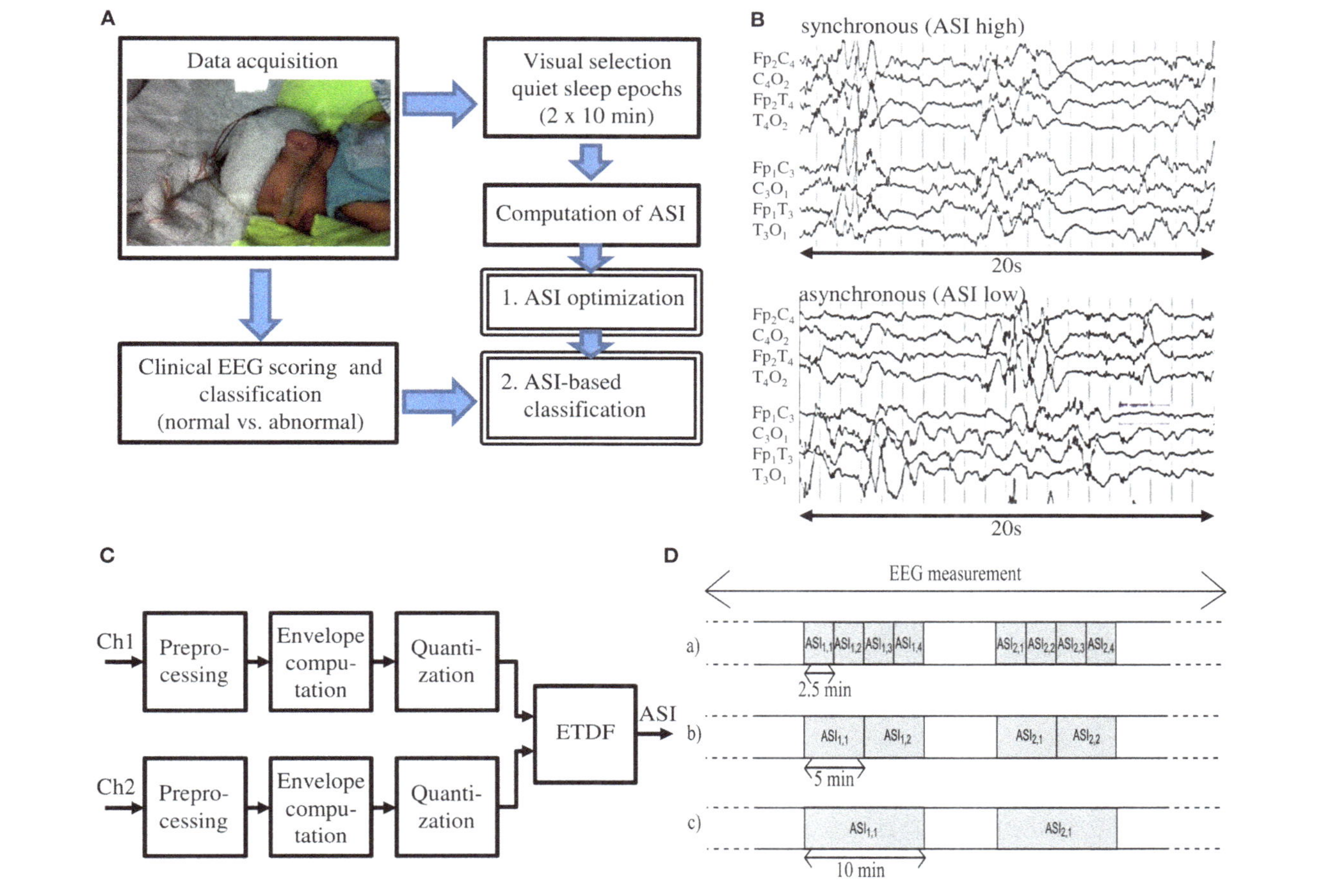

FIGURE 1 | (A) Schematic overview of the presented method. **(B)** EEG tracks with Normal and Abnormal synchrony. **(C)** Schematic view of the ASI algorithm (Räsänen et al., 2013). **(D)** Two 10-min quiet sleep epochs are subdivided into shorter epochs of 2.5, 5, and 10 min for analysis, which gives respectively *ASI2.5*, *ASI5*, and *ASI10* values.

the literature (Räsänen et al., 2013). However, it was not shown (1) how stable the ASI is technically and physiologically within an individual; (2) what window length would allow the most practical setting in clinical practice where selecting longer data epochs is always challenged by the intermittent, trivial artifacts; and (3) which of the bipolar EEG derivations would produce the best results.

Stability over time

It is commonly assumed by clinicians that IHS is a fairly stable property of a given brain function, at least at the scale of multiple hours. Thus, the IHS measure should be comparable between successive sleep cycles, and at least between few-minute epochs within a given QS period. Theoretically and physiologically thinking, it is also possible, and may even be more likely, that subtle fluctuations occur in the IHS over time. The clinically required intraindividual stability of our measure by a test-retest paradigm is technically straightforward, but the differences to be seen in repeated measures are affected by multiple factors. First, there is a numerical uncertainty in the measure itself when recorded from typically noisy neonatal recordings. Second, the feature quantified by ASI may change due to subtle fluctuations in brain state at multi-minute scale. The former possibility is typically tackled by using longer data epochs, while the latter possibility is better assessed by looking at multiple shorter data epochs. Hence, we decided to study the whole range of epoch lengths and numbers that we felt could be practical in future clinical implementations.

To this end, we divided the original 10-min data epochs into 10, 5, and 2.5-min epochs, and examined ASI in each. The aim was to define the epoch length with the smallest possible intra-patient deviations. This was assessed by searching for the lowest mean-squared difference (MSD) between the (average) ASI value of the first 10-min epoch (ASI_1) and the (average) ASI value of the second 10-min epoch (ASI_2). In formula 1 this difference is squared, summed and averaged over all patients, with n representing the number of patients.

$$MSD = \frac{1}{n}\sum_{i=1}^{n}(ASI_{1,i} - ASI_{2,i})^2 \qquad (1)$$

MSD measures the difference between the different ASI values within an individual. The optimal ASI parameters were expected to give the lowest MSD. In this way, a MSD minimization problem is solved as a function of different channel pair combinations and different ASI window lengths.

A further issue to investigate was the stability of ASI between different quiet sleep epochs. In clinical practice, it may not always be possible to find long epochs of undisturbed and good signal quality epochs of quiet sleep. Therefore, more data could be readily gathered from successive sleep cycles. Hence, we analyzed either continuous 20-min epochs from one cycle or two 10-min epochs from successive cycles.

ASI window length

ASI is a statistical estimate of synchrony, and its numerical accuracy ("technical reliability") will increase when the analysis epochs get longer. Our earlier work showed that an ASI estimate becomes more stable when the epochs grow longer than about 2 min (Räsänen et al., 2013). Longer EEG epochs are needed to statistically quantify temporal co-incidence of pseudoperiodic, intermittent cortical activity. In this work, we searched for the optimal window by calculating the ASI feature for window lengths of 2.5, 5, and 10 min. To have a fair comparison between different window lengths, we studied two manually-selected epochs of 10 min. First, we divided each epoch into 4 equal parts of 2.5 min from which we separately computed the ASI value (*ASI2.5*), and then averaged them (**Figure 1D** upper part). Similarly, the 10-min epoch was split into two equal parts of 5 min and the ASI values (*ASI5*) were estimated and averaged (**Figure 1D** middle part). These average ASI values were compared to the single ASI value from the 10-min analysis (*ASI10*) (**Figure 1D** lower part).

Channel pair combination

IHS is traditionally analyzed from bipolar derivations (Lombroso, 1979) rather than from individual EEG signals (Omidvarnia et al., 2014). To comply with this idea, we also analyzed ASI from symmetric bipolar derivations. We wanted to define the derivation with least intraindividual variability. Hence, we computed ASI from the following symmetric combinations; Fp_1C_3-Fp_2C_4, C_3O_1-C_4O_2, Fp_1O_1-Fp_2O_2, Fp_1T_3-Fp_2T_4, T_3O_1-T_4O_2.

CLASSIFICATION

After optimization of the ASI parameters, we examined the ability of ASI to distinguish normal and abnormal EEG recordings classified by clinical criteria. To this end, we used 20 min of data, channel pair combination C_3O_1-C_4O_2, and 2.5-min ASI analysis windows *(ASI2.5)*. This gave us two average ASI estimates in each patient, derived from the two 10-min epochs (**Figure 1D** upper part). The lower of these was used to represent the lowest possible synchrony level in the given patient (ASI_{class}).

$$ASI_{class} = minimum\,(mean_1\,ASI2.5,\ mean_2\,ASI2.5) \quad (2)$$

Next, we searched for a threshold that could distinguish normal and abnormal EEG records. The optimal ASI settings were found to yield nearly non-overlapping distributions of ASI values in the two groups, so the ASI threshold can be readily drawn between the distributions. However, we then wanted to see how much ASI-based classification would be compromised if the user has only a limited amount of data available for the ASI computation. In this situation, distributions between ASI values in the two groups are overlapping. Hence, all thresholds will have their own classifier performance, i.e., levels sensitivity and specificity. Their dependence on the threshold can be readily visualized using receiver operating characteristic (ROC) curves that were computed to assess the classifier performance as a function of thresholds.

AGE DEPENDENCE OF ASI

Finally, we studied the dependence of ASI on PMA to know whether it should be taken as a confounder in babies near term age. It is known that both anatomical and electrical cortico-cortical connectivity increases toward term age (Kostovic and Judas, 2010; Omidvarnia et al., 2014). The previous study with ASI showed a modest age-dependence in a much younger group of preterm babies compared to our present group of fullterm newborns (Räsänen et al., 2013). This could be a biological confounder when using ASI on babies with a wider age range.

RESULTS

OPTIMAL PARAMETERS FOR ASI STABILIZATION

In **Figure 2**, we show the ASI comparison of 10-min epochs for two clinically relevant channel pair combinations (Fp_1C_3-Fp_2C_4 and C_3O_1-C_4O_2). Visual inspection of the scatter plots shows that least scatter is found for C_3O_1-C_4O_2 in combination with smaller ASI windows (2.5 min). Quantitation of the scatter with MSD is summarized in **Table 1** for all channel pair combinations and ASI window lengths. Out of all channel pairs tested, C_3O_1-C_4O_2 yielded the lowest MSD values. Out of all combinations of ASI windows tested, the average over 4 windows of 2.5 min led to the lowest MSD.

Next, we tested how stable the ASI value is for different selections of epochs in the whole EEG recording. We could find uninterrupted 20-min epochs of "artifact-free" quiet sleep in only a few patients, while in most of them the EEG was interrupted by arousals, movements or care procedures. Therefore, a scatter plot is shown for the analysis of an epoch of the same quiet sleep period (20 min) and of two epochs of different quiet sleep periods (2 × 10 min) (**Figure 3**). There is no significant difference in the MSDs between the epochs taken from the same vs. different quiet sleep epochs (mean MSD_subsequent = 1.061 and mean MSD_separated = 1.066, respectively; $p = 0.12$; Mann–Whittney *U*-test).

CLASSIFICATION

Using the two epochs of 10 min, we plotted the ASI values using the best channel pair (C3O1-C4O2) and window lengths (4 × 2.5 min), and labeled them according to clinical EEG judgments. As shown in **Figure 4**, the distributions of ASI values in the two groups are distinct. Comparison of the smaller of the two ASI values in each baby shows that the difference is highly significant ($p < 0.001$, *t*-test). A tentative cut-off set at ASI = 3.6 gives only one misclassified normal baby (pt #28) having an ASI below that limit, yielding a very high classification accuracy (96.77%). This patient was clinically classified as normal due to age-specific transients interpreted as "borderline" for the PMA age of 37.6 weeks (i.e., "immaturity"), which as a clinical finding does not need to be associated with globally abnormal function detected by ASI.

After observing such high classification accuracy using 2 × 10 min EEG epochs, we finally wanted to do a *post-hoc* analysis to see how the classification accuracy is affected by reduction in EEG data. This is important for clinical studies where the ideal 20 min of good quality EEG from quiet sleep is usually not available. Hence, we systematically examined a range of EEG lengths (5, 10 or 20 min), ASI window lengths (2.5, 5, and 10 min), as well as the way of combining the ASI values from multiple windows. Instead of attempting formal statistical comparisons, we aimed to provide useful practical answers by visually analyzing how the ROC curves change when the underlying data and analysis settings are changed. As an expected finding in the visual comparison of ROC curves, using more EEG data led to a generally better overall classification (**Figure 5**). We also observed that the length of the ASI window made a difference such that shorter ASI windows tended to yield higher classification accuracy. Moreover, the way of combining ASI estimates of multiple windows (mean vs. minimum vs. maximum) also appeared to affect the classification accuracy. Taking the mean ASI value from several windows seemed to produce more accurate classifications. However, qualitative comparison of ROC curves based on subsequent 5-min epochs showed that the classification accuracy varies considerably.

AGE DEPENDENCE OF ASI

ASI was not found to significantly correlate with PMA in infants near term age (PMA >36 weeks) (**Figure 6**), and the slopes of the linear regression lines are very small. Hence, the same cut-off can

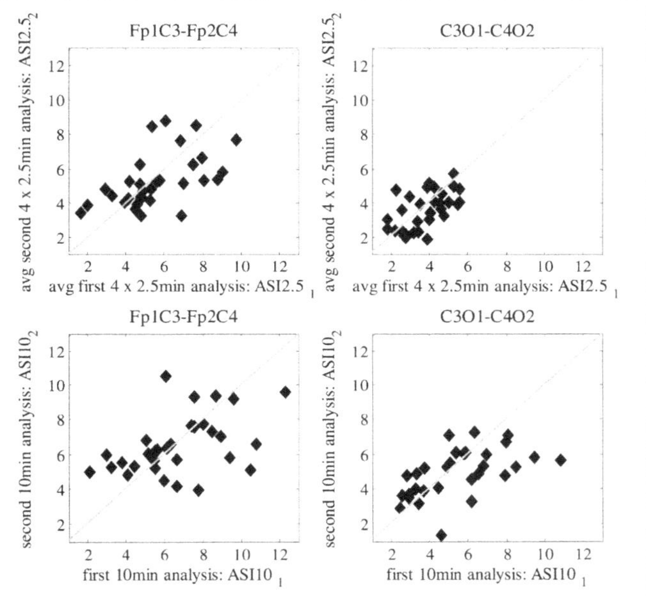

FIGURE 2 | Difference in mean-squared difference (MSD) between two analyzed periods of 10-min EEG, every dot representing a different patient. Results are shown for Frontal-Centro (Fp-C) and Centro-Occipital (C-O) derivations for different analyzing window lengths (2.5/10 min). Best result with lowest MSD is shown in the upper right plot, obtained for average ASI values over 4 × 2.5 min analysis on C-O derivations.

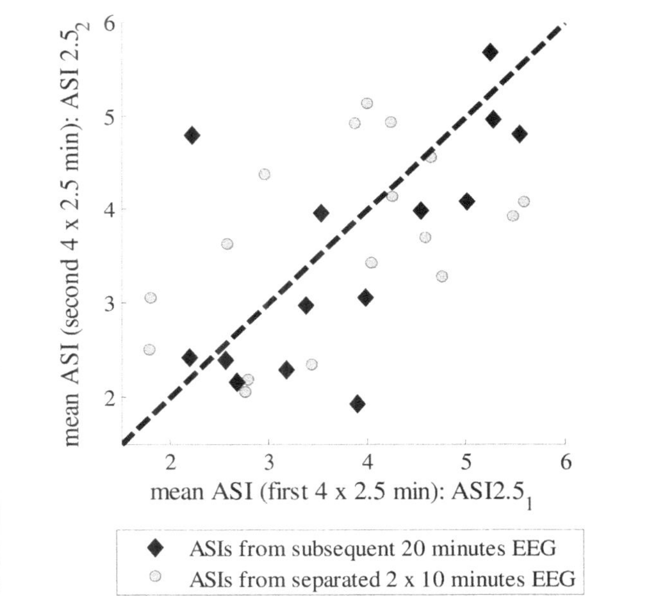

FIGURE 3 | ASIs for subsequent 10-min epochs from the same quiet sleep period or for separate 10-min epochs from two different quiet sleep periods.

Table 1 | Mean squared difference (MSD) for different channel pairs and different ASI analyzing window lengths shown as an average for all 31 patients.

	Fp_1C_3-Fp_2C_4	C_3O_1-C_4O_2	Fp_1O_1-Fp_2O_2	Fp_1T_3-Fp_2T_4	T_3O_1-T_4O_2	Mean MSD_ch
ASI_10 min	4.84	3.58	6.05	4.76	5.22	4.89
ASI avg_4 × 2.5min	2.99	1.06	1.63	1.15	2.02	1.77
ASI avg_2 × 5 min	9.90	4.23	8.60	5.51	5.25	6.70
ASI avg_2 × 2.5 min	3.21	2.22	3.82	2.91	3.74	3.18
ASI_5 min	7.59	4.71	5.71	5.38	9.05	6.49
Mean_MSD ASIwindows	5.71	316	5.16	3.94	5.06	

Grand averages of the MSD values over all channel pair combinations and window lengths are shown as well. Examples shown in ***Figure 2*** *are underlined in this table.*

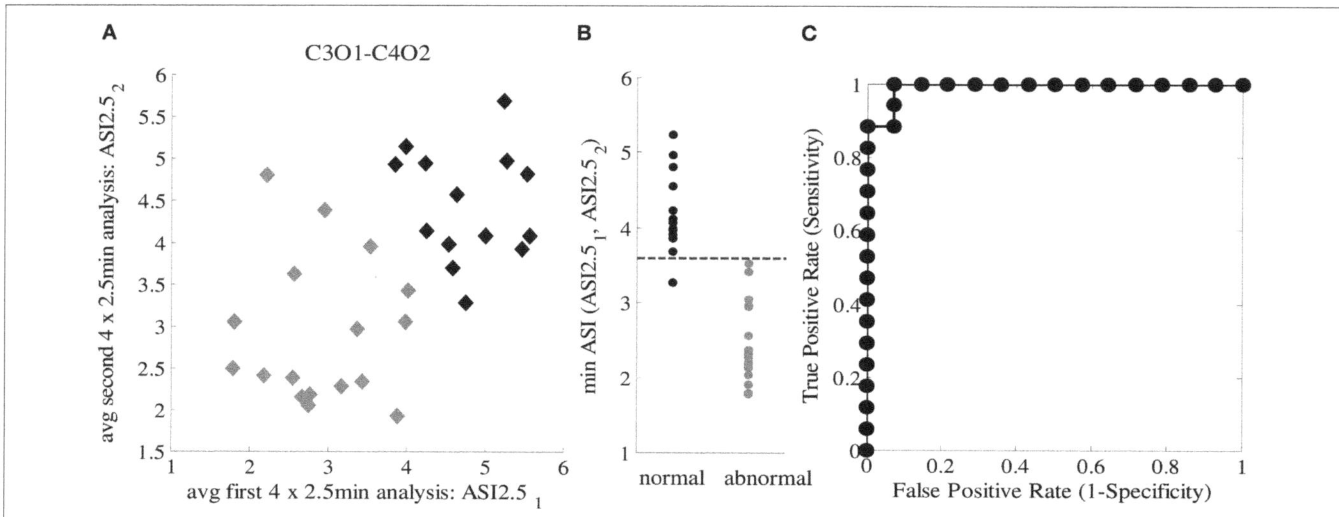

FIGURE 4 | (A) $ASI2.5_1$ and $ASI2.5_2$ for both 10-min EEG segments from 31 patients for C-O derivation with the lowest MSD value. Two groups are specified: normal patients (black labels) and abnormal patients (gray labels). **(B)** Discrimination between normal and abnormal ASI taking the minimum ASI of $ASI2.5_1$ and $ASI2.5_2$ and thresholding (Th_ASI = 3.6). **(C)** ROC curve for classification, AUC = 0.971.

be applied to distinguish normal and abnormal EEG throughout this age range, and no correction for PMA is needed.

DISCUSSION

Our study shows that IHS is a very robust feature of normal neonatal EEG, and that it can be readily quantified by using the novel metric ASI. We further show that ASI is able to reach the same classification that has been traditionally reached by a skilled EEG clinician when combining multiple visually-identified signal features. To the best of our knowledge, this study provides the first quantitative evidence in support of the old clinical thinking that disturbance of neonatal brain function is readily reflected in the interaction between hemispheres. We extend the earlier work with ASI by providing detailed assessment of how ASI performance is affected by variations in data length or analysis settings. As a conclusion, the results provide guidance for future employment of ASI in clinical work and research as well as in the development of automated EEG classifiers.

INTRAINDIVIDUAL STABILITY AND MEASUREMENT STABILITY: SELECTION OF SMALL EPOCHS

We found that the most stable ASI value was obtained by using the mean of multiple short-term ASI values, each estimated from a 2.5-min epoch. Physiologically, this observation suggests that long-range temporal correlations in the IHS are limited over time. Temporal correlations in amplitude fluctuations over several minutes have been shown in the adult brain (Linkenkaer-Hansen et al., 2001). Our recent observations in neonatal EEG datasets suggest, however, that only limited temporal correlations can be seen in the neonatal EEG signals (Matic et al., submitted), indirectly supporting the idea that ASI analyses may also best operate when using limited window lengths. Clinically and methodologically, using short segments offers several advantages in future studies and for possible implementation in brain monitoring algorithms. It is relatively easy to find several 2.5-min long undisturbed and sufficiently high quality (cf. Räsänen et al., 2013) EEG segments from neonatal recordings, while requesting longer (e.g., 10 min) continuous and undisturbed EEG epochs would pose a serious limitation in the future use of ASI. We suggest that the minimum duration of the recordings should be long enough to improve the statistical value and to overcome technical artifacts and subtle fluctuations in brain state at the multi-minute level. To this end, one should aim to collect a total of up to 20 min of quiet sleep data, which may come from successive sleep cycles. Reduction of the total data to 10 min will compromise individual diagnostic accuracy; however, it would only moderately decrease the utility of ASI at group level analyses (e.g., as an early biomarker).

CHANNEL PAIR COMBINATION AND CUT-OFF VALUE

We found that the best intraindividual stability is obtained from using central-occipital derivation. Despite decades of clinical visual assessment of IHS, there are no established practices as to which derivations should be used. A common clinical experience is that temporal co-incidence of activity bursts varies between brain areas, especially when the IHS is decreased in sick babies. It is also common to have disturbing movement and muscle artifacts in the frontal and temporal channels. Our finding suggests that ASI is optimally measured from a derivation that, by co-incidence, also happens to be usually clean of artifacts. This helps implementation of ASI in future studies. Physiologically, this finding is compatible with current knowledge of neonatal brain networks. It is well established that anatomical neonatal networks grow first in post-central regions (Kostovic and Judas, 2010), and that neonatal EEG activity mostly occurs in posterior regions (André et al., 2010). It was also shown recently that there is a prominent posterior-parietal network in the newborn brain created by long-range amplitude

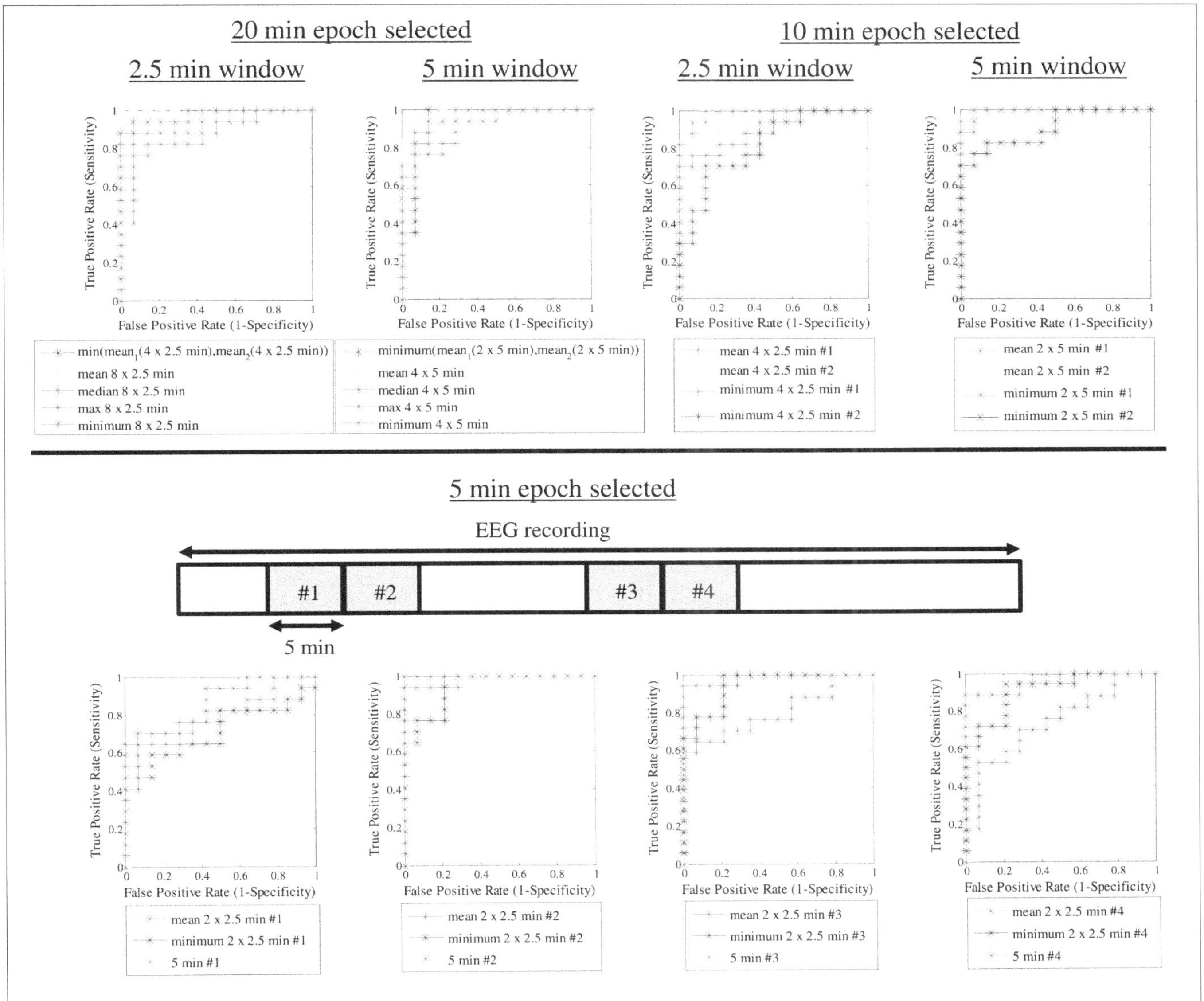

FIGURE 5 | ROC curves for different ASI window lengths and different epoch lengths.

correlations (Omidvarnia et al., 2014), which as a coupling mechanism comes close to what is measured by ASI. Taking these together, our observations suggest that the post-central networks may be the key driver of interhemispheric connectivity, and the traditionally observed loss of IHS in sick babies is probably due to changes in these posterior networks. Further studies are warranted to study whether different structural pathologies could give rise to altered IHS in a spatially selective manner.

AGE INDEPENDENCY OF ASI

We found a clear cut-off across the whole age range of babies, which suggests that future ASI implementation can disregard PMA when studying babies near term age. The younger infants in our group (PMA 36–38 weeks) showed more interindividual variability, which may reflect the as yet poorly established brain networks at that age. It has been shown that both the anatomical growth of callosal connections (Kostovic and Judas, 2010) and the appearance of visually observed IHS (Tharp et al., 1989; André et al., 2010) take place only a few weeks earlier, up to the 35th week of gestation. It is commonly seen in the clinic in these younger babies (data not shown) that the onset of quiet sleep may be markedly asynchronous and that synchrony increases within the quiet sleep period. Such dynamics could arise from functional instability in the young networks, which would readily explain a larger variability both within and between individuals.

FUTURE DIRECTIONS

Finding a high correlation between ASI and the traditional clinical visual EEG classification suggests that ASI may provide an objective and quantified global biomarker for neonatal

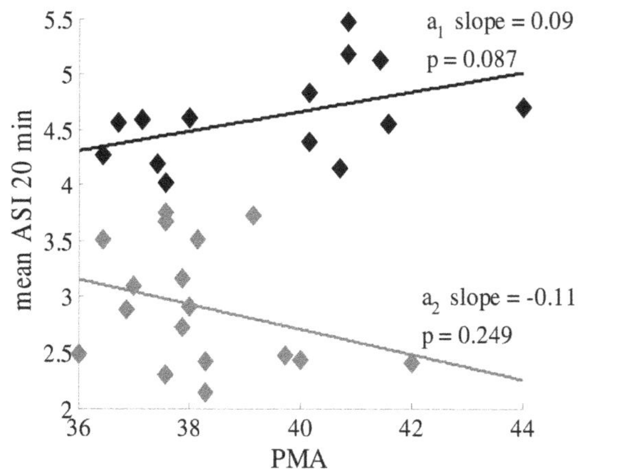

FIGURE 6 | ASI value is independent of postmenstrual age of the term infant (PMA >36 weeks). Black labels represent healthy patients with synchronous patterns; gray labels are patients with asynchronous patterns. The mean ASI value is calculated for manually-selected 20-min periods (8 × 2.5 min).

brain function. Its design makes it physiologically reasoned; our current work makes it clinically benchmarked; and its technical properties make it transparent and straightforward to implement. Hence, it holds promise for becoming a useful feature in future clinical work and research, as well as in the construction of automated classifiers of neonatal EEG. In this context, finding quiet sleep periods in an automated way would be beneficial.

This research has potential value, as prematurity-associated injury of the subplate, early extrauterine environmental stimulation, and acquired brain lesions may induce a structural adaptation of synapses and, consequently, alter the normal differentiation of cortical connectivity or even disruption of the cortical network development. These altered brain functions, expressed as levels of inter- and intrahemisperic synchrony, may reflect transiently or permanently disturbed connectivity of the cortico-cortical and cortico-basal ganglia connections, even in the absence of standard neuroimaging abnormalities. Further work for clinical research may include ASI as an outcome parameter in standardized neurodevelopment follow-up data and may also include quantitative analyses of synchrony in preterm and term infants, to identify normative and altered patterns of development.

ACKNOWLEDGMENTS

Research supported by Research Council KUL: GOA/10/09 MaNet, CoE PFV/10/002 (OPTEC); PhD/Postdoc grants; Flemish Government: FWO, IWT: projects: TBM 110697-NeoGuard; PhD/Postdoc grants; IWT project 110697; Belgian Federal Science Policy Office: IUAP P7/19/ (DYSCO); EU: ERC Advanced Grant: BIOTENSORS (n° 339804). Sampsa Vanhatalo and Okko Räsänen were supported by the Academy of Finland. Sampsa Vanhatalo was also supported by the European Community's Seventh Framework Programme European Community (FP7-PEOPLE-2009-IOF, grant agreement n°254235, as well as FP7-HEALTH-2009-4-2-1, grant agreement no. 241479, The NEMO Project).

REFERENCES

André, M., Lamblin, M.-D., d'Allest, A. M., Curzi-Dascalova, L., Moussalli-Salefranque, F. S., Nguyen The, T., et al. (2010). Electroencephalography in premature and full-term infants. Developmental features and glossary. *Clin. Neurophysiol.* 40, 59–124. doi: 10.1016/j.neucli.2010.02.002

Dudink, J., Kerr, J. L., Paterson, K., and Counsell, S. J. (2008). Connecting the developing preterm brain. *Early Hum. Dev.* 84, 777–782. doi: 10.1016/j.earlhumdev.2008.09.004

Hayashi-Kurahashi, N., Kidokoro, H., Kubota, T., Maruyama, K., Kato, Y., Kato, T., et al. (2012). EEG for predicting early neurodevelopment in preterm infants: an observational cohort study. *Pediatrics* 130, 891–897. doi: 10.1542/peds.2012-1115

Holmes, G. L., and Lombroso, C. T. (1993). Prognostic value of background patterns in the neonatal EEG. *Clin. Neurophysiol.* 10, 323–352.

Kostovic, I., and Jovanov-Milosevic, N. (2006). The development of cerebral connections during the first 20-45 weeks' gestation. *Semin. Fetal Neonatal Med.* 11, 415–422. doi: 10.1016/j.siny.2006.07.001

Kostovic, I., and Judas, M. (2010). The development of the subplate and thalamocortical connections in the human foetal brain. *Acta Paediatr.* 99, 1119–1127. doi: 10.1111/j.1651-2227.2010.01811

Linkenkaer-Hansen, K., Nikouline, V. V., Palva, J. M., and Ilmoniemi, R. J. (2001). Long-range temporal correlations and scaling behavior in human brain oscillations. *J. Neurosci.* 21, 1370–1377.

Lombroso, C. T. (1979). Quantified electrographic scales on 10 pre-term healthy newborns followed up to 40-43 weeks of conceptional age by serial polygraphic recordings. *Electroencephalogr. Clin. Neurophysiol.* 46, 460–474.

Lubsen, J., Vohr, B., Myers, E., Hampson, M., Lacadie, C., Schneider, K. C., et al. (2011). Microstructural and functional connectivity in the developing preterm brain. *Semin. Perinatol.* 35, 34–43. doi: 10.1053/j.semperi.2010.10.006

Omidvarnia, A., Fransson, P., Metsäranta, M., and Vanhatalo, S. (2014). Functional bimodality in the brain networks of preterm and term human newborns. *Cereb. Cortex* 24, 2657–2668. doi: 10.1093/cercor/bht120

Räsänen, O., Metsäranta, M., and Vanhatalo, S. (2013). Development of a novel robust measure for interhemispheric synchrony in the neonatal EEG: activation synchrony index (ASI). *Neuroimage* 69, 256–266. doi: 10.1016/j.neuroimage.2012.12.017

Scher, M. S., Turnbull, J., Loparo, K., and Johnson, M. W. (2005). Automated state analyses: proposed applications to neonatal neurointensive care. *Clin. Neurophysiol.* 22, 256–270. doi: 10.1097/01.WNP.0000161418.87923.10

Shellhaas, R. A., Chang, T., Tsuchida, T., Scher, M. S., Riviello, J. J., Abend, N. S., et al. (2011). The American clinical neurophysiology society's guideline on continuous electroencephalography monitoring in neonates. *Clin. Neurophysiol.* 28, 611–617. doi: 10.1097/WNP.0b013e31823e96d7

Tharp, B. R., Scher, M. S., and Clancy, R. R. (1989). Serial EEGs in normal and abnormal infants with birth weights less than 1200 grams–a prospective study with long term follow-up. *Neuropediatrics* 20, 64–72. doi: 10.1055/s-2008-1071267

Uhlhaas, P. J., Roux, F., Rodriguez, E., Rotarska-Jagiela, A., and Singer, W. (2010). Neural synchrony and the development of cortical networks. *Trends Cogn. Sci.* 14, 72–80. doi: 10.1016/j.tics.2009.12.002

10

Restricted nature of adult neural stem cells: re-evaluation of their potential for brain repair

Kirsten Obernier, Cheuk Ka Tong and Arturo Alvarez-Buylla*

Department of Neurological Surgery, The Eli and Edythe Broad Center of Regeneration Medicine and Stem Cell Research, University of California, San Francisco, San Francisco, CA, USA

Edited by:
Luca Bonfanti, University of Turin, Italy

Reviewed by:
Qin Shen, Albany Medical College, USA
Steven W. Levison, Rutgers New Jersey Medical School, USA

****Correspondence:***
Arturo Alvarez-Buylla, Department of Neurological Surgery, The Eli and Edythe Broad Center of Regeneration Medicine and Stem Cell Research, University of California, San Francisco, 35 Medical Center Way RMB, San Francisco, CA 94143, USA
e-mail: abuylla@stemcell.ucsf.edu

Neural stem cells (NSCs) in the walls of the lateral ventricles continue to produce new neurons and oligodendrocytes throughout life. The identification of NSCs, long-range neuronal migration, and the integration of new neurons into fully formed mature neural circuits—all in the juvenile or adult brain—has dramatically changed concepts in neurodevelopment and suggests new strategies for brain repair. Yet, the latter has to be seen in perspective: NSCs in the adult are heterogeneous and highly regionally specified; young neurons derived from these primary progenitors migrate and integrate in specific brain regions. Neurogenesis appears to have a function in brain plasticity rather than brain repair. If similar processes could be induced in regions of the brain that are normally not a target of new neurons, therapeutic neuronal replacement may one day reinstate neural circuit plasticity and possibly repair broken neural circuits.

Keywords: adult neural stem cells, V-SVZ, brain repair, circuit plasticity, specification

For many years, it was believed that once development is completed, no new nerve cells are added to the central nervous system. This view imposed a severe limitation on our thinking of possible mechanisms for neuronal replacement and brain repair. This dogma began to change with observations made by Joseph Altman in the 1960's: $[H]^3$-thymidine labeled progenitors gave rise to cells in several brain regions that had the morphology of neurons under the light microscope (Altman, 1962). However, the identity of these labeled cells remained highly controversial for many years (see: Rakic, 2002). Conclusive evidence for adult neurogenesis in homeotherms came from the work of Fernando Nottebohm and colleagues in the 1980's using electrophysiology, electron microscopy, and tracer methods. This work in adult songbirds, where seasonal changes in the size of song control nuclei had been previously documented, showed that new neurons continually replace older cells that have died (see: Nottebohm, 2002). Subsequent studies in mammals demonstrated that neurons are continually added to the adult olfactory bulb (OB) and the dentate gyrus during juvenile and adult life (for review see: Ihrie and Alvarez-Buylla, 2011; Gage and Temple, 2013).

New OB neurons are born postnatally within an extensive germinal zone lining the walls of the lateral ventricles. The ventricular-subventricular zone (V-SVZ) is the largest germinal niche in the adult mammalian brain. This germinal layer has been most extensively studied in rodents (Fuentealba et al., 2012; Tong and Alvarez-Buylla, 2014). Primary progenitor cells, which are frequently referred to as NSCs, generate new neurons and oligodendrocytes in the juvenile and adult brain. From the early observations in mammals and songbirds, to the more recent work in the mammalian hippocampus and the V-SVZ, adult neurogenesis has been proclaimed to offer a new hope for brain repair (Nottebohm, 1985; Gage and Temple, 2013). Certainly, the discovery of adult neurogenesis demonstrates that neuronal birth, migration over extremely long distances, and the integration of these cells into established brain circuitry *is indeed all possible*. However, as we discuss below, the NSCs, progenitors, and signaling that allow for new neurons to be born and the mechanisms that permit young neurons to migrate and integrate within the adult brain, do not seem to be intended for brain repair (summarized in **Table 1**). Instead, most of the evidence suggests that adult neurogenesis enables constant modification of neural circuits—likely related to unique forms of brain plasticity in which some key neurons are eliminated and replaced. Here we focus most of our discussion on the V-SVZ where NSCs, their lineages, and the migration of young neurons have been extensively characterized.

In the adult rodent V-SVZ a subpopulation of progenitors with astroglial characteristics, known as B1 cells, function as the NSCs. B1 cells generate young neurons that migrate long distances via the rostral migratory stream (RMS) to the OB where they differentiate into local circuit GABAergic interneurons. For potential brain repair, the understanding of the plasticity of these primary progenitors is key. If these cells are capable of generating a wide diversity of neuronal cell types they could potentially be directed to form nerve cells lost in a disease or following trauma. Earlier work suggested that NSCs could be plastic and that the environment played a key role in directing their differentiation into specific neuronal cell types (Fallon et al., 2000; Shihabuddin

Table 1 | Adult Neurogenesis in the V-SVZ: Challenges for Brain Repair.

Adult V-SVZ neurogenesis	Circuit plasticity	Brain repair?
Cell type specification	• Primary progenitors are regionally specified (Merkle et al., 2007) • Generation of GABAergic interneurons • Replacement of specific subsets of older neurons in the OB	• No confirmed evidence for differentiation into cell types required for replacement of lost neurons in different brain regions (Herrera et al., 1999; Raedt et al., 2009)
Migration of young neurons	• Mostly restricted to the V-SVZ and RMS, directed toward the OB (Lois and Alvarez-Buylla, 1994; Doetsch and Alvarez-Buylla, 1996)	• Requires exiting the V-SVZ and RMS • Requires migration and integration into the lesion site
New neuron integration	• Integration into defined circuits • Specialized synaptic contacts with mitral and tufted projection neurons (Whitman and Greer, 2009)	• Requires integration and survival of young neurons in environments that are normally non-neurogenic • Synaptic contacts with different neuronal partners depending on the types of circuit damaged
In context of human brain	• Mostly restricted to infants (Sanai et al., 2004, 2011; Bergmann et al., 2012)	• Limited evidence of neurogenesis under pathological conditions in the adult or aged human brain

et al., 2000). It was suggested that NSCs isolated from one brain region could function as those in another (e.g., hippocampal NSCs transplanted into the V-SVZ) (Brustle and McKay, 1996; Suhonen et al., 1996), whereas more recent work suggests that V-SVZ cells cannot acquire cortical, striatal or hippocampal properties following transplantation (Herrera et al., 1999; Raedt et al., 2009). Additional evidence indicates that NSCs under normal physiological conditions are highly specialized and regionally specified in a cell-autonomous manner to produce specific types of neurons destined for unique circuits within particular brain regions (Merkle et al., 2007). This limitation may be overcome by the trans-differentiation of the precursors using transcription factors (Chen et al., 2012), but in their default state their differentiation seems to be limited.

The specification of the neuroepithelium occurs early in development, restricting the potency of NSCs in the forebrain (Rubenstein, 2011) as well as the spinal cord (Jessell et al., 2011). In the developing murine embryonic brain early progenitors produce striatal, cortical, and septal neurons—possibly orchestrated by combinations of several transcription factors (Rubenstein, 2011)—but later progenitors fail to generate earlier fates (Shen et al., 2006). Whereas depending on their position within the VZ germinal zone embryonic NSCs generate both glutamatergic and GABAergic neurons for different forebrain regions, adult V-SVZ NSCs mostly generate GABAergic neurons destined for the OB. In the adult V-SVZ, NSCs are not only restricted to differentiate into OB interneurons but are heterogeneous and regionally specified (**Figure 1**). Adenovirus-mediated labeling of NSCs in different locations of the lateral, medial, and pallial wall has shown that dorsal NSCs generate mostly superficial granule cells (GCs) and dopaminergic tyrosine hydroxylase (TH)-positive (but not calbindin-positive) periglomerular cells (PGCs), while ventral NSCs produce deep GCs and calbindin-positive (but not TH-positive) PGCs and NSCs in the medial wall give rise to calretinin-positive PGCs and GCs. This positional specification seems to be primarily cell intrinsic, since labeled progenitors maintained their original phenotype *in vitro* and upon heterotopic grafting within the niche (Merkle et al., 2007). The positional identity of adult NSCs is likely inherited from the early embryonic differential expression of combinations of transcription factors by neuroepithelial and radial glia cells (for review see Kriegstein and Alvarez-Buylla, 2009; Rubenstein, 2011). Furthermore, transplantation of V-SVZ NSCs to non-neurogenic regions (outside the germinal niche) of the adult brain under normal physiological conditions is not permissive for neurogenesis; V-SVZ cells grafted into the cortex or striatum fail to migrate and produce few, if any, neurons (Herrera et al., 1999; Seidenfaden et al., 2006). For now it seems that NSCs and progenitor cells in the V-SVZ are highly restricted in their potential; this may 1 day be overcome by reprogramming.

An important obstacle for brain repair in the juvenile or adult brain is the long distances that frequently separate endogenous germinal niches, or sites of transplantation of progenitor cells, from the sites where new neurons would be required. Damaged areas are also frequently distributed over large volumes of brain tissue. Repair, therefore, requires long migrations of precursor cells through the complex postnatal brain parenchyma. NSCs (B1 and radial glia cells) are largely fixed to specific locations in the neuroepithelium. In contrast, young neurons derived from these specified locations need to migrate to their final destination, often very long distances. Consistently, neuroblasts derived from the adult V-SVZ, have an extraordinary capacity for long-range migration within the adult brain parenchyma (Lois and Alvarez-Buylla, 1994). In the context of brain repair, this migratory capacity could potentially allow young neurons to penetrate deep into a lesion and replace neurons where they are needed. However, under normal conditions, neuroblasts derived from the V-SVZ migrate within distinct corridors within the SVZ and the RMS (Doetsch and Alvarez-Buylla, 1996). This constrained migration mediated by chemotactic factors, glial ensheathment, and a vascular scaffold (Nguyen-Ba-Charvet et al., 2004; Sawamoto et al., 2006; Whitman et al., 2009; Kaneko et al., 2010) ensures the

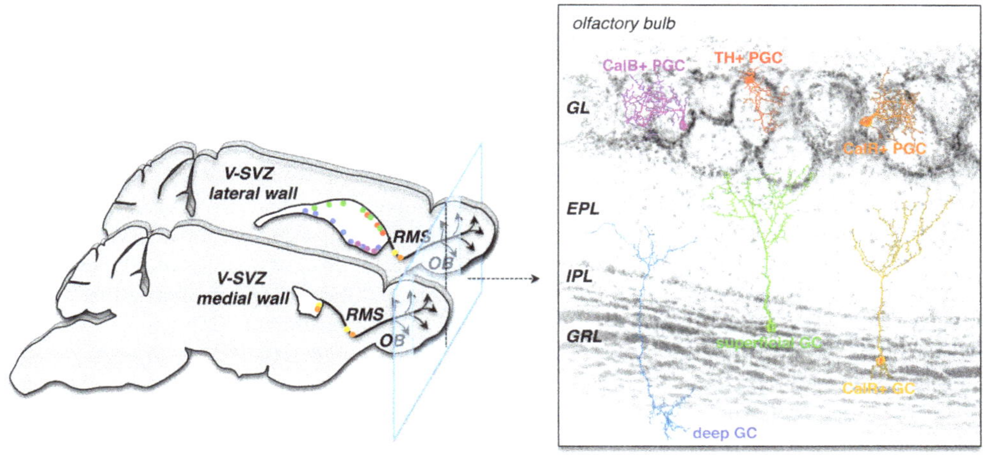

FIGURE 1 | V-SVZ NSCs are regionally specified and generate unique subtypes of OB interneurons depending on their location. This specified nature of primary progenitors sets limits to their direct use for brain repair; yet future strategies may exploit reprogramming to induce these NSCs to produce specific neuronal subsets required for brain repair. Left panel: the color dots in the medial (bottom) and lateral (top) walls of the lateral ventricles on the two sagittal views of the left mouse brain depict regions were specific subsets of olfactory bulb (OB) interneuron subtypes (right panel) are born. CalB, Calbindin; CalR, Calretinin; EPL, external plexiform layer; IPL, internal plexiform layer; GC, granule cell; GL, glomerular layer; GRL, granule cell layer; OB, olfactory bulb; PGC, periglomerular cell; RMS, rostral migratory stream; TH, tyrosine hydroxylase; V-SVZ, ventricular-subventricular zone (modified from Alvarez-Buylla et al., 2013).

delivery of these young neurons to the OB, where they then disperse radially into specific layers (Whitman and Greer, 2009; Ihrie and Alvarez-Buylla, 2011). Interestingly, there is some evidence that neuroblasts are able to leave the V-SVZ and RMS to invade the adjacent striatum. For example, following ischemia-induced activation of guidance molecules (e.g., CXCR4-SDF1) neuroblasts migrate toward the ischemic site but the ectopic migration may be due to aberrant expression of substrate and guidance molecules within the context of the lesions. It is also possible that the physical damage from these lesions could interfere with the normal migratory path, facilitating the derailment of neuroblasts into adjoining territories while they maintain their intrinsic differentiation potential and thus are rather misdirected OB interneurons (Liu et al., 2009). Although it has been suggested that few young neurons migrating toward the site of lesion can survive and possibly integrate (Arvidsson et al., 2002; Kokaia et al., 2006; Yamashita et al., 2006; Hou et al., 2008), most do not become mature neurons and do not survive long-term (Osman et al., 2011; Cui et al., 2013). Others have reported that intraventricular growth factor infusion may be necessary to promote regeneration (Kolb et al., 2007). In contrast to neurons, there is better evidence that oligodendrocyte progenitors derived from the V-SVZ can migrate into a demyelinated lesioned site and differentiate into new oligodendrocytes (Nait-Oumesmar et al., 1999; Picard-Riera et al., 2002; Menn et al., 2006). Upon brain injury some V-SVZ cells may also produce astrocytes that migrate to the injury site (Benner et al., 2013). Therefore, migration through the adult brain is limited to very specific paths and to specific subtypes of neurons and glial cells.

The ability to become synaptically incorporated into fully formed adult brain circuits is an essential characteristic of new neurons formed in the V-SVZ. While synaptic incorporation is a highly desired property for putative new neurons in the context of brain repair, these cells specifically integrate into the circuits of the OB. In the OB they mediate inhibition of mitral and tufted projection neurons and it is thought that their continual replacement into adulthood is associated to olfactory discrimination and plasticity (Gheusi et al., 2000; Cecchi et al., 2001; Sakamoto et al., 2011). Plasticity-related functions for adult-born neurons have also been proposed in songbirds (Alvarez-Buylla et al., 1990; Scharff et al., 2000) and in the rodent hippocampus (Kempermann, 2012; Gage and Temple, 2013). Therefore, the available evidence strongly suggests that the integration of newly formed neurons occurs within very specific circuits where ongoing plasticity requires new nerve cells. It is tempting to speculate that diseased or injured brain circuits could similarly present a permissive environment for the recruitment of new neurons, but this remains to be demonstrated. If the young neurons that are normally produced in the adult brain are so highly tuned to specific brain circuits, an important limitation might be their competence to differentiate into neuronal cell types that can migrate and integrate to reconstitute function in damaged circuits. Neuronal progenitors capable of differentiation, migration and integration within the environment of neurodegeneration or trauma may exist, but these cells do not seem to be the ones normally produced in the adult brain.

The above shows that the birth, migration, and integration of young neurons is fashioned for specific brain circuits with the demand for a special form of plasticity in the adult brain. This sets limits to the use of adult NSCs in brain repair. Species-specific differences in adult neurogenesis may also determine the potential use of NSCs in brain repair. For example, it has been known for sometime, that reptiles and amphibians can regenerate neuronal populations that are not repaired in mammals or birds (Polenov and Chetverukhin, 1993; Font et al., 2001; Garcia-Verdugo et al., 2002; Chapouton et al., 2007). However, there are also important differences among mammals. The human V-SVZ differs in its cytoarchitecture compared to the rodent germinal zone. While the human V-SVZ is also lined with a monolayer of ependymal cells at the apical side of the walls of the lateral ventricles, it basally consists of a hypocellular gap, an astrocytic ribbon that contains neural progenitor cells, and a transition zone into the parenchyma. In infant humans the V-SVZ is an important source of new neurons not only for the OB, but also for specific subregions of the anterior prefrontal cortex (Sanai et al., 2004, 2011; Yang et al., 2011). Unlike in rodents where neurogenesis persists throughout the animal's lifespan—though it is drastically reduced during aging—only very few migrating young neurons are observed in the adolescents or in adult human brains. Consistently, radiocarbon birth dating suggests that the vast majority of neurons in the OB are as old as the person, implying they are born during early development (Bergmann et al., 2012). Those neurons that are added to specific brain regions during early childhood could be key in understanding critical-period plasticity and postnatal developmental deficits. In the hippocampus, the story may be somewhat different when compared to the OB. It remains controversial how many new neurons continue to be added in the dentate gyrus in the adult human brain. Some studies suggest the presence of newly born hippocampal neurons in adults and a surprisingly stable birth rate from adolescence to aging (Eriksson et al., 1998; Spalding et al., 2013), yet other studies reveal very few cells expressing markers of young neurons in the hippocampus after birth (Knoth et al., 2010). In adult humans, in addition to the intrinsic limitations imposed by adult NSC specification, the possible low number of NSCs or their long-term quiescence pose further constraints, which may limit their potential use in cell replacement therapies. Even if the activation of resident quiescent NSCs—if they exist—is possible, the migration, survival, and integration into specific brain regions may be a greater challenge given the large size of the human brain.

While we have made significant progress in understanding the identity and lineages of adult NSCs, there is no evidence that these cells can repair neural circuits or replace diverse neuronal cell types. The function of adult neurogenesis remains unknown, but significant evidence points to processes of brain plasticity rather than brain repair. Regions of the postnatal brain that continue to receive new neurons may be plastic throughout life; they may not be constrained by defined critical-periods of plasticity that ends as their neuronal components mature (Southwell et al., 2010). The addition of new neurons may be seen as a constant infusion of youth into mature neural circuits. The more directed use of neuronal replacement for brain repair will likely require very specific types of progenitor cells that can navigate and appropriately integrate into target regions. Most likely this will involve the reprograming of embryonic or adult brain cells for the production of those specific neuronal cell types that can integrate and repair damaged neural circuits. Neural progenitor cells from the mouse embryonic MGE for example have been shown to migrate long distances upon transplantation and can contribute to neuronal replacement, although only with the generation of interneurons, not excitatory neurons (Wichterle et al., 1999; Alvarez-Dolado et al., 2006; Southwell et al., 2010). Human fetal cells transplanted into stroke-lesioned mice migrate long distances and differentiated into mature neurons in the lesioned striatum or cortex (Kelly et al., 2004; Darsalia et al., 2007). Also further efforts in the field of iPSC-derived neural progenitors may lead to neuronal replacement strategies. We also cannot exclude that very specific subsets of the heterogeneous population of endogenous adult V-SVZ NSCs may harbor the potential to function as precursors for neurons in different brain regions; this requires detailed analysis of the potential of individual NSCs located in different regions of the adult V-SVZ.

The identification of NSCs among astroglia and the abundance of glial cells suggest that the adult brain may contain a large reservoir of cells that could be target for such reprograming. Efforts along these lines have already begun (Guo et al., 2013; Niu et al., 2013), but further understanding of astrocyte heterogeneity is required (Hochstim et al., 2008; Tsai et al., 2012).

In the present perspective article we have focused mostly on adult neurogenesis in the V-SVZ, as this is the most extensive germinal region of the adult mammalian brain. Similar concepts of specification, confined migration, and integration probably also apply to neurogenesis in the adult hippocampus and avian forebrain (Scharff, 2000; Nottebohm and Liu, 2010; Ming and Song, 2011; Gage and Temple, 2013). This very high level of specification may suggest, to some, that adult neurogenesis is irrelevant to brain repair. However, this is not the case: one important lesson learned from studies of adult neurogenesis is that processes considered impossible three decades ago do indeed take place in the adult brain; young neurons can be produced and they can migrate, and most importantly integrate, into adult brain circuits. Their seamless migration and integration, whether in the song control circuits of birds, or in the OB and hippocampus of adult mammals, still has much to teach us about how to accomplish similar neuronal replacement for neurons lost during neurodegeneration or trauma.

ACKNOWLEDGMENTS

We thank Joseph Elsbernd for critical reading of the perspective. This work is funded by the US National Institutes of Health (NS28478 and HD032116). Arturo Alvarez-Buylla is the Heather and Melanie Muss Endowed Chair of Neurological Surgery at UCSF. Kirsten Obernier is supported by the German Research Foundation (Deutsche Forschungsgemeinschaft DFG). Cheuk Ka Tong is supported by the Singapore Agency for Science, Technology and Research.

REFERENCES

Altman, J. (1962). Are new neurons formed in the brains of adult mammals? *Science* 135, 1127–1128. doi: 10.1126/science.135.3509.1127

Alvarez-Buylla, A., Kirn, J. R., and Nottebohm, F. (1990). Birth of projection neurons in adult avian brain may be related to perceptual or motor learning. *Science* 249, 1444–1446. doi: 10.1126/science.1698312

Alvarez-Buylla, A., Merkle, F., and Fuentealba, L. (2013). "Neurogenesis in the postnatal VZ-SVZ and the origin of interneuron diversity," in *Patterning and Cell Type Specification in the Developing Cns and Pns*, ed J. L. R. Rubenstein (San Diego, CA: Comprehensive Developmental Neuroscience; Elsevier), 537–550. doi: 10.1016/B978-0-12-397265-1.00096-4

Alvarez-Dolado, M., Calcagnotto, M. E., Karkar, K. M., Southwell, D. G., Jones-Davis, D. M., Estrada, R. C., et al. (2006). Cortical inhibition modified by embryonic neural precursors grafted into the postnatal brain. *J. Neurosci.* 26, 7380–7389. doi: 10.1523/JNEUROSCI.1540-06.2006

Arvidsson, A., Collin, T., Kirik, D., Kokaia, Z., and Lindvall, O. (2002). Neuronal replacement from endogenous precursors in the adult brain after stroke. *Nat. Med.* 8, 963–970. doi: 10.1038/nm747

Benner, E. J., Luciano, D., Jo, R., Abdi, K., Paez-Gonzalez, P., Sheng, H., et al. (2013). Protective astrogenesis from the SVZ niche after injury is controlled by Notch modulator Thbs4. *Nature* 497, 369–373. doi: 10.1038/nature12069

Bergmann, O., Liebl, J., Bernard, S., Alkass, K., Yeung, M. S. Y., Steier, P., et al. (2012). The age of olfactory bulb neurons in humans. *Neuron* 74, 634–639. doi: 10.1016/j.neuron.2012.03.030

Brustle, O., and McKay, R. D. G. (1996). Neuronal progenitors as tools for cell replacement in the nervous system. *Curr. Opin. Neurobiol.* 6, 688–695. doi: 10.1016/S0959-4388(96)80104-8

Cecchi, G. A., Petreanu, L. T., Alvarez-Buylla, A., and Magnasco, M. O. (2001). Unsupervised learning and adaptation in a model of adult neurogenesis. *J. Comput. Neurosci.* 11, 175–182. doi: 10.1023/A:1012849801892

Chapouton, P., Jagasia, R., and Bally-Cuif, L. (2007). Adult neurogenesis in non-mammalian vertebrates. *Bioessays* 29, 745–757. doi: 10.1002/bies.20615

Chen, X., Lepier, A., Berninger, B., Tolkovsky, A. M., and Herbert, J. (2012). Cultured subventricular zone progenitor cells transduced with neurogenin-2 become mature glutamatergic neurons and integrate into the dentate gyrus. *PLoS ONE* 7:e31547. doi: 10.1371/journal.pone.0031547

Cui, L., Qu, H., Xiao, T., Zhao, M., Jolkkonen, J., and Zhao, C. (2013). Stromal cell-derived factor-1 and its receptor CXCR4 in adult neurogenesis after cerebral ischemia. *Restor. Neurol. Neurosci.* 31, 239–251. doi: 10.3233/RNN-120271

Darsalia, V., Kallur, T., and Kokaja, Z. (2007). Survival, migration and neuronal differentiation of human fetal striatal and cortical neural stem cells grafted I stroke-damaged rat striatum. *Eur. J. Neurosci.* 26, 605–614. doi: 10.1111/j.1460-9568.2007.05702.x

Doetsch, F., and Alvarez-Buylla, A. (1996). Network of tangential pathways for neuronal migration in adult mammalian brain. *Proc. Natl. Acad. Sci. U.S.A.* 93, 14895–14900. doi: 10.1073/pnas.93.25.14895

Eriksson, P. S., Perfilieva, E., Björk-Eriksson, T., Alborn, A. M., Nordborg, C., Peterson, D. A., et al. (1998). Neurogenesis in the adult human hippocampus. *Nat. Med.* 4, 1313–1317. doi: 10.1038/3305

Fallon, J., Reid, S., Kinyamu, R., Opole, I., Opole, R., Baratta, J., et al. (2000). *In vivo* induction of massive proliferation, directed migration, and differentiation of neural cells in the adult mammalian brain. *Proc. Natl. Acad. Sci. U.S.A.* 97, 14686–14691. doi: 10.1073/pnas.97.26.14686

Font, E., Desfilis, E., Perez-Canellas, M. M., and Garcia-Verdugo, J. M. (2001). Neurogenesis and neuronal regeneration in the adult reptilian brain. *Brain Behav. Evol.* 58, 276–295. doi: 10.1159/000057570

Fuentealba, L. C., Obernier, K., and Alvarez-Buylla, A. (2012). Adult neural stem cells bridge their niche. *Cell Stem Cell* 10, 698–708. doi: 10.1016/j.stem.2012.05.012

Gage, F. H., and Temple, S. (2013). Neural stem cells: generating and regenerating the brain. *Neuron* 80, 588–601. doi: 10.1016/j.neuron.2013.10.037

Garcia-Verdugo, J. M., Ferron, S., Flames, N., Collado, L., Desfilis, E., and Font, E. (2002). The proliferative ventricular zone in adult vertebrates: a comparative study using retiles, birds, and mammals. *Brain Res. Bull.* 57, 765–775. doi: 10.1016/S0361-9230(01)00769-9

Gheusi, G., Cremer, H., McLean, H., Chazal, G., Vincent, J. D., and Lledo, P. M. (2000). Importance of newly generated neurons in the adult olfactory bulb for odor discrimination. *Proc. Natl. Acad. Sci. U.S.A.* 97, 1823–1828. doi: 10.1073/pnas.97.4.1823

Guo, Z., Zhang, L., Wu, Z., Chen, Y., Wang, F., and Chen, G. (2013). *In vivo* direct reprogramming of reactive glial cells into functional neurons after brain injury and in an Alzheimer's disease model. *Cell Stem Cell* 14, 188–202. doi: 10.1016/j.stem.2013.12.001

Herrera, D. G., Garcia-Verdugo, J. M., and Alvarez-Buylla, A. (1999). Adult-derived neural precursors transplanted into multiple regions in the adult brain. *Ann. Neurol.* 46, 867–877.

Hochstim, C., Deneen, B., Lukaszewicz, A., Zhou, Q., and Anderson, D. J. (2008). Identification of positionally distinct astrocyte subtypes whose identities are specified by a homeodomain code. *Cell* 133, 510–522. doi: 10.1016/j.cell.2008.02.046

Hou, S. W., Wang, Y. Q., Xu, M., Shen, D. H., Wang, J. J., Huang, F., et al. (2008). Functional integration of newly generated neurons into striatum after cerebral ischemia in the adult rat brain. *Stroke* 39, 2837–2844. doi: 10.1161/STROKEAHA.107.510982

Ihrie, R. A., and Alvarez-Buylla, A. (2011). Lake-front property: a unique germinal niche by the lateral ventricles of the adult brain. *Neuron* 70, 674–686. doi: 10.1016/j.neuron.2011.05.004

Jessell, T. M., Sürmeli, G., and Kelly, J. S. (2011). Motor neurons and the sense of place. *Neuron* 72, 419–424. doi: 10.1016/j.neuron.2011.10.021

Kaneko, N., Marin, O., Koike, M., Hirota, Y., Uchiyama, Y., Wu, J. Y., et al. (2010). New neurons clear the path of astrocytic processes for their rapid migration in the adult brain. *Neuron* 67, 213–223. doi: 10.1016/j.neuron.2010.06.018

Kelly, S., Bliss, T. M., Shah, A. K., Sun, G. H., Ma, W., Foo, W. C., et al. (2004). Transplanted human fetal neural stem cells survive, migrate, and differentiate in ischemic rat cerebral cortex. *Proc. Natl. Acad. Sci. U.S.A.* 101, 11839–11844. doi: 10.1073/pnas.0404474101

Kempermann, G. (2012). New neurons for survival of the fittest. *Nat. Rev. Neurosci.* 13, 727–736. doi: 10.1038/nrn3319

Knoth, R., Singec, I., Ditter, M., Pantazis, G., Capetian, P., Meyer, R. P., et al. (2010). Murine features of neurogenesis in the human hippocampus across the lifespan from 0 to 100 years. *PLoS ONE* 5:e8809. doi: 10.1371/journal.pone.0008809

Kokaia, Z., Thored, P., Arvidsson, A., and Lindvall, O. (2006). Regulation of stroke-induced neurogenesis in adult brain–recent scientific progress. *Cereb. Cortex* 16(Suppl. 1), i162–i167. doi: 10.1093/cercor/bhj174

Kolb, B., Morshead, C., Gonzalez, C., Kim, M., Gregg, C., Shingo, T., et al. (2007). Growth factor-stimulated generation of new cortical tissue and functional recovery after stroke damage to the motor cortex of rats. *J. Cereb. Blood Flow Metab.* 27, 983–997. doi: 10.1038/sj.jcbfm.9600402

Kriegstein, A., and Alvarez-Buylla, A. (2009). The glial nature of embryonic and adult neural stem cells. *Ann. Rev. Neurosci.* 32, 149–184. doi: 10.1146/annurev.neuro.051508.135600

Liu, F., You, Y., Li, X., Ma, T., Nie, Y., Wei, B., et al. (2009). Brain injury does not alter the intrinsic differentiation potential of adult neuroblasts. *J. Neurosci.* 29, 5075–5087. doi: 10.1523/JNEUROSCI.0201-09.2009

Lois, C., and Alvarez-Buylla, A. (1994). Long-distance neuronal migration in the adult mammalian brain. *Science* 264, 1145–1148. doi: 10.1126/science.8178174

Menn, B., Garcia-Verdugo, J. M., Yaschine, C., Gonzalez-Perez, O., Rowitch, D., and Alvarez-Buylla, A. (2006). Origin of oligodendrocytes in the subventricular zone of the adult brain. *J. Neurosci.* 26, 7907–7918. doi: 10.1523/JNEUROSCI.1299-06.2006

Merkle, F. T., Mirzadeh, Z., and Alvarez-Buylla, A. (2007). Mosaic organization of neural stem cells in the adult brain. *Science* 317, 381–384. doi: 10.1126/science.1144914

Ming, G., and Song, H. (2011). Adult neurogenesis in the mammalian brain: significant answers and significant questions. *Neuron* 70, 687–702. doi: 10.1016/j.neuron.2011.05.001

Nait-Oumesmar, B., Decker, L., Lachapelle, F., Avellana-Adalid, V., Bachelin, C., and Baron-van Evercooren, A. (1999). Progenitor cells of the adult mouse subventricular zone proliferate, migrate and differentiate into oligodendrocytes after demyelination. *Eur. J. Neurosci.* 11, 4357–4366. doi: 10.1046/j.1460-9568.1999.00873.x

Nguyen-Ba-Charvet, K. T., Picard-Riera, N., Tessier-Lavigne, M., Baron-van Evercooren, A., Sotelo, C., and Chédotal, A. (2004). Multiple roles for slits in the control of cell migration in the rostral migratory stream. *J. Neurosci.* 24, 1497–1506. doi: 10.1523/JNEUROSCI.4729-03.2004

Niu, W., Zang, T., Zou, Y., Fang, S., Smith, D. K., Bachoo, R., et al. (2013). *In vivo* reprogramming of astrocytes to neuroblasts in the adult brain. *Nat. Cell Biol.* 15, 1164–1175. doi: 10.1038/ncb2843

Nottebohm, F. (1985). Neuronal replacement in adulthood. *Ann. N.Y. Acad. Sci.* 457, 143–161. doi: 10.1111/j.1749-6632.1985.tb20803.x

Nottebohm, F. (2002). Neuronal replacement in adult brain. *Brain Res. Bull.* 57, 737–749. doi: 10.1016/S0361-9230(02)00750-5

Nottebohm, F., and Liu, W.-C. (2010). The origins of vocal learning: new sounds, new circuits, new cells. *Brain Lang.* 115, 3–17. doi: 10.1016/j.bandl.2010.05.002

Osman, A. M., Prorritt, M. J., Nilsson, M., and Kuhn, G. (2011). Long-term stimulation on neural progenitor cell migration after cortical ischemia in mice. *Stroke* 42, 3559–3565. doi: 10.1161/STROKEAHA.111.627802

Picard-Riera, N., Decker, L., Delarasse, C., Goude, K., Nait-Oumesmar, B., Liblau, R., et al. (2002). Experimental autoimmune encephalomyelitis mobilizes neural progenitors from the subventricular zone to undergo oligodendrogenesis in adult mice. *Proc. Natl. Acad. Sci. U.S.A.* 99, 13211–13216. doi: 10.1073/pnas.192314199

Polenov, A. L., and Chetverukhin, V. K. (1993). Ultrastructural radioautographic analysis of neurogenesis in the hypothalamus of the adult frog, Rana temporaria, with special reference to physiological regeneration of the preoptic nucleus. II. Types of neuronal cells produced. *Cell Tissue Res.* 271, 351–362. doi: 10.1007/BF00318622

Raedt, R., van Dycke, A., Waeytens, A., Wyckhuys, T., Vonck, K., Wadman, W., et al. (2009). Unconditioned adult-derived neurosphere cells mainly differentiate towards astrocytes upon transplantation in sclerotic rat hippocampus. *Epilepsy Res.* 87, 148–159. doi: 10.1016/j.eplepsyres.2009.08.009

Rakic, P. (2002). Adult neurogenesis in mammals: an identity crisis. *J. Neurosci.* 22, 614–618.

Rubenstein, J. L. R. (2011). Annual research review: development of the cerebral cortex: implications for neurodevelopmental disorders. *J. Child Psychol. Psychiatry* 52, 339–355. doi: 10.1111/j.1469-7610.2010.02307.x

Sakamoto, M., Imayoshi, I., Ohtsuka, T., Yamaguchi, M., Mori, K., and Kageyama, R. (2011). Continuous neurogenesis in the adult forebrain is required for innate olfactory responses. *Proc. Natl. Acad. Sci. U.S.A.* 108, 8479–8484. doi: 10.1073/pnas.1018782108

Sanai, N., Nguyen, T., Ihrie, R. A., Mirzadeh, Z., Tsai, H.-H., Wong, M., et al. (2011). Corridors of migrating neurons in the human brain and their decline during infancy. *Nature* 478, 382–386. doi: 10.1038/nature10487

Sanai, N., Tramontin, A. D., Quinones-Hinojosa, A., Barbaro, N. M., Gupta, N., Kunwar, S., et al. (2004). Unique astrocyte ribbon in adult human brain contains neural stem cells but lacks chain migration. *Nature* 427, 740–744. doi: 10.1038/nature02301

Sawamoto, K., Wichterle, H., Gonzalez-Perez, O., Cholfin, J. A., Yamada, M., Spassky, N., et al. (2006). New neurons follow the flow of cerebrospinal fluid in the adult brain. *Science* 311, 629–632. doi: 10.1126/science.1119133

Scharff, C. (2000). Chasing fate and function of new neurons in adult brains. *Curr. Opin. Neurobiol.* 10, 774–783. doi: 10.1016/S0959-4388(00)00155-0

Scharff, C., Kirn, J. R., Grossman, M., Macklis, J. D., and Nottebohm, F. (2000). Targeted neuronal death affects neuronal replacement and vocal behavior in adult songbirds. *Neuron* 25, 481–492. doi: 10.1016/S0896-6273(00)80910-1

Seidenfaden, R., Desoeuvre, A., Bosio, A., Virard, I., and Cremer, H. (2006). Glial conversion of SVZ-derived committed neuronal precursors after ectopic grafting into the adult brain. *Mol. Cell Neurosci.* 32, 187–198. doi: 10.1016/j.mcn.2006.04.003

Shen, Q., Wang, Y., Dimos, J. T., Fasano, C. A., Phoenix, T. N., Lemischka, I. R., et al. (2006). The timing of cortical neurogenesis is encoded within lineages of individual progenitor cells. *Nat. Neurosci.* 9, 143–151. doi: 10.1038/nn1694

Shihabuddin, L. S., Horner, P. J., Ray, J., and Gage, F. H. (2000). Adult spinal cord stem cells generate neurons after transplantation in the adult dentate gyrus. *J. Neurosci.* 20, 8727–8735.

Southwell, D. G., Froemke, R. C., Alvarez-Buylla, A., Stryker, M. P., and Gandhi, S. P. (2010). Cortical plasticity induced by inhibitory neuron transplantation. *Science* 327, 1145–1148. doi: 10.1126/science.1183962

Spalding, K. L., Bergmann, O., Alkass, K., Bernard, S., Salehpour, M., Huttner, H. B., et al. (2013). Dynamics of hippocampal neurogenesis in adult humans. *Cell* 153, 1219–1227. doi: 10.1016/j.cell.2013.05.002

Suhonen, J. O., Peterson, D. A., Ray, J., and Gage, F. H. (1996). Differentiation of adult hippocampus-derived progenitors into olfactory neurons *in vivo*. *Nature* 383, 624–627. doi: 10.1038/383624a0

Tong, C. K., and Alvarez-Buylla, A. (2014). SnapShot: adult neurogenesis in the V-SVZ. *Neuron* 81, 220–220. doi: 10.1016/j.neuron.2013.12.004

Tsai, H.-H., Li, H., Fuentealba, L. C., Molofsky, A. V., Taveira-Marques, R., Zhuang, H., et al. (2012). Regional astrocyte allocation regulates CNS synaptogenesis and repair. *Science* 337, 358–362. doi: 10.1126/science.1222381

Whitman, M. C., Fan, W., Rela, L., Rodriguez-Gil, D. J., and Greer, C. A. (2009). Blood vessels form a migratory scaffold in the rostral migratory stream. *J. Comp. Neurol.* 516, 94–104. doi: 10.1002/cne.22093

Whitman, M. C., and Greer, C. A. (2009). Adult neurogenesis and the olfactory system. *Prog. Neurobiol.* 89, 162–175. doi: 10.1016/j.pneurobio.2009.07.003

Wichterle, H., Garcia-Verdugo, J. M., Herrera, D. G., and Alvarez-Buylla, A. (1999). Young neurons from medial ganglionic eminence disperse in adult and embryonic brain. *Nat. Neurosci.* 2, 461–466. doi: 10.1038/8131

Yamashita, T., Ninomiya, M., Hernández Acosta, P., Garcia-Verdugo, J. M., Sunabori, T., Sakaguchi, M., et al. (2006). Subventricular zone-derived neuroblasts migrate and differentiate into mature neurons in the post-stroke adult striatum. *J. Neurosci.* 26, 6627–6636. doi: 10.1523/JNEUROSCI.0149-06.2006

Yang, Z., Ming, G.-L., and Song, H. (2011). Postnatal neurogenesis in the human forebrain: from two migratory streams to dribbles. *Cell Stem Cell* 9, 385–386. doi: 10.1016/j.stem.2011.10.007

11

Oxotremorine treatment reduces repetitive behaviors in BTBR T+ tf/J mice

Dionisio A. Amodeo[1], Julia Yi[1], John A. Sweeney[2] and Michael E. Ragozzino[1]*

[1] Laboratory of Integrative Neuroscience, Department of Psychology, University of Illinois at Chicago, Chicago, IL, USA
[2] Department of Psychiatry, University of Texas Southwestern Medical Center, Dallas, TX, USA

Edited by:
Sukumar Vijayaraghavan, University of Colorado Health Science Center, USA

Reviewed by:
Susan Powell, University of California at San Diego (UCSD), USA
Mark H. Lewis, University of Florida, USA

***Correspondence:**
Michael E. Ragozzino, Laboratory of Integrative Neuroscience, Department of Psychology, University of Illinois at Chicago, 1007 West Harrison Street, Chicago, IL 60607-7137, USA
e-mail: mrago@uic.edu

Repetitive behaviors with restricted interests is one of the core criteria for the diagnosis of autism spectrum disorder (ASD). Current pharmacotherapies that target the dopaminergic or serotonergic systems have limited effectiveness in treating repetitive behaviors. Previous research has demonstrated that administration of muscarinic cholinergic receptor (mAChR) antagonists can exacerbate motor stereotypies while mAChR agonists reduce stereotypies. The present study determined whether the mAChR agonist, oxotremorine affected repetitive behaviors in the BTBR T+ tf/J (BTBR) mouse model of autism. To test the effects of oxotremorine on repetitive behaviors, marble burying and grooming behavior were measured in BTBR mice and compared to that in C57BL/6J (B6) mice. The effects of oxotremorine on locomotor activity was also measured. Thirty minutes before each test, mice received an intraperitoneal (ip) injection of saline, 0.001 mg or 0.01 mg of oxotremorine methiodide. Saline- treated BTBR mice exhibited increased marble burying and self-grooming behavior compared to that of saline-treated B6 mice. Oxotremorine significantly reduced marble burying and self-grooming behavior in BTBR mice, but had no significant effect in B6 mice. In addition, oxotremorine did not affect locomotor activity in BTBR mice, but significantly reduced locomotor activity in B6 mice at the 0.01 mg dose. These findings demonstrate that activation of mAChRs reduces repetitive behavior in the BTBR mouse and suggest that treatment with a mAChR agonist may be effective in reducing repetitive behaviors in ASD.

Keywords: acetylcholine, muscarinic receptors, autism, repetitive behaviors, marble burying, grooming

INTRODUCTION

Autism spectrum disorders (ASDs) represent a cluster of neurodevelopmental disorders characterized by social and communicative impairments, as well restricted interests and repetitive behaviors (RRBs). RRBs are subdivided into lower-order and high-order behaviors (Lam and Aman, 2007). Lower order RRBs involve repetitive manipulation of objects, stereotyped movements or repetitive self-injurious behavior (Lam and Aman, 2007). Higher order RRBs are characterized by an insistence on sameness, or rigid adherence to a rule or routine (Turner, 1999; Szatmari et al., 2006). RRBs are reported to be the most distressing aspect of ASD for patients and families that profoundly impact daily living (Bishop et al., 2007).

Current treatments for RRBs have limited effectiveness (Boyd et al., 2012). Most pharmacotherapies in ASD focus on treating symptoms by principally modifying dopaminergic and serotonergic signaling (McPheeters et al., 2011). Atypical antipsychotics have food and drug administration (FDA) indications for treating irritability but not the core features of ASD (McPheeters et al., 2011). Selective serotonin reuptake inhibitor (SSRI) medications, used to reduce restricted interest symptoms, have resulted in mixed improvements with irritability observed in some individuals (Hollander et al., 2005; Owley et al., 2005, 2010; Henry et al., 2006; King et al., 2009). An alternative possibility is to treat RRBs by targeting the cholinergic system. Accumulating evidence suggests that brain cholinergic abnormalities could explain some of the pathophysiology in ASD. Post-mortem studies indicate that there is altered expression of muscarinic and nicotinic cholinergic receptors (Perry et al., 2001; Deutsch et al., 2010). Recent gene networks that confer risk for ASD include genes related to cholinergic transmission and these are also highly expressed in the brain (Voineagu et al., 2011; Ben-David and Shifman, 2012; Lee et al., 2012). Moreover, anti-psychotic treatments which have significant muscarinic receptor antagonism, e.g., quetiapine, can exacerbate symptoms in ASD (Martin et al., 1999; Hardan et al., 2005). Thus, treatments that increase muscarinic cholinergic receptor (mAChR) transmission may reduce core symptoms in ASD.

Animal models are often an important initial step in evaluating new treatment approaches. The BTBR T+ tf/J (BTBR) mouse is one preclinical model employed to better understand ASD because the mouse exhibits a phenotype that is comparable to the core symptoms in ASD (see Meyza et al., 2013 for review). Compared to B6 mice, BTBR mice exhibit deficits in social interactions and communication (McFarlane et al., 2008; Scattoni et al., 2008, 2011; Pobbe et al., 2010; Silverman et al., 2010;

Chadman, 2011); restricted interests and behavioral inflexibility (Moy et al., 2008; Pearson et al., 2011; Amodeo et al., 2012; Karvat and Kimchi, 2012; Guariglia and Chadman, 2013); as well as repetitive or stereotyped behaviors, e.g., increased self-grooming and marble burying (McFarlane et al., 2008; Silverman et al., 2010; Amodeo et al., 2012; Babineau et al., 2013; McTighe et al., 2013; Reynolds et al., 2013). Grooming and digging can be viewed as part of the common behavioral repertoire exhibited by rodents (Garner and Mason, 2002). Studying these behaviors in BTBR mice is of particular interest related to ASD because of the excessive quantity in which these behaviors are expressed (Yang et al., 2007, 2009; McFarlane et al., 2008; Pobbe et al., 2010; Pearson et al., 2011; Amodeo et al., 2012), as well as being exhibited in various contexts and with repeated testing (Yang et al., 2007, 2009; McFarlane et al., 2008; Pobbe et al., 2010). For example, Yang et al. (2007) found that BTBR mice showed higher levels of repetitive grooming than B6 mice when raised with either a biological BTBR mother, a foster BTBR mother, or a low grooming B6 mother, demonstrating that excessive self-grooming in BTBR mice is not attenuated by an environmental influence such as caregiver.

In addition, recent findings indicate that BTBR mice exhibit decreased brain acetylcholine levels (McTighe et al., 2013) and infusion of an acetylcholinestase inhibitor into the dorsomedial striatum can alleviate a reversal learning deficit in BTBR mice (Karvat and Kimchi, 2014). However, unknown is whether cholinergic treatments may also be effective in reducing repetitive motor behaviors in BTBR mice. A past study reported that treatment with a mAChR agonist can reduce stereotyped behaviors in rodents (Wang and McGinty, 1997). Moreover, post-mortem studies report reduced mAChR signaling in various brain regions of ASD patients (Deutsch et al., 2010). Thus, treatment with a mAChR agonist may be effective in reducing repetitive behaviors in ASD.

To determine whether treatment with a mAChR agonist reduces repetitive behaviors, the present experiments examined whether the mAChR agonist, oxotremorine methoidine alleviates elevated self-grooming and marble burying in BTBR mice compared to that in B6 mice. To understand whether oxotremorine treatment has a more general effect on motor behavior, the effect of oxotremorine on horizontal locomotor activity was also measured in BTBR and B6 mice.

MATERIALS AND METHODS

ANIMALS

Male C57BL/6J and BTBR mice, 7–8 weeks old, were obtained from the Jackson Laboratory (Bar Harbor, ME). Mice were singly housed in plastic cages (28 cm wide × 17 cm long × 12 cm high) in humidity (30%) and temperature (22°C) controlled room with a 12-h light/dark cycle (lights on at 07:00 am). Ten to fourteen days after arrival behavioral testing procedures began. Animal care and use was in accordance with the National Institutes of Health Guide for the Care and Use of Laboratory Animals, and was approved by the Institutional Laboratory Animal Care and Use Committee at the University of Illinois at Chicago.

DRUGS

Oxotremorine methoidine (Tocris, Ellisville, MO) 0.001 and 0.01 mg/kg was dissolved in 0.9% physiological saline. Mice received an intraperitoneal (ip) injection at 10 ml/kg volume.

SPONTANEOUS SELF-GROOMING

The procedure used to measure spontaneous self-grooming behavior was modified from McFarlane et al. (2008). Mice were individually placed in a clear plastic cage (28 cm wide × 17 cm long × 12 cm high) for a total of 20 min. Twenty minutes before being placed in the plastic cage mice received an ip injection of either vehicle, 0.001 or 0.01 mg/kg of oxotremorine. The treatment groups included the following: B6-vehicle (n = 8), B6-0.001oxotremorine (n = 8), B6-0.01oxotremorine (n = 8), BTBR-vehicle (n = 9), BTBR-0.001oxotremorine (n = 9), BTBR-0.01oxotremorine (n = 9). These doses were chosen based on past studies measuring the effects of oxotremorine on activity in rodents (Yano et al., 2009; Koda et al., 2011). The plastic cage was placed in a room separate from the mouse housing room. Subjects were allowed to freely explore the cage for the entirety of the test. The first 10 min served as a habituation period. Therefore mice received injections 30 min prior to measurement of grooming behavior. During the second 10 min of testing a trained observer sat approximately 1.6 m from the test cage and recorded cumulative time spent grooming all body regions in real time with a stopwatch. Grooming behavior included head washing, body grooming, genital/tail grooming and paw and leg licking. Experimenters were blind to treatment but were not blind to strain because BTBR mice are dark brown with a cream colored ventral patch while B6 do not have this patch. After each mouse was tested, the cage was thoroughly cleaned with a 2% ammonium chloride solution.

MARBLE BURYING

Subjects tested for grooming behavior were also tested for marble burying. The marble burying test occurred 8 days following the grooming test to ensure there were no potential residual effects from the initial drug treatment (Birdsall et al., 1978). Subjects received a different treatment before marble burying from that administered during the spontaneous self-grooming experiment, with the exception of three B6 mice. One B6 received vehicle in both tests and two B6 mice received oxotremorine 0.01 mg in both tests. For all other mice, approximately half from each treatment group in the self-grooming test were assigned to one of the other two treatment groups. For example, for mice receiving 0.001 mg oxotremorine in the self-grooming test, approximately half were assigned to the vehicle group and half assigned to the 0.01 mg oxotremorine group. With this experimental design, half of the mice in the oxotremorine treatment groups (low or high dose) were receiving the drug for the first time. Seven days after the grooming test, mice were habituated to the plastic container used for the marble burying test. The same marble burying test procedure was used as in Amodeo et al. (2012). Mice were individually placed in a plastic container (46 cm long by 24 cm wide by 21 cm deep) with 3 cm of clean woodchip bedding (Northeastern Products, NY). The plastic container was placed in a room used for behavioral testing. Mice were allowed to freely explore a container for 30 min undisturbed. This served to habituate mice to the chamber. Twenty-four hours later, 20 glass marbles (1.5 cm in diameter) were arranged in five rows of four. The marbles were placed on top of 3 cm of clean woodchip bedding. A template was used to ensure that there was a consistent positioning of marbles. Thirty minutes before being placed into the test container, mice received an injection of either vehicle, 0.001, or 0.01 mg of oxotremorine in 0.9% physiological saline. The treatment groups included the following: B6-vehicle (n = 8), B6-0.001oxo (n = 8), B6-0.01oxo (n = 8), BTBR-vehicle (n = 9), BTBR-0.001oxo (n = 9), BTBR-0.01oxo (n = 9). As in the grooming test, experimenters were blind to treatment but were not blind to strain. Once a mouse was placed into the test container a wire lid was placed on top. Mice were allowed to explore the container and marbles for 30 min. After 30 min, each mouse was removed from the testing container and returned to their home cage. Marbles were considered buried if ≥2/3 of the surface area was covered in woodchip bedding. The total number of buried marbles was recorded. Between testing, marbles were thoroughly cleaned and new bedding was used for each mouse.

LOCOMOTOR ACTIVITY

A separate group of naïve mice were used to measure locomotor activity. Testing of locomotor activity was conducted in a black acrylic rectangular-shaped chamber (76 cm long × 50 cm wide × 30 cm high). Mice were injected with vehicle, 0.001 or 0.01 mg of oxotremorine 30 min before being placed in the test chamber. Before mice were introduced to the testing chamber, the entire apparatus was cleaned with 2% ammonium chloride solution. Treatment groups included the following: B6-vehicle (n = 8), B6-0.001oxo (n = 8), B6-0.01oxo (n = 8), BTBR-vehicle (n = 8), BTBR-0.001oxo (n = 8), BTBR-0.01oxo (n = 8). The bottom of the chamber was divided into nine (25 × 16.5 cm) equally sized rectangles. After a mouse was placed into the chamber the experimenter exited the testing room for 20 min. Once the session ended mice were removed from the test chamber and returned to the vivarium. Locomotor activity was recorded via camcorder (Sony Handycam, model DCR-DVD650) stationed above the chamber. Once the testing session was complete, locomotor activity was measured by an observer blind to treatment conditions. The number of lines crossed was calculated. A line cross was defined as a mouse having all four paws cross a line. The number of lines crossed was calculated in two separate 10-min blocks.

STATISTICAL ANALYSIS

Separate two-way analysis of variance ANOVAs (*strain*: B6, BTBR × *treatment*: vehicle, 0.001, 0.01 mg/kg oxotremorine) were conducted for self-grooming and marble burying. A significant interaction was followed by Tukey HSD *post hoc* tests to determine significant treatment differences in both strains. A three-way ANOVA with repeated measures (*strain* × *treatment* × *block*) was conducted for locomotor activity. A significant interaction was followed by Tukey HSD *post hoc* tests.

RESULTS

SPONTANEOUS SELF-GROOMING

Figure 1 illustrates the findings for spontaneous self-grooming in BTBR and B6 mice. Vehicle-treated BTBR mice spent approximately 180 s grooming compared to 20 s in B6 mice. Oxotremorine decreased self-grooming behavior in BTBR mice with the largest effect at the 0.01 mg dose which reduced the time self-grooming to half that observed in vehicle-treated BTBR mice. In contrast, oxotremorine treatment tended to increase self-grooming behavior in B6 mice. The main effect of strain was significant ($F_{(1,45)} = 48.26, p < 0.01$), but there was no significant treatment effect ($F_{(2,45)} = 1.78, p > 0.05$). However there was a significant strain × treatment interaction ($F_{(2,45)} = 6.99, p < 0.01$). *Post hoc* tests indicated that in the vehicle-treated groups,

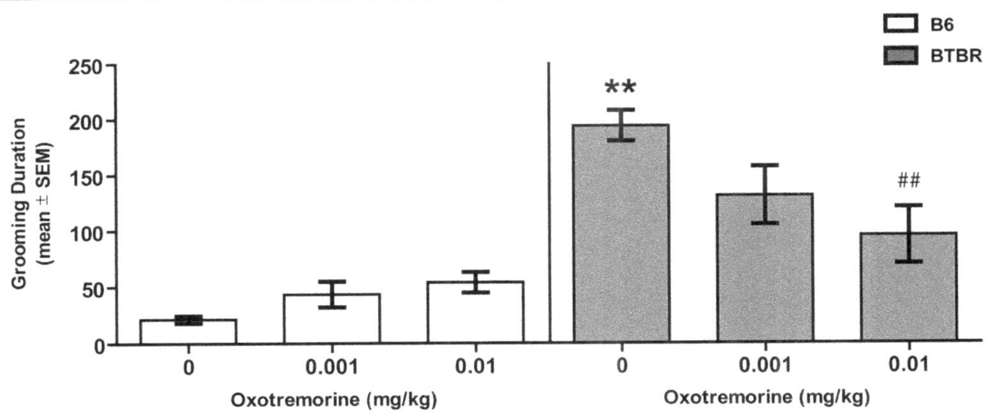

FIGURE 1 | Oxotremorine treatment attenuates spontaneous self-grooming behavior in BTBR mice. Mean (±SEM) time spent grooming all body regions. Self-grooming behavior was measured in BTBR and B6 mice. Each mouse received an i.p. injection of vehicle, 0.001 or 0.01 mg of oxotremorine 30 min before grooming behavior was measured. BTBR mice spent significantly more time grooming compared to that of B6 mice. Vehicle or oxotremorine treatment did not affect spontaneous grooming behavior in B6 mice. Oxotremorine at 0.01 mg significantly decreased spontaneous grooming in BTBR mice. B6: vehicle (n = 8), 0.001 (n = 8), 0.01 (n = 8), BTBR: vehicle (n = 9), 0.001 oxo (n = 9), 0.01 oxo (n = 9). ** $p < 0.01$ vs. B6-vehicle, ## $p < 0.01$ vs. BTBR-vehicle.

BTBR mice spent significantly more time self-grooming than that of B6 mice ($p < 0.01$). Oxotremorine 0.001 treatment in BTBR mice reduced self-grooming time, but the difference was not significantly different from that of vehicle-treated BTBR mice ($p > 0.05$). In contrast, oxotremorine 0.01 treatment significantly reduced self-grooming time compared to that of vehicle treatment in BTBR mice ($p < 0.01$). In B6 mice, oxotremorine treatment tended to increase in self-grooming time, but self-grooming time for both doses compared to that of vehicle treatment was not significant (p's > 0.05). Thus, oxotremorine treatment reduced self-grooming behavior in BTBR mice in a dose-dependent fashion.

MARBLE BURYING

The effects of oxotremorine treatment on marble burying behavior in BTBR and B6 mice are shown in **Figure 2**. Vehicle-treated BTBR buried approximately 10 marbles compared to 3 in B6 mice. Oxotremorine dose-dependently decreased marbles buried in BTBR mice. The oxotremorine 0.001 mg dose reduced marbles buried to approximately seven. The higher dose of oxotremorine reduce marble burying to approximately three. There was a significant main effect for strain ($F_{(1,42)} = 35.87$, $p < 0.01$) and treatment ($F_{(2,42)} = 13.12$, $p < 0.01$). Similarly, there was a significant strain × treatment interaction, ($F_{(2,42)} = 3.92$, $p < 0.05$). *Post hoc* tests indicated that in the vehicle-treated groups, BTBR mice buried significantly more marbles than that of B6 mice ($p < 0.01$). In BTBR mice, oxotremorine 0.001 mg treatment reduced marble burying, but the difference was not significantly different from that of vehicle treatment ($p > 0.05$). In contrast, oxotremorine 0.01 mg treatment significantly reduced marble burying compared to that of vehicle treatment in BTBR mice ($p < 0.01$). In B6 mice, there was a trend for oxotremorine treatment to reduce marble burying, although neither dose compared to that of vehicle treatment was significant (p's > 0.05). Thus, oxotremorine treatment reduced marble burying in BTBR mice in a dose-dependent manner.

One possibility is that the prior treatment received in the self-grooming test interacted with the treatment received in the marble burying test to affect performance. As each treatment group in marble burying included mice that received a mixture of treatments this could be examined within each treatment group. In both the low-dose and high-dose oxotremorine group, BTBR mice that previously received vehicle treatment compared to mice that previously received the drug exhibited comparable marble burying performance. Specifically, in the oxotremorine 0.001 mg group, mice that previously received vehicle had a mean marble burying score of 6.75 ± 2.7 SEM while mice that previously received the drug had a mean score of 7.75 ± 1.3. In the oxotremorine 0.01 mg group, previous vehicle treatment led to a mean score of 3.0 ± 1.5 while previous drug treatment led to a mean score of 2.5 ± 0.9. In the vehicle-treated group, mice that previously received the low dose of oxotremorine had a mean score of 11.0 ± 1.3 while mice that previously received the high dose of oxotremorine had a mean score of 10.75 ± 0.6. Thus, previous treatment in the self-grooming test did not affect performance in the vehicle-treated group or drug groups during the marble burying test.

A similar pattern was observed for B6 mice. In the oxotremorine 0.001 mg group, mice that previously received vehicle had a mean marble burying score of 2.33 ± 0.58 SEM while mice that previously received the drug had a mean score of 2.25 ± 1.44. In the oxotremorine 0.01 mg group, previous vehicle treatment led to a mean score of 1.0 ± 0.41 while previous drug treatment led to a mean score of 1.33 ± 1.15. In the vehicle-treated group, mice that previously received the low dose of oxotremorine had a mean score of 3.25 ± 0.53 while mice that previously received the high dose of oxotremorine had a mean score of 3.67 ± 0.38.

LOCOMOTOR ACTIVITY

Figures 3A,B illustrates the findings for locomotor activity in B6 and BTBR mice, respectively. The locomotor activity was analyzed

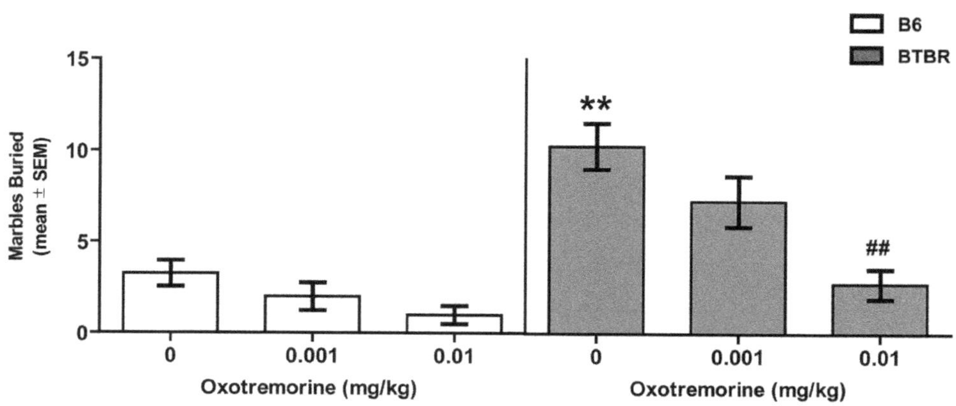

FIGURE 2 | Oxotremorine treatment attenuates marble burying in BTBR mice. Mean (±SEM) marbles buried. Marble burying was measured in BTBR and B6 mice. Each mouse received an i.p. injection of vehicle, 0.001 or 0.01 mg of oxotremorine 30 min prior to marble exposure. BTBR mice buried significantly more marbles compared to that of B6 mice. Vehicle or oxotremorine treatment did not significantly affect marble burying in B6 mice. Oxotremorine at 0.01 mg significantly decreased marble burying in BTBR mice. B6: vehicle ($n = 9$), 0.001 oxo ($n = 8$), 0.01 oxo ($n = 8$), BTBR: vehicle ($n = 9$), 0.001 oxo ($n = 9$), 0.01 oxo ($n = 9$). ** $p < 0.01$ vs. B6-vehicle, ## $p < 0.01$ vs. BTBR vehicle.

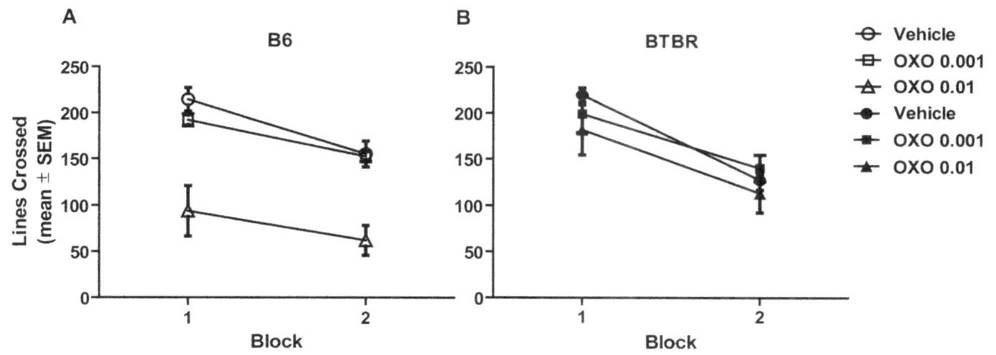

FIGURE 3 | Oxotremorine treatment did not affect locomotor activity in BTBR mice across two consecutive 10-min blocks. Mean (±SEM) lines crossed. Locomotor activity was measured in B6 and BTBR mice. Each mouse received an i.p. injection of vehicle, 0.001 or 0.01 mg of oxotremorine 30 min before locomotor activity was measured. **(A)** Locomotor activity in B6 mice. Activity decreased in the second 10-min block compared to the first. Oxotremorine 0.01 mg significantly reduced locomotor activity compared to that of other treatment groups. B6: vehicle (n = 8), 0.001 oxo (n = 8), 0.01 oxo (n = 8). **(B)** Locomotor activity in BTBR mice. Activity decreased in the second 10-min block compared to the first. Oxotremorine treatment did not affect activity compared to that of vehicle treatment. BTBR: vehicle (n = 8), 0.001 oxo (n = 8), 0.01 oxo (n = 8).

across two 10 min blocks. All groups exhibited similar locomotor activity, with the exception of oxotremorine 0.01 mg in B6 mice. There was a significant effect of treatment ($F_{(2,42)} = 18.82$, $p < 0.001$), but there was no significant strain effect ($F_{(1,42)} = 2.65$, $p > 0.05$). However, the strain × treatment interaction was significant ($F_{(2,42)} = 8.31$, $p < 0.01$). *Post hoc* analysis revealed that in B6 mice, the oxotremorine 0.01 mg treatment significantly lowered activity compared to that of all other treatment groups (p's < 0.05). The analysis further revealed that there was a significant effect for block ($F_{(1,40)} = 110.01$, $p < 0.001$), reflecting that mice decreased their activity in the second block compared to the first block. There was also a significant block × strain interaction ($F_{(1,40)} = 5.88$, $p < 0.05$). *Post hoc* tests revealed that block 2 activity in B6 mice was significantly reduced compared to block 1 activity in B6 and BTBR mice (p's < 0.05). In addition, block 2 activity was significantly reduced compared to block 1 activity in BTBR mice ($p < 0.05$). No other interactions were significant.

DISCUSSION

Individuals with ASD exhibit repetitive, stereotyped behaviors and cognitive inflexibility that can severely limit daily living (Bishop et al., 2007; Lam and Aman, 2007; D'Cruz et al., 2013). Comparable to that observed in ASD, BTBR mice exhibited increased repetitive behaviors compared to that of B6 mice. The increased repetitive behaviors in BTBR mice included both elevated self-grooming and marble burying as observed in past studies (Yang et al., 2007; Silverman et al., 2010; Gould et al., 2011; Pearson et al., 2011; Amodeo et al., 2012). Because past studies in rats indicated that mAChR antagonists increase stereotyped behavior while mAChR agonists reduce stereotyped behavior (Wang and McGinty, 1997; Laviolette et al., 2000; Aliane et al., 2011), these studies investigated whether treatment with the non-specific, mAChR agonist, oxotremorine reduced repetitive behaviors in BTBR mice. Acute oxotremorine treatment, dose-dependently, attenuated the elevated self-grooming and marble-burying behavior in BTBR mice. These findings suggest that activation of mAChR can attenuate certain repetitive behaviors.

A past study examined the self-grooming microstructure in BTBR mice (Pearson et al., 2011). This analysis showed that BTBR mice exhibit an increase in almost all grooming subtypes with the exception of paw licking. Examination of the self-grooming microstructure also revealed that BTBR mice display a decrease in the percentage of incorrect transitions across the different grooming subtypes. Mice commonly groom in a cephalocaudal fashion starting with head washing and concluding with tail/genital licking. The present study did not examine the self-grooming microstructure or the grooming sequence. Thus, unknown is whether oxotremorine preferentially affected grooming subtypes or broadly decreased grooming subtypes. Further, unclear from the present study is whether oxotremorine altered the grooming sequence in BTBR mice in any way. Future studies investigating the effects of mAChR treatment on repetitive behaviors can address how mAChR agonists may alter self-grooming subtypes and self-grooming sequence. However, the present results indicate that oxotremorine treatment decreases self-grooming duration in BTBR mice without the highest dose of oxotremorine having an effect on locomotor activity. Taken together, the results suggest that mAChR agonist treatment may be effective in reducing lower-order repetitive behaviors in ASD.

In contrast to BTBR mice, B6 mice exhibited minimal grooming behavior as reported previously (Yang et al., 2007; McFarlane et al., 2008; Silverman et al., 2010; Pearson et al., 2011; Amodeo et al., 2012). Oxotremorine treatment actually showed a trend toward increasing grooming behavior in B6 mice. This increase in grooming behavior may explain why an oxotremorine injection in B6 mice tended to decrease marble burying and locomotor activity. The opposite effects of oxotremorine on grooming behavior in BTBR and B6 mice may suggest that there is an inverted U-shaped curve for mAChR activation to minimize grooming behavior. In particular, B6 mice may typically exhibit the "optimal level" of mAChR activity, but when treated with a mAChR agonist, i.e., oxotremorine, this increases mAChR activation above the optimal levels leading to increased grooming. Conversely, BTBR mice may have lower levels of mAChR activation leading to increased grooming, but treatment with oxotremorine brings mAChR activity into the optimal range that then decreases grooming behavior. Therefore, either too little or too great mAChR activation may lead to increased grooming behavior.

Comparable to that observed with self-grooming, oxotremorine 0.01 mg significantly reduced marble burying in BTBR mice. In B6 mice, there was a trend for oxotremorine 0.01 mg to reduce marble burying. Relative to BTBR mice, B6 mice display low levels of marble burying. The lower level of marble burying in B6 mice is consistent with previous studies (Amodeo et al., 2012; Schwartzer et al., 2013). However, because B6 mice exhibit a low level of marble burying this may obscure a drug effect in reducing marble burying. Another potential issue in interpreting the marble burying results is that mice were tested on marble burying following a self-grooming test. One possibility is that a previous treatment in the self-grooming test affected marble burying behavior. However, examination of the previous treatment received indicated that this did not influence marble burying behavior. This was the case for both BTBR mice and B6 mice. Also worth noting is that the number of marbles buried by vehicle-treated BTBR mice was comparable to that buried by drug-naïve BTBR mice in previous studies (Gould et al., 2011, 2012; Amodeo et al., 2012; Schwartzer et al., 2013). Thus, despite vehicle-treated BTBR mice in the marble burying test receiving either the low or high dose of oxotremorine in the self-grooming test, this did not alter their marble burying behavior compared to past observations in BTBR mice. Again, because oxotremorine treatment had no effect on locomotor activity in BTBR mice, the drug-induced reduction in marble burying behavior can not be explained by a more general reduction in activity. Instead, the results suggest that activation of mAChRs selectively modulated repetitive behaviors in BTBR mice.

The current findings complements a recent study that demonstrated treatment with the acetylcholinesterase inhibitor, donepezil, can improve behavioral rigidity as measured by reversal learning in BTBR mice (Karvat and Kimchi, 2014). Because acetylcholinesterase inhibitors leads to a non-specific increase in acetylcholine levels unknown is whether specific cholinergic receptors mediate these behavioral effects. The current experiments investigating the effects of oxotremorine demonstrate that activation of mAChRs is sufficient to attenuate repetitive behaviors in BTBR mice. Although stimulation of mAChRs was able to attenuate repetitive behaviors, this does not rule out that nicotinic cholinergic receptors may also play a role in affecting repetitive behaviors. Nicotine treatment in rats has shown to reduce certain stereotyped or repetitive behaviors (Zarrindast et al., 1999; Tizabi et al., 2002). Moreover, oxotremorine is a non-specific mAChR agonist, therefore still to be determined is whether specific mAChR subtypes may be sufficient to alleviate repetitive behaviors.

Previous studies investigated the effects of a M1 mAChR agonist on drug-induced or spontaneous grooming behavior in rodents (Bhattacharya and Sen, 1991; Inan et al., 2011). In both studies, McN-A-343 significantly reduced grooming behavior. Unclear is whether other muscarinic receptor subtypes may also be sufficient to reduce repetitive behaviors. There is evidence that targeting M5 mAChR can affect locomotion (Wang et al., 2004; Steidl and Yeomans, 2009), but unknown is whether this is restricted to general ambulation or also to motor stereotyped behavior. Repetitive behaviors in ASD have been separated into lower-order and higher-order repetitive behaviors (Bodfish et al., 2000; Lam and Aman, 2007). Lower order repetitive behaviors can include stereotyped movements or repetitive self-injurious behavior. Higher order RRBs instead are characterized by an "insistence on sameness" or rigid adherence to a rule or routine (Lam and Aman, 2007; Boyd et al., 2012). The findings with McN-343 suggest that treatment with a M1 mAChR agonist may be effective in treating lower-order repetitive behaviors in ASD. However, a recent study reported that the partial M1 mAChR agonist, CDD-102A, enhances set-shifting in rats (Ragozzino et al., 2012). Thus, treatment with a M1 mAChR agonist may be effective in treating both lower-order and higher-order repetitive behaviors.

The present studies indicated that a systemic injection of oxotremorine reduced repetitive behaviors in BTBR mice. The dorsomedial striatum may be a key anatomical site in which oxotremorine acts to affect repetitive behaviors. This is because drug treatments that increase stereotyped behaviors decrease acetylcholine output from this region (Aliane et al., 2011). Furthermore, destruction of cholinergic interneurons or injection of a mAChR antagonist in the dorsomedial striatum leads to increased repetitive behaviors that is alleviated by drug treatments that increase dorsomedial striatal acetylcholine output (Aliane et al., 2011). Cholinergic signaling in the dorsomedial striatum may not only be important for minimizing repetitive motor behaviors, but also for enabling cognitive flexibility. Karvat and Kimchi (2014) showed that donepezil injections into the dorsomedial striatum also improved reversal learning in BTBR mice. This effect of donepezil is consistent with past results showing that enhancing acetylcholine efflux in the rat dorsomedial striatum improves reversal learning while blocking acetylcholine efflux in this region impairs reversal learning (Palencia and Ragozzino, 2006; Ragozzino et al., 2009). Moreover, recent findings suggest that activation of M1 mAChRs in the dorsomedial striatum may mediate acetylcholine effects on cognitive flexibility (Tzavos et al., 2004; McCool et al., 2008; Ragozzino et al., 2012). Thus, treatment with a mAChR agonist may be effective in alleviating stereotyped motor behaviors and cognitive flexibility deficits.

To date, there exists some evidence, but not extensive findings, suggesting altered brain cholinergic transmission in ASD. In particular, there are results from gene networks that confer risk of ASD that include genes related to cholinergic transmission (Voineagu et al., 2011; Ben-David and Shifman, 2012; Lee et al., 2012) and post-mortem studies indicating reduced brain mAChR expression in ASD individuals (Deutsch et al., 2010). However, there is not a definitive understanding of whether pathophysiology of the brain cholinergic system exists in ASD. Related, unknown is whether there are specific brain cholinergic systems that are altered in the disorder and/or if a brain acetylcholine pathophysiology exists and how it may relate to particular symptoms in ASD. Addressing these issues can further our understanding of the etiology of ASD and help develop new effective therapeutics. The employment of animal models can help address these issues. The present findings in the BTBR mouse, a model of idiopathic autism, reveal that the non-specific mAChR agonist, oxotremorine attenuates repetitive motor behaviors without affecting general ambulation. Thus, treatment with a mAChR agonist may be effective in reducing repetitive behaviors in ASD.

ACKNOWLEDGMENTS

This research was supported by NIH grant P50 HD055751. John A. Sweeney has served as a consultant for Takeda Pharmaceutical Company, Bristol-Myers Squibb and Roche Pharmaceuticals for the past two years.

REFERENCES

Aliane, V., Pérez, S., Bohren, Y., Deniau, J. M., and Kemel, M. L. (2011). Key role of striatal cholinergic interneurons in processes leading to arrest of motor stereotypies. *Brain* 134, 110–118. doi: 10.1093/brain/awq285

Amodeo, D. A., Jones, J. H., Sweeney, J. A., and Ragozzino, M. E. (2012). Differences in BTBR T+ tf/J and C57BL/6J mice on probabilistic reversal learning and stereotyped behaviors. *Behav. Brain Res.* 227, 64–72. doi: 10.1016/j.bbr.2011.10.032

Babineau, B. A., Yang, M., Berman, R. F., and Crawley, J. N. (2013). Low home cage social behaviors in BTBR T+ tf/J mice during juvenile development. *Physiol. Behav.* 114, 49–54. doi: 10.1016/j.physbeh.2013.03.006

Ben-David, E., and Shifman, S. (2012). Networks of neuronal genes affected by common and rare variants in autism spectrum disorders. *PLoS Genet.* 8:e1002556. doi: 10.1371/journal.pgen.1002556

Bhattacharya, S. K., and Sen, A. P. (1991). Effects of muscarinic receptor agonists and antagonists on dopamine-mediated behavioural paradigms. *J. Neural Transm. Gen. Sect.* 84, 241–246. doi: 10.1007/bf01244975

Birdsall, N. J., Burgen, A. S., and Hulme, E. C. (1978). The binding of agonists to brain muscarinic receptors. *Mol. Pharmacol.* 14, 723–736.

Bishop, S. L., Richler, J., Cain, A. C., and Lord, C. (2007). Predictors of perceived negative impact in mothers of children with autism spectrum disorder. *Am. J. Ment. Retard.* 112, 450–461. doi: 10.1352/0895-8017(2007)112[450:popnii]2.0.co;2

Bodfish, J. W., Symons, F. J., Parker, D. E., and Lewis, M. H. (2000). Varieties of repetitive behavior in autism: comparisons to mental retardation. *J. Autism Dev. Disord.* 30, 237–243. doi: 10.1023/A:1005596502855

Boyd, B. A., McDonough, S. G., and Bodfish, J. W. (2012). Evidence-based behavioral interventions for repetitive behaviors in autism. *J. Autism Dev. Disord.* 42, 1236–1248. doi: 10.1007/s10803-011-1284-z

Chadman, K. K. (2011). Fluoxetine but not risperidone increases sociability in the BTBR mouse model of autism. *Pharmacol. Biochem. Behav.* 97, 586–594. doi: 10.1016/j.pbb.2010.09.012

D'Cruz, A. M., Ragozzino, M. E., Mosconi, M. W., Shrestha, S., Cook, E. H., and Sweeney, J. A. (2013). Reduced behavioral flexibility in autism spectrum disorders. *Neuropsychology* 27, 152–160. doi: 10.1037/a0031721

Deutsch, S. I., Urbano, M. R., Neumann, S. A., Burket, J. A., and Katz, E. (2010). Cholinergic abnormalities in autism: is there a rationale for selective nicotinic agonist interventions? *Clin. Neuropharmacol.* 33, 114–120. doi: 10.1097/wnf.0b013e3181d6f7ad

Garner, J. P., and Mason, G. J. (2002). Evidence for a relationship between cage stereotypies and behavioural disinhibition in laboratory rodents. *Behav. Brain Res.* 136, 83–92. doi: 10.1016/s0166-4328(02)00111-0

Gould, G. G., Hensler, J. G., Burke, T. F., Benno, R. H., Onaivi, E. S., and Daws, L. C. (2011). Density and function of central serotonin (5-HT) transporters, 5-HT1A and 5-HT2A receptors and effects of their targeting on, BTBR T+tf/J mouse social behavior. *J. Neurochem.* 116, 291–303. doi: 10.1111/j.1471-4159.2010.07104.x

Gould, G. G., Seillier, A., Weiss, G., Giuffrida, A., Burke, T. F., Hensler, J. G., et al. (2012). Acetaminophen differentially enhances social behavior and cortical cannabinoid levels in inbred mice. *Prog. Neuropsychopharmacol. Biol. Psychiatry* 38, 260–269. doi: 10.1016/j.pnpbp.2012.04.011

Guariglia, S. R., and Chadman, K. K. (2013). Water T-maze: a useful assay for determination of repetitive behaviors in mice. *J. Neurosci. Methods* 220, 24–29. doi: 10.1016/j.jneumeth.2013.08.019

Hardan, A. Y., Jou, R. J., and Handen, B. L. (2005). Retrospective study of quetiapine in children and adolescents with pervasive developmental disorders. *J. Autism Dev. Disord.* 35, 387–391. doi: 10.1007/s10803-005-3306-1

Henry, C. A., Steingard, R., Venter, J., Guptill, J., Halpern, E. F., and Bauman, M. (2006). Treatment outcome and outcome associations in children with pervasive developmental disorders treated with selective serotonin reuptake inhibitors: a chart review. *J. Child Adolesc. Psychopharmacol.* 16, 187–195. doi: 10.1089/cap.2006.16.187

Hollander, E., Phillips, A., Chaplin, W., Zagursky, K., Novotny, S., Wasserman, S., et al. (2005). A placebo controlled crossover trial of liquid fluoxetine on repetitive behaviors in childhood and adolescent autism. *Neuropsychopharmacology* 30, 582–589. doi: 10.1038/sj.npp.1300627

Inan, S., Dun, N. J., and Cowan, A. (2011). Investigation of gastrin-releasing peptide as a mediator for 5′-guanidinonaltrindole-induced compulsive scratching in mice. *Peptides* 32, 286–292. doi: 10.1016/j.peptides.2010.11.022

Karvat, G., and Kimchi, T. (2012). Systematic autistic-like behavioral phenotyping of 4 mouse strains using a novel wheel-running assay. *Behav. Brain Res.* 233, 405–414. doi: 10.1016/j.bbr.2012.05.028

Karvat, G., and Kimchi, T. (2014). Acetylcholine elevation relieves cognitive rigidity and social deficiency in a mouse model of autism. *Neuropsychopharmacology* 39, 831–840. doi: 10.1038/npp.2013.274

King, B. H., Hollander, E., Sikich, L., McCracken, J. T., Scahill, L., Bregman, J. D., et al. (2009). Lack of efficacy of citalopram in children with autism spectrum disorders and high levels of repetitive behavior: citalopram ineffective in children with autism. *Arch. Gen. Psychiatry* 66, 583–590. doi: 10.1001/archgenpsychiatry.2009.30

Koda, K., Ago, Y., Yano, K., Nishimura, M., Kobayashi, H., Fukada, A., et al. (2011). Involvement of decreased muscarinic receptor function in prepulse inhibition deficits in mice reared in social isolation. *Br. J. Pharmacol.* 162, 763–772. doi: 10.1111/j.1476-5381.2010.01080.x

Lam, K. S. L., and Aman, M. G. (2007). The repetitive behavior scale—revised: independent validation in individuals with autism spectrum disorders. *J. Autism Dev. Disord.* 37, 855–866. doi: 10.1007/s10803-006-0213-z

Laviolette, S. R., Priebe, R. P., and Yeomans, J. S. (2000). Role of the laterodorsal tegmental nucleus in scopolamine- and amphetamine-induced locomotion and stereotypy. *Pharmacol. Biochem. Behav.* 65, 163–174. doi: 10.1016/s0091-3057(99)00195-1

Lee, T. L., Raygada, M. J., and Rennert, O. M. (2012). Integrative gene network analysis provides novel regulatory relationships, genetic contributions and susceptible targets in autism spectrum disorders. *Gene* 496, 88–96. doi: 10.1016/j.gene.2012.01.020

Martin, A., Koenig, K., Scahill, L., and Bregman, J. (1999). Open-label quetiapine in the treatment of children and adolescents with autistic disorder. *J. Child Adolesc. Psychopharmacol.* 9, 99–107. doi: 10.1089/cap.1999.9.99

McCool, M. F., Patel, S., Talati, R., and Ragozzino, M. E. (2008). Differential involvement of M1-type and M4-type muscarinic cholinergic receptors in the dorsomedial striatum in task switching. *Neurobiol. Learn. Mem.* 89, 114–124. doi: 10.1016/j.nlm.2007.06.005

McFarlane, H. G., Kusek, G. K., Yang, M., Phoenix, J. L., Bolivar, V. J., and Crawley, J. N. (2008). Autism-like behavioral phenotypes in, BTBR T+tf/J mice. *Genes Brain Behav.* 7, 152–163. doi: 10.1111/j.1601-183x.2007.00330.x

McPheeters, M. L., Warren, Z., Sathe, N., Bruzek, J. L., Krishnaswami, S., Jerome, R. N., et al. (2011). A systematic review of medical treatments for children with autism spectrum disorders. *Pediatrics* 127, e1312–e1321. doi: 10.1542/peds.2011-0427

McTighe, S. M., Neal, S. J., Lin, Q., Hughes, Z. A., and Smith, D. G. (2013). The BTBR mouse model of autism spectrum disorders has learning and attentional impairments and alterations in acetylcholine and kynurenic acid in prefrontal cortex. *PLoS One* 8:e62189. doi: 10.1371/journal.pone.0062189

Meyza, K. Z., Defensor, E. B., Jensen, A. L., Corley, M. J., Pearson, B. L., Pobbe, R. L., et al. (2013). The BTBR T+ tf/J mouse model for autism spectrum disorders-in search of biomarkers. *Behav. Brain Res.* 251, 25–34. doi: 10.1016/j.bbr.2012.07.021

Moy, S. S., Nadler, J. J., Poe, M. D., Nonneman, R. J., Young, N. B., Koller, B. H., et al. (2008). Development of a mouse test for repetitive, restricted behaviors: relevance to autism. *Behav. Brain Res.* 188, 178–194. doi: 10.1016/j.bbr.2007.10.029

Owley, T., Brune, C. W., Salt, J., Walton, L., Guter, S., Ayuyao, N., et al. (2010). A pharmacogenetic study of escitalopram in autism spectrum disorders. *Autism Res.* 3, 1–7. doi: 10.1002/aur.109

Owley, T., Walton, L., Salt, J., Guter, S. J. Jr., Winnega, M., Leventhal, B. L., et al. (2005). An open-label trial of escitalopram in pervasive developmental disorders. *J. Am. Acad. Child Adolesc. Psychiatry* 44, 343–348. doi: 10.1097/01.chi.0000153229.80215.a0

Palencia, C. A., and Ragozzino, M. E. (2006). The effect of N-methyl-D-aspartate receptor blockade on acetylcholine efflux in the dorsomedial striatum during response reversal learning. *Neuroscience* 143, 671–678. doi: 10.1016/j.neuroscience.2006.08.024

Pearson, B. L., Pobbe, R. L. H., Defensor, E. B., Oasay, L., Bolivar, V. J., Blanchard, D. C., et al. (2011). Motor and cognitive stereotypies in the BTBR T+tf/J mouse model of autism. *Genes Brain Behav.* 10, 228–235. doi: 10.1111/j.1601-183x.2010.00659.x

Perry, E. K., Lee, M. L., Martin-Ruiz, C. M., Court, J. A., Volsen, S. G., Merrit, J., et al. (2001). Cholinergic activity in autism: abnormalities in the cerebral cortex and basal forebrain. *Am. J. Psychiatry* 158, 1058–1066. doi: 10.1176/appi.ajp.158.7.1058

Pobbe, R. L. H., Pearson, B. L., Defensor, E. B., Bolivar, V. J., Blanchard, D. C., and Blanchard, R. J. (2010). Expression of social behaviors of C57BL/6J versus BTBR inbred mouse strains in the visible burrow system. *Behav. Brain Res.* 214, 443–449. doi: 10.1016/j.bbr.2010.06.025

Ragozzino, M. E., Artis, S., Singh, A., Twose, T. M., Beck, J. E., and Messer, W. S. Jr. (2012). The selective M1 muscarinic cholinergic agonist CDD-0102A enhances working memory and cognitive flexibility. *J. Pharmacol. Exp. Ther.* 340, 588–594. doi: 10.1124/jpet.111.187625

Ragozzino, M. E., Mohler, E. G., Prior, M., Palencia, C. A., and Rozman, S. (2009). Acetylcholine activity in selective striatal regions supports behavioral flexibility. *Neurobiol. Learn. Mem.* 91, 13–22. doi: 10.1016/j.nlm.2008.09.008

Reynolds, S., Urruela, M., and Devine, D. P. (2013). Effects of environmental enrichment on repetitive behaviors in the BTBR T+ tf/J mouse model of autism. *Autism Res.* 6, 337–343. doi: 10.1002/aur.1298

Scattoni, M. L., Gandhy, S. U., Ricceri, L., and Crawley, J. N. (2008). Unusual repertoire of vocalizations in the BTBR T+tf/J mouse model of autism. *PLoS One* 3:e3067. doi: 10.1371/journal.pone.0003067

Scattoni, M. L., Ricceri, L., and Crawley, J. N. (2011). Unusual repertoire of vocalizations in adult BTBR T+tf/J mice during three types of social encounters. *Genes Brain Behav.* 10, 44–56. doi: 10.1111/j.1601-183x.2010.00623.x

Schwartzer, J. J., Careaga, M., Onore, C. E., Rushakoff, J. A., Berman, R. F., and Ashwood, P. (2013). Maternal immune activation and strain specific interactions in the development of autism-like behaviors in mice. *Transl. Psychiatry* 3:e240. doi: 10.1038/tp.2013.16

Silverman, J. L., Tolu, S. S., Barkan, C. L., and Crawley, J. N. (2010). Repetitive self-grooming behavior in the BTBR mouse model of autism is blocked by the mGluR5 antagonist MPEP. *Neuropsychopharmacology* 35, 976–989. doi: 10.1038/npp.2009.201

Steidl, S., and Yeomans, J. S. (2009). M5 muscarinic receptor knockout mice show reduced morphine-induced locomotion but increased locomotion after cholinergic antagonism in the ventral tegmental area. *J. Pharmacol. Exp. Ther.* 328, 263–275. doi: 10.1124/jpet.108.144824

Szatmari, P., Georgiades, S., Bryson, S., Zwaigenbaum, L., Roberts, W., Mahoney, W., et al. (2006). Investigating the structure of the restricted, repetitive behaviours and interests domain of autism. *J. Child Psychol. Psychiatry* 47, 582–590. doi: 10.1111/j.1469-7610.2005.01537.x

Tizabi, Y., Louis, V. A., Taylo, C. T., Waxman, D., Culver, K. E., and Szechtman, H. (2002). Effect of nicotine on quinpirole-induced checking behavior in rats: implications for obsessive-compulsive disorder. *Biol. Psychiatry* 51, 164–171. doi: 10.1016/s0006-3223(01)01207-0

Turner, M. (1999). Annotation: repetitive behaviour in autism: a review of psychological research. *J. Child Psychol. Psychiatry* 40, 839–849. doi: 10.1111/1469-7610.00502

Tzavos, A., Jih, J., and Ragozzino, M. E. (2004). Differential effects of M1 muscarinic receptor blockade and nicotinic receptor blockade in the dorsomedial striatum on response reversal learning. *Behav. Brain Res.* 154, 245–253. doi: 10.1016/j.bbr.2004.02.011

Voineagu, I., Wang, X., Johnston, P., Lowe, J. K., Tian, Y., Horvath, S., et al. (2011). Transcriptomic analysis of autistic brain reveals convergent molecular pathology. *Nature* 474, 380–384. doi: 10.1038/nature10110

Wang, J. Q., and McGinty, J. F. (1997). Intrastriatal injection of a muscarinic receptor agonist and antagonist regulates striatal neuropeptide mRNA expression in normal and amphetamine-treated rats. *Brain Res.* 748, 62–70. doi: 10.1016/s0006-8993(96)01244-9

Wang, H., Ng, K., Hayes, D., Gao, X., Forster, G., Blaha, C., et al. (2004). Decreased amphetamine-induced locomotion and improved latent inhibition in mice mutant for the M5 muscarinic receptor gene found in the human 15q schizophrenia region. *Neuropsychopharmacology* 29, 2126–2139. doi: 10.1038/sj.npp.1300502

Yang, M., Clarke, A. M., and Crawley, J. N. (2009). Postnatal lesion evidence against a primary role for the corpus callosum in mouse sociability. *Eur. J. Neurosci.* 29, 1663–1677. doi: 10.1111/j.1460-9568.2009.06714.x

Yang, M., Zhodzishsky, V., and Crawley, J. N. (2007). Social deficits in BTBR T+tf/J mice are unchanged by cross-fostering with C57BL/6J mothers. *Int. J. Dev. Neurosci.* 25, 515–521. doi: 10.1016/j.ijdevneu.2007.09.008

Yano, K., Koda, K., Ago, Y., Kobayashi, H., Kawasaki, T., Takuma, K., et al. (2009). Galantamine improves apomorphine-induced deficits in prepulse inhibition via muscarinic ACh receptors in mice. *Br. J. Pharmacol.* 156, 173–180. doi: 10.1111/j.1476-5381.2008.00037.x

Zarrindast, M. R., Shekarchi, M., and Rezaya, T. M. (1999). Effect of nicotine on apomorphine-induced licking behaviour in rats. *Eur. Neuropsychopharmacol.* 9, 235–238. doi: 10.1016/s0924-977x(98)00027-3

12

Fetal autonomic brain age scores, segmented heart rate variability analysis, and traditional short term variability

Dirk Hoyer[1]*, Eva-Maria Kowalski[1,2], Alexander Schmidt[1] Florian Tetschke[1], Samuel Nowack[1], Anja Rudolph[1,3], Ulrike Wallwitz[1,3], Isabelle Kynass[1,3], Franziska Bode[1,3], Janine Tegtmeyer[1,3], Kathrin Kumm[1,3], Liviu Moraru[1], Theresa Götz[1], Jens Haueisen[2], Otto W. Witte[1], Ekkehard Schleußner[3] and Uwe Schneider[3]

[1] *Biomagnetic Center, Hans Berger Department of Neurology, Jena University Hospital, Friedrich Schiller University, Jena, Germany*
[2] *Institute of Biomedical Engineering and Informatics, Ilmenau University of Technology, Ilmenau, Germany*
[3] *Department of Obstetrics, Jena University Hospital, Friedrich Schiller University, Jena, Germany*

Edited by:
Silvia Comani, Università degli Studi "G. d'Annunzio", Italy

Reviewed by:
Dirk Cysarz, Witten/Herdecke University, Germany
Kathleen M. Gustafson, University of Kansas Medical Center, USA

***Correspondence:**
Dirk Hoyer, Biomagnetic Center, Hans Berger Department of Neurology, Jena University Hospital, Friedrich Schiller University, Erlanger Allee 101, D-07747 Jena, Germany
e-mail: Dirk.Hoyer@med.uni-jena.de

Disturbances of fetal autonomic brain development can be evaluated from fetal heart rate patterns (HRP) reflecting the activity of the autonomic nervous system. Although HRP analysis from cardiotocographic (CTG) recordings is established for fetal surveillance, temporal resolution is low. Fetal magnetocardiography (MCG), however, provides stable continuous recordings at a higher temporal resolution combined with a more precise heart rate variability (HRV) analysis. A direct comparison of CTG and MCG based HRV analysis is pending. The aims of the present study are: (i) to compare the fetal maturation age predicting value of the MCG based fetal Autonomic Brain Age Score (fABAS) approach with that of CTG based Dawes-Redman methodology; and (ii) to elaborate fABAS methodology by segmentation according to fetal behavioral states and HRP. We investigated MCG recordings from 418 normal fetuses, aged between 21 and 40 weeks of gestation. In linear regression models we obtained an age predicting value of CTG compatible short term variability (STV) of $R^2 = 0.200$ (coefficient of determination) in contrast to MCG/fABAS related multivariate models with $R^2 = 0.648$ in 30 min recordings, $R^2 = 0.610$ in active sleep segments of 10 min, and $R^2 = 0.626$ in quiet sleep segments of 10 min. Additionally segmented analysis under particular exclusion of accelerations (AC) and decelerations (DC) in quiet sleep resulted in a novel multivariate model with $R^2 = 0.706$. According to our results, fMCG based fABAS may provide a promising tool for the estimation of fetal autonomic brain age. Beside other traditional and novel HRV indices as possible indicators of developmental disturbances, the establishment of a fABAS score normogram may represent a specific reference. The present results are intended to contribute to further exploration and validation using independent data sets and multicenter research structures.

Keywords: prenatal diagnosis, fetal autonomic brain age, magnetocardiography, cardiotocography

INTRODUCTION

Prenatal risk factors can permanently change the fetal brain development and are associated with diseases in later age. Adverse influences during fetal development that became permanently programmed can increase the postnatal risk for cardiovascular, metabolic, hyperkinetic, cognitive, learning and behavioral disorders (e.g., Barker, 1998, 2002; Barker et al., 2002; O'Keeffe et al., 2003; Van den Bergh et al., 2005).

Prenatal functional diagnosis is limited and requires innovative concepts. In that context, the fetal autonomic (neuro-vegetative) control plays a key role since it provides valuable information about several control systems that are mediated by the autonomic nervous system. The associated heart rate patterns (HRP) are one of the few signals that can be obtained non-invasively from the fetus, and hence, heart rate variability (HRV) analysis is uniquely suited to assess the fetal functional autonomic brain development. Fetal HRP provide quantitative information about sympathetic and vagal activation, fetal behavioral states, and fetal movements (Nijhuis et al., 1982; Van Leeuwen et al., 1999; David et al., 2007; Hoyer et al., 2009; Schmidt et al., 2014).

In order to obtain normal values of maturation indices in healthy fetuses and deviations due to risk factors, a sophisticated analysis of fetal HRP is required. Finally, the association between prenatal and postnatal autonomic control and disturbances needs to be investigated in that context.

Antepartum cardiotocography (CTG) is a predominant established method that contributes to fetal surveillance and risk assessment both antenatal and during labor based on the analysis of fetal HRP age (Nijhuis et al., 2000; Pardey et al., 2002; Serra et al., 2008, 2009). FIGO (International Federation of Gynaecology and Obstetrics) risk score as well as the fluctuation indices short term variability (STV) and long term variability (LTV) are realized in Dawes-Redman methodology (Pardey et al., 2002). The fetal HRP displayed in CTG depends on gestational age, fetal activity and a variety of other factors, but classification of recordings primarily aimed on distinguishing the healthy from the distressed fetus rather than precisely assessing maturation. Hence, the resulting question to be followed in this study is, to which extent CTG methodology allows a fetal autonomic brain age assessment in comparison to the higher quality MCG methodology.

Universal characteristics of evolution and development in non-living and living nature are increasing fluctuation amplitude, increasing complexity and pattern formation. Those characteristics similarly apply in the phylogenetic and the ontogenetic development. The fetal HRP reflect corresponding characteristics of the maturating fetal autonomic brain activity. All of those characteristics can be interpreted as reflecting autonomous influences of the sympathetic and parasympathetic nervous systems, influenced by the superordinate medullary centers. In a previous study, using continuous magnetocardiographic (MCG) recordings at 1 ms temporal resolution, we designed a resulting "fetal autonomic brain age score" (fABAS; Hoyer et al., 2013b).

However, a certain part of variance could not be explained by the score and the question arises how and to which extent a more sophisticated model may improve the performance. In that context, segmentation of the measured HRP under consideration of behavioral states as well as of the particular exclusion of acceleration (AC) and deceleration (DC) patterns may provide information about different aspects of autonomic modulations in more detail.

The aims of the present study are: (i) to compare the fetal maturation age predicting value of the MCG based fABAS approach with that of Dawes-Redman methodology; and (ii) to elaborate fABAS methodology by segmentation of the recordings according to behavioral states and HRP.

MATERIALS AND METHODS

SUBJECTS AND DATA AQUISITION

From the study database of the Biomagnetic Center, Department of Neurology, and Department of Obstetrics, both Jena University Hospital, recordings of 418 normal singleton fetuses, aged between 21 and 40 weeks of gestation (WGA), healthy according to standard obstetric observation methods, single recording in a non-stress situation were included. The study was approved by the Local Ethics Committee of the Friedrich Schiller University. All women signed a written, informed consent form.

All measurements were taken in a magnetically shielded room at the Biomagnetic Center, Department of Neurology, Jena University Hospital using the vector-magnetograph ARGOS 200 (ATB, Chieti, Italy). Pregnant women were positioned supine or with a slight twist to either side to prevent compression of the inferior vena cava. The dewar was positioned as close as possible above the fetal heart determined by sonographic localization, but without contact to the maternal abdominal wall. The MCG signal was recorded over a period of 30 min with a sampling rate of 1024 Hz. The fetal heart beats were detected using a newly developed independent component analysis based strategy (Schmidt et al., 2014). The fetal body movements were reconstructed from the fMCG signal (for details see Schmidt et al., 2014).

CTG COMPATIBLE ANALYSIS ACCORDING TO DAWES-REDMAN

In the present work the heart beat intervals (MCG sampling period $\approx$1 ms) were integrated over 3.75 s epochs in order to obtain a CTG compatible signal of the identical recording. Analyzable 1 min sections were considered as those that contain neither large decelerations nor more than 50% artifacts (not detected beats/beat intervals; Pardey et al., 2002).

- STV is calculated as mean difference between consecutive heart beat interval epochs in all analyzable 1 min sections. The results of all analyzed 1 min sections are averaged.
- LTV is calculated as fluctuation range of heart beat interval epochs in analyzable 1 min sections. The fluctuation range is calculated as a sum between maximal deviation above baseline and maximal deviation below baseline. The fluctuation ranges of all analyzed 1 min sections are averaged.

Furthermore, the Dawes-Redman criteria for normality from 26 WGA upwards, that require up to 60 min recordings, were formally applied to the 30 min recordings of the fetuses aged at least 26 WGA (n = 313). The following criteria have to be met (adapted from Pardey et al., 2002):

- The recording must contain at least one episode of high variation.
- STV >3.0 ms, but if it is <4.5 ms LTV averaged across all episodes of high variation must be >3rd percentile for WGA.
- No evidence of a high-frequency sinusoidal rhythm.
- At least one AC, or a fetal movement rate of ≥20 per hour and a LTV averaged across all episodes of high variation >10th percentile for WGA.
- At least one fetal movement or three AC.
- No DC of >20 lost beats if the recording is <30 min, no more than one DC of 21–100 lost beats if it is >30 min, and no DC at all >100 lost beats.
- The basal fetal heart rate must be 116–160 beats/min if the recording is <30 min.
- LTV within 3 SD of its estimated value or (a) STV >5.0 ms; (b) an episode of high variation with ≥0.5 fetal movements per minute; (c) the basal fHR ≥120 beats/min; and (d) the signal loss <30%.
- The final epoch of the recording must not be part of a DC.
- No suspected artifacts at the end of the recording if the recording is <60 min.

In that context, an AC is defined as an increase in heart rate for more than 15 s with a minimum deviation from baseline exceeding 10 bpm. A DC is defined as a decrease below the baseline for more than 30 s and a deviation >20 bpm or 60 s and >10 bpm, respectively (Pardey et al., 2002).

Table 1 | Heart rate variability indices.

Parameter	Meaning, Interpretation	Calculation
Dawes-Redman		
STV	**Short Term Variability** Integrative sympatho-vagal modulations, fluctuation periods of seconds	Mean difference between consecutive heart beat interval epochs of 3.75 s, w/o DC and artifacts <50%
LTV	**Long Term Variability** Fluctuation periods of minutes	Mean fluctuation range of heart beat interval epochs in 1 min sections, w/o DC and artifacts <50%
fABAS		
AMP	**Fluctuation range** of heart beat intervals, overall sympatho-vagal modulations	20–95 inter-quantile distance of detrended NN interval series
gMSE3	**Complexity** of sympatho-vagal rhythms	Generalized Mutual Information at coarse graining level 3 of beat interval series, see Hoyer et al. (2013a)
skewness	**Asymmetry**, contribution of vagal and sympathetic activity with their different time constants, decline of DC and formation of AC	skewness of instantaneous heart rate series
pNN5	**Fast, vagal** Mainly vagally modulated rhythms	Percentage of differences between adjacent NN intervals that are >5 ms.
lnVLF/LF	**Baseline fluctuation** in relation to sympatho-vagal modulations	Ratio between very low (0.02–0.08 Hz) and low (0.08–0.2 Hz) frequency band power
Pattern segmented		
gMSE3 w/o DC		
gMSE3 basic	**w/o DC** - parameters under exclusion of DC	Mean of parameter of subsegments without DC
skewness w/o DC		
skewness basic		
pNN5 w/o DC	**basic** - parameters of basic rhythm	Mean of parameter of subsegments w/o DC and w/o AC
pNN5 basic		
lnVLF/LF w/o DC		
lnVLF/LF basic		

** Segmented analysis of fluctuation range (AMP) was not performed due to lacking significance in quiet sleep. Partly adapted from Hoyer et al. (2013b), further details in TaskForce (1996), Pardey et al. (2002), Hoyer et al. (2013a).*

MCG BASED HEART RATE VARIABILITY ANALYSIS—FETAL AUTONOMIC BRAIN AGE SCORE

The fABAS was previously proposed by the authors using a calculation precision of ≈1 ms according to the MCG sampling rate (Hoyer et al., 2013b). Fetal autonomic brain age score based on particular HRV parameters that were selected according to universal developmental characteristics, namely increasing fluctuation amplitude (assessed by AMP), increasing complexity (assessed by gMSE3), and pattern formation (assessed by skewness, pNN5, lnVLF/LF, see **Table 1**). In that previous work, the fetal age was predicted by multivariate linear regression models (forward procedure: stepwise inclusion of variables while $P(F) < 0.05$; backward procedure: stepwise exclusion of variables while $P(F) > 0.1$) for each sleep state independently. The resulting models for quiet and active sleep were considered fABAS. While [gMSE3, skewness, VLF/LF, pNN5] contributed in the quiet sleep model, [AMP, skewness, gMSE3, pNN5, VLF/LF] contributed in the active sleep model. Here, an additional model was built for the entire 30 min recordings that can include only one or several behavioral states. The resulting additional model constitutes a third branch of fABAS. Furthermore, the linear regression models were supplemented with quadratic term regression models that were built using the same HRV parameters.

SLEEP STATE SEGMENTATION

From the entire 30 min recordings 10 min segments according to quiet and active sleep related HRP I, HRP II were selected following a consensus decision by three independent obstetricians according to an advanced version of standard criteria (Nijhuis et al., 1982; Schneider et al., 2009; Hoyer et al., 2013b).

- HRP I (quiet state, correlated to quiet sleep 1F): stable fetal heart rate (fHR) (variation of visually determined floating baseline <10 bpm/3 min) with a small oscillation bandwidth (< ±5 bpm from floating baseline fHR), isolated (maximum 2 per 10 min) AC (>15 bpm over >15 s) and a floating baseline fHR that does not exceed 160 bpm.
- HRP II (active state, correlated to active sleep 2F): fluctuating fHR with an oscillation bandwidth exceeding +/− 5 bpm from floating baseline, frequent (at least 3 per 10 min) AC (>15 bpm, >15 s), and the fHR exceeding 160 bpm only during AC.
- HRP III (active state, correlated to active awakeness 4F): fHR patterns with long-lasting AC exceeding 160 bpm, frequently fused into a sustained tachycardia.

Based on the classification results we selected 10 min sections of quiet sleep ($n = 137$) and active sleep ($n = 344$). Consequently, in 63 of the 418 recordings, sections of both, HRP I and HRP

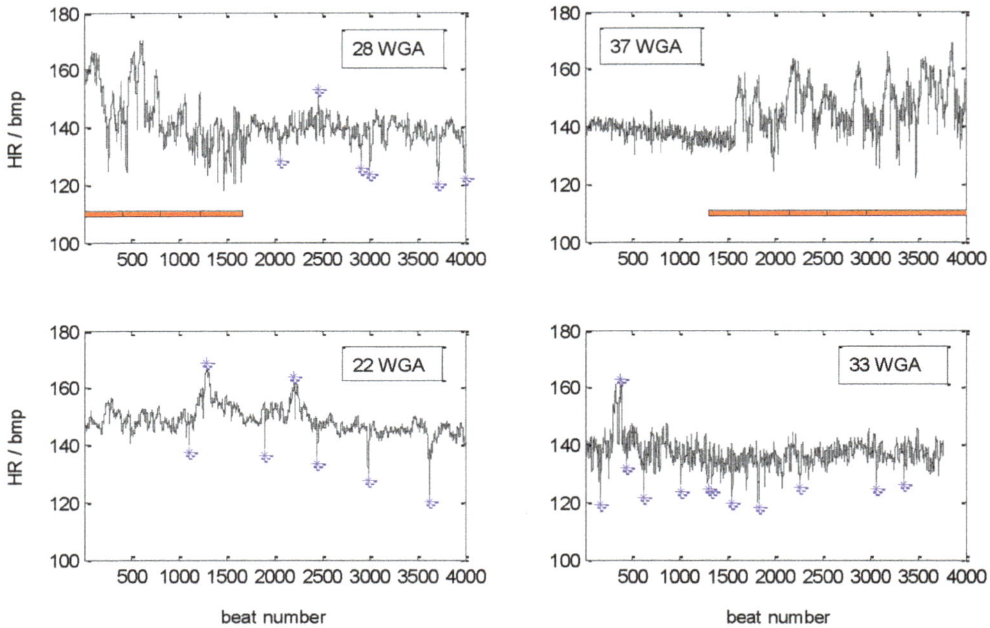

FIGURE 1 | Tachograms of 30 min recordings of four different fetuses. Upper part: changes between sections of active (marked by red horizontal bar) and quiet sleep related heart rate patterns in a younger (28 WGA) and an older (37 WGA) fetus. Lower part: quiet sleep related heart rate patterns at 22 and 33 WGA. DC and AC (>10 bpm deviation from floating baseline, marked by blue *) are identified in the quiet sleep sections only.

II, were classified. Active awakeness classified recordings were not analyzed because of their small sample size ($n = 29$).

PATTERN SEGMENTATION–PARTIAL EXCLUSION OF HEART RATE ACCELERATIONS AND DECELERATIONS

In addition, periods without DC and segments of basic activity (with neither DC nor AC), respectively, were analyzed in the HRP I segments. The methodology of the here proposed MCG based segmented HRV analysis is different from the CTG—Dawes-Redman methodology used above. In the present context, the definitions of AC and DC were modified according to the following rules:

- Sections without DC were identified in moving 3 min windows (shifted by 1 min over 10 min segment) if there were no deviations below the baseline (estimated for each 3 min window) > 10 bpm;
- Sections of basic activity were identified in moving 3 min windows (shifted by 1 min over 10 min segment) if there were no deviations below or above the baseline (estimated for each 3 min window) > 10 bpm.

The baseline was estimated according to original Dawes-Redman methodology (Pardey et al., 2002). From all identified windows the HRV parameters were calculated and averaged.

This kind of pattern segmentation was performed for all significantly age predicting HRV parameters of fABAS (see **Table 1**).

The example recordings shown in **Figure 1** demonstrate the diversity of the recorded pattern. In the upper part a change between active and quiet state in a premature age of 28 WGA is compared with a clear change from quiet to active state in the mature age of 37 WGA. In the part underneath, recordings classified as quiet sleep at 22 and 33 WGA are shown. Please notice partly unstable baseline, AC and DC are marked in the quiet sleep section. There are neither periods of incorrect heart beat detections (beat intervals) nor periods of dropouts.

STATISTICAL ANALYSIS

The predictive value of the HRV parameters was assessed by univariate and multivariate, linear and quadratic term regression models over the entire investigated maturation period (corrected coefficient of determination R^2). The cases were weighted to approximate equal distribution over gestational age. $P < 0.05$ was considered significant. Since most of the predictors were significant, only non-significant results are marked by "n.s.". For better reading, predictors with $R^2 > 0.3$ were marked by bold letters. All statistical analyses were carried out using IBM SPSS Statistics 21.

RESULTS

30 MIN RECORDINGS

Traditional STV and LTV were calculated from analyzable periods according to CTG methodology like outlined above. Short term variability predicted the maturation age with a low coefficients of determination ($R^2 = 0.200$, 206, linear and quadratic model, **Table 2**). The Dawes-Redman criteria were met with increasing frequency between 26 and 32 WGA and were consistently met from 32 WGA onwards (**Figure 2**).

From the fABAS related HRV parameters, AMP, skewness, and pNN5 and provided strong univariate linear age predictors

Table 2 | Analyses of 30 min recordings: univariate and multivariate, linear and quadratic term regression models, coefficients of determination R^2, parameters selected according to CTG (Dawes-Redman related (Pardey et al., 2002)) and MCG based fABAS related (Hoyer et al., 2013b), $R^2 > 0.3$ in bold, all cases significant.

Parameter	30 min recording	
	Linear	Quadratic
CTG compatible		
STV (ms)	0.200	0.206
LTV (ms)	0.085	0.116
fMCG based, fABAS related		
Time domain		
AMP	**0.312**	**0.321**
skewness	**0.458**	**0.502**
pNN5	**0.347**	**0.367**
Power spectra		
lnVLF/LF	0.034	0.060
Complexity		
gMSE3	0.226	0.231
Multivariate model, fABAS		
[AMP, skewness, pNN5, lnVLF/LF, gMSE3]	**0.648**	**0.656**
Multivariate model, fABAS + STV		
[AMP, skewness, pNN5, lnVLF/LF, gMSE3, STV]	**0.649**	**0.657**

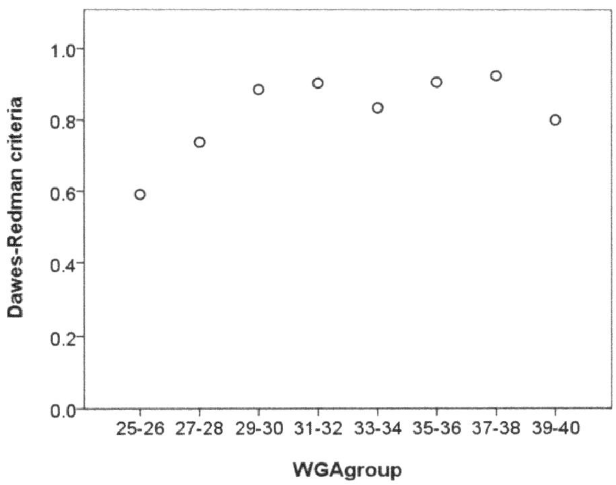

FIGURE 2 | Relative frequency of recordings that meet the Dawes-Redman criteria (1 = 100%) vs. chronological age (in weeks GA) of 30 min recordings. In absolute values, 134 of 167 cases met the criteria in the subset of ≤32 WGA and 130 of 146 in the subset of >32 WGA, respectively.

(R^2 = 0.312, 0.458, 0.347). They were partly improved by including a quadratic term (R^2 = 0.321, 0.502, 0.367). In the multivariate models all parameters significantly contributed leading to R^2 = 0.648 and R^2 = 0.656, respectively (**Table 2**, **Figure 3**). In contrast, STV and LTV did not provide additional predictive value to the multivariate models.

SEGMENTED RECORDINGS

Active sleep 10 min segments

In the active sleep data, AMP (R^2 = 0.392 and 0.430, linear and quadratic), skewness (R^2 = 0.352 and 0.431) and pNN5

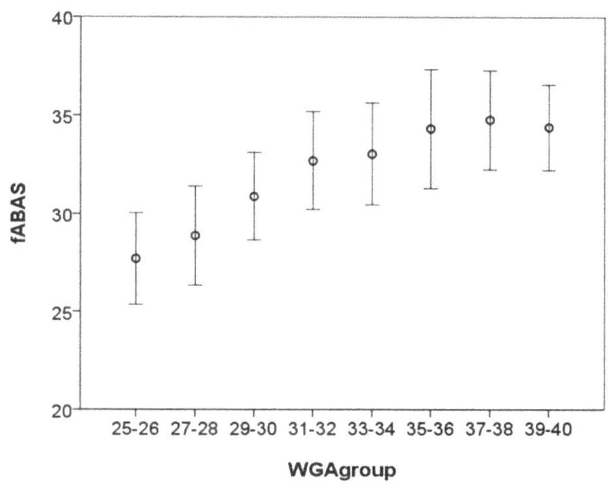

FIGURE 3 | Fetal autonomic brain age score [AMP, skewness, pNN5, lnVLF/LF, gMSE3] vs. chronological age (in WGA) of 30 min recordings, mean ± standard deviation.

Table 3 | Analyses of 10 min segments in active sleep: linear and quadratic regression models, coefficients of determination R^2, parameters selected according to fABAS (Hoyer et al., 2013b), $R^2 > 0.3$ in bold.

Predictor	R^2	
	Linear	Quadratic
Time domain		
AMP	**0.392**	**0.430**
Skewness	**0.352**	**0.431**
pNN5	**0.350**	**0.376**
Power spectra		
lnVLF/LF	0.098	0.103
Complexity		
gMSE3	0.128	0.130
Multivariate model	-	-
[AMP, Skewness, gMSE3, pNN5, lnVLF/LF]	**0.610**	**0.636**

(R^2 = 0.350 and 0.376) clearly predicted the fetal maturation age. In the multivariate models, additionally gMSE3 and lnVLF/LF contributed leading to R^2 = 0.610 and 0.636 in the linear and quadratic, respectively, models (**Table 3**).

Quiet sleep 10 min segments

In the quiet sleep data, gMSE3 (R^2 = 0.542 and 0.565), but also pNN5 (R^2 = 0.320 and 0.338) and skewness (R^2 = 0.316 and 0.320) were stronger predictors than lnVLF/LF (R^2 = 0.147 and 0.159). AMP did not provide predictive value. The stepwise built multivariate model included [skewness, gMSE3, pNN5] (R^2 = 0.626 and 0.641; **Table 4**).

Further pattern segmentation in quiet sleep

Further pattern segmentation, namely the exclusion of DC and AC removed the predictive value of skewness. This result is consistent with the fact that skewness mainly reflects asymmetries due to DC and AC which are important maturation characteristics. Other aspects of behavior are basic activity, i.e., the basic rhythm

Table 4 | Analyses of 10 min segments in quiet sleep: additional pattern segmentation (without decelerations: w/o DC; basic activity, neither DC nor AC: basic), linear and quadratic regression models, coefficients of determination R^2, parameters according to Table 2, $R^2 > 0.3$ in bold.

Predictor	R^2	
	Linear	Quadratic
Time domain		
AMP	n.s.	n.s.
Skewness	**0.316**	**0.320**
skewness w/o DC	0.123	0.127
skewness basic	0.032	0.038
pNN5	**0.320**	**0.338**
pNN5 w/o DC	**0.396**	**0.451**
pNN5 basic	**0.374**	**0.428**
Power spectra		
lnVLF/LF	0.147	0.159
lnVLF/LF w/o DC	0.192	0.201
lnVLF/LF basic	0.195	0.206
Complexity		
gMSE3	**0.542**	**0.565**
gMSE3 w/o DC	**0.609**	**0.627**
gMSE3 basic	**0.632**	**0.657**
Multivariate model, fABAS indices		
[Skewness, gMSE3, pNN5]	**0.626**	**0.641**
Multivariate model, pattern segmented		
[Skewness, gMSE3, gMSE3w/oDC, gMSE3basic]	**0.706**	**0.714**

containing neither AC nor DC, and activity under exclusion of DC. Concerning those aspects, the predictive value of pNN5, gMSE3 and lnVLF/LF was increased. The gMSE3 related indices were the strongest univariate predictors (gMSE, gMSEw/oDC, gMSE3basic: $R^2 = 0.542$, 0.609. 0.632 in the linear models, and $R^2 = 0.565$, 0.627. 0.657 in the quadratic models, see **Table 4**).

The stepwise built multivariate model resulted on the inclusion of [skewness, gMSE3, gMSEw/oDC, gMSE3basic] with $R^2 = 0.706$ in the linear and $R^2 = 0.714$ quadratic model. This result indicates a relevant advantage compared to the consideration of data that are classified as quiet sleep as a total without further pattern segmentation.

DISCUSSION

Traditional HRV indices reflect: (i) vagal activity during quiet sleep; (ii) sympathetic activity during active sleep; and (iii) integrative control in longer recordings with changing states. In a recent study, we have demonstrated a strong relationship between those HRV indices and fetal maturation age (Hoyer et al., 2009). Compared to those traditional HRV indices, we newly developed a fABAS based on universal developmental characteristics assessing maturation age with a high precision in active and quiet sleep (Hoyer et al., 2013b). In this study we show that fABAS based methodology significantly improves fetal maturation age assessment compared to established CTG. Those results are based on our comprehensive database obtained from MCG measurements.

The particular aims of the present study were: (i) to compare the fetal maturation age predicting value of the MCG based fABAS approach with that of CTG (Dawes-Redman) compatible STV; and (ii) to elaborate fABAS methodology by segmentation according to behavioral states (overall recording, active and quiet sleep segments) and HRP.

30 MIN RECORDINGS

The maturation age predicting value of STV ($R^2 = 0.200$, linear model) was significantly lower in comparison to fABAS.

Interestingly, using the indices of fABAS applied to the entire 30 min recordings, the maturation age was clearly predictable ($R^2 = 0.648$, linear model), although the signals were very heterogeneous due to the occurrence of only one or several behavioral states. The increased R^2 in the quadratic models, moreover, may reflect the saturating maturation after 32 WGA mainly expressed in skewness (see **Figure 3**). This characteristic curve is in line with previous results of power spectral analysis (Van Leeuwen et al., 2003).

ACTIVE AND QUIET SLEEP 10 MIN SEGMENTS

The predictive value of the fABAS related models in active and quiet sleep ($R^2 = 0.610$, 0.626, linear models) was slightly lower in comparison to the 30 min recordings. However, it should be noticed that state dependent aspects of autonomic control, such as vagal and sympathetic dominance, provided an almost similar predictive value. Saturating maturation after 32 WGA considered in quadratic models of vagal HRV (pNN5) in quiet sleep and mainly sympathetic/overall HRV (AMP, skewness) in active sleep may have also contributed to increased R^2 in the quadratic models.

FURTHER PATTERN SEGMENTATION IN QUIET SLEEP

Further segmentation in quiet sleep focused on the differential contribution of basic activity and AC as well as DC of at least 10 bpm deviation from baseline. The resulting independent factors of the novel model, namely skewness, gMSE3, gMSE3w/oDC, gMSE3basic, may highlight the role of complex adjustments between sympatho-vagally mediated fluctuations in connection with AC and DC patterns. The predictive value ($R^2 = 0.706$, linear model) was clearly higher than that of fABAS. This result indicates that the essential universal developmental characteristics, namely increasing complexity and pattern formation which go hand in hand with fetal development, also apply for the particular pattern during quiet sleep. Furthermore, the result implies that a consideration of the respective physiological pattern in detail, might even improve the maturation assessment. Therefore, fABAS may serve as classification tool for the general condition, whereas further pattern segmentation provides a more detailed focus on an observed abnormality.

Fetal autonomic brain age score indices in combination with the novel pattern segmentation based on our comprehensive MCG database can serve as a representative norm-sample of the normal fetal autonomic maturation age (see **Figures 3**, **4**). With that it will be easy to detect even minor deviations from the normal fetal development.

METHODOLOGICAL ISSUES

In principle, the application of the Dawes-Redman criteria and LTV as a traditional CTG methodology to MCG based HRV

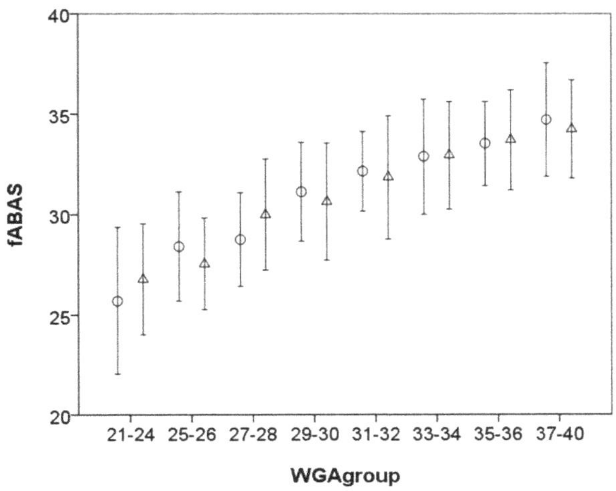

FIGURE 4 | Fetal autonomic brain age score [Skewness, gMSE3, pNN5] for quiet sleep segments ○ and [AMP, Skewness, gMSE3, pNN5, lnVLF/LF] for active sleep segments △ vs. chronological age (in WGA), mean ± standard deviation, notice that 21–24 WGA and 37–40 WGA, respectively, are merged due to the small number of samples.

analysis was possible. During a period of 60 min, which is recommended for the application of the Dawes-Redman criteria, at least one active pattern is statistically expected to occur. However, since only 30 min recordings were analyzed, a number of subjects did not meet the criteria. Recordings of 60 min length would allow direct consideration of FIGO Dawes-Redman criteria. Even longer observations would furthermore lead to a better evaluation of sleep state dynamics. However, due to patient compliance and the possibly increasing number of artifacts in longer measurements, the performance in shorter recordings is of particular interest.

The segmentation according to behavioral state classification is the result of a consensus decision of three experts based on HRP that furthermore slightly change with maturation age between 21–40 WGA. This classification is not always unequivocal, but it reflects the heterogeneity of recordings and the state of the art.

The present results are mainly representative for the investigated 30 min recordings and 10 min segments. A next necessary step would be the validation and improvement of the presented methodology in recordings from different measurement sites.

For a fair evaluation of the here proposed methodology and search for the optimum, other HRV indices should also be taken into consideration. The here presented methodology allows the inclusion of further precise MCG HRV indices as well of FIGO recommended CTG compatible indices.

In the subsequent steps, multifactorial models are required to consider both, maturation age and developmental disorders.

CONCLUSION

Heart rate variability indices selected according to fABAS using 30 min fMCG recordings and segmented HRV analysis provide a promising tool for the estimation of the fetal autonomic brain age that is superior to CTG based indices. Resulting normograms of normal autonomic brain maturation may constitute significant references for the identification of developmental disturbances. The presented methodology is intended to contribute to further exploration and validation with regard to the early identification of developmental disorders using independent data sets in multicenter studies.

ACKNOWLEDGMENTS

This work was supported by the German Research Foundation (Deutsche Forschungsgemeinschaft, HO 1634 12-2, Schn 775/2-3) and the Curie Intra-European Fellowship IEF-2009-237290. We thank Stefan Claus for editing the manuscript.

REFERENCES

Barker, D. J. (1998). In utero programming of chronic disease. *Clin. Sci. (Lond)* 95, 115–128. doi: 10.1042/cs19980019

Barker, D. J. (2002). Fetal programming of coronary heart disease. *Trends Endocrinol. Metab.* 13, 364–368. doi: 10.1016/s1043-2760(02)00689-6

Barker, D. J., Eriksson, J. G., Forsén, T., and Osmond, C. (2002). Fetal origins of adult disease: strength of effects and biological basis. *Int. J. Epidemiol.* 31, 1235–1239. doi: 10.1093/ije/31.6.1235

David, M., Hirsch, M., Karin, J., Toledo, E., and Akselrod, S. (2007). An estimate of fetal autonomic state by time-frequency analysis of fetal heart rate variability. *J. Appl. Physiol. (1985)* 102, 1057–1064. doi: 10.1152/japplphysiol.00114.2006

Hoyer, D., Heinicke, E., Jaekel, S., Tetschke, F., Di Pietro Paolo, D., Haueisen, J., et al. (2009). Indices of fetal development derived from heart rate patterns. *Early Hum. Dev.* 85, 379–386. doi: 10.1016/j.earlhumdev.2009.01.002

Hoyer, D., Nowack, S., Bauer, S., Tetschke, F., Rudolph, A., Wallwitz, U., et al. (2013a). Fetal development of complex autonomic control evaluated from multiscale heart rate patterns. *Am. J. Physiol. Regul. Integr. Comp. Physiol.* 304, R383–R392. doi: 10.1152/ajpregu.00120.2012

Hoyer, D., Tetschke, F., Jaekel, S., Nowack, S., Witte, O. W., Schleußner, E., et al. (2013b). Fetal functional brain age assessed from universal developmental indices obtained from neuro-vegetative activity patterns. *PLoS One* 8:e74431. doi: 10.1371/journal.pone.0074431

Nijhuis, J. G., Prechtl, H. F., Martin, C. B. Jr., and Bots, R. S. (1982). Are there behavioural states in the human fetus?. *Early Hum. Dev.* 6, 177–195. doi: 10.1016/0378-3782(82)90106-2

Nijhuis, I. J., ten Hof, J., Mulder, E. J., Nijhuis, J. G., Narayan, H., Taylor, D. J., et al. (2000). Fetal heart rate in relation to its variation in normal and growth retarded fetuses. *Eur. J. Obstet. Gynecol. Reprod. Biol.* 89, 27–33. doi: 10.1016/s0301-2115(99)00162-1

O'Keeffe, M. J., O'Callaghan, M., Williams, G. M., Najman, J. M., and Bor, W. (2003). Learning, cognitive and attentional problems in adolescents born small for gestational age. *Pediatrics* 112, 301–317. doi: 10.1542/peds.112.2.301

Pardey, J., Moulden, M., and Redman, C. W. (2002). A computer system for the numerical analysis of nonstress tests. *Am. J. Obstet. Gynecol.* 186, 1095–1103. doi: 10.1067/mob.2002.122447

Schmidt, A., Schneider, U., Witte, O. W., Schleussner, E., and Hoyer, D. (2014). Developing fetal motor-cardiovascular coordination analysed from multi-channel magnetocardiography. *Physiol. Meas.* 35, 1943–1959. doi: 10.1088/0967-3334/35/10/1943

Schneider, U., Schleussner, E., Fiedler, A., Jaekel, S., Liehr, M., Haueisen, J., et al. (2009). Fetal heart rate variability reveals differential dynamics in the intrauterine development of the sympathetic and parasympathetic branches of the autonomic nervous system. *Physiol. Meas.* 30, 215–226. doi: 10.1088/0967-3334/30/2/008

Serra, V., Bellver, J., Moulden, M., and Redman, C. W. (2009). Computerized analysis of normal fetal heart rate pattern throughout gestation. *Ultrasound Obstet. Gynecol.* 34, 74–79. doi: 10.1002/uog.6365

Serra, V., Moulden, M., Bellver, J., and Redman, C. W. (2008). The value of the short-term fetal heart rate variation for timing the delivery of growth-retarded fetuses. *BJOG* 115, 1101–1117. doi: 10.1111/j.1471-0528.2008.01774.x

TaskForce. (1996). Heart rate variability: standards of measurement, physiological interpretation and clinical use. Task Force of the European Society of Cardiology and the North American Society of Pacing and Electrophysiology. *Circulation* 93, 1043–1065. doi: 10.1161/01.CIR.93.5.1043

Van den Bergh, B. R., Mulder, E. J., Mennes, M., and Glover, V. (2005). Antenatal maternal anxiety and stress and the neurobehavioural development of the fetus and child: links and possible mechanisms. A review. *Neurosci. Biobehav. Rev.* 29, 237–258. doi: 10.1016/j.neubiorev.2004.10.007

Van Leeuwen, P., Geue, D., Lange, S., Hatzmann, W., and Gronemeyer, D. (2003). Changes in the frequency power spectrum of fetal heart rate in the course of pregnancy. *Prenat. Diagn.* 23, 909–916. doi: 10.1002/pd.723

Van Leeuwen, P., Lange, S., Bettermann, H., Grönemeyer, D., and Hatzmann, W. (1999). Fetal heart rate variability and complexity in the course of pregnancy. *Early Hum. Dev.* 54, 259–269. doi: 10.1016/s0378-3782(98)00102-9

13

Abiotic-biotic characterization of Pt/Ir microelectrode arrays in chronic implants

Abhishek Prasad[1]*, Qing-Shan Xue[2], Robert Dieme[3], Viswanath Sankar[3], Roxanne C. Mayrand[4], Toshikazu Nishida[3], Wolfgang J. Streit[2] and Justin C. Sanchez[1,4,5]

[1] Department of Biomedical Engineering, University of Miami, Coral Gables, FL, USA
[2] Department of Neuroscience, University of Florida, Gainesville, FL, USA
[3] Department of Electrical and Computer Engineering, University of Florida, Gainesville, FL, USA
[4] Department of Neuroscience, University of Miami, Coral Gables, FL, USA
[5] Miami Project to Cure Paralysis, University of Miami, Miami, FL, USA

Edited by:
Ulrich G. Hofmann, Albert-Ludwigs-University Freiburg, Germany

Reviewed by:
Sofyan H. H. Hammad, Aalborg University, Denmark
Susanne Löffler, Karolinska Institute, Sweden

***Correspondence:**
Abhishek Prasad, Department of Biomedical Engineering, B91 University of Miami, 1251 Memorial Drive, McArthur Engineering Annex #219A, Coral Gables, FL 33146, USA
e-mail: a.prasad@miami.edu

Pt/Ir electrodes have been extensively used in neurophysiology research in recent years as they provide a more inert recording surface as compared to tungsten or stainless steel. While floating microelectrode arrays (FMA) consisting of Pt/Ir electrodes are an option for neuroprosthetic applications, long-term *in vivo* functional performance characterization of these FMAs is lacking. In this study, we have performed comprehensive abiotic-biotic characterization of Pt/Ir arrays in 12 rats with implant periods ranging from 1 week up to 6 months. Each of the FMAs consisted of 16-channel, 1.5 mm long, and 75 μm diameter microwires with tapered tips that were implanted into the somatosensory cortex. Abiotic characterization included (1) pre-implant and post-explant scanning electron microscopy (SEM) to study recording site changes, insulation delamination and cracking, and (2) chronic *in vivo* electrode impedance spectroscopy. Biotic characterization included study of microglial responses using a panel of antibodies, such as Iba1, ED1, and anti-ferritin, the latter being indicative of blood-brain barrier (BBB) disruption. Significant structural variation was observed pre-implantation among the arrays in the form of irregular insulation, cracks in insulation/recording surface, and insulation delamination. We observed delamination and cracking of insulation in almost all electrodes post-implantation. These changes altered the electrochemical surface area of the electrodes and resulted in declining impedance over the long-term due to formation of electrical leakage pathways. In general, the decline in impedance corresponded with poor electrode functional performance, which was quantified via electrode yield. Our abiotic results suggest that manufacturing variability and insulation material as an important factor contributing to electrode failure. Biotic results show that electrode performance was not correlated with microglial activation (neuroinflammation) as we were able to observe poor performance in the absence of neuroinflammation, as well as good performance in the presence of neuroinflammation. One biotic change that correlated well with poor electrode performance was intraparenchymal bleeding, which was evident macroscopically in some rats and presented microscopically by intense ferritin immunoreactivity in microglia/macrophages. Thus, we currently consider intraparenchymal bleeding, suboptimal electrode fabrication, and insulation delamination as the major factors contributing toward electrode failure.

Keywords: Pt/Ir microelectrodes, neural interface, blood brain barrier (BBB), neuroinflammation, abiotic, biotic, floating microelectrode arrays (FMA), impedance

INTRODUCTION

The development of clinically viable microelectrode arrays for humans has produced multiple engineering design and neurophysiological requirements that are believed to be necessary for facilitating high performance (Jackson and Zimmermann, 2012). These include the ability to target and access the activity in ensembles of neurons located in cortical and deep brain structures for treating a variety of neurological problems including paralysis (Ethier et al., 2012; Hochberg et al., 2012; Collinger et al., 2013), stroke (Iosa et al., 2012), movement disorders (Andrews, 2010; Rouse et al., 2011), epilepsy (Morrell, 2011; Truccolo et al., 2011), and neuropsychiatric disorders (Maling et al., 2012). Not only is short-term access of these neurons important but also the microelectrode arrays should be able to sense and stimulate targeted neurons reliably, which could be of the order of tens of years. From a materials science perspective, there are differences in the design considerations between sensing and stimulation but in general, it is desirable to have stable electrodes that do not corrode (Sanchez et al., 2006; Prasad et al., 2012), produce stable impedance (Ward et al., 2009; Prasad and Sanchez, 2012), and are robust after repeated delivery of current through them (Johnson et al., 2005; Otto et al., 2005, 2006; Koivuniemi and Otto, 2011; Lempka et al., 2011). A variety of materials including tungsten, platinum, platinum-iridium, and iridium oxide coatings have been used to improve the reliability of recordings (Geddes and Roeder, 2003; Cogan, 2008; Ward et al., 2009). Closely coupled to the abiotic materials aspects are the biotic responses to chronically implanted microelectrode arrays. The biotic effects include the disruption of the blood-brain barrier (BBB) (Prasad et al., 2011; Karumbaiah et al., 2013; Saxena et al., 2013), tissue inflammatory response involving astroglial and microglial reactions occurring at/around the implanted site, and macrophage recruitment to the implanted site (Schmidt et al., 1976; Stensaas and Stensaas, 1978; Edell et al., 1992; Kam et al., 1999; Turner et al., 1999; Szarowski et al., 2003; Biran et al., 2005; Lee et al., 2005; Polikov et al., 2005; Biran et al., 2007; McConnell et al., 2009b; Winslow and Tresco, 2010; Thelin et al., 2011; Prasad et al., 2012). The abiotic effects include the changes occurring at the electrode recording sites such as corrosion and insulation delamination and cracking that alters the electrochemical properties of the electrode recording surface area (Geddes and Roeder, 2003; Patrick et al., 2011; Prasad and Sanchez, 2012; Prasad et al., 2012; Streit et al., 2012; Kane et al., 2013). Both these effects are dynamic in nature, occur concurrently, and cannot be isolated from one another. Therefore, high-performance arrays should produce minimal tissue reactivity including disruption of the blood-brain-barrier (Prasad et al., 2012), glial response (Frampton et al., 2010; Winslow and Tresco, 2010; Prasad et al., 2012), and neuronal damage (McConnell et al., 2009b). Finding the optimal balance of all of these design considerations is challenging and various electrode tip geometries (Andrei et al., 2012) and multiple array solutions have been proposed including microwire arrays, floating planar silicon arrays, floating 2-D silicon arrays, and floating microwire arrays (Drake et al., 1988; Rousche and Normann, 1998; Williams et al., 1999a,b; Rousche et al., 2001; Csicsvari et al., 2003; Kipke et al., 2003; Nicolelis et al., 2003; Vetter et al., 2004; Patrick et al., 2006; Jackson and Fetz, 2007; Musallam et al., 2007; Kozai et al., 2012a; Kim et al., 2013; Richter et al., 2013). Unique among these available solutions is the "floating" aspect of the array design. It is believed that floating arrays can mitigate many of the challenges of chronic implantation as they have been shown to cause reduced lesions due to electrode array micro-movements in the brain tissue (Biran et al., 2007). Systematic and quantitative study of each of these array types is necessary to prove their benefits and weaknesses in the context of electrode performance and failure.

In this work, floating microelectrode arrays (FMA) fabricated by Microprobes (Gaithersburg, MD) are studied. These electrodes are made of Pt/Ir which provide a more stable and inert electrode-recording site that is less prone to corrosion and surface changes compared to other metals such as tungsten and stainless steel (Geddes and Roeder, 2003; Cogan, 2008; Patrick et al., 2011; Prasad et al., 2012; Kane et al., 2013). In addition, they are laser cut with a conical tip to reduce the trauma during insertion. Unlike the Utah array, which is the only other commercial design that is similar, the FMA can be custom cut for both deep brain and cortical targets. The arrays are fabricated on a planar substrate and connected via a thin flexible cable, which allows the array to float with the brain. While FMAs have been used in a variety of cortical and spinal applications for basic neurophysiological and neuroprosthetic applications, they have not undergone comprehensive characterization to quantify their electrophysiological properties over long-durations (weeks to months) *in vivo*. We have recently developed an *in vivo* testbed (Prasad and Sanchez, 2012; Prasad et al., 2012; Streit et al., 2012) to quantify the failure mechanisms of microelectrodes and have shown that there are a variety of biotic and abiotic aspects that contribute to electrode performance. Since microelectrode array design is so diverse among the available options (Utah, FMA, microwires, Michigan), each design needs to be evaluated independently using a common set of relevant metrics. Toward developing a comprehensive characterization of FMA performance and failure, this study performs an *in vivo* long-term abiotic and biotic analysis with an aim to build a quality control system for microelectrodes. FMAs were implanted into the rat somatosensory cortex for implant duration ranging from 7 days up to 6 months. Abiotic analysis included (1) pre-implant and post-explant SEM imaging for qualitative comparison of the changes that occur at the electrode recording surface, and (2) chronic *in vivo* impedance spectroscopy for studying the changes in the electrode impedance chronically. Biotic analysis was assessed using microglial activation and degeneration and BBB disruption. Chronic electrode performance was quantified via array yield. The array yield, specified by the number of recording sites producing single neuron recordings, provides insight to the overall health of the array. High-performance electrode arrays produce single neuron recordings from a maximal number of recording sites. Likewise, failing electrode arrays produce low yields. It has been shown that impedance spectroscopy provides insight to the fundamental aspects of biotic and abiotic interactions that affect array performance (Grill and Mortimer, 1994; Merrill and Tresco, 2005; Ludwig et al., 2006, 2011; Williams et al., 2007; McConnell et al., 2009a; Karumbaiah et al., 2013). Combining standard electrophysiological measurements with abiotic and biotic analysis can produce comprehensive insight to electrode failure.

METHODS

All procedures were approved by the University of Miami Institutional Animal Care and Use Committee (IACUC). Twelve age-matched adult male Sprague–Dawley rats, all weighing between 300 and 350 grams (at implant time) were used in this study. Animals were divided into short-term implant group ($\leq$2 weeks) (Turner et al., 1999; Winslow and Tresco, 2010) and chronic groups ($\leq$6 months) (Williams et al., 1999b; Polikov et al., 2005; Winslow and Tresco, 2010). In this study, 3 animals were implanted for up to 7 days, 2 for 15 days, 1 for 3 weeks, 3 for up to 3 months, and 3 for 6 months, respectively. The 7-days and 15-days animals were classified in the short-term implant group whereas the remaining animals were classified in the chronic group. All animals were euthanized at the end of their prospective study period intentionally and the brain tissue was harvested for histological analysis. **Table 1** summarizes the pre-implant and post-explant SEM observations, functional performance, and histopathological summary for all 12 animals included in the study.

Table 1 | Summary of all animals used in this study.

Animal groups	Rat no.	Days post-implant	Scanning electron microscopy (SEM) imaging		Electrophysiology			Histopathology	
			Pre-implant	Post-explant	Impedance (MΩ) on day 1	Impedance (MΩ) at euthanasia	Average array array yield (%)	Activated microglia (Yes/No)	Degenerated microglia (Yes/No)
Short-term implants($\leq$15 days)	F11	15	Non-uniform insulation, cracks in insulation near recording tips	Bent tips, insulation delamination and cracks in insulation	0.45 ± 0.14	0.689 ± 0.17	39.3 ± 32.8	Y	Y
	F12	7	Crack in no. 1, some wires not straight, non-uniform insulation along wires	Cracks in insulation, insulation delamination, recessed insulation	0.37 ± 0.12	0.504 ± 0.29	65 ± 28.1	Y	Y
	F13	15	Electrode tip not straight for no. 13, cracks along wire shank, some wires not straight	Insulation delamination in some electrodes, cracks in insulation	0.41 ± 0.12	1.27 ± 0.43	78.1 ± 19.6	Y	Y
	F14	7	Electrode tip not straight for no. 16, cracks in insulation along shank	Broken tip, insulation delamination	0.51 ± 0.68	0.494 ± 0.23	33.3 ± 20	Y	Y
	F15	6	No. 2 crack on recording surface, cracks in insulation along shanks, no. 8 wire tip not straight	Electrode tip not straight, some deinsulation	0.4 ± 0.11	0.593 ± 0.22	81.2 ± 22.2	Y	Y
Chronic implants ($\leq$6 months)	F9	71	Majorly flawed: cracks in insulation at recording tips for most electrodes, non-uniform insulation	Cracks in insulation, insulation delamination, recessed insulation	1.44 ± 0.59	0.947 ± 0.26	16.8 ± 22.4	Y	Y
	F10	21	Cracks on electrode shanks, cracks in insulation at recording tips	Cracks, delamination, insulation damage	0.47 ± 0.14	0.594 ± 0.19	4.8 ± 13.7	Y	Y
	F2	180	Non-uniform insulation on all wires, some wires not straight	Some bent tips, two electrodes have cracks in insulation	0.61 ± 0.65	1.96 ± 0.71	74.3 ± 13.9	Y	Y
	F4	180	Irregular insulation, some wires not straight, tip missing for no. 6, bent recording tip no. 9	Bent tips, insulation delamination	0.397 ± 0.134	1.43 ± 0.49	40.5 ± 22.5	N	N
	F6	180	Bent tips for nos. 3, 4, 5, 9, and 13, some wires not straight, cracks in insulation	Insulation delamination on some wires, bent tips	0.43 ± 0.2	0.7 ± 0.3	35.1 ± 19.6	N	N
	F7	90	Moderately flawed: bent tip no. 16, non-uniform insulation at recording tips, crack in insulation at tips	Insulation delamination in some electrodes, cracks, bent tips	0.59 ± 0.7	1.47 ± 0.81	12 ± 8.6	N	Y
	F8	91	Majorly flawed: crack in recording tip no. 5, cracks in insulation of 8 electrodes, some wires not straight	Insulation delamination	1.08 ± 0.24	2.14 ± 0.43	19.5 ± 21.4	Y	Y

Animals are divided into short-term implants ($\leq$2 week) and long-term implants ($\leq$6 months). The table provides summarizes general abiotic and biotic observations.

ELECTRODE

We characterized 16-channel FMA (MicroProbes, Inc, MD) for our implants in all animals (Musallam et al., 2007; Mollazadeh et al., 2011). The microelectrode array consisted of 16 microwires [Pt/Ir (70/30%) 75 μm diameter at the base which tapered to a fine tip] attached to a ceramic substrate (**Figure 1A**). Each of the microwires were 1.5 mm long and separated by 400 μm. The microwires were insulated with parylene-C, the thickness of which was 3 μm along the wire shaft and the microwires were laser cut at the tip, which produced a conical recording surface. The microwires were soldered to gold wires, which were bundled together and soldered to a 16-channel Omnetics connector that was fixed on the skull. The wire bundle was coated with medical grade silicone to provide insulation.

SCANNING ELECTRON MICROSCOPY (SEM) IMAGING

In order to evaluate the structural changes in chronically implanted microelectrode arrays, all arrays were imaged before implantation and after explantation using a variable pressure scanning electron microscope (Hitachi S-3000N VP-SEM). The environmental mode in the VP-SEM was chosen for imaging the arrays to enable direct placement of the samples into the SEM chamber without the use of carbon or conductive coating. This is very critical especially for pristine electrodes as they will be implanted into an animal after the SEM imaging procedure. Such a method was used so as to cause no damage to the arrays from the imaging process for both pre-implant as well as explanted arrays. When the pre-implant images were taken, electrode arrays were handled with care to prevent any damage to the microwires. The post-explant images were taken on the electrode arrays extracted from the implanted tissue. The post-explant arrays were carefully placed on a holder positioned on to the SEM stage. The following parameters were used to take the pre- and post-implant images: (1) environmental secondary electron detector (ESED) mode with an acceleration potential of 12 kV, (2) working distance range was set between 18 and 40 mm, and (3) magnification was varied according to need and the minimum magnification was set at 20X.

IMPEDANCE TESTING PROCEDURE

Electrode impedance spectroscopy was performed using NanoZ (TDT, Alachua, FL) using procedures described in detail elsewhere (Prasad and Sanchez, 2012). Briefly, NanoZ measures impedance by applying a small sinusoidal voltage of 4 mVpp at specific frequencies of 1 Hz, 2 Hz, 5 Hz, 10 Hz, 20 Hz, 50 Hz, 100 Hz, 200 Hz, 500 Hz, 1 kHz, and 2 kHz, respectively. The small amount of voltage applied by NanoZ causes a maximum test current of 1.4 nA RMS to flow through the measuring circuit. The impedance measurement protocol was approved by the electrode manufacturer. We combined repeated impedance measurements following the above protocol with scanning electron microscopy (SEM) imaging to verify that electrode recording surfaces were not altered due to the measurement process itself. Impedance spectroscopy *in vitro* was performed for electrode arrays with respect to a low impedance stainless steel reference wire prior to implantation in 0.9% phosphate buffered saline (PBS) for obtaining baseline values for each array. The two-electrode method has been deemed suitable for measuring microelectrode impedance owing to the large difference in impedance between the electrode being tested and the distant low impedance reference wire (Brett and Brett, 1993; Geddes, 1997; Williams et al., 2007). *In vivo* measurements were made with respect to the same stainless steel wire tied to the skull screw while the animals were lightly anesthetized during impedance measurements. *In vivo*, impedance was measured 3–4 times a week before electrophysiological recordings. In our testing, the NanoZ calculated the impedance values for each electrode by repeating the process 20 times and reported the average of those values to reduce errors due to measurement.

SURGICAL PROCEDURE

Electrodes were individually sterilized using ethylene oxide gas prior to implantation and sterile surgical techniques were followed for all implant surgeries. Animals were anesthetized with an induction of isoflurane (4%) and O_2 (2 L/min) and deep anesthesia level was maintained for the entire duration of the surgical procedure using isoflurane (1.5%) and 1 L/min O_2. Xylazine (5 mg/kg, subcutaneous) was used to maintain an even plane of anesthesia and as a muscle relaxant. Upon fixing the animal's head in a stereotaxic frame (Kopf Instruments, Tujunga, CA) to stabilize the skull, a midline incision was made on the skin from between the eyes up to the ears and the periosteum was scraped from on top of the skull. The skull surface was cleaned and the bregma and lambda landmarks were identified. Four stainless steel screws were manually drilled into the skull. Using stereotaxic coordinates, the craniotomy location (1 mm lateral and 1.8 mm caudal to the bregma) was marked which correspond to the somatosensory cortex. A 5 mm diameter circular craniotomy was drilled at the above marked location (**Figure 1B**) and the dura was then cut using microscissors to expose the cortical surface. The setup shown in **Figure 1C** was used to hold the electrode connector and position the electrode array using a vacuum pump wand. The electrode array was slowly (~0.1 mm/min) lowered into the cortex using the micropositioner (Kopf Instruments, Tujunga, CA). Slow speed of insertion was used for these FMA as recommended by the manufacturer and similar to studies that have shown success in recording single neurons with a slow insertion speed for microwire arrays (Nicolelis, 1999). A small piece of gelfoam soaked in sterile saline was used to cover the craniotomy and dental acrylic (A-M Systems, Carlsborg, CA) was placed on and around the craniotomy. Extreme care was taken such that none of the acrylic entered the craniotomy. The ground and reference wires were tied to the skull screw and the entire area was filled with acrylic. Animals were placed under supervision in a recovery box kept on a heating pad post-surgery and housed individually upon recovery. Bupivacaine was used around the wound site after the surgery and Carprofen (5 mg/kg, subcutaneous) was used as the analgesic. No antibiotics or any other drugs were used in this study.

RECORDING PROCEDURE

Animals were recorded 3–4 times each week. Electrode impedance spectroscopy was performed prior to each recording session. The animal was connected to a preamplifier that was optically isolated from a real-time digital signal processor (RZ2, TDT, FL).

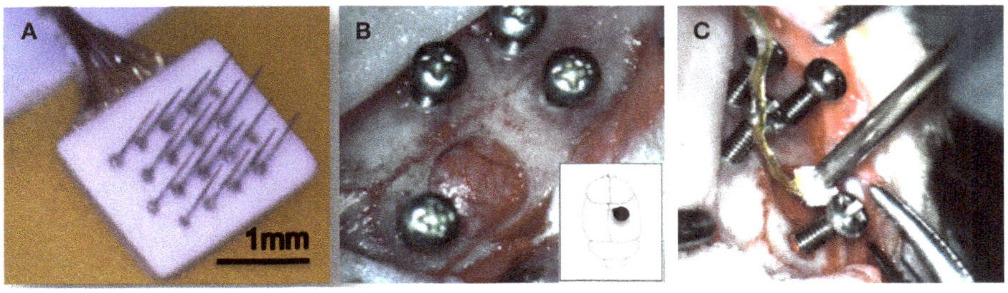

FIGURE 1 | Experimental setup. A 16-channel Pt/Ir floating microelectrode array (FMA) consisting of 1.5 mm long and 75 μm diameter with tapered microwires tips was used for all implants **(A)**. Surgical implantation procedure in the rat somatosensory cortex is shown **(B,C)**.

A custom made program (RPvDx, TDT, FL) was used to acquire neural signals sampled at 24414.06 Hz. Signals were band-pass filtered between 0.5 and 6 kHz and online spike sorting based on boxes and thresholding as determined by the experimenter was used to isolate neuronal waveforms. Offline spike sorting was then performed to verify isolated single units and remove other artifacts. Waveforms were classified as single units based upon the repeatability of waveform shape and peak-to-peak amplitude with respect to the background noise (Suner et al., 2005). Electrophysiological recordings were quantified via array yield, which was defined as the percentage of electrodes within an array that were able to isolate at least one neuron during a recording session. Array yield was used as a functional measure for electrode assessment. An electrode was said to isolate a neuron (single unit) when at least 100 reproducible biphasic waveforms could be collected during a session.

Signal-to-Noise ratio (SNR) was calculated using the formula: $SNR = \frac{V}{2*\sigma}$, where V is the peak-to-peak amplitude of the mean waveform and σ is the standard deviation of the noise. These methods have been described in detail elsewhere (Suner et al., 2005). **Figure 2A** provides a general measure of the signal quality where offline sorted waveforms from four isolated neurons is shown with SNR value calculated for each neuron. The neuron waveforms shown are for animal F6 and are from different electrodes and different sessions. All waveforms were collected and shown within a 1.2 ms time-window. Weekly signal-to-noise levels are shown for four animals (F6–9) during their respective implant durations in **Figure 2B**. In general, SNR values ranged between 3 and 6 and were comparable to those reported earlier by other studies (Suner et al., 2005; Ward et al., 2009). We found that SNR values were not dependent upon implant durations or daily changes in impedance values and also not correlated to the electrode performance.

IMMUNOHISTOCHEMICAL PROCEDURES

Immunohistochemical procedures have been described in detail elsewhere (Prasad et al., 2012). Briefly, microglial cells in brain sections were examined immunohistochemically using the rabbit polyclonal primary antibody Iba1 (Wako, 019–19741, diluted at 1:800). Phagocytic microglia were identified using ED1 antibody (mouse anti-rat monocytes/macrophages (CD68), Chemicon; MAB1435, diluted at 1:300). Immunolabeling for the iron storage protein was performed using antiferritin polyclonal antibody (rabbit anti-horse spleen ferritin, Sigma, F6136, diluted at 1:800). Ferritin, an iron storage protein that becomes expressed in some microglia in the human brain are often dystrophic rather than activated (Dijkstra et al., 1985). Ferritin staining of microglia seems to be induced under certain injury/disease conditions when the blood–brain barrier is disturbed and there is a need for iron sequestration. The ferritin antibody also binds to oligodendrocytes in the normal uninjured central nervous system (Lopes et al., 2008). Quantitative analysis of antigen expression was conducted on images using Image J program (NIH, Bethesda, MD). The total positive area of an antigen expression per unit section area (i.e., per microscopic field ×20; total area size 267320.12 μm^2) were scored in an image captured from each side of rat brain by using Image J program. The mean values and standard deviation of the counts were computed. An intact microglial cell was defined as a cell with a cell body area larger than 30 μm^2 and less than 300 μm^2 for Iba1 and ferritin labeling. The ED1 positive particle was defined as areas from 1 to 10 μm^2. The difference between the electrode implant side and the contralateral side was interpreted to reflect an approximation of microglial cell function.

RESULTS

SEM IMAGING OBSERVATIONS

A comparison of the pre-implant and post-explant SEM images of the electrode arrays was made to analyze qualitatively the changes at the electrode recording surface morphology for all animals. All electrodes prior to implantation were imaged to observe any pre-implant defects in the electrodes due to the manufacturing process. We observed several defects occurring as a result of manufacturing most commonly present in the recording surfaces and the interface between the recording surface and the insulation. The manufacturing defects most commonly present were cracks in the insulation material, non-uniform insulation, bent and broken recording tips, cracks on the recording tips, and non-uniform deinsulation (**Figure 3**). **Figure 3** shows examples of electrodes with pre-implant manufacturing imperfections for 4 of the longest term animals (3–6 months implant period). These images were taken prior to electrode implants. Note that not all the electrodes within an array had issues but approximately 25% or more electrodes tend to have one or the other issue as described above. Thus, there was a large variation between electrodes within an array with some electrodes with no issues whereas others with

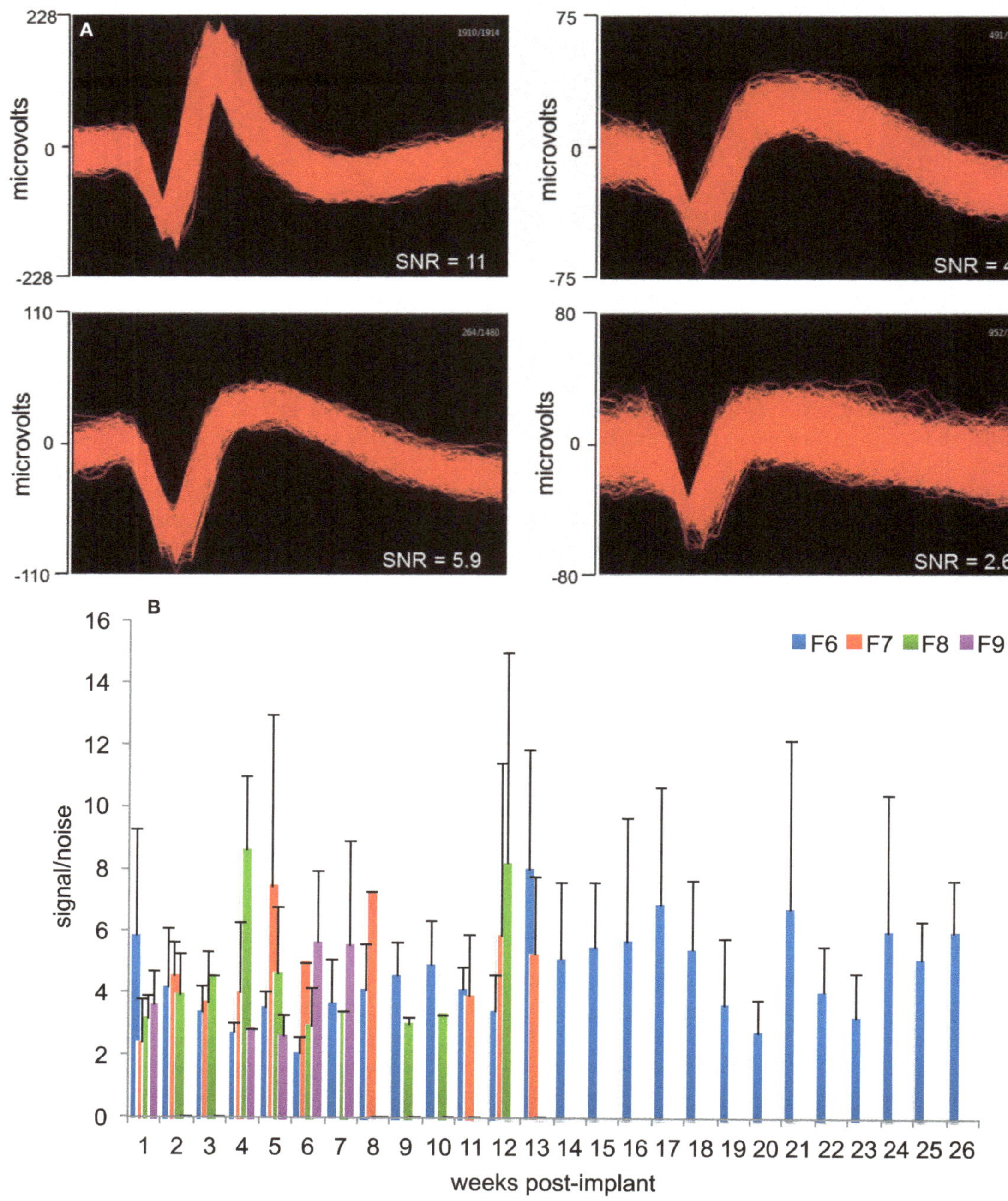

FIGURE 2 | Signal quality and SNR. (A) Representative offline sorted waveforms isolated from individual electrodes to depict signal quality. High (>5), medium (3–5), and low SNR (<3) waveforms are shown. In general, SNR values were in the range 3–6. Waveforms are shown within a 1.2 ms time-window. **(B)** Weekly signal-to-noise levels for animals F6, F7, F8, and F9 are shown. SNR values were comparable to those reported earlier by other studies. SNR values were not dependent upon implant durations or daily changes in impedance values.

pre-implant imperfections. Pre-implant and post-explant SEM images were taken for qualitative comparison of the changes that occur at the electrode recording surface and insulation material. **Figure 4A** shows such changes occurring after chronic implantation in animals where the electrodes underwent moderate to minimal changes at the recording surfaces. We observed that Pt/Ir undergoes little corrosion for implants up to 6 months. However, there was a great variability among individual electrodes even within the same array with regard to corrosion and/or insulation deterioration. While electrode corrosion did not appear to be a significant problem with Pt/Ir, we observed severe delamination and cracking of insulation material. Gross morphological

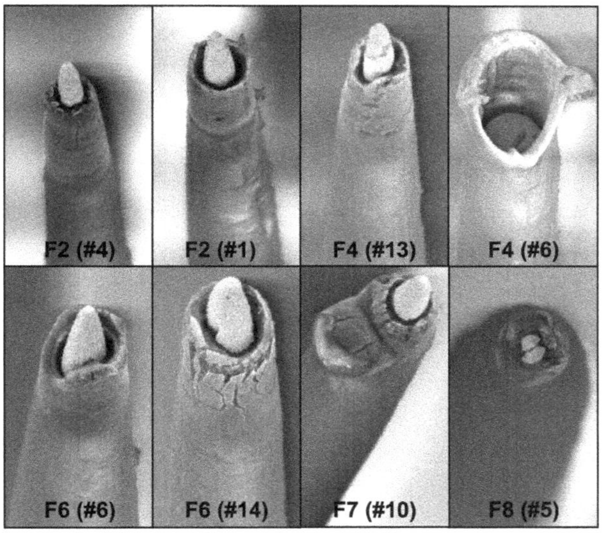

FIGURE 3 | Manufacturing variability. We observed large variation between electrodes within the same Pt/Ir array. Shown here are 8 wires from four arrays pre-implant with imperfections as a result of manufacturing process. One of the wires is missing the recording tip whereas others have cracks in the insulation/recording tip, and uneven insulation at the interface of the recording surface/insulation.

changes occurred at the recording surface in the form of bent tips, cracks appearing in the insulation material, and insulation delamination. **Figure 4B** show 12 representative electrodes from 7 long-term animals (3–6 months) where severe damage to the insulation material was observed. Insulation damage and delamination resulted in a decrease in electrode impedance during the chronic lifetime and affected functional performance (**Figure 5**). **Figure 5** shows such an example for 4 electrodes from 3 long-term animals (F4 and F6: 6 months; F9: 71 days) where electrode impedance declined during the latter part of the implant period. Interestingly, as the electrode was undergoing these morphological changes, the functional performance (electrode yield) became poor.

IMPEDANCE AND ELECTROPHYSIOLOGICAL OBSERVATIONS

To study general trends in impedance magnitude, 1 kHz impedance was chosen throughout this study as this is the fundamental frequency of an action potential and the value commonly used to report impedance in other studies (Ward et al., 2009). **Figure 6** shows the 1 kHz impedance trends and the array yield during the implant period for 4 long-term animals (F2, F4, F6: 6 months; F8: 3 months). The figure plots the average array yield (red bars) and average impedance (blue trace) from 16 electrodes on each of the recording days. Impedance values increased progressively to 2–3 times the post-implant values by the 1-week period. In general, impedance values continued to increase until the 3–4 week period with values in the range 1.5–2.5 MΩ after which they decreased. There was also greater variation in the daily impedance values as suggested by the large error bars. The impedance values generally decreased after the 15-day period with occasional fluctuations in the chronic period thereafter. These general impedance magnitude trends with large daily variations were consistent among all animals. Array yield generally was high post-implantation and declined in the days following surgery. In general, an inverse relationship between the daily impedance measurements and the array yield was observed for all our long-term animals.

HISTOPATHOLOGY OBSERVATIONS

Light microscopic examination of sections stained with microglial markers revealed a rather heterogeneous picture of histopathological changes (**Figure 7**), but some clear trends were apparent. In general microglial activation, as judged by cell hypertrophy and cell density on Iba1-stained preparations was strongest during early survival times and tended to decrease with increasing survival post-implantation, that is the intensity of neuroinflammation declined over time. Expression of ED1 antigen, indicative of ongoing phagocytic activity, was variable and showed no apparent correlation with post-implant survival times. The ED1 antigen was always present in microglia/macrophages. Expression of ferritin was not related to post-implantation survival times but instead was variable and likely related directly to the extent of vascular damage and hemorrhage (**Figure 8**). Dense encapsulation of electrodes was not observed in many of the animals and at most involved two cell layers surrounding electrode tracks (**Table 2**). The extent of encapsulation was not correlated with electrode performance, e.g., F8 (**Figure 7**; **Table 2**).

COMBINED ABIOTIC-BIOTIC ANALYSIS

One or more metrics can be used for predicting electrode failure through modeling approaches that would provide us with a reliable estimate of electrode failure. A combined analysis that included histopathological and morphological evaluation combined with functional assessment of these arrays was performed to support our hypothesis of the various abiotic and biotic failure modes that contributes to electrode failure (**Figure 9**). All histopathological markers (Iba1, ED1, and Ferritin) were normalized across all animals for comparison. We used the following measures to define functional performance: poor (<25% array yield), moderate (25–70% array yield), and good (>70% array yield). All the longest term animals (6-months implant: F2, F4, F6) had moderate to good performance with low histopathology marker levels. Among animals that had good performance, 4 out of 7 animals had very low levels of ferritin expression. The animals (F11, F12, F15) which had higher ferritin levels were very short-term implants. It is likely that ferritin along with other markers were upregulated due to surgical trauma. Even then, the ferritin levels in these animals were much lower than other animals (F7, F9, F10). Therefore, low levels of ferritin was correlated with better functional performance. Electrodes that were poorly manufactured to begin with underwent gross morphological changes overall and had poor functional performance (F7, F8, F9, F10). This supports our hypothesis that insulation delamination/cracking and manufacturing variability leads to reduced impedance over time and degradation in functional performance. There were animals (F11, F12, F15) that had good performance with high

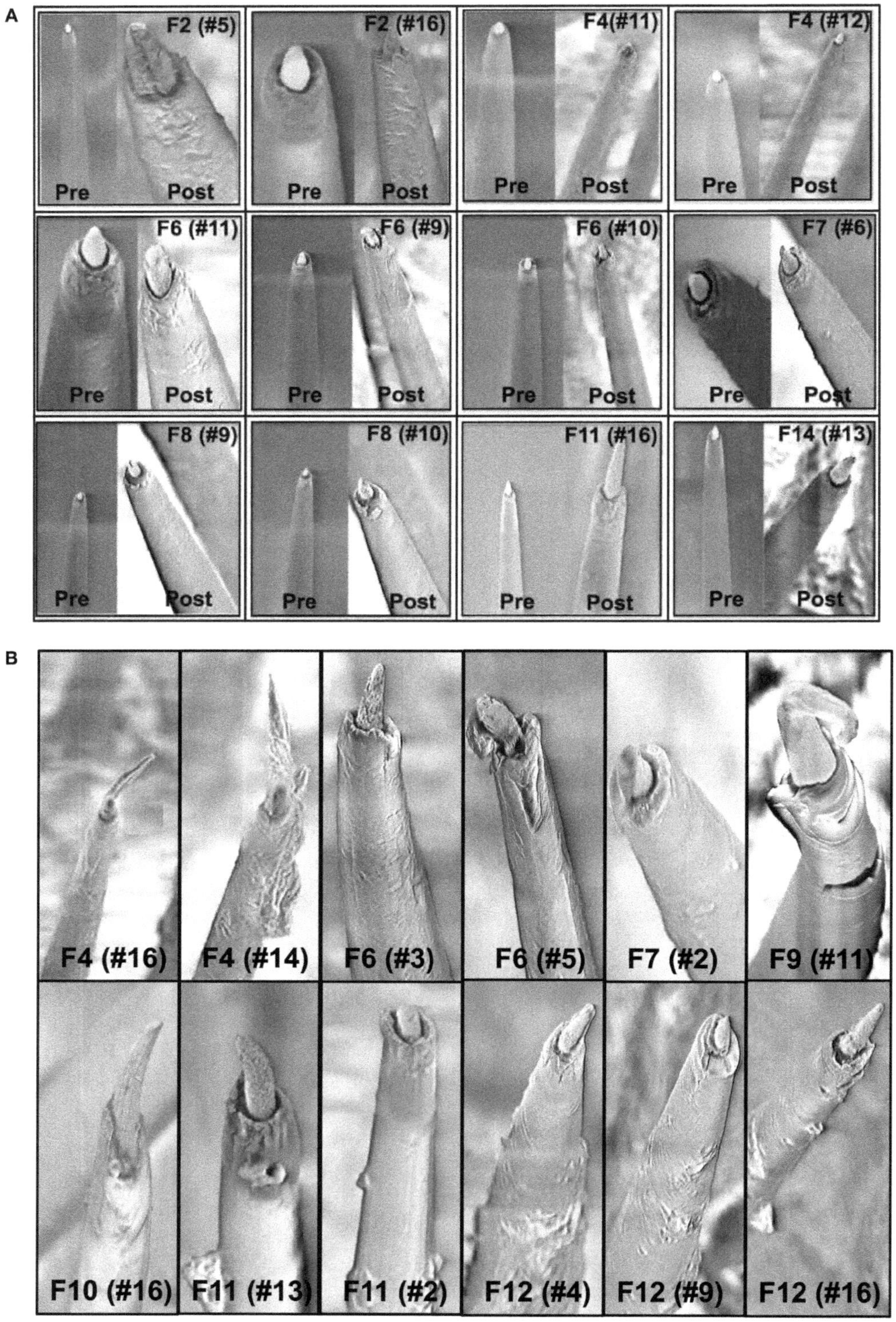

FIGURE 4 | (A) Pre-implant and post-explant SEM. Pre-implant and post-explant SEM images to show minimal to moderate changes at the recording site structure for the longest term animals. However, recording site changes occur as a result of corrosion of the recording surface for long-term implants. Shown here are three 6-month implants (F2, F4, F6), two 3-month animals (F7, F8), one 15-day animal (F11), and one 7-day animal (F14), respectively. A crack at the recording site can be observed to be developing in the electrode F2 (no. 5). **(B)** Insulation deterioration post-explant SEM. Post-explant SEM of individual microwire to indicate deterioration in electrode insulation for parylene-C coated Pt/Ir microwires. The deterioration occurs in the form of delamination and cracks. While the insulation deterioration varies among microwires even with the same array, we observed it to be present in all the wires across animals for all implant durations (7 days–6 months).

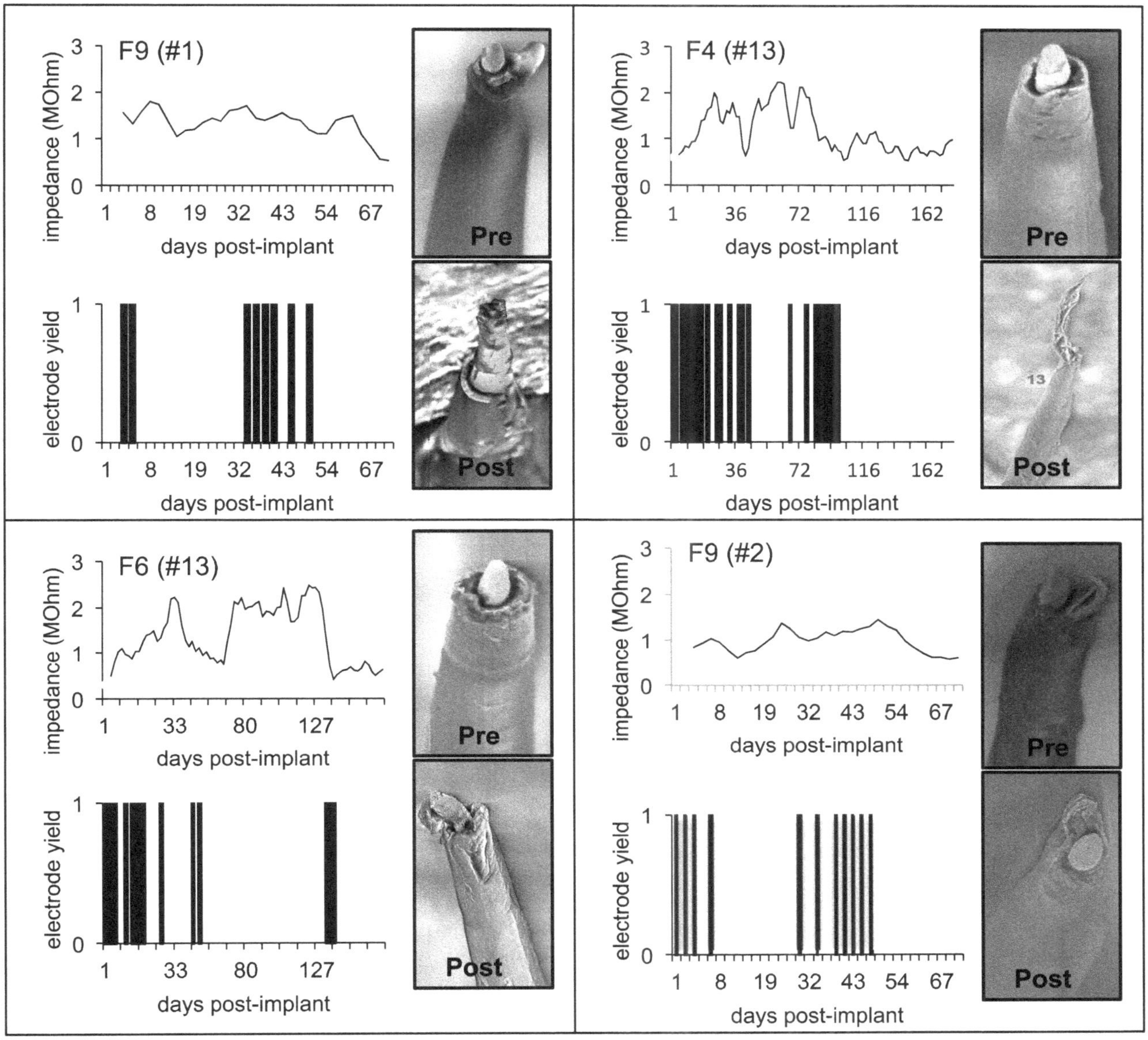

FIGURE 5 | Effect of insulation damage. Pre-implant and post-explant SEM images are shown for four Pt/Ir electrodes in three chronic animals that undergoes delamination during their respective implant durations. Insulation delamination results in a decline in 1 KHz electrode impedance combined with poor functional performance (low yield). Functional performance is characterized by electrode yield on each of the recording days. A zero yield suggests that the respective electrode was not able to record a single unit whereas a 1 suggests that the electrode was able to record a single unit.

histopathology markers which is consistent with our hypothesis that neuroinflammation was not correlated with electrode performance.

DISCUSSION

We presented in this study an *in vivo* abiotic and biotic characterization approach for Pt/Ir microelectrode arrays in chronic implants. The study combined SEM imaging, impedance spectroscopy, histopathology with electrode functional performance so that better understanding of long-term microelectrode performance can be achieved. Abiotic and biotic measurements were performed over 6-months of implant duration revealing changes that occurred at the electrode-tissue interface affecting functional performance of the microelectrodes. This study was predicated on the hypothesis that failure of this electrode type occurred as a result of both abiotic and biotic factors. Pre-implant SEM imaging showed significant variation between electrodes even within the same array indicating manufacturing imperfections. Post-explant SEM imaging indicated that Pt/Ir electrodes did not suffer from deterioration due to corrosion

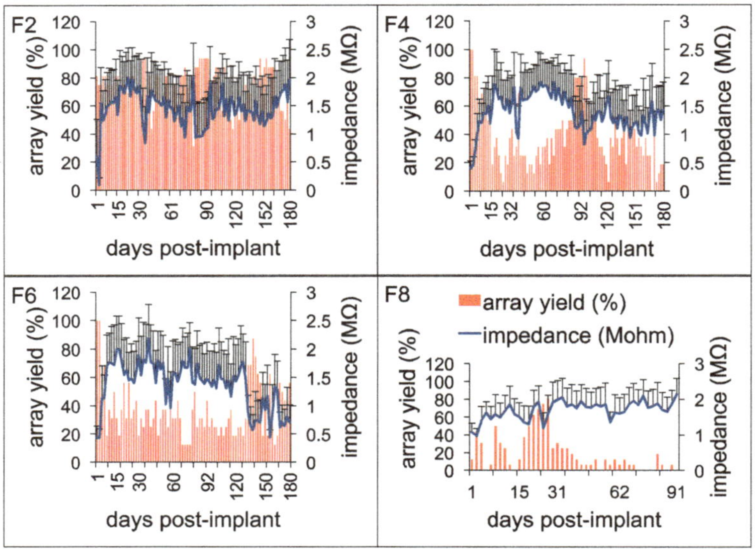

FIGURE 6 | Electrode impedance and electrophysiology trends. Daily array yield (red) and average 1 KHz impedance trends (blue) for four long-term animals (F2, F4, F6: 6-months; F8: 3-months) to show the large daily variations in electrode impedance that result in low array yield. Array yield was defined as the percentage of electrodes out of 16 electrodes in an array that was able to isolate at least a single neuron during a recording session. Error bars depict standard deviations among the impedance values recorded from 16 electrodes during a recording session.

like tungsten (Prasad et al., 2012), however electrodes exhibited deformation of the recording sites such as bent or cracked tips. In addition, deterioration of insulation material was observed among all electrodes in all animals in the form of insulation delamination and cracking. Generally, electrode impedance reduced chronically in electrodes that had insulation deterioration and poor functional performance. Histopathological evaluation suggested modest elevation of microglial markers for longest-term animals. In contrast, we show evidence in this study that the insulation deterioration, manufacturing, and corrosion were the likely abiotic factors contributing to the electrode failure. In addition to the chronic abiotic and biotic effects, we provide evidence that vascular disruption and concurrent intraparenchymal hemorrhaging during brain implantation is a major biotic factor that likely contributes to electrode failure.

The results of this study indicate a need for precision and consistency of manufacturing of microelectrode arrays, an improvement that will likely play a major role in the long-term performance (Prasad and Sanchez, 2012; Prasad et al., 2012; Streit et al., 2012; Barrese et al., 2013). Of particular interest is the recording site itself and interface between that site and the surrounding insulation. Pre-implant variations such as those depicted in **Figure 3** provide a weak or fault site on the microelectrodes that will lead to an accelerated deterioration of the recording surface of individual electrodes. We observed that electrodes with imperfections prior to implantation were more susceptible to morphological changes during the implant period (**Figure 5**). Manufacturing defects at the recording sites provided fault sites where accelerated deterioration happened resulting in a decreased electrode impedance and poor functional performance (**Figure 5**). Therefore, to mitigate the variability arising out of the manufacturing process, greater quality control measures should be employed pre-implant to ensure that implanted electrodes are all of good quality. The manufacturer of the FMAs manipulated the amount of deinsulation for each microwire during the laser cutting process to control the impedance. For this study, FMAs were custom-ordered with 100–150 KΩ as the impedance for each microwire. That value of impedance was chosen based upon our experience with tungsten microwires that had the best electrode yield for the impedance range 40–150 KΩ (Prasad and Sanchez, 2012). Pre-implant baseline impedance measurements for these Pt/Ir FMAs were in the range 100–400 KΩ at 1 kHz measured in PBS. While the intent of the deinsulation process was to control impedance, observations from the electrodes used in this study revealed that the process is not as precise as would be desired and there is inconsistency in the manufacturing process (**Figure 3**). Variance in the starting impedance and manufacturing is compounded by changes in impedance following surgery, which were approximately 2–3 times compared to that measured *in vitro*. The impedance increased progressively over the next 4-week period reaching up to 2–3 MΩ. We observed larger increase in impedance value for these microwires in the first 2–3 weeks as compared to tungsten microwires during the same time period (Williams et al., 2007; Ward et al., 2009; Prasad et al., 2012). While in general, impedance value for tungsten microwires was in the range 30–400 KΩ (Prasad and Sanchez, 2012), the impedance of Pt/Ir microwires were in the order of 1–3 MΩ for most electrodes during the course of chronic implant. This may be attributed to the sharp recording surfaces (smaller geometric surface area) of the Pt/Ir microwires compared to blunt cut recording tips (larger geometric surface area) of tungsten microwires. We and

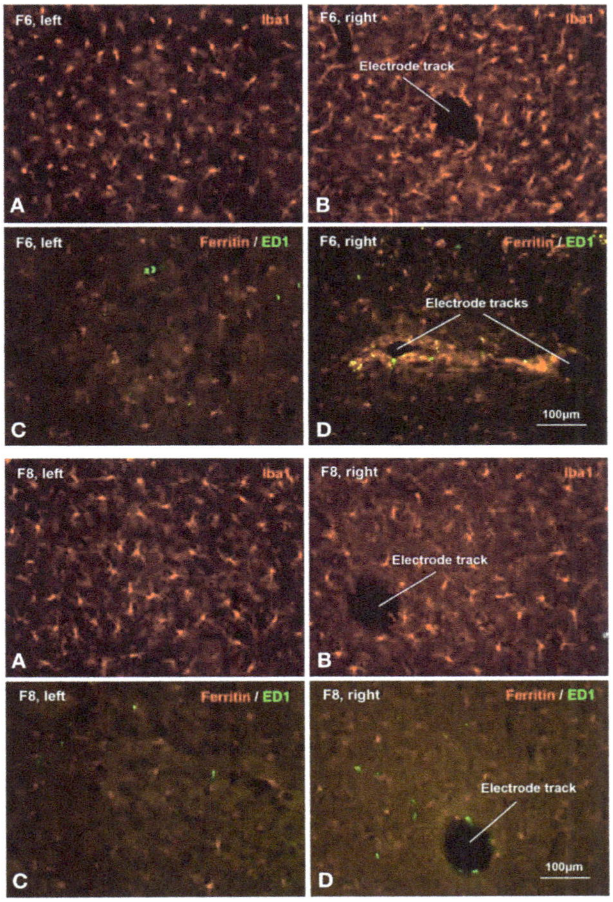

FIGURE 7 | Histopathology. Histopathological staining of microglial cells in two chronically implanted animals, F8 (91 days, top panel) and F6 (180 days, bottom panel). In F8, poor electrode array yield was correlated with minimal microglial activation. Comparing Iba1 labeling on the non-implanted contralateral side **(A)** with the implanted side **(B)** it is evident that microglia display a characteristic resting morphology as well as similar density on both sides. There was only modest upregulation of ED1 and ferritin expression in F8, as seen in **Table 2** and in panels **(C,D)**. In F6, a moderate-to-good array yield correlated with minimal microglial activation. Comparing panels **(A,B)** microglia appear slightly hypertrophic and somewhat increased in number. Ferritin expression was upregulated modestly and to a similar extent as in F8 (**Table 2**). Panel **(D)** shows an example of the maximal ferritin upregulation observed around electrode tracks in this animal.

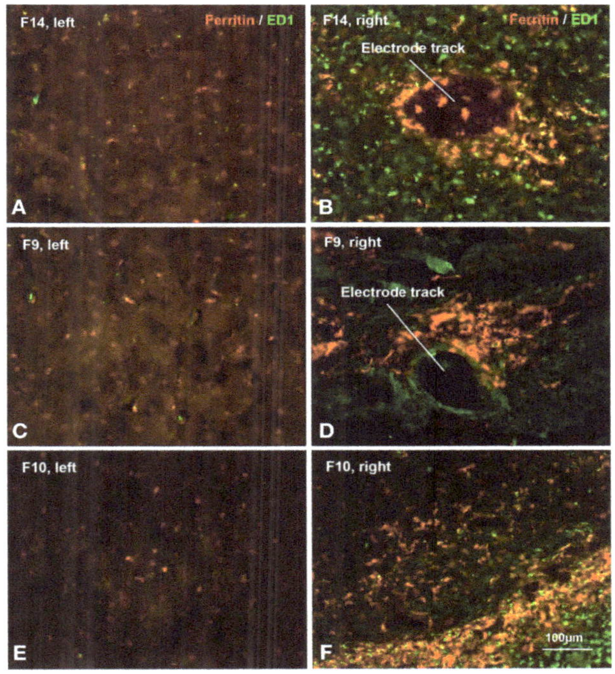

FIGURE 8 | Hemorrhage. Increased ferritin expression in animals with poor electrode performance. Shown are micrographs from three different rats all illustrating dramatic upregulation of ferritin (see also **Table 2**). **(A,B)** F14 is 7 dpi (days post-implantation) and shows a 20-fold increase; **(C,D)** F9 is 71 dpi and shows a 48-fold increase; **(E,F)** F10 is 21 dpi and shows a 91-fold increase in ferritin expression over the control (left) side. The animals also show strong upregulation of both Iba1 and ED1 markers (**Table 2**). These histopathological findings are indicative of significant tissue damage, hemorrhage, and BBB disruption.

others have reported for tungsten microwires large daily variation in impedance values within an array during the first 3–4 weeks after which the impedance reduced and there were smaller daily variations in the chronic period (Ward et al., 2009; Prasad and Sanchez, 2012; Prasad et al., 2012). In comparison, there was greater day-to-day variability in impedances for Pt/Ir microwires during the entire implant duration as suggested by large error bars (**Figure 6**). In addition to the abiotic factors affecting electrode impedance, the trends in impedance during the chronic lifetime of the electrodes also suggest the involvement of biotic factors. The cellular changes occurring in the local environment of the electrode tips is a likely contributor of the daily changes in the observed electrode impedance (Williams et al., 2007).

In addition to the electrode insulation interface, our results strongly suggest the bulk insulation itself is an important contributor leading to electrode failure. We have evaluated two of the most commonly used insulation materials in neural electrodes: Polyimide coated tungsten wires (Prasad et al., 2012) and Parylene-C coated Pt/Ir wires (in this study). Insulation delamination and cracking was evident among all wires across all animals for both insulation types (**Figure 4B**). However, there was a large variation in the extent of the insulation deterioration even between electrodes in the same array. We observed electrodes that had insulation damage pre-implant were more prone to undergo insulation deterioration during the chronic implant (**Figure 5**). Insulation damage results in leakage resistance and parasitic capacitance (Kane et al., 2013) and continuous decrease in impedance, which leads to an accelerated damage causing decrease in electrode functional performance (**Figure 5**). These results indicate that electrode delamination and cracking to be a significant failure mode and steps must be taken in order to evaluate better electrode insulation materials in future.

Material differences should also be considered while choosing electrode metals for recording purposes. In previous studies, we

Table 2 | Histopathology.

Animal groups	Rat No.	Days post-implant	Iba1		ED1		Ferritin	
			Left	Right	Left	Right	Left	Right
Short-term implants (≤15 days)	F11	15	2819	10,901	66	826	487	7104
	F12	7	2226	14,248	74	998	745	18,330
	F13	15	4219	14,747	78	687	288	2685
	F14	7	1731	15,941	131	881	248	4974
	F15	6	4761	17,966	19	999	367	5925
Chronic implants (≤6 months)	F9	71	850	16,137	16	253	64	3094
	F10	21	1555	15,149	59	1157	78	7106
	F2	180	3519	4133	594	280	911	2273
	F4	180	2402	3158	260	385	976	2481
	F6	180	1836	2647	125	125	950	2839
	F7	90	4058	4727	35	429	299	4893
	F8	91	1495	2225	24	74	493	1401

Total positive areas of each of the stains for all animals with Pt/Ir array implants. Right refers to the implanted tissue and left refers to the contralateral control tissue.

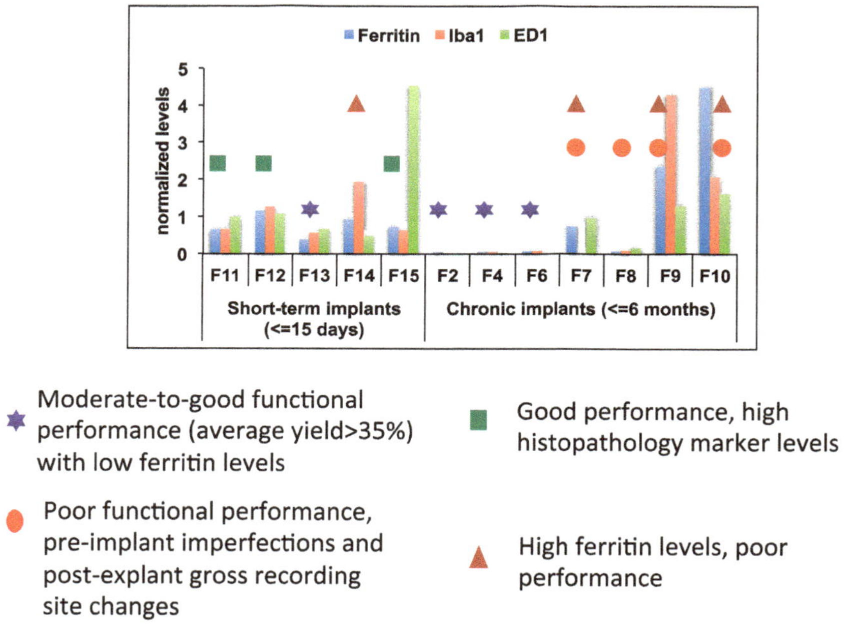

FIGURE 9 | Combined analysis. Combined abiotic-biotic analysis to include histological, morphological, and functional performance for all animals to indicate contributing failure modes.

have observed that tungsten undergoes rapid corrosion *in vitro* (Patrick et al., 2011) and *in vivo* for implants as early as 1-week following surgery (Prasad et al., 2012). We reported that deterioration of tungsten continued in the chronic phase in the form of recording sites becoming more recessed. Therefore, choice of recording material was one of the contributing abiotic failure modes for tungsten electrodes. However, we observed in this study that Pt/Ir provides better recording surfaces and corrosion was not as big of an issue as with tungsten. **Figure 4A** shows various Pt/Ir electrodes both pre-implant and post-explant for varying implant durations (7 days–6 months). We can observe that corrosion was not a significant problem. We did not observe recessed recording sites like tungsten in any of the electrodes and across animals. Even for electrodes, which underwent large morphological changes at the electrode recording sites (**Figure 4B**), electrodes were not as much affected by corrosion. Therefore, corrosion does not appear to be a significant contributing factor to electrode failure for Pt/Ir electrodes.

One of the experimental design factors that enabled deeper insight to electrode failure is that we coupled electrode array functional performance with impedance spectroscopy to study if there was a functional relationship between them. Electrode array functional performance was quantified by array yield which was defined as the percentage of electrodes in an array that were able to isolate single units. Higher array yield are desirable for a neuroprosthetic application. In general for these floating arrays, 1 kHz impedance magnitude trends were similar for long-term animals where impedance increased progressively in the first 2–3 weeks and then decreased in the subsequent weeks with occasional increases and decreases in the chronic period (**Figure 6**). We observed that array yield generally declined during this initial 2–3 week period following implant attributed as a result of surgical trauma in other studies (Biran et al., 2005). Poor array yield (<25% yield) was observed when impedance was high (>1.5 MΩ) and yield increased when impedance was low during the late chronic period (>12 weeks) for long-term animals (**Figure 6**). The daily variations observed in average impedance magnitude corresponded with moderate (25–70% yield) to poor (<25% yield) functional yield from these Pt/Ir MEAs among all animals (**Table 1**).

There is a cascade of biological reactions that occur following an electrode implant surgery that in brief includes activation and recruitment of astrocytes, microglia, and macrophages at the implant site in order to isolate the implanted device and repair the damaged tissue (Polikov et al., 2005; Thelin et al., 2011; Kozai et al., 2012b). Several studies have pointed out the time course of such biological reactions occurring at the tissue-electrode interface that begin as early as right after insertion and continue as long as the implant is in the neural tissue (Szarowski et al., 2003; Freire et al., 2011; Prasad et al., 2012). Of course, the most obvious and inevitable biological consequence of intracerebral electrode insertion, or for that matter any type of traumatic brain injury, is a neuroinflammatory response. Neuroinflammation is mediated primarily by activated microglial cells which is why we have focused our attention on these cells in this and prior studies (Prasad et al., 2011, 2012; Streit et al., 2012). Our findings with regard to activated microglia were as expected in that electrode implantation elicited widespread microglial activation at the implantation site, which in most cases became somewhat attenuated over time. However, we also studied microglial degeneration, evident as cytoplasmic fragmentation, which we believe is a direct consequence of oxidative stress brought about by influx of free iron through intracerebral bleeding. In contrast to our prior study with tungsten microwires where microglial degeneration was observed only during early survival times, the current study shows that microglial degeneration can also occur during relatively late time points (**Figure 8**), especially in animals where there was significant intracerebral bleeding thus supporting our belief that microglial cytoplasmic fragmentation occurs as a direct consequence of iron-mediated oxidative stress.

In conclusion, the results of our study serve to further illuminate the problem of electrode failure by focusing attention on two major failure modes, one abiotic and the other one biotic. Future efforts geared toward prolonging the functional lifetime of electrodes should thus be focused on further improving electrode manufacturing practices and on innovative ways of minimizing intracerebral bleeding and associated oxidative stress.

ACKNOWLEDGMENTS

This work was sponsored by the Defense Advanced Research Projects Agency (DARPA) Microsystems Technology Office under the auspices of Dr. Jack Judy (jack.judy@darpa.mil) through the Space and Naval Warfare Systems Center, Pacific Grant No. N66001-11-1-4009.

REFERENCES

Andrei, A., Welkenhuysen, M., Nuttin, B., and Eberle, W. (2012). A response surface model predicting the *in vivo* insertion behavior of micromachined neural implants. *J. Neural Eng.* 9:016005. doi: 10.1088/1741-2560/9/1/016005

Andrews, R. J. (2010). Neuromodulation: advances in the next five years. *Ann. N.Y. Acad. Sci.* 1199, 204–211. doi: 10.1111/j.1749-6632.2009.05379.x

Barrese, J. C., Rao, N., Paroo, K., Triebwasser, C., Vargas-Irwin, C., Franquemont, L., et al. (2013). Failure mode analysis of silicon-based intracortical microelectrode arrays in non-human primates. *J. Neural Eng.* 10:066014. doi: 10.1088/1741-2560/10/6/066014

Biran, R., Martin, D. C., and Tresco, P. A. (2005). Neuronal cell loss accompanies the brain tissue response to chronically implanted silicon microelectrode arrays. *Exp. Neurol.* 195, 115–126. doi: 10.1016/j.expneurol.2005.04.020

Biran, R., Martin, D. C., and Tresco, P. A. (2007). The brain tissue response to implanted silicon microelectrode arrays is increased when the device is tethered to the skull. *J. Biomed. Mater. Res.* 82, 169–178. doi: 10.1002/jbm.a.31138

Brett, M. A. C., and Brett, A. M. O. (1993). *Electrochemistry: Principles, Methods and Applications.* New York, NY: Oxford Science.

Cogan, S. F. (2008). Neural stimulation and recording electrodes. *Annu. Rev. Biomed. Eng.* 10, 275–309. doi: 10.1146/annurev.bioeng.10.061807.160518

Collinger, J. L., Wodlinger, B., Downey, J. E., Wang, W., Tyler-Kabara, E. C., Weber, D. J., et al. (2013). High-performance neuroprosthetic control by an individual with tetraplegia. *Lancet* 381, 557–564. doi: 10.1016/S0140-6736(12) 61816-9

Csicsvari, J., Henze, D. A., Jamieson, B., Harris, K. D., Sirota, A., Barthó, P., et al. (2003). Massively parallel recording of unit and local field potentials with silicon-based electrodes. *J. Neurophysiol.* 90, 1314–1323. doi: 10.1152/jn.00116.2003

Dijkstra, C. D., Dopp, E. A., Joling, P., and Kraal, G. (1985). The Heterogeneity of mononuclear phagocytes in lymphoid organs - distinct macrophage subpopulations in the rat recognized by monoclonal antibody-Ed1, antibody-Ed2 and antibody-Ed3. *Immunology* 54, 589–599.

Drake, K. L., Wise, K. D., Farraye, J., Anderson, D. J., and Bement, S. L. (1988). Performance of planar multisite microprobes in recording extracellular single-unit intracortical activity. *IEEE Trans. Biomed. Eng.* 35, 719–732. doi: 10.1109/10.7273

Edell, D. J., Vo Van, T., McNeil, V. M., and Clark, L. D. (1992). Factors influencing the biocompatibility of insertable silicon microshafts in cerebral cortex. *IEEE Trans. Biomed. Eng.* 39, 635–643. doi: 10.1109/10.141202

Ethier, C., Oby, E. R., Bauman, M. J., and Miller, L. E. (2012). Restoration of grasp following paralysis through brain-controlled stimulation of muscles. *Nature* 485, 368–371. doi: 10.1038/nature10987

Frampton, J. P., Hynd, M. R., Shuler, M. L., and Shain, W. (2010). Effects of glial cells on electrode impedance recorded from neuralprosthetic devices *in vitro*. *Ann. Biomed. Eng.* 38, 1031–1047. doi: 10.1007/s10439-010-9911-y

Freire, M. A., Morya, E., Faber, J., Santos, J. R., Guimaraes, J. S., Lemos, N. A., et al. (2011). Comprehensive analysis of tissue preservation and recording quality from chronic multielectrode implants. *PLoS ONE* 6:e27554. doi: 10.1371/journal.pone.0027554

Geddes, L. A. (1997). Historical evolution of circuit models for the electrode-electrolyte interface. *Ann. Biomed. Eng.* 25, 1–14. doi: 10.1007/BF02738534

Geddes, L. A., and Roeder, R. (2003). Criteria for the selection of materials for implanted electrodes. *Ann. Biomed. Eng.* 31, 879–890. doi: 10.1114/1.1581292

Grill, W. M., and Mortimer, J. T. (1994). Electrical properties of implant encapsulation tissue. *Ann. Biomed. Eng.* 22, 23–33. doi: 10.1007/BF02368219

Hochberg, L. R., Bacher, D., Jarosiewicz, B., Masse, N. Y., Simeral, J. D., Vogel, J., et al. (2012). Reach and grasp by people with tetraplegia using a neurally controlled robotic arm. *Nature* 485, 372–375. doi: 10.1038/nature11076

Iosa, M., Morone, G., Fusco, A., Bragoni, M., Coiro, P., Multari, M., et al. (2012). Seven capital devices for the future of stroke rehabilitation. *Stroke Res. Treat.* 2012:187965. doi: 10.1155/2012/187965

Jackson, A., and Fetz, E. E. (2007). Compact movable microwire array for long-term chronic unit recording in cerebral cortex of primates. *J. Neurophysiol.* 98, 3109–3118. doi: 10.1152/jn.00569.2007

Jackson, A., and Zimmermann, J. B. (2012). Neural interfaces for the brain and spinal cord-restoring motor function. *Nat. Rev. Neurol.* 8, 690–699. doi: 10.1038/nrneurol.2012.219

Johnson, M. D., Otto, K. J., and Kipke, D. R. (2005). Repeated voltage biasing improves unit recordings by reducing resistive tissue impedances. *IEEE Trans. Neural Syst. Rehabil. Eng.* 13, 160–165. doi: 10.1109/TNSRE.2005.847373

Kam, L., Shain, W., Turner, J. N., and Bizios, R. (1999). Correlation of astroglial cell function on micro-patterned surfaces with specific geometric parameters. *Biomaterials* 20, 2343–2350. doi: 10.1016/S0142-9612(99)00163-5

Kane, S. R., Cogan, S. F., Ehrlich, J., Plante, T. D., McCreery, D. B., and Troyk, P. R. (2013). Electrical performance of penetrating microelectrodes chronically implanted in cat cortex. *IEEE Trans. Biomed. Eng.* 60, 2153–2160. doi: 10.1109/TBME.2013.2248152

Karumbaiah, L., Saxena, T., Carlson, D., Patil, K., Patkar, R., Gaupp, E. A., et al. (2013). Relationship between intracortical electrode design and chronic recording function. *Biomaterials* 34, 8061–8074. doi: 10.1016/j.biomaterials.2013.07.016

Kim, B. J., Kuo, J. T., Hara, S. A., Lee, C. D., Yu, L., Gutierrez, C. A., et al. (2013). 3D Parylene sheath neural probe for chronic recordings. *J. Neural Eng.* 10:045002. doi: 10.1088/1741-2560/10/4/045002

Kipke, D. R., Vetter, R. J., Williams, J. C., and Hetke, J. F. (2003). Silicon-substrate intracortical microelectrode arrays for long-term recording of neuronal spike activity in cerebral cortex. *IEEE Trans. Neural Syst. Rehabil. Eng.* 11, 151–155. doi: 10.1109/TNSRE.2003.814443

Koivuniemi, A. S., and Otto, K. J. (2011). Asymmetric versus symmetric pulses for cortical microstimulation. *IEEE Trans. Neural Syst. Rehabil. Eng.* 19, 468–476. doi: 10.1109/TNSRE.2011.2166563

Kozai, T. D. Y., Langhals, N. B., Patel, P. R., Deng, X. P., Zhang, H. N., Smith, K. L., et al. (2012a). Ultrasmall implantable composite microelectrodes with bioactive surfaces for chronic neural interfaces. *Nat. Mater.* 11, 1065–1073. doi: 10.1038/nmat3468

Kozai, T. D., Vazquez, A. L., Weaver, C. L., Kim, S. G., and Cui, X. T. (2012b). *In vivo* two-photon microscopy reveals immediate microglial reaction to implantation of microelectrode through extension of processes. *J. Neural Eng.* 9:066001. doi: 10.1088/1741-2560/9/6/066001

Lee, H., Bellamkonda, R. V., Sun, W., and Levenston, M. E. (2005). Biomechanical analysis of silicon microelectrode-induced strain in the brain. *J. Neural Eng.* 2, 81–89. doi: 10.1088/1741-2560/2/4/003

Lempka, S. F., Johnson, M. D., Moffitt, M. A., Otto, K. J., Kipke, D. R., and McIntyre, C. C. (2011). Theoretical analysis of intracortical microelectrode recordings. *J. Neural Eng.* 8:045006. doi: 10.1088/1741-2560/8/4/045006

Lopes, K. O., Sparks, D. L., and Streit, W. J. (2008). Microglial dystrophy in the aged and Alzheimer's disease brain is associated with ferritin immunoreactivity. *Glia* 56, 1048–1060. doi: 10.1002/glia.20678

Ludwig, K. A., Langhals, N. B., Joseph, M. D., Richardson-Burns, S. M., Hendricks, J. L., and Kipke, D. R. (2011). Poly(3,4-ethylenedioxythiophene) (PEDOT) polymer coatings facilitate smaller neural recording electrodes. *J. Neural Eng.* 8:014001. doi: 10.1088/1741-2560/8/1/014001

Ludwig, K. A., Uram, J. D., Yang, J., Martin, D. C., and Kipke, D. R. (2006). Chronic neural recordings using silicon microelectrode arrays electrochemically deposited with a poly(3,4-ethylenedioxythiophene) (PEDOT) film. *J. Neural Eng.* 3, 59–70. doi: 10.1088/1741-2560/3/1/007

Maling, N., Hashemiyoon, R., Foote, K. D., Okun, M. S., and Sanchez, J. C. (2012). Increased thalamic gamma band activity correlates with symptom relief following deep brain stimulation in humans with tourette's syndrome. *PLoS ONE* 7:e44215. doi: 10.1371/journal.pone.0044215

McConnell, G. C., Butera, R. J., and Bellamkonda, R. V. (2009a). Bioimpedance modeling to monitor astrocytic response to chronically implanted electrodes. *J. Neural Eng.* 6:055005. doi: 10.1088/1741-2560/6/5/055005

McConnell, G. C., Rees, H. D., Levey, A. I., Gutekunst, C. A., Gross, R. E., and Bellamkonda, R. V. (2009b). Implanted neural electrodes cause chronic, local inflammation that is correlated with local neurodegeneration. *J. Neural Eng.* 6:056003. doi: 10.1088/1741-2560/6/5/056003

Merrill, D. R., and Tresco, P. A. (2005). Impedance characterization of microarray recording electrodes *in vitro*. *IEEE Trans. Biomed. Eng.* 52, 1960–1965. doi: 10.1109/TBME.2005.856245

Mollazadeh, M., Aggarwal, V., Davidson, A. G., Law, A. J., Thakor, N. V., and Schieber, M. H. (2011). Spatiotemporal Variation of Multiple Neurophysiological Signals in the Primary Motor Cortex during Dexterous Reach-to-Grasp Movements. *J. Neurosci.* 31, 15531–15543. doi: 10.1523/JNEUROSCI.2999-11.2011

Morrell, M. J. (2011). Responsive cortical stimulation for the treatment of medically intractable partial epilepsy. *Neurology* 77, 1295–1304. doi: 10.1212/WNL.0b013e3182302056

Musallam, S., Bak, M. J., Troyk, P. R., and Andersen, R. A. (2007). A floating metal microelectrode array for chronic implantation. *J. Neurosci. Methods* 160, 122–127. doi: 10.1016/j.jneumeth.2006.09.005

Nicolelis, M. A. L. (1999). *Methods for Neural Ensemble Recordings.* Boca Raton, FL: CRC Press.

Nicolelis, M. A. L., Dimitrov, D., Carmena, J. M., Crist, R., Lehew, G., Kralik, J. D., et al. (2003). Chronic, multisite, multielectrode recordings in macaque monkeys. *Proc. Natl. Acad. Sci. U.S.A.* 100, 11041–11046. doi: 10.1073/pnas.1934665100

Otto, K. J., Johnson, M. D., and Kipke, D. R. (2006). Voltage pulses change neural interface properties and improve unit recordings with chronically implanted microelectrodes. *IEEE Trans. Biomed. Eng.* 53, 333–340. doi: 10.1109/TBME.2005.862530

Otto, K. J., Rousche, P. J., and Kipke, D. R. (2005). Cortical microstimulation in auditory cortex of rat elicits best-frequency dependent behaviors. *J. Neural Eng.* 2, 42–51. doi: 10.1088/1741-2560/2/2/005

Patrick, E., Orazem, M. E., Sanchez, J. C., and Nishida, T. (2011). Corrosion of tungsten microelectrodes used in neural recording applications. *J. Neurosci. Methods* 198, 158–171. doi: 10.1016/j.jneumeth.2011.03.012

Patrick, E., Ordonez, M., Alba, N., Sanchez, J. C., and Nishida, T. (2006). Design and fabrication of a flexible substrate microelectrode array for brain machine interfaces. *Conf. Proc. IEEE Eng. Med. Biol. Soc.* 1, 2966–2969. doi: 10.1109/IEMBS.2006.260581

Polikov, V. S., Tresco, P. A., and Reichert, W. M. (2005). Response of brain tissue to chronically implanted neural electrodes. *J. Neurosci. Methods* 148, 1–18. doi: 10.1016/j.jneumeth.2005.08.015

Prasad, A., and Sanchez, J. C. (2012). Quantifying long-term microelectrode array functionality using chronic *in vivo* impedance testing. *J. Neural Eng.* 9:026028. doi: 10.1088/1741-2560/9/2/026028

Prasad, A., Sankar, V., Dyer, A. T., Knott, E., Xue, Q. S., Nishida, T., et al. (2011). Coupling biotic and abiotic metrics to create a testbed for predicting neural electrode performance. *Conf. Proc. IEEE Eng. Med. Biol. Soc.* 2011, 3020–3023. doi: 10.1109/IEMBS.2011.6090827

Prasad, A., Xue, Q. S., Sankar, V., Nishida, T., Shaw, G., Streit, W. J., et al. (2012). Comprehensive characterization and failure modes of tungsten microwire arrays in chronic neural implants. *J. Neural Eng.* 9:056015. doi: 10.1088/1741-2560/9/5/056015

Richter, A., Xie, Y., Schumacher, A., Loffler, S., Kirch, R. D., Al-Hasani, J., et al. (2013). A simple implantation method for flexible, multisite microelectrodes into rat brains. *Front. Neuroeng.* 6:6. doi: 10.3389/fneng.2013.00006

Rousche, P. J., and Normann, R. A. (1998). Chronic recording capability of the utah intracortical electrode array in cat sensory cortex. *J. Neurosci. Methods* 82, 1–15. doi: 10.1016/S0165-0270(98)00031-4

Rousche, P. J., Pellinen, D. S., Pivin, D. P. Jr., Williams, J. C., Vetter, R. J., and Kipke, D. R. (2001). Flexible polyimide-based intracortical electrode arrays with bioactive capability. *IEEE Trans. Biomed. Eng.* 48, 361–371. doi: 10.1109/10.914800

Rouse, A. G., Stanslaski, S. R., Cong, P., Jensen, R. M., Afshar, P., Ullestad, D., et al. (2011). A chronic generalized bi-directional brain-machine interface. *J. Neural Eng.* 8:036018. doi: 10.1088/1741-2560/8/3/036018

Sanchez, J. C., Alba, N., Nishida, T., Batich, C., and Carney, P. R. (2006). Structural modifications in chronic microwire electrodes for cortical neuroprosthetics: a case study. *IEEE Trans. Neural Syst. Rehabil. Eng.* 14, 217–221. doi: 10.1109/TNSRE.2006.875581

Saxena, T., Karumbaiah, L., Gaupp, E. A., Patkar, R., Patil, K., Betancur, M., et al. (2013). The impact of chronic blood-brain barrier breach on intracortical electrode function. *Biomaterials* 34, 4703–4713. doi: 10.1016/j.biomaterials.2013.03.007

Schmidt, E. M., Bak, M. J., and McIntosh, J. S. (1976). Long term chronic recording from cortical neurons. *Exp. Neurol.* 52, 496–506. doi: 10.1016/0014-4886(76)90220-X

Stensaas, S. S., and Stensaas, L. J. (1978). Histopathological evaluation of materials implanted in the cerebral cortex. *Acta Neuropathol.* 41, 145–155. doi: 10.1007/BF00689766

Streit, W., Xue, Q. S., Prasad, A., Sankar, V., Knott, E., Dyer, A., et al. (2012). Electrode failure: tissue, electrical, and material responses. *IEEE Pulse* 3, 30–33. doi: 10.1109/MPUL.2011.2175632

Suner, S., Fellows, M. R., Vargas-Irwin, C., Nakata, G. K., and Donoghue, J. P. (2005). Reliability of signals from a chronically implanted, silicon-based electrode array in non-human primate primary motor cortex. *IEEE Trans. Neural Syst. Rehabil. Eng.* 13, 524–541. doi: 10.1109/TNSRE.2005.857687

Szarowski, D. H., Andersen, M. D., Retterer, S., Spence, A. J., Isaacson, M., Craighead, H. G., et al. (2003). Brain responses to micro-machined silicon devices. *Brain Res.* 983, 23–35. doi: 10.1016/S0006-8993(03)03023-3

Thelin, J., Jorntell, H., Psouni, E., Garwicz, M., Schouenborg, J., Danielsen, N., et al. (2011). Implant size and fixation mode strongly influence tissue reactions in the CNS. *PLoS ONE* 6:e16267. doi: 10.1371/journal.pone.0016267

Truccolo, W., Donoghue, J. A., Hochberg, L. R., Eskandar, E. N., Madsen, J. R., Anderson, W. S., et al. (2011). Single-neuron dynamics in human focal epilepsy. *Nat. Neurosci.* 14, 635–641. doi: 10.1038/nn.2782

Turner, J. N., Shain, W., Szarowski, D. H., Andersen, M., Martins, S., Isaacson, M., et al. (1999). Cerebral astrocyte response to micromachined silicon implants. *Exp. Neurol.* 156, 33–49. doi: 10.1006/exnr.1998.6983

Vetter, R. J., Williams, J. C., Hetke, J. F., Nunamaker, E. A., and Kipke, D. R. (2004). Chronic neural recording using silicon-substrate microelectrode arrays implanted in cerebral cortex. *IEEE Trans. Neural Syst. Rehabil. Eng.* 51, 896–904. doi: 10.1109/TBME.2004.826680

Ward, M. P., Rajdev, P., Ellison, C., and Irazoqui, P. P. (2009). Toward a comparison of microelectrodes for acute and chronic recordings. *Brain Res.* 1282, 183–200. doi: 10.1016/j.brainres.2009.05.052

Williams, J. C., Hippensteel, J. A., Dilgen, J., Shain, W., and Kipke, D. R. (2007). Complex impedance spectroscopy for monitoring tissue responses to inserted neural implants. *J. Neural Eng.* 4, 410–423. doi: 10.1088/1741-2560/4/4/007

Williams, J. C., Rennaker, R. L., and Kipke, D. R. (1999a). Long-term neural recording characteristics of wire microelectrode arrays implanted in cerebral cortex. *Brain Res. Protoc.* 4, 303–313. doi: 10.1016/S1385-299X(99)00034-3

Williams, J. C., Rennaker, R. L., and Kipke, D. R. (1999b). Stability of chronic multichannel neural recordings: Implications for a long-term neural interface. *Neurocomputing* 26–27, 1069–1076. doi: 10.1016/S0925-2312(99)00106-X

Winslow, B. D., and Tresco, P. A. (2010). Quantitative analysis of the tissue response to chronically implanted microwire electrodes in rat cortex. *Biomaterials* 31, 1558–1567. doi: 10.1016/j.biomaterials.2009.11.049

14

The importance of systemic response in the pathobiology of blast-induced neurotrauma

Ibolja Cernak*

Biomedicine Business Area, National Security Technology Department, Johns Hopkins University Applied Physics Laboratory, Laurel, MD, USA

Edited by:
Marten Risling, Karolinska Institutet, Sweden

Reviewed by:
Marten Risling, Karolinska Institutet, Sweden
Hans Lindå, Karolinska Institutet, Sweden

****Correspondence:***
Ibolja Cernak, Johns Hopkins University Applied Physics Laboratory, 11100 Johns Hopkins Road, Mail Stop MP2 N108, Laurel, MD 20723, USA.
e-mail: ibolja.cernak@jhuapl.edu

Due to complex injurious environment where multiple blast effects interact with the body parallel, blast-induced neurotrauma is a unique clinical entity induced by systemic, local, and cerebral responses. Activation of autonomous nervous system; sudden pressure increase in vital organs such as lungs and liver; and activation of neuroendocrine–immune system are among the most important mechanisms that contribute significantly to molecular changes and cascading injury mechanisms in the brain. It has been hypothesized that vagally mediated cerebral effects play a vital role in the early response to blast: this assumption has been supported by experiments where bilateral vagotomy mitigated bradycardia, hypotension, and apnea, and also prevented excessive metabolic alterations in the brain of animals exposed to blast. Clinical experience suggests specific blast–body–nervous system interactions such as (1) direct interaction with the head either through direct passage of the blast wave through the skull or by causing acceleration and/or rotation of the head; and (2) via hydraulic interaction, when the blast overpressure compresses the abdomen and chest, and transfers its kinetic energy to the body's fluid phase, initiating oscillating waves that traverse the body and reach the brain. Accumulating evidence suggests that inflammation plays important role in the pathogenesis of long-term neurological deficits due to blast. These include memory decline, motor function and balance impairments, and behavioral alterations, among others. Experiments using rigid body- or head protection in animals subjected to blast showed that head protection failed to prevent inflammation in the brain or reduce neurological deficits, whereas body protection was successful in alleviating the blast-induced functional and morphological impairments in the brain.

Keywords: blast, traumatic brain injury, autonomous nervous system, inflammation

INTRODUCTION

The history of blast injuries coincides with the history of explosives and modern warfare. Blast effects from high explosives have been described in the World Wars I and II as well as in the military actions of the twentieth and current centuries. For several reasons, the wars of the twenty-first century brought a new injury pattern: (1) the overwhelming majority of injuries are caused by explosions or blasts by rocket-propelled grenades, improvised explosive devices (IEDs), and land mines (Ritenour et al., 2010); (2) the mortality caused by explosion is relatively low due to improved interceptive properties of body armors, effectiveness of treatments, and promptness of medical evacuation, among others; and (3) due to increased survivability, the rate of severe, long-term deficits shows increasing trend. Based on the U.S. Defense and Veterans Brain Injury Center (DVBIC) analysis, approximately 180,000 U.S. military service members had a diagnosis of traumatic brain injury (TBI) in the period of 2001–2010. The overwhelming distribution of mild TBI (mTBI) was caused by blast. Because many servicemen with potential TBI remain undiagnosed or have delayed diagnosis, this number could be potentially higher (Terrio et al., 2009).

The complexity of the injurious environment generated by an explosion has been long recognized (Zuckerman, 1940). The injuries caused by multiple effects of the blast wave have been identified as: (a) primary blast injury cased by the blast wave itself; (b) secondary injury caused by the fragments of debris propelled by the explosion; (c) tertiary injury due to the acceleration of the body or part of the body by the blast wind and the sudden deceleration when it hits a ground or surrounding object; and (d) flash burns or toxic gas inhalation due to the intense heat of the explosion (Owen-Smith, 1981). It has been long posited that primary blast, e.g., blast overpressure generated during an explosion typically affects gas-containing organs through main mechanisms such as spalling, implosion, inertia, and pressure differences. On the other hand, the possibility of blast-induced neurotrauma (BINT) remained underestimated due to an outdated dogma that neurologic impairments caused by primary blasts are rare since the skull provides excellent protection for the brain (Rossle, 1950). Interestingly, despite several detailed reports published in 1940s portraying neurological symptoms in soldiers exposed to blast and describing underlying clinical findings and morphological changes in the brain not seen before (Stewart and Russel, 1941; Garai, 1944), the medical community ignored the pre-existing knowledge and attributed neurologic impairments due to blast to rare cases of air emboli in cerebral blood vessels (Clemedson, 1956).

While many servicemen with TBI experience remission of their symptoms, over one-third suffers at least one mTBI-related symptom at the post-deployment health assessment (Terrio et al., 2009). Immediately after exposure, individuals exposed to blast reported memory loss for events before and after explosion, confusion, impaired sense of reality, and reduced decision-making ability (Cernak et al., 1999a,b; Martin et al., 2008; Warden et al., 2009). Later, sometimes months and years after blast exposure, patients with BINT may experience irritability; memory and speech problems (reduced verbal fluency, working memory, and executive functioning; Nelson et al., 2009); headache; dizziness and balance problems (Hoffer et al., 2010); as well as psychological impairments such as depression and post-traumatic stress disorder (Terrio et al., 2009; Peskind et al., 2010). While many question the possibility that primary blast could have damaging effects to the brain, there is a higher-level agreement about the aspects of BINT that sets aside this pathological condition from civilian TBI, including high rates of sensory impairment, increased sensitivity toward pain issues, multiple organ involvement, and strong emotional context in which the injury occurred (French, 2010).

Thus, to be able to develop reliable and accurate diagnostic tools, efficient and timely treatments, and successful preventive measures, we have to identify what makes BINT potentially different from civilian TBI, and specify the main elements involved in the complexity of BINT.

BASIC MECHANISMS OF BINT

Traumatic brain injury of all types and etiologies is caused by mechanical factors interacting with the brain either directly or indirectly. It is a complex process that consists of four overlapping phases: primary injury; evolution of the primary injury; secondary or additional injury; and regeneration (Reilly, 2001; Cernak, 2005). In civilian, non-blast TBI, the primary injury develops as a consequence of a direct interaction between the mechanical force and the head. The predominate injury causes are (1) direct contusion of the brain from the skull as a consequence of a direct hit; (2) brain contusion caused by a movement against rough interior surfaces of the skull, and/or indirect contusion of the brain opposite to the sate of the impact, i.e., coup–contrecoup; (3) shearing and stretching of the brain tissue due to a motion of the brain structures relative to each other or the skull; and (4) vascular consequences of the impact such as subdural hematoma originating from ruptured bridging blood vessels between brain and dura mater; reduced cerebral blood flow caused by intracranial pressure or infarction (Greve and Zink, 2009); and brain edema developing as a consequence of increased permeability of cerebral vasculature.

In BINT, these primary injury categories can be induced by: (a) fragments of the environment generated by explosion (so called "secondary blast effect") and impacting the head causing either blunt or penetrating head trauma; or (b) when explosion propels (i.e., accelerates) the body through the air and the brain is contused either due to the acceleration/deceleration (coup–contrecoup), or a hit from the surrounding objects or ground (so called "tertiary blast effect"). Nevertheless, in addition to these primary injury categories seen in civilian environment, primary blast is a unique injurious factor that is exclusively generated by explosion. The shockwave or blast wave, comprised of a high-pressure front that compresses the surrounding air and is followed by a negative pressure phase, is the major determinant of primary blast-induced injury. It travels with a high velocity, often thousands km/h (Owen-Smith, 1981), and damages its surroundings in few milliseconds. Primary blast envelops the whole body, and interacts with all organs and organ systems, including the brain, simultaneously (Cernak and Noble-Haeusslein, 2010). The main mechanisms by which primary blast may cause brain injury can be direct or indirect. A direct passage of the blast wave through the skull might cause bruising, acceleration, or rotation of the brain. On the other hand, as the front of the blast wave connects with the elastic body wall, it compresses the abdomen and chest transferring its kinetic energy inside the body, to the body's fluid phase (i.e., blood). The resulting "rippling" effect generates oscillating waves in the blood that traverse the body delivering the kinetic energy of the blast wave to organs, including the brain, remote from the initial point of coupling. Once delivered, that kinetic energy initiates functional and morphological alterations in distinct, mainly deep brain structures (Cernak et al., 1999a; Warden et al., 2009; Peskind et al., 2010). This second, indirect interactive pathway is unique for BINT, and underlies its immense complexity as compared to non-blast TBI.

SYSTEMIC EFFECTS OF BINT

Blast-induced neurotrauma is caused by multiple, interwoven mechanisms of systemic, local, and cerebral responses to blast exposure, often interacting with the body simultaneously (Cernak et al., 1991, 1996b; Cernak and Noble-Haeusslein, 2010; **Figure 1**). While the importance of multi-system, multi-organ response to blast exposure is more obvious in moderate-to-severe brain injuries, it is often neglected in the case of mild BINT. Nevertheless, accumulating clinical and experimental evidence show that systemic and local alterations initiated by blast significantly influence the brain's response, thus contribute to the pathobiology of acute and/or chronic deficits due to blast.

IMMEDIATE ACTIVATION OF THE AUTONOMOUS NERVOUS SYSTEM

In the experiments using rabbits, the animals were exposed to a blast overpressure generated by a compressed air-driven shock tube and causing mild-to-moderate blast lung injury. Aiming to analyze the effects of instantaneous activation of parasympathetic nervous system (PSNS) on the early response to blast, one subset of the animals was subjected to pulmonary deafferentation performed by bilateral dissection of the vagus 2 h before a blast exposure. Measured 30 min after blast exposure, brain edema and significant metabolic disturbances were found in the brain including decreased glucose and adenosine-triphosphate (ATP) concentrations (Cernak et al., 1996b); increased calcium and reduced magnesium concentrations as well as reduced magnesium/calcium ratio (Cernak et al., 1995). Bilateral vagotomy successfully mitigated bradycardia, hypotension, and apnea caused by blast; prevented extreme metabolic alterations and brain edema; but failed to eliminate oxidative stress in the brain due to blast (Cernak et al., 1996b).

It was hypothesized that hyperinflation of the lungs caused by blast overpressure stimulates the juxtacapillary J-receptors located in the alveolar interstitium and innervated by vagal fibers, triggering a vago-vagal reflex that leads to apnea followed by tachypnea, bradycardia, and hypotension (Zuckerman, 1940; Cernak et al., 1996b). In addition, hypoxia/ischemia caused by the pulmonary vagal reflex stimulates chemoreceptors in the left ventricle and subsequently activates a cardiovascular decompressor Bezold–Jarish reflex leading to significant parasympathetic efferent discharge to the heart

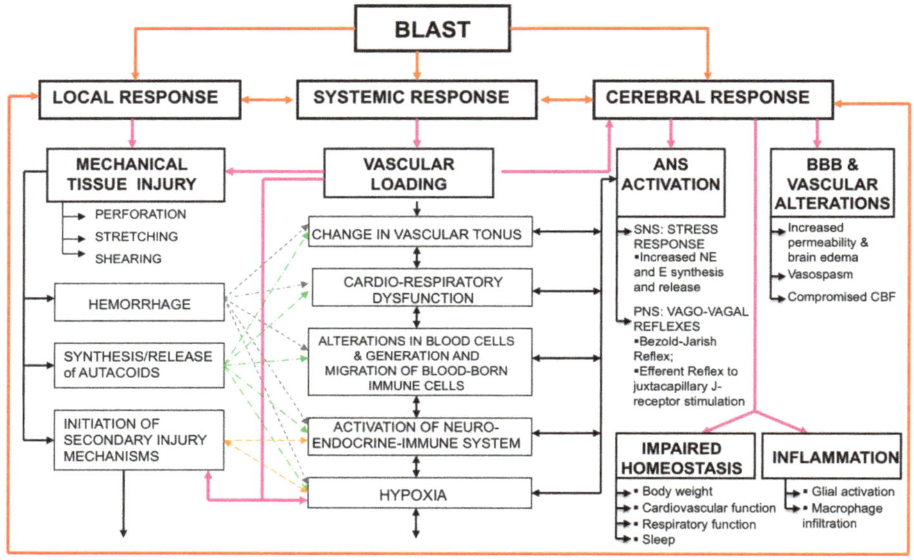

FIGURE 1 | Simultaneous activation of systemic, local, and cerebral responses to blast exposure, and interactive mechanisms causing or contributing to the pathobiology of BINT. Abbreviations: ANS, autonomous nervous system; BBB, blood brain barrier; BINT, blast-induced neurotrauma; CBF, cerebral blood flow; E, epinephrine; NE, norepinephrine; SNS, sympathetic nervous system; PNS, parasympathetic nervous system.

(Zucker, 1986). This, in turn, further deepens heart rate reduction (bradycardia) and peripheral blood vessel dilatation resulting in lowering blood pressure and eventually contributing to cerebral hypoxemia (Cernak et al., 1996a).

Na^+, K^+-ATPASE DURING EARLY POST-TRAUMATIC PHASE

Based on previous studies showing that blast exposure induces distinct pathological alterations in the brain including impaired energy metabolism (Cernak et al., 1995, 1996b), the activity of sodium–potassium ATPase (Na^+, K^+-ATPase; E.C.3.6.1.3.) was measured in the brainstem and erythrocyte membranes of rabbits exposed to blast. The aim was to establish the comparability of the enzyme changes as an indirect measure of systemic-cerebral response interaction during the early post-traumatic period after blast (Cernak et al., 1997). The Na^+, K^+-ATPase, i.e., sodium pump, is a ubiquitous plasma membrane enzyme that catalyzes the movement of K^+ into cells in exchange for Na^+, sustaining a gradient for Na^+ in to and for K^+ out of the cell (Skou and Esmann, 1992). The resulting gradient is used as an energy source for the de- and re-polarization of the membrane potential, regulation of cytoplasmic ionic composition, and for transepithelial transport. The sodium pump is regulated by numerous factors including several circulating hormones (Lopina, 2000; Lima et al., 2008). Since Na^+, K^+-ATPase is very sensitive to free radical reactions (Petrushanko et al., 2007) and impairments of energy metabolism (Silver and Erecinska, 1997), its activity can indicate membrane response to an insult indirectly giving insight into the efficiency of compensatory mechanisms and the level of membrane dysfunction.

Adult male rabbits were randomly assigned to three groups: control, mild-to-moderate, and moderate-to-severe blast injury groups. The blast injury groups were anesthetized and subjected to a blast overpressure generated by a compressed air-driven shock tube. During the early post-traumatic period (i.e., 30 min post-exposure), arterial pressure, electrocardiogram (ECG) and electroencephalogram (EEG) activities were measured. At the end of the 30-min observation period, arterial blood samples were collected, the animals sacrificed, and brain structures harvested. Light-microscopy examinations of brain samples stained with Hematoxylin–Eosin, Trichrom Masson, and van Gieson Elastica were also performed. Erythrocyte plasma membranes (Dodge et al., 1963; Mrsulja et al., 1993) and brainstem homogenates (Enseleit et al., 1984; Cernak et al., 1997) for the Na^+, K^+-ATPase assays were prepared as previously described. Briefly, the reaction mixture for the Na^+, K^+-ATPase assay contained 5.0 mM/L $MgCl_2$, 130.0 mM/L NaCl, 20.0 mM/L KCl, and 45.0 mM/L Tris–HCl buffer, pH 7.4. The reaction was started by the addition of ATP (disodium salt, vanadium free) to a final concentration of 0.1, 0.5, 1.0, 1.5, 3.0, and 5.0 mM, and stopped after a 60 min incubation period with the addition of the ice cold $HClO_4$. The activity obtained in the presence of 2 mM ouabain (without the NaCl and KCl) was attributed to Mg^{2+}-ATPase. Na^+, K^+-ATPase activity was calculated as a difference between the total ATPase activity (Na^+, K^+, Mg^{2+}-dependent) and Mg^{2+}-ATPase activity. Released inorganic phosphate (P_i) was measured by the method of Fiske and Subbarow (1925). Enzyme specific activity was expressed as nmol P_i released per mg of protein per min. All assays were performed in duplicate and the mean was used for statistical analysis. In this experiment, protein was measured by the method of (Lowry et al., 1951), with bovine serum albumin used as standard. The Michaelis–Menten constant (K_m) and the maximum reaction rate (V_{max}) of Na^+, K^+-ATPase were calculated using the Lineweaver–Burk double reciprocal plot.

Blast exposure caused the characteristic fall in mean arterial pressure, bradycardia, fast and shallow respiration, and significant increases in both frequency and amplitude of the EEG activity as compared to control animals (25 versus 15–18 Hz, and 22 versus 10 μV, respectively). The neuropathology analysis showed no hemorrhages or areas of contused brain tissue. The development of brain edema as well as the sodium pump changes demonstrated a graded response to the shockwave intensity, i.e., more prominent in the moderate-to-severe blast group as compared to the animals subjected to mild-to-moderate intensity blast. In all tested groups Na^+, K^+-ATPase activity in plasma membrane was substrate (ATP) dependent, such that the lowest activity was obtained at 0.1 mM, whereas the highest activity was at 1–1.5 mM concentrations of the substrate, ATP. At these substrate concentrations, the activity of the Na^+, K^+-ATPase was significantly increased in the erythrocyte membranes and the brainstem as compared to control values.

Changes in Na^+, K^+-ATPase have been shown being time-dependent (Sztriha et al., 1987), and in the present study the activity Na^+, K^+-ATPase was measured at the time when significant neuro-endocrine changes occur in the brain with TBI. Indeed, complex alterations such as the over-activation or inhibition of neurotransmitter synthesis, release, or transport have been reported during the early period after TBI (McIntosh et al., 1994). Among the most important neuro-endocrine changes, an increase in norepinephrine (NE) synthesis and metabolism have been reported in animal experiments inducing transient cerebral ischemia (Globus et al., 1989; Bhardwaj et al., 1990), focal cortical lesions (Pappius, 1991), and fluid-percussion TBI (McIntosh et al., 1994) during the first hours after the insult. Several mechanisms have been suggested to explain the NE activation of the enzyme: one involves specific receptors or a nonspecific chelating action related to the catechol group that would relieve the inhibition by divalent cations such as Ca^{2+} (Godfraind et al., 1974; Adam-Vizi et al., 1979; Phillis and Wu, 1981), while the other describes a possibility that NE removes an endogenous inhibitory factor present in the cytoplasm (Hernandez, 1992). A dose-dependent response of the Na^+, K^+-ATPase to dopamine and NE concentrations in mouse brain synaptosomes have been confirmed by Desaiah and Ho (1977) reporting that these catecholamines modified the behavior of the enzyme kinetics against ATP, producing an increase in V_{max}. Our previous studies have shown a direct relationship between injury severity and blood concentrations of epinephrine and NE in soldiers with military gunshot or missile (thus explosive) injuries (Savic et al., 1995) as well as in the brain of rats exposed to whole-body blast during the early post-traumatic phase.

Taken together, we hypothesize that the increased activity and V_{max} of the Na^+, K^+-ATPase in our study may be related to the catecholamine surge in the brain. Additionally, the edema formation developed in the brainstem parallel with the increase in the Na^+, K^+-ATPase activity could be explained as a result of Na^+-influx, bearing in mind that abrupt increase of cytoplasmic Na^+ in the brain tissue has been shown after trauma both *in vitro* (Young et al., 1986; Sheldon et al., 2004; Wang et al., 2009) and *in vivo* (Young et al., 1986). Moreover, the role of the Na^+-influx in the pathobiology of acute vasogenic edema was demonstrated by *in vivo* sodium MRI imaging in both clinical and experimental studies of brain edema development compared with signal in health brain tissue (Turski et al., 1986).

IMPORTANCE OF THE INDIRECT BLAST–BRAIN INTERACTING PATHWAY IN LONG-TERM NEUROLOGICAL DEFICITS

In an attempt to link systemic and cerebral inflammation as one of the potential mechanisms leading to long-term neurological deficits caused by blast, we performed real-time, *in vivo* imaging of myeloperoxidase (MPO) activity of activated phagocytes in mice exposed to mild intensity blast, during a 1-month post-injury period. Namely, migration and accumulation of polymorphonuclear leukocytes (PMNs) are among the major hallmarks of the host response to injuries (Maslinska and Gajewski, 1998; Toft et al., 2003; Menezes et al., 2008). Locally, activated PMNs release antimicrobial and inflammatory mediators, such as MPO, among others. MPO is a key inflammatory enzyme secreted by activated PMNs and macrophages/microglia, capable of generating highly reactive oxygen species to cause additional damage in various pathological conditions such as cerebral ischemia (Weston et al., 2007; Breckwoldt et al., 2008); ischemic heart conditions (Loria et al., 2008); inflammatory bowel disease (Naito et al., 2007); and kidney (Malle et al., 2003) and lung (Kinnula, 2005) pathologies, among others. Based on its importance in inflammatory processes and as a reliable indicator of PMN presence in tissues (Arnhold and Flemmig, 2010), MPO has been widely used as an inflammatory marker of both acute and chronic conditions (Werner and Szelenyi, 1992; Breckwoldt et al., 2008; Faith et al., 2008).

Briefly, mice were anesthetized, mounted in supine position to the animal holder secured inside the driven section of the helium-driven shock tube, and exposed to mild intensity shock wave (measured rupture pressure: 183 ± 14 kPa, i.e., 26.5 ± 2.1 psig; measured total pressure: 103 kPa, i.e., 14.9 psig) causing 5% mortality (Cernak et al., 2010). Subsets of animals ($n = 5$) were exposed to: (1) whole-body blast; (2) blast with torso (chest and abdomen) protection using a custom-made rigid Plexiglas "body armor," while the head exposed; or (3) blast with head protection using a custom-made Plexiglas "helmet" covering skull, face, and the neck of the animal while the torso exposed (**Figure 2**). Ten minutes before imaging, mice were injected with XenoLight Rediject Inflammation probe (Caliper Life Sciences; Hopkinton, MA, USA) at 200 mg/kg (150 μL/mouse) intraperitoneally. The XenoLight Rediject Inflammation probe is a chemiluminescent reagent in a ready-to-use format that allows for longitudinal tracking of MPO level and inflammation status, *in vivo*, in a variety of disease models. Bioluminescence imaging (BLI) was performed using the IVIS® Imaging System 3-D Series (Caliper Life Sciences, Hopkinton, MA, USA). During the imaging, the animals were anesthetized with a gas mixture (isoflurane:nitrous oxide:oxygen at 1:66:33% proportions, respectively) using the integrated system for gas anesthesia. The duration of imaging was 5 min. To validate substrate injection quality, fluorescence images were taken right before BLI, using the 745-nm excitation and 800-nm emission filter set, and exposure time between 1 and 5 s. Photons were quantified using Living Image software (Caliper Life Sciences, Hopkinton, MA, USA). Sham control animals did show only low-intensity localized bioluminescence at the injection site (results not shown).

Figure 3 shows the distribution of increased bioluminescence in mice subjected to whole-body blast exposure imaged during the 1-month observation period. One day after blast exposure, the

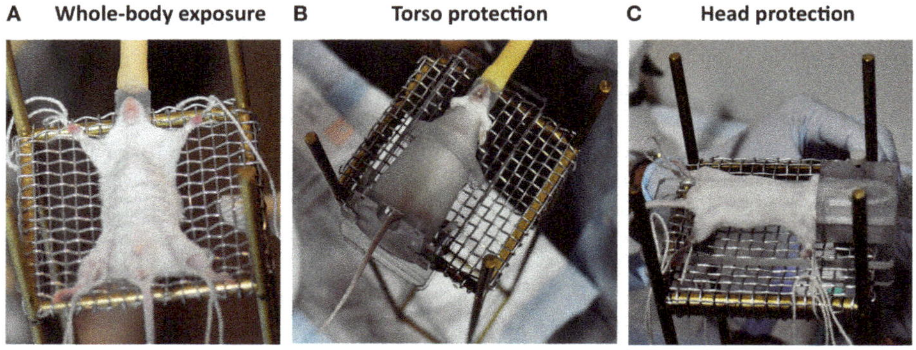

FIGURE 2 | Experimental setting for establishing the importance of blast-head and blast–body interactive pathways in the pathobiology of BINT. **(A)** whole-body blast exposure without protection; **(B)** head blast exposure with torso (chest and abdomen) protection; and **(C)** torso blast exposure with head protection.

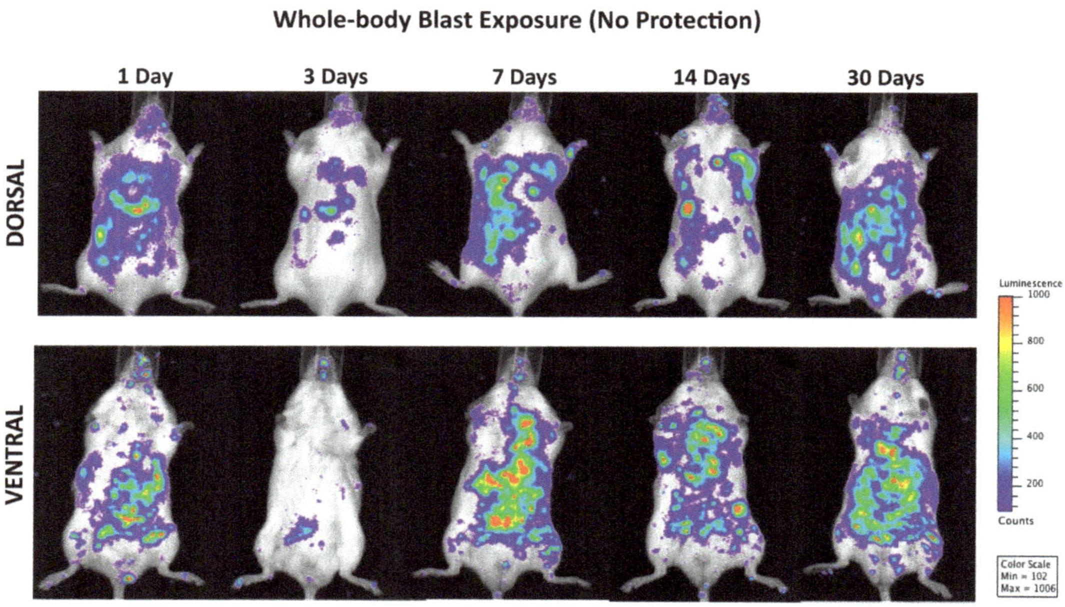

FIGURE 3 | Distribution of increased bioluminescence showing MPO activity in mice subjected to whole-body blast exposure, imaged during the 1-month observation period. The representative photographs show the same animal imaged in both dorsal and ventral positions at the given time point after blast exposure. The intensity of bioluminescence was scaled based on the photon counts. The nose cone that can be discerned on the photos is part of the anesthesia device that is the integral part of the IVIS® imaging system 3-D series, and does not represent a head cover.

highest MPO activity is found in the gastrointestinal tract, with clearly outlined transverse and descending colon. Additionally, enhanced signal is observed bilaterally in diaphragmal mediastinal parts of the lungs as well as in the brain. Interestingly, the PMNs activation showed a declining trend 3 days post-exposure followed by intensified MPO activity in lungs, gastrointestinal tract and the brain measured at 7, 14, and 30 days after blast. It is noteworthy that the most intense bioluminescence signal measured in the brain was found 1 month after injury.

Figure 4 demonstrates MPO activity in animals subjected to blast with head protection. Because the torso was exposed to blast, the finding of the activation of PMNs in lungs and gastrointestinal tract, similar to the changes observed in animals with whole-body blast exposure, is not surprising. The temporal and spatial profiles of MPO activity were also comparable, i.e., a declining trend at 3 days post-trauma followed by progressively increasing signal peaking at 1 month after blast. However, regardless of the head protection, MPO was significantly increased in the brain, with the highest activity at 14 and 30 days post-injury suggesting chronic inflammation. Importantly, the increase in MPO activity observed in mice with head protection was equal to corresponding changes found in the brain of animals exposed to whole-body blast without head protection, suggesting that head protection did not prevent inflammation in the brain and implying the importance of inflammatory cells of systemic origin in the pathobiology of blast-induced inflammatory processes in the brain.

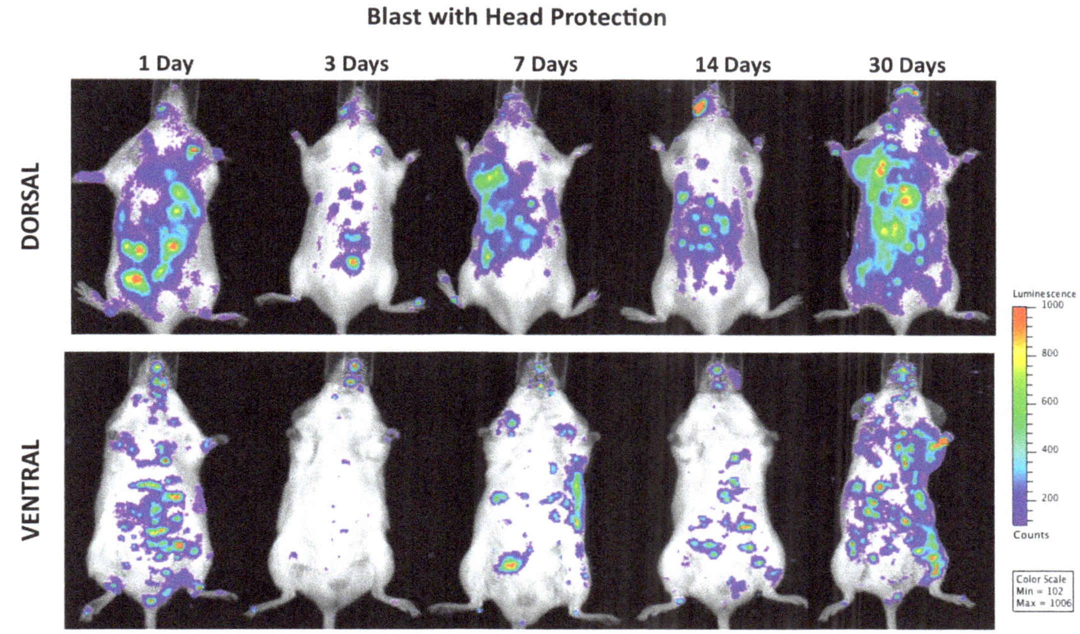

FIGURE 4 | Distribution of increased bioluminescence showing MPO activity in mice subjected to blast with head protection, imaged during the 1-month observation period. The representative photographs show the same animal imaged in both dorsal and ventral positions at the given time point after blast exposure. The intensity of bioluminescence was scaled based on the photon counts. The nose cone that can be discerned on the photos is part of the anesthesia device that is the integral part of the IVIS® imaging system 3-D series, and does not represent a head cover.

It is also noteworthy that while head protection did not prevent inflammation in the brain, it did reduce MPO activity in the gastrointestinal tract. It is well known that vagal afferent neurons play an important role in gut–brain communication (Berthoud and Neuhuber, 2000; Danzer et al., 2004) responding to a variety of physiological stimuli relevant not only to food intake and regulation of digestive activity, but in the response to immunological and noxious stimuli also (Gaykema et al., 2007). Indeed, direct and indirect pathways that originate in the caudal brainstem and propagate immune-related information from the periphery have been shown to play important role in the integration of brain responses to infection and injury (Gaykema et al., 2007). Additionally, it has been suggested that part of the peripheral immune information can be conveyed *via* vagal pathway to the catecholaminergic neurons in the medullary visceral zone from where it is transferred to the central amygdaloid nucleus (Ge et al., 2001). Such an approach suggests a complex interaction of the autonomous nervous system components with immune system elements in the response to injury-induced inflammation. Thus, we hypothesize that protecting the head reduced the susceptibility of the brain toward incoming vagal information and subsequently decreased the intensity of the efferent feedback response to peripheral injury; this in turn led to diminished inflammation in the gastrointestinal tract and lungs after blast as compared to animals with whole-body blast exposure.

Figure 5 shows progressive development of inflammation in both peripheral organs/organ systems and the brain of animals subjected to blast with torso protection. Systemic inflammation and the intensity of MPO activation in the brain were significantly reduced throughout the 1 month post-injury period as compared to mice either with whole-body exposure to blast or those with head protection. Moreover, while the inflammation in the brain was evident at 24 h post-exposure and still present at the end of the observation period, its intensity was significantly less than in animals with whole-body exposure or with head protection.

The fact that there was still MPO activation in the lungs regardless of the torso protection could be explained by pulmonary complications of the head injury such as neurogenic lung edema, seen both experimentally (Baumann et al., 2007; Irwin et al., 2008) and clinically (Dettbarn and Davidson, 1989; Fontes et al., 2003) after TBI. The roles of systemic sympathetic discharge, changes in intracranial pressure, and inflammation in central nervous system trigger zones have been suggested as essential mechanisms underlying the etiopathogenesis of neurogenic pulmonary edema (Sedy et al., 2008).

Taken together, the results of our study clearly demonstrate the importance of the indirect, i.e., blast–body interaction as well as the decisive role of autonomous nervous–neuroendocrine–immune systems interaction in the pathogenesis of BINT.

DISCUSSION AND CONCLUSIONS

Our findings demonstrate a multi-phase and multi-factorial nature of BINT where the mechanisms essential for the injury development and progress show significantly different phase-dependent trends. While acute alterations reflect compensatory attempts (such as increased activation of the sodium pump to potentially compensate for injury-induced impairments in electrolyte milieu or

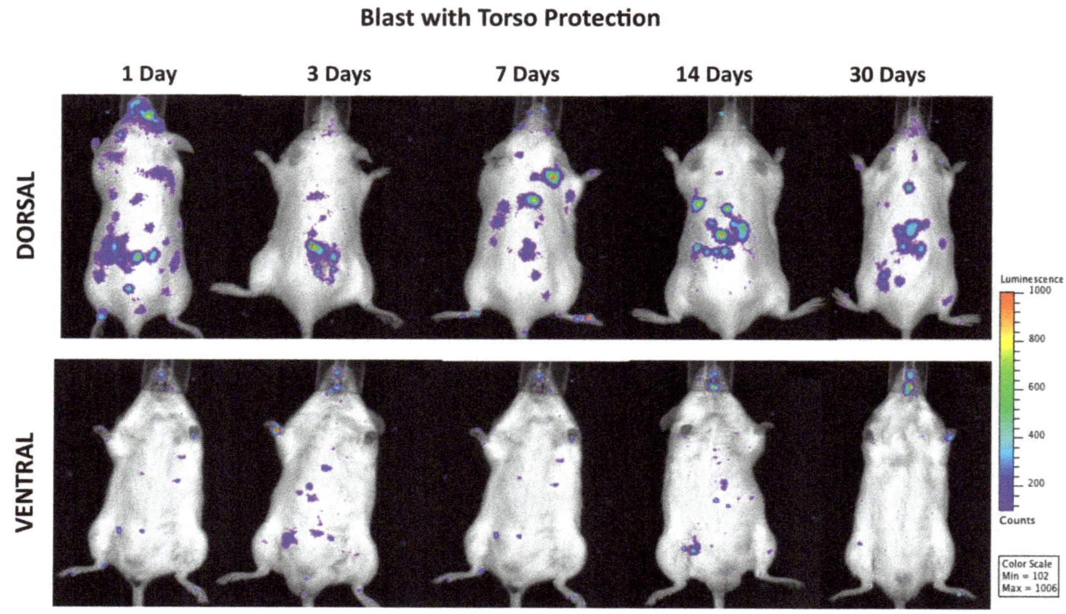

FIGURE 5 | Distribution of increased bioluminescence showing MPO activity in mice subjected to blast with torso protection while the head exposed, imaged during the 1-month observation period. The representative photographs show the same animal imaged in both dorsal and ventral positions at the given time point after blast exposure. The intensity of bioluminescence was scaled based on the photon counts. The nose cone that can be discerned on the photos is part of the anesthesia device that is the integral part of the IVIS® imaging system 3-D series, and does not represent a head cover.

parasympathetic stimulation to counteract the sudden pressure increase in the lungs and heart), chronic changes such as inflammation can lead to irreversible degenerative pathologies. Thus, to establish reliable diagnostic tools capable of identifying BINT and its progress, we should fully understand and characterize the multiple phases of the brain response to blast exposure.

The Na^+, K^+-ATPase activity change is an excellent example demonstrating the duality of response mechanisms to injury where increased and reversible activity after various brain insults in animals during the acute (<3 h) post-injury period (MacMillan, 1982; Goldberg et al., 1984; Sztriha et al., 1987) is followed by reduced activity during the chronic post-injury period (Jovicic et al., 2008; Crema et al., 2010) potentially leading to irreversible neurodegenerative central nervous system disorders (Seddik et al., 1991; Kumar and Kurup, 2002; Lima et al., 2008). While the Na^+, K^+-ATPase activity is not disease specific, its phase-dependent activity change as well as its kinetic profile to ATP might be a useful indicator of the BINT development and progress. The fact that the sodium pump changes correspond well to the changes in the erythrocyte membranes makes measurements of the Na^+, K^+-ATPase even more feasible as diagnostic parameters for BINT. There is a long list of research tasks ahead of us that concerns the importance of the Na^+, K^+-ATPase in the pathobiology of the BINT including establishing temporal and spatial profile characterization of its activity and kinetic pattern in the brain structures parallel with the changes in the erythrocyte membrane, and testing the diagnostic values of identified alterations in predicting functional neurological (memory, cognition, motor, and behavior) deficits, among others.

The results showing that head protection does not prevent chronic inflammation and neurological deficits suggest the vital importance of the blast–body interactive pathway in the etiopathogenesis of BINT. This fact is extremely important in designing effective protective equipment for servicemen that would prevent blast-body coupling, thus prevent the systemically induced mechanisms of BINT, as well as protect the brain from the direct impact caused by blast.

We need well-organized studies that begin in the field and identify the blast environment in relation to immediate and delayed mTBI symptoms in servicemen. Further, those data should be shared with the basic and applied research community to understand the uniqueness of this injury and to develop adequate and sensitive diagnostic tools and successful treatment. Without knowing what and how the blast injury occurred, it will be difficult to develop timely, reliable and specific diagnosis, and treatments for our servicemen. This multifaceted task is extremely challenging, and its successful solution is possible only through highly synchronized multi-institutional and international research efforts.

ACKNOWLEDGMENTS

Dr. Farid A. Ahmed significantly contributed to the Section "Importance of the Indirect Blast–Brain Interacting Pathway in Long-term Neurological Deficits" study. The study described in Section "Importance of the Indirect Blast–Brain Interacting Pathway in Long-term Neurological Deficits" was supported by the Johns Hopkins University Applied Physics Laboratory internal research and development (IR&D) funds. The sponsor did not influence the study design; data collection, analysis and interpretation of data; or the writing of the article.

REFERENCES

Adam-Vizi, V., Vizi, E. S., and Horvath, I. (1979). Stimulation by noradrenaline of Na^+K^+ ATPasein different fractions of rat brain cortex. *J. Neural Transm.* 46, 59–69.

Arnhold, J., and Flemmig, J. (2010). Humanmyeloperoxidaseininnateand acquired immunity. *Arch. Biochem. Biophys.* 500, 92–106.

Baumann,A.,Audibert, G., McDonnell, J., and Mertes, P. M. (2007). Neurogenic pulmonary edema. *Acta Anaesthesiol. Scand.* 51, 447–455.

Berthoud, H. R., and Neuhuber, W. L. (2000). Functional and chemical anatomy of the afferent vagal system. *Auton. Neurosci.* 85, 1–17.

Bhardwaj, A., Brannan, T., Martinez- Tica, J., and Weinberger, J. (1990). Ischemia in the dorsal hippocampus is associated with acute extracellular release of dopamine and norepine- phrine. *J. Neural Transm. Gen. Sect.* 80, 195–201.

Breckwoldt, M. O., Chen, J. W., Stangenberg,L.,Aikawa,E.,Rodriguez, E., Qiu, S., Moskowitz, M. A., and Weissleder, R. (2008). Tracking the inflammatory response in stroke in vivo by sensing the enzyme mye- loperoxidase. *Proc. Natl. Acad. Sci. U.S.A.* 105, 18584–18589.

Cernak, I. (2005). Animal models of head trauma. *NeuroRx* 2, 410–422.

Cernak, I., Ignjatovic, D., Andelic, G., and Savic, J. (1991). Metabolic changes as part of the general response of the body to the effect of blast waves. *Vojnosanit. Pregl.* 48, 515–522.

Cernak,I.,Malicevic,Z.,Prokic,V.,Zunic, G.,Djurdjevic,D.,Ilic,S.,and Savic,J. (1997). Indirect neurotrauma caused by pulmonary blast injury: develop- ment and prognosis. *Int. Rev. Armed Forces Med. Serv.* 52, 114–120.

Cernak, I., Merkle, A. C., Koliatsos, V. E., Bilik, J. M., Luong, Q. T., Mahota, T. M., Xu,L.,Slack,N.,Windle,D.,andAhmed, F. A. (2010). The pathobiology of blast injuriesandblast-inducedneurotrauma as identifi d using a new experimental modelofinjuryinmice. *Neurobiol. Dis.* doi: 10.1016/j.nbd.2010.10.025. [Epub ahead of print].

Cernak, I., and Noble-Haeusslein, L. J. (2010). Traumatic brain injury: an overview of pathobiology with emphasis on military populations. *J. Cereb. Blood Flow Metab.* 30, 255–266.

Cernak,I.,Radosevic,P.,Malicevic,Z.,and Savic,J. (1995). Experimental magne- sium depletion in adult rabbits caused by blast overpressure. *Magnes. Res.* 8, 249–259.

Cernak, I., Savic, J., Ignjatovic, D., and Jevtic, M. (1999a). Blast injury from explosive munitions. *J. Trauma.* 47, 96–103; discussion 103–104.

Cernak, I., Savic, J., Zunic, G., Pejnovic, N., Jovanikic, O., and Stepic, V. (1999b). Recognizing, scoring, and predict- ing blast injuries. *World J. Surg.* 23, 44–53.

Cernak, I., Savic, J., Malicevic, Z., Zunic, G., Radosevic, P., and Ivanovic, I. (1996a). Leukotrienes in the patho- genesis of pulmonary blast injury. *J. Trauma* 40, S148–S151.

Cernak, I., Savic, J., Malicevic, Z., Zunic, G., Radosevic, P., Ivanovic, I., and Davidovic, L. (1996b). Involvement of the central nervous system in the general response to pulmonary blast injury. *J. Trauma* 40, S100–S104.

Clemedson, C. J. (1956). Blast injury. *Physiol. Rev.* 36, 336–354.

Crema, L., Schlabitz, M., Tagliari, B., Cunha, A., Simao, F., Krolow, R., Pettenuzzo, L., Salbego, C., Vendite, D., Wyse, A. T., and Dalmaz, C. (2010). Na^+, K^+ ATPase activity is reduced in amygdala of rats with chronic stress-induced anxiety- like behavior. *Neurochem. Res.* 35, 1787–1795.

Danzer, M., Jocic, M., Samberger, C., Painsipp, E., Bock, E., Pabst, M. A., Crailsheim, K., Schicho, R., Lippe, I. T., and Holzer, P. (2004). Stomach-brain communication by vagal afferents in response to luminal acid backdiffu- sion, gastrin, and gastric acid secre- tion. *Am. J. Physiol. Gastrointest. Liver Physiol.* 286, G403–G411.

Desaiah, D., and Ho, I. K. (1977). Kinetics of catecholamine sensitive Na^+-K^+ ATPase activity in mouse brain syn- aptosomes. *Biochem. Pharmacol.* 26, 2029–2035.

Dettbarn, C. L., and Davidson, L. J. (1989). Pulmonary complications in the patient with acute head injury: neurogenic pulmonary edema. *Heart Lung* 18, 583–589.

Dodge, J. T., Mitchell, C., and Hanahan, D. J. (1963). The preparation and chemi- cal characteristics of hemoglobin-free ghosts of human erythrocytes. *Arch. Biochem. Biophys.* 100, 119–130.

Enseleit,W. H., Domer, F. R., Jarrott, D. M., and Baricos, W. H. (1984). Cerebral phospholipid content and Na^+, K^+-ATPase activity during ischemia and postischemic reperfusion in the mongolian gerbil. *J. Neurochem.* 43, 320–327.

Faith, M., Sukumaran, A., Pulimood, A. B., and Jacob, M. (2008). How reli- able an indicator of inflammation is myeloperoxidaseactivity? *Clin. Chim. Acta* 396, 23–25.

Fiske, C. H., and Subbarow,Y. (1925). The colorimetric determination of phos- phorus. *J. Biol. Chem.* 66, 375–400.

Fontes, R. B., Aguiar, P. H., Zanetti, M. V., Andrade, F., Mandel, M., and Teixeira, M. J. (2003). Acute neurogenic pulmo- nary edema: case reports and litera- ture review. *J. Neurosurg. Anesthesiol.* 15, 144–150.

Gaykema, R. P., Chen, C. C., and Goehler, L. E. (2007). Organization of immune-responsive medullary projections to the bed nucleus of the stria terminalis, central amygdala, and paraventricu- lar nucleus of the hypothalamus: evidence for parallel viscerosensory pathways in the rat brain. *Brain Res.* 1130, 130–145.

Ge, X., Yang, Z., Duan, L., and Rao, Z. (2001). Evidence for involvement of the neural pathway containing the peripheral vagus nerve, medullary visceral zone and central amygdaloid nucleus in neuroimmunomodulation. *Brain Res.* 914, 149–158.

Globus, M. Y., Busto, R., Dietrich, W. D., Martinez, E., Valdes, I., and Ginsberg, M. D. (1989). Directevidenceforacute and massive norepinephrine release in the hippocampus during transient ischemia. *J. Cereb. Blood Flow Metab.* 9, 892–896.

Godfraind, T., Koch, M. C., and Verbeke, N. (1974). The action of EGTA on the catecholamines stimulation of rat brain Na-K-ATPase. *Biochem. Pharmacol.* 23, 3505–3511.

Goldberg, W. J., Watson, B. D., Busto, R., Kurchner, H., Santiso, M., and Ginsberg, M. D. (1984). Concurrent measurement of (Na^+, K^+)-ATPase activity andlipidperoxidesinratbrain following reversible global ischemia. *Neurochem. Res.* 9, 1737–1747.

Greve, M. W., and Zink, B. J. (2009). Pathophysiology of traumatic brain injury. *Mt. Sinai J. Med.* 76, 97–104.

Hernandez, R. J. (1992). $Na^+/K^{(+)}$-ATPase regulation by neurotransmitters. *Neurochem. Int.* 20, 1–10.

Hoffer, M. E., Balaban, C., Gottshall, K., Balough, B. J., Maddox, M. R., and Penta, J. R. (2010). Blast exposure: vestibular consequences and associ- ated characteristics. *Otol. Neurotol.* 31, 232–236.

Irwin, D. C., Subudhi, A. W., Klopp, L., Peterson, D., Roach, R., and Monnet, E. (2008). Pulmonary edema induced by cerebral hypoxic insult in a canine model. *Aviat. Space Environ. Med.* 79, 472–478.

Jovicic, M. E., Popovic, M., Nesic, K. J., Popovic, N., Pavlovic, S. J., and Rakic, L. (2008). Aging, aluminium and basal forebrain lesions modify substrate kinetics of erythrocyte membrane Na, K-ATPase in the rat. *J. Alzheimers Dis.* 14, 85–93.

Kinnula, V. L. (2005). Production and deg- radation of oxygen metabolites during inflory states in the human lung. *Curr. Drug Targets Inflamm. Allergy* 4, 465–470.

Kumar, A. R., and Kurup, P. A. (2002). Inhibition of membrane Na^+-K^+ ATPase activity: a common pathway in central nervous system disorders. *J. Assoc. Physicians India* 50, 400–406.

Lima, F. D., Souza, M. A., Furian, A. F., Rambo, L. M., Ribeiro, L. R., Martignoni, F. V., Hoffmann, M. S., Fighera, M. R., Royes, L. F., Oliveira, M. S., and de Mello, C. F. (2008). Na^+, K^+-ATPase activity impairment after experimental traumatic brain injury: relationship to spatial learning defi its andoxidativestress. *Behav. Brain Res.* 193, 306–310.

Lopina, O. D. (2000). Na^+, K^+-ATPase: structure, mechanism, and regulation. *Membr. Cell Biol.* 13, 721–744.

Loria,V.,Dato,I.,Graziani,F.,and Biasucci, L. M. (2008). Myeloperoxidase: a new biomarker of inflammation in ischemic heart disease and acute coro- nary syndromes. *Mediators Infl* 2008, 135625.

Lowry, O. H., Rosebrough, N. J., Farr, A. L., and Randall, R. J. (1951). Protein measurement with the Folin phenol reagent. *J. Biol. Chem.* 193, 265–275.

MacMillan, V. (1982). Cerebral Na^+, K^+-ATPase activity during exposure toand recovery from acute ischemia. *J. Cereb. Blood Flow Metab.* 2, 457–465.

Malle, E., Buch, T., and Grone, H. J. (2003). Myeloperoxidase in kidney disease. *Kidney Int.* 64, 1956–1967.

Martin, E. M., Lu, W. C., Helmick, K., French, L., and Warden, D. L. (2008). Traumatic brain injuries sustained in the Afghanistan and Iraq wars. *Am. J. Nurs.* 108, 40–47.

Maslinska, D., and Gajewski, M. (1998). Some aspects of the inflamma- tory process. *Folia Neuropathol.* 36, 199–204.

McIntosh, T. K., Yu, T., and Gennarelli, T. A. (1994). Alterations in regional brain catecholamine concentrations after experimental brain injury in the rat. *J. Neurochem.* 63, 1426–1433.

Menezes, G. B., Rezende, R. M., Pereira- Silva, P. E., Klein, A., Cara, D. C., and Francischi, J. N. (2008). Differential involvement of cyclooxygenase iso- forms in neutrophil migration in vivo and in vitro. *Eur. J. Pharmacol.* 598, 118–122.

Mrsulja, B. B., Stojadinovic, N., Maletic- Savatic, M., Stojanovic, T., Cvejic, V., Nenadovic, M., Paunovic, V. R., Marinkovic,D.,and Kostic,V.S. (1993). Substrate erythrocyte membrane Na, K-ATPase: a potentially ubiquitous mechanism reflecting central nervous system pathology. *Iugoslav. Physiol. Pharmacol. Acta* 29, 115–119.

Naito, Y., Takagi, T., and Yoshikawa, T. (2007). Molecular fingerprints of neutrophil-dependent oxidative stress in inflory bowel disease. *J. Gastroenterol.* 42, 787–798.

Nelson, L. A., Yoash-Gantz, R. E., Pickett, T. C., and Campbell, T. A. (2009).

Relationship between processing speed and executive functioning performance amongOEF/OIFveterans:implications for postdeployment rehabilitation. *J. Head Trauma Rehabil.* 24, 32–40.

Owen-Smith, M. S. (1981). Explosive blast injury. *Med. Bull. US Army Eur.* 38, 36–43.

Pappius, H. M. (1991). Brain injury: new insights into neurotransmitter and receptor mechanisms. *Neurochem. Res.* 16,941–949.

Peskind, E. R., Petrie, E. C., Cross, D. J., Pagulayan, K., McCraw, K., Hoff, D., Hart, K., Yu, C. E., Raskind, M. A., Cook,D.G.,and Minoshima,S.(2010). Cerebrocerebellar hypometabolism associated with repetitive blast expo- sure mild traumatic brain injury in 12 Iraq war Veterans with persistent post- concussive symptoms. *Neuroimage.* doi:10.1016/j.neuroimage.2010.04.008. [Epub ahead of print].

Petrushanko, I. Y., Bogdanov, N. B., Lapina, N., Boldyrev,A.A., Gassmann, M., and Bogdanova, A. Y. (2007). Oxygen-induced regulation of Na/K ATPase in cerebellar granule cells. *J. Gen. Physiol.* 130, 389–398.

Phillis, J. W., and Wu, P. H. (1981). Catecholamines and the sodium pump in excitable cells. *Prog. Neurobiol.* 17, 141–184.

Reilly, P.L. (2001). Brain injury: the patho- physiology of the first hours. "Talk and die revisited"*J. Clin. Neurosci.* 8, 398–403.

Ritenour, A. E., Blackbourne, L. H., Kelly, J. F., McLaughlin, D. F., Pearse, L. A., Holcomb, J. B., and Wade, C. E. (2010). Incidence of primary blast injury in US military overseas contingency operations:a retrospective study.*Ann. Surg.* 251, 1140–1144.

Rossle,R.(1950)."Pathologyof blasteffects," in*GermanAviationMedicine,WorldWar IIed.* USAFSchoolof AviationMedicine, (Washington, DC: Department of the Air Force), 1260–1273.

Savic, J., Lazarov,A., Malicevic, Z., Nikolic, J., and Vujinov, S. (1995). Relationship between early neuroendocrine response and severity of war injury according to the red cross classifica- tion. *Vojnosanit. Pregl.* 52, 107–117.

Seddik, Z., Habib, Y. A., and el Shamy, E. (1991). The prognostic value of the brain sodium-potassium ATPase enzyme concentration in head injury. *Childs Nerv. Syst.* 7, 135–138.

Sedy, J., Zicha, J., Kunes, J., Jendelova, P., and Sykova, E. (2008). Mechanisms of neurogenic pulmonary edema devel- opment.*Physiol. Res.* 57,499–506.

Sheldon, C., Diarra, A., Cheng, Y. M., and Church, J. (2004). Sodium infl pathways during and after anoxia in rat hippocampal neurons. *J. Neurosci.* 24, 11057–11069.

Silver, I. A., and Erecinska, M. (1997). Energetic demands of the Na^+/K^+ ATPasein mammalian astrocytes.*Glia* 21, 35–45.

Skou, J. C., and Esmann, M. (1992). The Na, K-ATPase. *J. Bioenerg. Biomembr.* 24, 249–261.

Stewart, O. W., and Russel, C. K. (1941). Injury to the central nervous system by blast.*Lancet* 1, 172–174.

Sztriha, L., Joo, F., Dux, L., and Boti, Z. (1987). Effects of systemic kainic acid administration on regional Na^+, K^+-ATPase activity in rat brain. *J. Neurochem.* 49, 83–87.

Terrio, H., Brenner, L.A., Ivins, B. J., Cho, J. M., Helmick, K., Schwab, K., Scally, K., Bretthauer, R., and Warden, D. (2009). Traumatic brain injury screening: pre- liminaryfi s in a US army brigade combatteam.*J. Head Trauma Rehabil.* 24, 14–23.

Toft, P., Andersen, S. K., and Tonnesen, E. K. (2003). The systematic inflam- matory response after major trauma. *Ugeskr. Laeg.* 165, 669–672.

Turski, P. A., Perman, W. H., Hald, J. K., Houston, L. W., Strother, C. M., and Sackett, J. F. (1986). Clinical and experimental vasogenic edema: in vivo sodium MR imaging. Work in progress.*Radiology* 160,821–825.

Wang, J. A., Lin, W., Morris, T., Banderali, U., Juranka, P. F., and Morris, C. E. (2009). Membrane trauma and Na^+ leak from Nav1.6 channels. *Am. J. Physiol., Cell Physiol.* 297, C823–C834.

Warden, D. L., French, L. M., Shupenko, L.,Fargus,J.,Riedy,G.,Erickson,M.E., Jaffee, M. S., and Moore, D. F. (2009). Case report of a soldier with pri- mary blast brain injury. *Neuroimage* 47(Suppl. 2), T152–T153.

Werner, U., and Szelenyi, I. (1992). Measurement of MPO activity as model for detection of granulocyte infi ration in different tissues. *Agents Actions* Spec No. C101–C103.

Weston, R. M., Jones, N. M., Jarrott, B., and Callaway, J. K. (2007). Inflammatory cell infiltration after endothelin-1-induced cerebral ischemia: histochemical and myeloperoxidase correlation with temporal changes in brain injury. *J. Cereb. Blood Flow Metab.* 27, 100–114.

Young, W., DeCrescito, V., Flamm, E. S., Hadani, M., Rappaport, H., and Cornu, P. (1986). Tissue Na, K, and Ca changes in regional cerebral ischemia: their measurement and interpreta- tion. *Cent. Nerv. Syst. Trauma* 3, 215–234.

Zucker, I. H. (1986). Left ventricular receptors: physiological controllers or pathological curiosities? *Basic Res. Cardiol.* 81, 539–557.

Zuckerman,S.(1940).Experimentalstudy of blast injuries to the lungs. *Lancet* 236, 219–224.

Pivotal role of anterior cingulate cortex in working memory after traumatic brain injury in youth

Fabienne Cazalis[1,2]*, Talin Babikian[1], Christopher Giza[3], Sarah Copeland[3], David Hovda[3] and Robert F. Asarnow[1]

[1] Psychiatry and Biobehavioral Sciences, University of California Los Angeles David Geffen School of Medicine, Los Angeles, CA, USA
[2] Department of Anatomy, Ross University School of Medicine, Roseau, Commonwealth of Dominica
[3] Department of Neurosurgery, University of California Los Angeles David Geffen School of Medicine, Los Angeles, CA, USA

Edited by:
Marten Risling, Karolinska Institutet, Sweden

Reviewed by:
Hans Lindå, Karolinska Institutet, Sweden
Frank Krueger, George Mason University, USA

***Correspondence:**
Fabienne Cazalis, Department of Anatomy, Ross University School of Medicine, P.O. Box 266, Roseau, Commonwealth of Dominica.
e-mail: fcazalis@rossu.edu

In this fMRI study, the functions of the anterior cingulate cortex (ACC) were studied in a group of adolescents who had sustained a moderate to severe traumatic brain injury (TBI). A spatial working memory task with varying working memory loads, representing experimental conditions of increasing difficulty, was administered. In a cross-sectional comparison between the patients and a matched control group, patients performed worse than Controls, showing longer reaction times and lower response accuracy on the spatial working memory task. Brain imaging findings suggest a possible double-dissociation: activity of the ACC in the TBI group, but not in the Control group, was associated with task difficulty; conversely, activity of the left sensorimotor cortex (lSMC) in the Control group, but not in the TBI group, was correlated with task difficulty. In addition to the main cross-sectional study, a longitudinal study of a group of adolescent patients with moderate to severe TBI was done using fMRI and the same spatial working memory task. The patient group was studied at two time-points: one time-point during the post-acute phase and one time-point 12 months later, during the chronic phase. Results indicated that patients' behavioral performance improved over time, suggesting cognitive recovery. Brain imaging findings suggest that, over this 12-month period, patients recruited less of the ACC and more of the lSMC in response to increasing task difficulty. The role of ACC in executive functions following a moderate to severe brain injury in adolescence is discussed within the context of conflicting models of the ACC functions in the existing literature.

Keywords: traumatic brain injury, diffuse axonal injury, functional MRI, working memory, anterior cingulate cortex, executive functions, adolescent

INTRODUCTION

Anterior cingulate cortex (ACC) activity is reportedly related to task difficulty, in healthy subjects (Botvinick et al., 2004) as well as in clinical populations, such as patients with post-traumatic stress disorder (Shaw et al., 2009) or patients with traumatic brain injury (TBI) (Rasmussen et al., 2008; Kohl et al., 2009). The exact role of the ACC in executive functions is still debated, with most prominent theories suggesting a role in cognitive control, including error detection, conflict monitoring, and/or task switching (Botvinick et al., 2004; Kerns et al., 2004; Ullsperger and Von Cramon, 2004; Carter and van Veen, 2007; Hyafil et al., 2009).

Executive function is affected by TBI, independently of the presence/absence of cortical lesions (Metting et al., 2007; Sanchez-Carrion et al., 2008). It has been suggested that it is diffuse axonal injury – commonly observed after TBI – that disrupts integrative networks and that is the main cause of executive functions impairment following TBI (Ghajar and Ivry, 2008; Niogi et al., 2008). This makes TBI a very interesting neuropsychological model for studying the role of ACC in executive functions.

In this study, we investigated ACC activation in relation to task difficulty, using a working memory task in adolescent patients with moderate to severe TBI. Our hypotheses were consistent with the literature: we expected that patients in the cross-sectional study would present lower performance than controls, notably with longer reaction times, and an alteration of their pattern of cerebral activation as compared to controls. We also expected patients in the longitudinal study to exhibit improvement of performance at Time 2 as compared to Time 1, as well as a change in brain imaging.

MATERIALS AND METHODS

This fMRI study of working memory in adolescents with TBI was conducted in two stages. First, a cross-sectional design compared youth with TBI to matched Controls. Secondly, a longitudinal study was conducted on a subset of the adolescent TBI patients who were reevaluated 12 months after their initial exam.

The spatial working memory task was parametrically designed in order to allow study of the effect of working memory load (WML) on brain activation.

PATIENTS

Participants included in this study presented with the following characteristics: 13–18 years of age; normal vision (contact lenses were accepted); right handedness; English skills sufficient enough to understand instructions; no previous history of major neurological, developmental, or psychiatric disorders (as stated by the parents of the patients during the inform consent process); and safety compliance to MRI. Recruitment and consent processes were approved by the UCLA Institutional Review Board (IRB).

Traumatic brain injury patients were recruited from two Pediatric ICUs within Los Angeles County (UCLA Medical Center and Harbor-UCLA Medical Center) as well as a local rehabilitation facility. Patients presented with moderate to severe non-penetrating TBI. Glasgow Coma Scale score (at intake at Emergency Department or post-resuscitation) was between 3 and 12, although three patients with GCS > 12 were included, since they presented with abnormalities on clinical imaging and therefore were classified as having moderate TBI. Severe TBI was defined by a GCS of 8 or less. All TBI patients exhibited diffuse axonal injury, as identified on FLAIR and T2 star MRI sequences. **Tables 1 and 2** describe the study groups.

PARADIGM DESCRIPTION

During the functional MRI exam, subjects performed a parametric cognitive task in an event-related design. They received instructions for the task prior to the exam. Participants responded by pressing a four-button keyboard that was placed under the subject's right hand. Responses and response times (RTs) were recorded.

The task was an original non-verbal spatial working memory task that required participants to reproduce visual sequences (**Figure 1**). A set of four positions was presented on the screen, as shown in **Figure 1**. Photographs of fruits and vegetables appeared sequentially, forming a spatio-temporal sequence that subjects were instructed to reproduce using the keyboard. Each picture was sufficiently detailed to be identifiable but sufficiently complex to prevent verbal description (Pepin Press, 2006a,b). The use of non-verbal material was *sine qua non* to avoid bilingualism being a confound, since exclusion of bilingual children was not a reasonable option (more than half of the children of Los Angeles, California, are bilingual, according to http://www.mla.org). The task was programmed using Matlab (The MathWorks Inc.).

Table 1 | Description of TBI and Control groups for the cross-sectional study.

	TBI	Controls
Number of subjects (males/females)	11 (9/2)	12 (4/8)
Mean age (years) ± SD (range)	16.0 ± 1.5 (14–18)	15.4 ± 1.5 (13–18)
Mean delay post-injury (months) ± SD (range)	7.0 ± 2 (3–17)	
Mean Glasgow coma scale score ± SD (range)	9.0 (3–15)	

Table 2 | Description of TBI group for the longitudinal study.

	Longitudinal TBI
Number of subjects (males/females)	6 (5/1)
Mean age (years) ± SD (range) at Time 1	16.7 ± 0.7 (15.8–17.4)
Mean age (years) ± SD (range) at Time 2	17.7 ± 0.8 (16.7–18.5)
Mean delay post-injury (months) ± SD (range) at Time 1	4.5 ± 1.0 (3–6)
Mean delay post-injury (months) ± SD (range) at Time 2	16.5 ± 3.1 (14–22)
Mean Glasgow coma scale score ± SD (range)	9.4 ± 5.1 (3–14)

The task included four conditions that were defined by the number of items to be manipulated in working memory, i.e., WML: Baseline (1 item); Low WML (3 items); Intermediate WML (4 items); High WML (5 items). There were 30 trials per condition. Conditions were alternated pseudo-randomly.

MRI EXAM

The MRI exam was conducted on a 3-T scanner (Siemens, Allegra) and included the following sequences:

- Structural T2 (TE = 56; TR = 4040 ms; FOV = 200 mm; voxel size = 0.8 mm × 0.8 mm × 5.0 mm; 25 slices of 5 mm; distance of 1.3 mm; axial orientation; order of acquisition = interleaved)
- EPI BOLD (TE = 30 ms; TR = 2000 ms; FOV = 200 mm; voxel size = 3.125 mm × 3.125 mm × 3 mm; 33 slices; axial orientation; order of acquisition = interleaved; 500 volumes acquired)
- T2* 3D flash (48 slices, voxel size = 1 mm × 0.5 mm × 2 mm; FOV = 256 mm; TR = 57 ms; TE = 20 ms; flip angle = 20°)
- A 3D volume structural sequence was acquired on a 1.5-T scanner (Siemens, Sonata) on the same day as functional scanning: MP-RAGE sequence (180 sagittal slices; FOV = 256 mm, voxel size = 1 mm × 1 mm × 1 mm; TR = 1900 ms; TE = 4.4 ms; TI = 1100 ms; flip angle = 15°)

BEHAVIORAL DATA PROCESSING

Two behavioral measures were used for statistical analyses: response accuracy and RT. Performance on both of these measures was recorded for each of the four conditions, representing WML [1-3-4-5]. Two groups were compared in the cross-sectional study: TBI and Control groups. For the Control group, behavioral

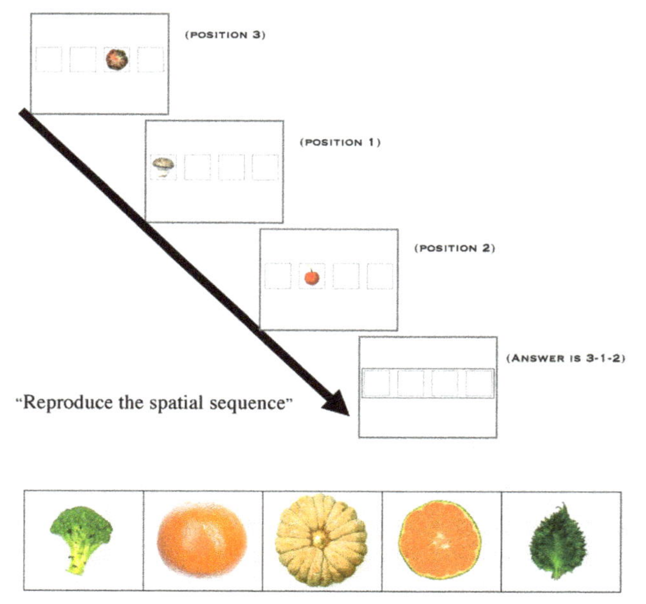

FIGURE 1 | Working memory task and examples of pictures used in the task.

data was available for 11 subjects. A subset of the TBI subjects, for whom data was available at two time-points, was included in the longitudinal study.

Cross-sectional study

Non-parametric Spearman correlations (two-tailed) were used to determine associations between the behavioral measures of response accuracy and RT with WML. A linear mixed model with *post hoc* (LSD) analyses were used to characterize case/control differences, with the between subject factor of Group (TBI or Control) and the within-subject factor of WML [1-3-4-5].

Longitudinal study

Because of the small sample size of the subgroup of the subjects for whom longitudinal data was acquired, simple paired *t*-tests were used for within-group comparison between Time 1 and Time 2.

MRI DATA PROCESSING

Functional MRI data were preprocessed and processed using the FSL package (Smith et al., 2004; Woolrich et al., 2009).

Preprocessing

Preprocessing included motion correction, brain extraction, spatial smoothing (FWHM = 5 mm), and high pass temporal filtering (66 s).

Processing: first-level analysis

Data were processed at the individual level according to their event-related design, for a total of five events-lists. Correct trials constituted the first four events, corresponding to the number of items loaded in working memory (WML): WML = 1 ("Baseline"); WML = 3 ("Low WML"); WML = 4 ("Intermediate WML"); WML = 5 ("High WML"). Failed and missed trials were assembled together in a fifth event that was excluded from analysis. Whitening was appended to data estimation, after convolution with double Gamma hemodynamic response function. Temporal derivative was applied, as well as temporal filtering. Four contrasts were used for this study:

- "Low WML" (Low WML versus Baseline)
- "Intermediate WML" (Intermediate WML versus Baseline)
- "High WML" (High WML versus Baseline)
- "WML increase" (High WML versus Low WML)

Individual activation maps were registered on the standard MNI space through the following steps: structural T2 was the initial image (linear – normal search – 7 DOF), 3D structural volume was the main structural image (linear – normal search – 12 DOF) and the MNI template ("avg152T1_brain" in FSL) was the standard space (linear – normal search – 12 DOF).

Processing: higher-level analysis

Higher-level analyses were processed at the group level (TBI and Control), using a fixed effects model. The measures for the cross-sectional study were: "mean Control group" and "mean TBI group" for the above-mentioned four contrasts. The contrasts for the longitudinal study were "mean TBI group Time 1" and "mean TBI group Time 2." In addition to a voxel threshold of $p = 0.05$, all maps were thresholded at the cluster level ($Z = 1.8$) in order to correct for multiple comparison. The template space was used as background for rendering.

Qualitative analysis

A complete list of all activated areas was compiled, using anatomical atlases (Mai et al., 2004; Ratiu and Talos, 2006) for correct determination of areas.

Quantitative analysis: regions of interest

Our choice for the regions of interest (ROI), determined by our working hypothesis, included the ACC. In an ideally large study, we would have compared the ACC activity with all the areas reportedly involved in spatial working memory processing (Wager and Smith, 2003; D'Esposito, 2008). However, because of the sample size of our study, we focused on the comparison of ACC with the left sensorimotor cortex (lSMC) because involvement of this later area has been well demonstrated in spatial working memory studies (Shaw et al., 2009) as well as in studies of mental imagery (Fiehler et al., 2008; Hanakawa et al., 2008; Sack et al., 2008).

We defined two spherical ROI according to their MNI coordinates and radius length (mm):

- Left sensorimotor cortex: $x = -40$; $y = -32$; $z = 56$; $r = 20$
- Anterior cingulate cortex : $x = 0$; $y = 34$; $z = 28$; $r = 14$

Regions of interests were used as masks in order to retrieve individual time-series values within these areas, using the "avwmeants" function included in the FSL package, hence obtaining the intensity of the betas based on the GLM model.

Statistical analyses were conducted for each ROI:

- Within-subjects differences between contrasts were explored using repeated measures ANOVAs. One-tailed *t*-tests were used for *post hoc* analyses.
- Within-subjects correlations between each ROI's levels of activation and WML (3, 4, or 5 items) were calculated using non-parametric Spearman correlations.
- Between subjects differences for each ROI were assessed using one-tailed *t*-tests.
- For the longitudinal study, within-subjects changes over time for each ROI were assessed using paired *t*-tests.

RESULTS

The first part of this section describes the cross-sectional study (TBI group versus Control group); the second part describes the longitudinal study (TBI group at Time 1 versus Time 2).

CROSS-SECTIONAL STUDY

Behavioral results: within-group analysis

Spearman correlation coefficients indicated a decline in both accuracy and RT with increasing WML in the control group. A decline in accuracy with increasing WML was observed for the TBI group, but no such effects were noted for RT (**Table 3**).

Behavioral results: between-groups analysis

Linear mixed model analyses for response accuracy indicated significant main effects of Group ($F = 9.635$, $p = 0.003$) and WML ($F = 17.356$, $p < 0.001$). There were no Group by WML interactions ($F = 1.213$, $p = 0.321$). *Post hoc* analyses with LSD corrections using one-tailed statistics suggested statistically significant effects (all $p < 0.10$) between all pairwise comparisons of WML. This suggests that our spatial working memory task is not only sensitive in detecting case/control differences but also shows the expected dose–response relationship between response accuracy and WML, with less accurate responding observed with increasing WML.

Similarly, linear mixed model analyses for RT indicated significant main effects of Group ($F = 28.188$, $p < 0.001$) and WML ($F = 2.767$, $p = 0.052$). There were no Group by WML interactions ($F = 0.173$, $p = 0.914$). *Post hoc* analyses with LSD corrections using one-tailed statistics suggested statistically significant effects (all $p < 0.10$) between the following pairwise comparisons of WML: 1 versus 4 and 5; 3 versus 4 and 5, indicating significant differences in RT from the baseline and easy conditions (load of 1 and 3) compared to the harder and more demanding conditions (load of 4 and 5). The Control group performed faster than the TBI group, regardless of WML. Also, across groups, participants were faster on the higher, and thus more difficult, WML trials (4 and 5) compared to the easier trials (1 and 3), with the longest time taken on the Baseline condition (WML of 1) in both groups. Results are summarized in **Figure 2**.

Post hoc analysis (see **Table 4**) show groups differences for accuracy and RTs in all conditions, with the exception of accuracy during the Baseline condition (WML = 1). Both groups were indeed close to 100% accuracy on the Baseline condition (96 and 99%, respectively for TBI and Controls).

Table 3 | Within-groups performance effects.

	TBI group	Control group
Correlation between WML and accuracy	$r = -0.645$; $p < 0.001$*	$r = -0.843$; $p < 0.001$*
Correlation between WML and response time	$r = -0.179$; $p = 0.244$	$r = -0.403$; $p = 0.007$*

**Statistically significant result.*

Imaging results and qualitative analysis: network recruited by the spatial working memory task

Differences between groups were visible on statistical maps for each condition. In all cases, however, a common network of activated areas was observed in both groups, as follows: cingulate cortex (anterior and posterior); frontal cortex, including: frontal gyri (superior, middle, and inferior) and precentral gyrus; parietal cortex, including: supramarginal gyrus, angular gyrus, parietal lobule, and post-central gyrus; temporal cortex (medial and inferior temporal gyri); occipital cortex; subcortical structures, including: head of caudate nucleus, parahippocampal gyrus, putamen, thalamus and insula.

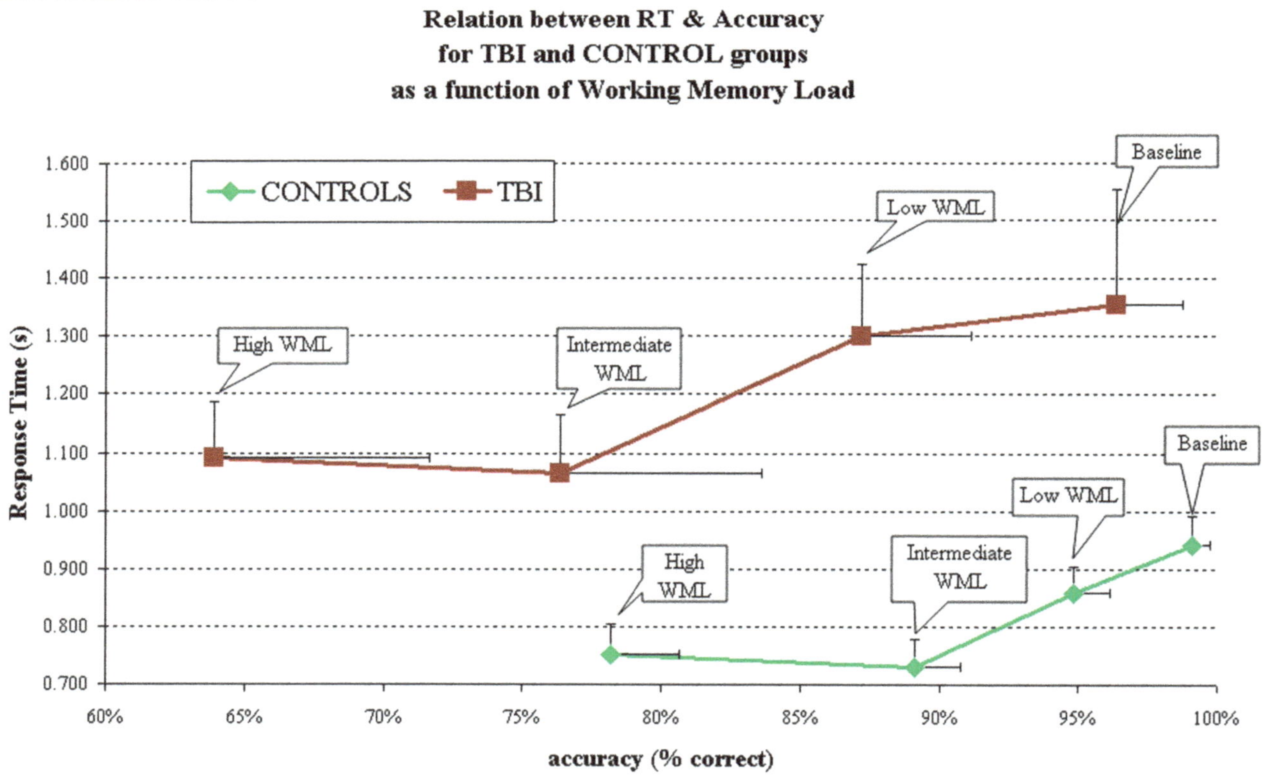

FIGURE 2 | Behavioral results for the cross-sectional study.

Imaging results and quantitative analysis of regions of interest: within-subjects effect of working memory load

Two ROI, ACC and lSMC, were defined as described in the section "Materials and Methods" and compared with regards for WML. Comparison of "Low WML" to "High WML" contrasts for the TBI group showed significant difference for the ACC ($p = 0.049$) but not for the lSMC ($p = 0.127$). The opposite was observed in the Control group, where the comparison of "Low WML" to "High WML" showed no difference for the ACC ($p = 0.387$) but a significant difference was observed for the lSMC ($p = 0.005$). **Figure 3** illustrates these results.

In the TBI group, activity in the ACC was associated (as a trend) with WML ($r = 0.327$; $p = 0.06$) but activity in lSMC was not ($r = -0.210$; $p = 0.24$). In the Control group, the opposite was observed: activity in the ACC was not correlated with WML ($r = 0.052$; $p = 0.76$) but correlation of the activity in the lSMC was significant, albeit in a negative direction ($r = -0.462$; $p = 0.005$).

Table 4 | *p* values for TBI and Control groups comparisons on the behavioral measures.

	Baseline	Low WML	Intermediate WML	High WML
Accuracy	0.139	0.040*	0.051	0.048*
RT	0.028*	0.002*	0.004*	0.003*

**Statistically significant result.*

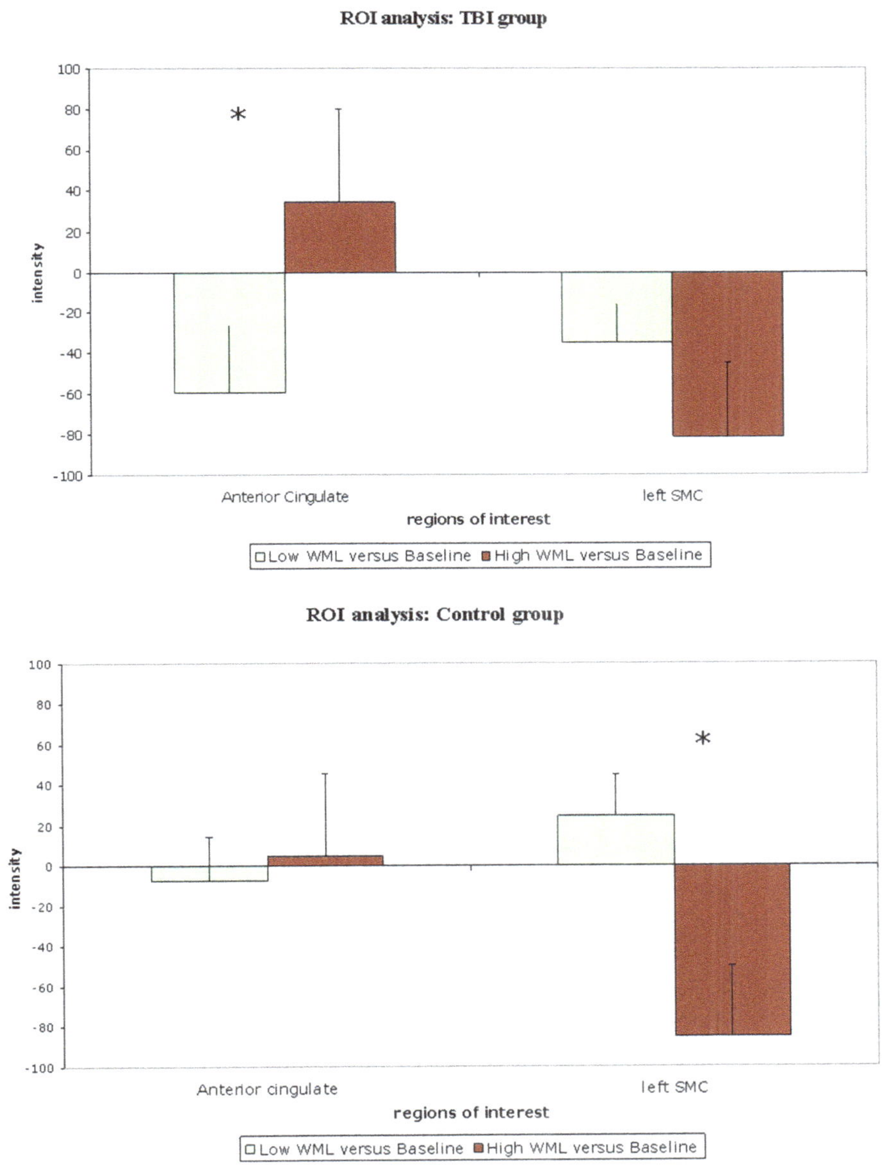

FIGURE 3 | Comparison of activation in regions of interest for "Low WML" (green) and "High WML" (brown) contrasts in traumatic brain injury group and Control group respectively.

Imaging results and quantitative analysis of regions of interest: between-subjects effect of working memory load

The use of a parametric task allowed us to examine the effect of WML by analyzing the contrast "WML increase" (WML = 5 items versus WML = 3 items). For the ACC region, a significant group difference was observed ($p = 0.038$), with the TBI group exhibiting more activation than the Control group. There was no observed group difference for this contrast, however, for the lSMC region ($p = 0.356$).

LONGITUDINAL STUDY

Behavioral results

As summarized in **Table 5** and **Figure 4**, the TBI patients' performances were compared between Time 1 and Time 2 (approximately 12 months apart).

Imaging results

Activation was observed in the ACC and the head of caudate nucleus for the "Time 1 versus Time 2" contrast, while activation of lSMC was observed for the contrast "Time 2 versus Time 1," as shown in **Figure 5**.

Table 5 | *p* values for Time 1 versus Time 2 behavioral data for the TBI patients.

	Accuracy	RT
Baseline	0.394	0.103
Low WML	0.117	0.047*
Intermediate WML	0.263	0.049*
High WML	0.289	0.032*

**Statistically significant result.*

Between Time 1 and Time 2, the change of activation in ACC was not significant ($p = 0.321$) but the activation of lSMC was significantly increased at Time 2 as compared to Time 1 ($p = 0.032$).

DISCUSSION

CROSS-SECTIONAL STUDY: PERFORMANCE

Adolescent TBI patients showed worse behavioral performance (higher RTs and poorer accuracy) than Controls on the spatial working memory task. This finding is consistent with an extended literature of cognition after brain injury, which reports that pediatric patients with moderate to severe TBI experience psychomotor slowing and impaired working memory (see Babikian and Asarnow, 2009 for a review). It is important to note that the composition of the groups may have influence this result because gender was not equally distributed across the TBI and Control groups. Education level was not tested and difference of education level between groups cannot be excluded.

CROSS-SECTIONAL STUDY: BRAIN IMAGING

In both groups, the spatial working memory task activated a broadly distributed network involving the prefrontal cortex, the cingulate cortex, the pre and post-central gyri, wide areas of the parietal and occipital cortices, medial and inferior temporal gyri, as well as subcortical structures, notably the head of the caudate nucleus. These findings are consistent with literature of spatial working memory (Wager and Smith, 2003; D'Esposito, 2008). Quantitative differences between groups were observed, and this also is consistent with the literature on brain imaging of TBI (Hillary et al., 2002; Cazalis et al., 2006; Niogi et al., 2008).

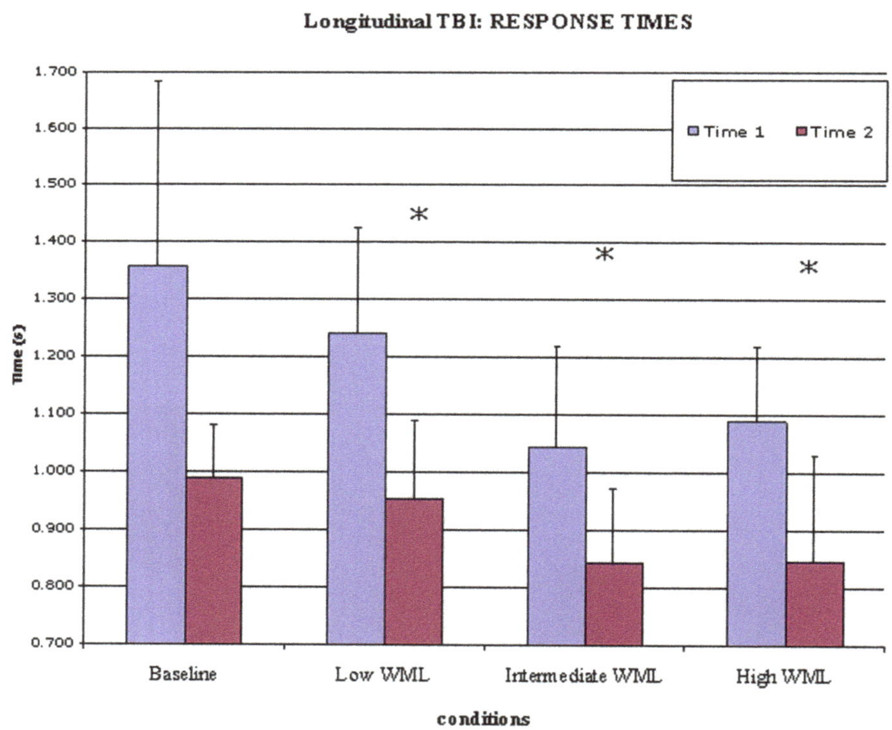

FIGURE 4 | Significant decrease of response times at Time 2 versus Time 1 in TBI patients.

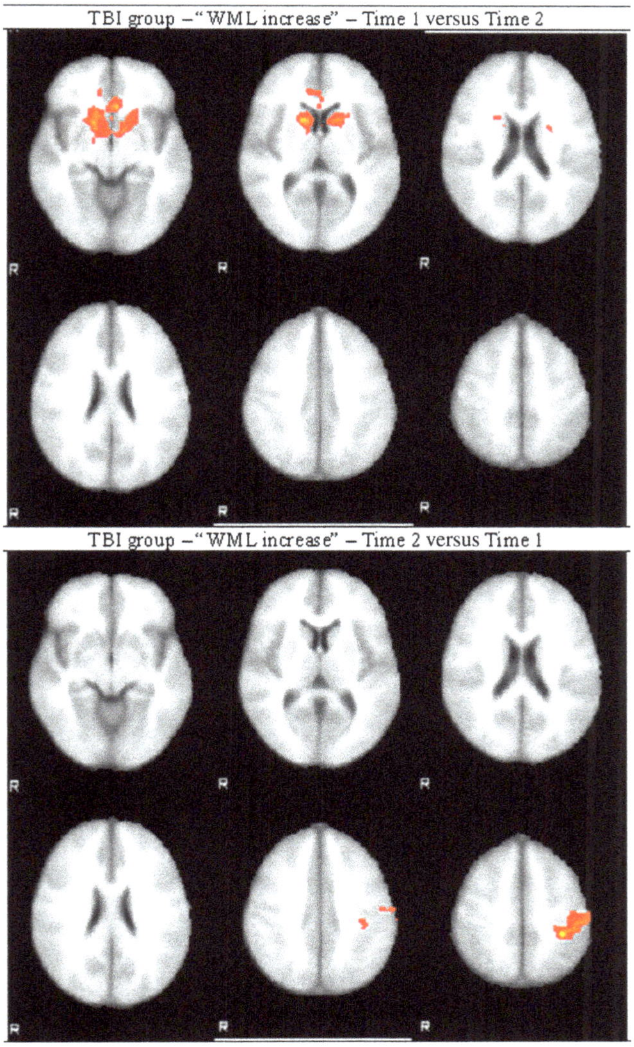

FIGURE 5 | Longitudinal contrasts for TBI patients.

The region of interest analysis was focused on the ACC, in order to understand its role in executive functions after moderate to severe TBI, and on the lSMC as well, because of its established role in spatial working memory.

Quantitative within-subject analyses of ROI activity in response to WML showed that, in the TBI group, ACC was significantly more activated when WML increased, while there was no change of lSMC activation. In the Control group, the opposite was observed: there was no change in ACC activation between conditions while lSMC activation decreased when WML increased. Our interpretation of those results is that Control subjects and TBI patients do not rely on recruiting the same cortical areas in response to increasing WML: Control subjects showed decreased activation of lSMC while TBI patients showed increased activation of ACC. Corroborating this result, correlation analysis showed that ACC activation was associated (as a trend) with WML in TBI patients but not in Controls, and that lSMC activation was correlated (inversely) in Controls but not in TBI patients. This double dissociation suggests that ACC activation depends on WML in TBI patients but not in Controls, while lSMC activation depends on WML in Controls but not in TBI patients.

Between-subject analysis, that compared TBI and Control groups for "WML increase," showed that ACC activation was significantly increased in the TBI group as compared to the Control group. In contrast, there was no difference between groups regarding lSMC activation. These results brought supplementary precisions to the findings above: ACC activation in TBI significantly increased in response to task difficulty as compared to Controls. Control subjects apparently responded to difficulty by decreasing activation of lSMC, while such decrease could not be observed in TBI patients who showed very low lSMC activation from the beginning.

Our interpretation of these results is that, although TBI patients and Control subjects seemed to use similar cognitive processes and neural networks in order to solve a spatial working memory task, there were notable differences between groups in the way these networks were recruited in response to difficulty, i.e., increasing WML in our case. Such differences, which were strongly suggested by the differences of performance during task solving, were revealed by comparing activation of two of the areas composing this network: ACC and lSMC.

While measure of clear differences between TBI and Control groups is an encouraging finding, we are aware that this may be only one part of a larger picture and that further research should be done with larger samples in order to determine the behavior of other areas involved in processing of items in spatial working memory, such as intraparietal cortex and dorsolateral prefrontal cortex.

LONGITUDINAL STUDY: PERFORMANCE

Six TBI patients were able to return for a second experimental session an average of 12 months after Time 1. While they did not show improvement in accuracy, their RTs were significantly decreased at Time 2. Recovery of cognitive functions after TBI has been extensively studied and our results are highly consistent with the existing literature. A recent meta-analysis of cognitive outcome after TBI (Babikian and Asarnow, 2009) showed that there is substantial recovery of processing speed in TBI patients over time, while recovery of working memory was noted in patients presenting with the most severe TBI.

LONGITUDINAL STUDY: BRAIN IMAGING

Within-subject analysis was a comparison of "WML increase" (WML of 5 items versus WML of 3 items) between Time 1 and Time 2. ACC and the head of caudate nucleus were more activated post-acutely as compared to the chronic phase, while lSMC was more activated in the chronic phase as compared to the post-acute phase; that is after a period of time allowing for recovery. These results, despite the small sample size, confirm our cross-sectional findings suggesting that prior to recovery, TBI patients significantly recruit ACC region for working memory, but they switch to lSMC recruitment following a period of recovery. Quantitative analyses of ROI activation in response to difficulty confirmed the increase of lSMC recruitment after recovery. This should be interpreted with regard to the cross-sectional study, which demonstrated a decreased recruitment of lSMC in response to difficulty (WML increase) in Controls while lSMC activation was consistently low in the TBI group. The fact that we observed more lSMC activation in TBI patients at Time 2 as compared to Time 1 suggests that they recovered the ability to use this area, although it is unclear if it follows the activation pattern observed in Controls. Moreover, it is important to note that because there was no longitudinal control group, we cannot exclude that such changes would not be due to recovery but simply to the fact that patients were one year older at Time 2, or may even have emerged by chance. This limitation, as well as the low number of subjects, makes the results of this longitudinal study difficult to interpret, but nevertheless encouraging, because they do show a change of activation pattern overtime, which parallels improvement in behavioral performance. It is reasonable to postulate that the changes of brain activation and behavioral performance observed in the TBI group between Time 1 and Time 2 result in the TBI group resembling the Control group over time, suggesting normalization and recovery.

FUNCTIONS OF ANTERIOR CINGULATE CORTEX

Over the last decade, several theories of ACC functions have been proposed, with some overlapping and some contradicting elements. Activation in ACC is observed in solving of difficult problem, multiple response management, conflict management, attention monitoring, and error detection (Botvinick et al., 2004; Ullsperger and Von Cramon, 2004; Declerck et al., 2006; Carter and van Veen, 2007; Hyafil et al., 2009; Ursu et al., 2009). In our study, only correct trials were included in brain imaging processing, therefore activation of the ACC cannot be attributed to error detection. In their study, Ursu et al. (2009) showed that there may be activation of ACC in presence of conflict even if the subject is not aware of such a conflict. Due to the structure of the task used in our study, it is not likely that the observed ACC activation was due to response override or conflict management. Magno et al. (2006) have indeed suggested that ACC activity is not related to error but to evaluation of difficulty. Furthermore, another study has shown that increased ACC activity was independent of anticipated error or conflict (Aarts et al., 2008). Finally, a study of TBI patients showed that ACC activity is increased with cognitive fatigue as experienced during effortful tasks (Kohl et al., 2009). This suggests that models of ACC functioning should include the broader concept of task difficulty – also described as challenging, effortful or demanding cognitive tasks –, thus encompassing concepts of error detection and conflict management.

Botvinick et al. (2004) have proposed an integrative hypothesis of ACC monitoring attention that applies to our results. According to their theory, activation of the ACC is associated with compensatory adjustment in response to tasks "experienced as cognitively difficult," considering that "conflict might serve as an index of the demand for mental effort," but that difficulty can occur in absence of conflict. While TBI subjects in our study did not perform as well as Controls despite exhibiting the highest ACC activation, this is not sufficient to exclude a compensatory adjustment. The compensatory adjustment theory, however, is used to explain studies showing that ACC activation is associated with higher performance (Botvinick et al., 2001; Garavan et al., 2002; Kerns et al., 2004). The results of our study apparently contradict those results, since TBI patients exhibited worse performance than Controls. However, in a previous fMRI study, we have shown that adult patients with severe TBI who perform very poorly on a planning task with working memory components exhibited reduced activation of the ACC as compared to severe TBI patients who were able to perform as well as Control subjects (Cazalis et al., 2006). Similar results were described by Kohl et al. (2009) as a coping mechanism. It is therefore reasonable to assume that those TBI patients in our current study, who were able to complete the task, may have recruited ACC in a compensatory adjustment fashion, in order to avoid poorer performance.

Alternatively, other studies of individual performance and cortical activation variability suggest that activity in ACC could reflect the ability of the individual to succeed at the task, in which case ACC activation could be seen as a predictor of performance. In a review of PET studies, Paus et al. (1998) argued that ACC activation positively reflects the level of difficulty of a task, which is itself indicative of the level of performance. In a study of a planning task, Cazalis et al. (2003) showed that subjects with poorer performance exhibited greater activation of the ACC than subjects with better performance. Hahn et al. (2007) have shown that ACC activity is dependent on performance (RTs). In two studies of verbal working memory, Osaka et al. (2003, 2004) found greater ACC activation in individuals with higher verbal working memory spans. Although it is difficult to transpose verbal WM and spatial WM, these studies interestingly confirm the dependence of ACC activation on performance. Furthermore, another study of anatomical variation of ACC demonstrated an association between a specific (leftward) morphological pattern of paracingulate sulcus folding and higher performance in demanding cognitive tasks (Fornito et al., 2004).

Such accumulation of results, including conflicting data, may lead the reader to a broad vision of ACC as a backup system that takes over problem solving when the executive system is overloaded. In simple words, ACC could be the ace up the prefrontal cortex's sleeve, meant to be used when executive functions are impaired or overloaded, whether by physical disconnection as in TBI or simply by a high level of difficulty. As a backup system, its efficiency would be limited, but would be involved in improving performance up to a certain limit, and would remain activated after this limit has been reached. This hypothesis is compatible with the concept of compensatory adjustment and would explain why some studies show that individuals with ACC lesions are still able to solve difficult problems (di Pellegrino et al., 2007). Furthermore, as suggested by our results, a double dissociation between ACC and lSMC activation in response to difficulty could account for the conflicting literature regarding the role of ACC.

CONCLUSION

While our study provides yet another small brick to the construction of ACC understanding, it is noteworthy that the ACC is involved in so many apparently distinct functions that one may have to reconsider the existing theoretical framework before one can reach firm conclusions. One aspect that deserves further consideration is the structure–function relationship that exists at the level of the ACC (Koski and Paus, 2000; Margulies et al., 2007; Orr and Weissman, 2009) as it exists in other regions. For example, one appealing model has been proposed that connects the structure of dorsolateral prefrontal cortex to its functions, with concrete action planning being closer to motor areas and more abstract planning being more rostral (Koechlin and Jubault, 2006; Badre and D'Esposito, 2007), consistently with the perception–action model that was developed by Fuster (2005). A similarly innovative proposition was made by Postle (2006), stating that working memory is an emergent function rather than an embedded function, a theory also supported by Zimmer (2008). The ACC occupies a strategic location in the brain and therefore has the capacity of integrating of a wide variety of inputs. Indeed, ACC activity has been associated with a wide variety of mental functions, such as attention (Brocki et al., 2009), motivation (Ullsperger and Von Cramon, 2004), sexuality (Stoléru et al., 1999), pain (Robinson et al., 2009), executive functions (Mansouri et al., 2009), among others.

Most models, deeply influenced by Cartesian heritage, draw a scientific line between emotional and intellectual processes, despite our knowledge that these functions are highly interdependent. In order to fully understand how one cerebral area can process such diverse information, we may have to rethink those categories and investigate their potential interconnections. A neurophenomenological approach would suggest that all inputs processed by one area have to share either a common architecture or require a common processing (Allman et al., 2001). Therefore, seeking the common ground of these inputs would provide essential information on the fundamental roles of the ACC. It is likely that such an integrative theory would help unifying the current models of ACC functions.

ACKNOWLEDGMENTS

We want to thank Bernard Mendiburu for Matlab programming and support, Russell Poldrack for help with study design, Trent Thixton for help with brain imaging, Tarman Aziz for proofreading, Claudia Kernan and Nina Newman for patients' assessment and consenting, all the RAPBI members for discussion and feedback. This work was supported by the UCLA Brain Injury Research Center (Christopher Giza, Robert F. Asarnow), The Della Martin Foundation, Winokur Family Foundation/Child Neurology Foundation (Christopher Giza), UCLA Faculty Grants Program.

REFERENCES

Aarts, E., Roelofs, A., and van Turennout, M. (2008). Anticipatory activity in anterior cingulate cortex can be independent of conflict and error likelihood. *J. Neurosci.* 28,4671–4678.

Allman, J. M., Hakeem, A., Erwin, J. M., Nimchinsky, E., and Hof, P. (2001). The anterior cingulate cortex: the evolution of an interface between emotion and cognition. *Ann. N. Y. Acad. Sci.* 935,107–117.

Babikian, T., and Asarnow, R. (2009). Neurocognitive outcomes and recovery after pediatric TBI: meta- analytic review of the literature. *Neuropsychology* 23,283–296.

Badre, D., and D'Esposito, M. (2007). FMRI evidence for a hierarchical organization of the prefrontal cortex. *J. Cogn. Neurosci.* 19, 1–18. Botvinick, M. M., Braver, T. S., Barch, D. M., Carter, C. S., and Cohen, J. D. (2001). Conflict monitoring and cognitive control. *Psychol. Rev.* 108, 624–652.

Botvinick, M. M., Cohen, J. D., and Carter, C. S. (2004). Conflict moni- toring and anterior cingulate cor- tex: an update. *Trends in Cogn. Sci.* 8, 539–546.

Brocki, K., Clerkin, S. M., Guise, K. G., Fan, J., and Fossella, J. A. (2009). Assessing the molecular genetics of the devel- opment of executive attention in children: focus on genetic pathways related to the anterior cingulate cor- tex and dopamine. *Neuroscience* 164, 241–246.

Carter, C. S., and van Veen, V. (2007). Anterior cingulate cortex and con- flict detection: an update of theory anddata. *Cogn. Affect. Behav. Neurosci.* 7, 367–379.

Cazalis, F., Feydy, A., Valabregue, R., Pelegrini-Issac, M., Pierot, L., and Azouvi, P. (2006). fMRI study of prob- lem-solvingafterseveretraumaticbrain injury. *Brain Inj.* 20,1019–1028.

Cazalis, F., Valabregue, R., Pelegrini-Issac, M., Asloun, S., Robbins, T. W., and Granon, S. (2003). Individual differ- ences in prefrontal cortical activation on the Tower of London planning task: implication for effortful processing. *Eur. J. Neurosci.* 17,2219–2225.

Declerck, C. H., Boone, C., and De Brabander, B. (2006). On feeling in control: a biological theory for indi- vidual differences in control percep- tion. *Brain Cogn.* 62,143–176.

D' Esposito, M. (2008). "Working memory," in *Handbook of Clinical Neurology*, eds P. J. Vinken and G. W. Bruyn (Amsterdam: Elsevier), 237–247.

di Pellegrino, G., Ciaramelli, E., and Ladavas, E. (2007). The regulation of cognitive control following ros- tral anterior cingulate cortex lesion in humans. *J. Cogn. Neurosci.* 19, 275–286.

Fiehler, K., Burke, M., Engel, A., Bien, S., and Rösler, F. (2008). Kinesthetic Working Memory and Action Control within the Dorsal Stream. *Cereb. Cortex* 18, 243–253.

Fornito, A., Yucel, M., Wood, S., Stuart, G. W., Buchanan, J. A., Proffitt, T., Anderson, V., Velakoulis, D., and Pantelis, C. (2004). Individual dif- ferences in anterior cingulate/parac- ingulate morphology are related to executive functions in healthy males. *Cereb. Cortex* 14, 424–431.

Fuster, J. M. (2005). *Cortex and Mind: Unifying Cognition.* New York: Oxford University Press.

Garavan, H., Ross, T. J., Murphy, K., Roche, R. A. P., and Stein, E. A. (2002). Dissociable executive functions in the dynamic control of behavior: inhibi- tion, error detection, and correction. *Neuroimage* 17, 1820–1829.

Ghajar, J., and Ivry, R. B. (2008). The pre- dictive brainstate: timingdeficiencyin traumatic brain injury? *Neurorehabil. Neural. Repair* 22, 217–227.

Hahn, B., Ross, T. J., and Stein, E.A. (2007). Cingulate activation increases dynam- ically with response speed under stim- ulus unpredictability. *Cereb. Cortex* 17, 1664–1671.

Hanakawa, T., Dimyan, M.A., and Hallett, M. (2008). Motor planning, imagery, and execution in the distributed motor network: a time-course study with functional MRI. *Cereb. Cortex.* 18,2775–2788.

Hillary, F., Steffener, J., Biswal, B., Lange, G., DeLuca, J., and Ashburner, J. (2002). Functional magnetic reso- nance imaging technology and trau- matic brain injury rehabilitation: guidelines for methodological and conceptual pitfalls. *J. Head Trauma Rehabil.* 17, 411–430.

Hyafi A., Summerfi ld, C., and Koechlin, E. (2009). Two mechanisms for task switching in the prefrontal cortex. *J. Neurosci.* 29, 5135–5142.

Kerns, J. G., Cohen, J. D., MacDonald, A. W. III, Cho, R. Y., Stenger, V. A., and Carter, C. S. (2004).Anterior cingulate confl t monitoring and adjustments in control. *Science* 303, 1023–1026.

Koechlin, E., and Jubault, T. (2006). Broca's area and the hierarchical organiza- tion of human behavior. *Neuron* 50, 963–974.

Kohl, A. D., Wylie, G. R., Genova, H. M., Hillary, F.G., and DeLuca, J. (2009). The neuralcorrelatesofcognitivefatiguein traumaticbraininjuryusingfunctional MRI. *Brain Inj.* 2,420–432.

Koski, L., and Paus, T. (2000). Functional connectivity of the anterior cingulate cortex within the human frontal lobe: a brain-mapping meta-analysis. *Exp. Brain Res.* 133, 55–65.

Magno, E., Foxe, J. J., Molholm, S., Robertson, I. H., and Garavan, H. (2006). The anterior cingulate and error avoidance. *J. Neurosci.* 26, 4769–4773.

Mai, J. K., Paxinos, G., and Assheuer, J. K. (2004). Atlas of the Human Brain, 2nd Edn. San Diego, CA: Academic Press. Mansouri, F. A., Tanaka, K., and Buckley, M. J. (2009). Confl t-induced behav- ioural adjustment: a clue to the execu- tive functions of the prefrontal cortex. *Nat. Rev. Neurosci.* 10, 141–152.

Margulies, D. S., Kelly, A. M., Uddin, L. Q., Biswal, B. B., Castellanos, F. X., and Milham, M. P. (2007). Mapping the functional connectivity of ante- rior cingulate cortex. *Neuroimage* 37, 579–588.

Metting, Z., Rödiger, L. A., De Keyser, J., and van der Naalt, J. (2007). Structural and functional neuroimaging in mild- to-moderate head injury. *Lancet Neurol.* 6,699–710.

Niogi, S. N., Mukherjee, P., Ghajar, J., Johnson, C. E., Kolster, R., Lee, H., Suh, M., Zimmerman, R. D., Manley, G. T., and McCandliss, B. D. (2008). Structural dissociation of attentional control and memory in adults with and without mild traumatic brain injury. *Brain* 131,3209–3221.

Orr, J. M., and Weissman, D. H. (2009). Anterior cingulate cortex makes 2 con- tributions to minimizing distraction. *Cereb. Cortex* 19,703–711.

Osaka, M., Osaka, N., Kondo, H., Morishita, M., Fukuyama, H., Aso, T., and Shibasaki, H. (2003). The neural basis of individual differences in working memory capacity: an fMRI study. *Neuroimage* 18, 789–797.

Osaka, N., Osaka, M., Kondo, H., Morishita, M., Fukuyama, H., and Shibasaki, H. (2004). The neural basis of executive function in work- ing memory: an fMRI study based on individual differences. *Neuroimage* 21, 623–631.

Paus, T., Koski, L., Caramanos, Z., and Westbury, C. (1998). Regional dif- ferences in the effects of task dif- ficulty and motor output on blood flow response in the human anterior cingulate cortex: a review of 107 PET activation studies. *Neuroreport* 9, R37–R47.

Pepin Press. (2006a). *The Agile Rabbit Visual Dictionary of Vegetables*, Agile Rabbit Editions. Amsterdam: Pepin Press.

Pepin Press. (2006b). *The Agile Rabbit Visual Dictionary of Fruits*, Agile Rabbit Editions. Amsterdam: Pepin Press.

Postle, B. R. (2006). Working memory as an emergent property of the mind and brain. *Neuroscience* 139, 23–38.

Rasmussen, I.-A., Xu, J., Antonsen, I. K., Brunner, J., Skandsen, T., Axelson, D. E., Berntsen, E. M., Lydersen, S., and Håberg, A. (2008). Simple dual tasking recruits prefrontal cortices in chronic severe traumatic brain injury patients, but not in controls. *J. Neurotrauma* 25, 1057–1070.

Ratiu, P., and Talos, I.-F. (2006). *Cross- Sectional Atlas of the Brain*. Cambridge, MA: Cambridge Harvard University Press.

Robinson, M., Edwards, S., Iyengar, S., Bymaster, F., Clark, M., and Katon, W. (2009). Depression and pain. *Front. Biosci.* 1, 5031–5051.

Sack, A. T., Jacobs, C., Martino, F. D., Staeren, N., Goebel, R., and Formisano, E. (2008). Dynamic premotor-to-parietal interactions during spatial imagery. *J. Neurosci.* 28, 8417–8429.

Sanchez-Carrion, R., Fernandez-Espejo, D., Junque, C., Falcon, C., Bargallo, N., Roig, T., Bernabeu, M., Tormos, J. M., and Vendrell, P. (2008). A lon- gitudinal fMRI study of working memory in severe TBI patients with diffuse axonal injury. *Neuroimage* 43, 421–429.

Shaw, M. E., Moores, K. A., Clark, R. C., McFarlane, A. C., Strother, S. C., Bryant, R.A., Brown, G. C., and Taylor, J. D. (2009). Functional connectivity reveals inefficient working memory systems in post-traumatic stress disor- der. *Psychiatry Res.* 172, 235–241.

Smith, S. M., Jenkinson, M., Woolrich, M. W., Beckmann, C. F., Behrens, T. E. J., Johansen-Berg, H., Bannister, P. R., De Luca, M., Drobnjak, I., Flitney, D. E., Niazy, R. K., Saunders, J., Vickers, J., Zhang, Y., De Stefano, N., Brady, J. M., and Matthews, P. M. (2004). Advances in functional and structural MR image analysis and implementa- tion as FSL. *Neuroimage* 23(Suppl. 1), S208–S219.

Stoléru, S., Grégoire, M., Gérard, D., Decety, J., Lafarge, E., Cinotti, L., Lavenne, F., Le Bars, D., Vernet-Maury, E., Rada, H., Collet, C., Mazoyer, B., Forest, M. G., Magnin, F., Spira, A., and Comar, D. (1999). Neuroanatomical correlates of visually evoked sexual arousal in human males. *Arch. Sex. Behav.* 28, 1–21.

Ullsperger, M., and Von Cramon, D. Y. (2004). Neuroimaging of perform- ance monitoring: error detection and beyond. *Cortex* 40, 593–604.

Ursu, S., Clark, K. A., Aizenstein, H. J., Stenger, V. A., and Carter, C. S. (2009). Conflict-related activity in the cau- dal anterior cingulate cortex in the absence of awareness. *Biol. Psychol.* 80, 279–286.

Wager, T. D., and Smith, E. E. (2003). Neuroimaging studies of working memory: a meta-analysis. *Cogn. Affect. Behav. Neurosci.* 3, 255–274.

Woolrich, M., Jbabd, S., Patenaude, B., Chappell, M., Makni, S., Behrens, T., Beckmann, C., Jenkinson, M., and Smith, S. M. (2009). Bayesian analysis of neuroimaging data in FSL. *Neuroimage* 45(Suppl.), S173–S186.

Zimmer, H. D. (2008). Visual and spatial working memory: from boxes to networks. *Neurosci. Biobehav. Rev.* 32, 1373–1395..

Smaller, softer, lower-impedance electrodes for human neuroprosthesis: a pragmatic approach

Elisa Castagnola[1], Alberto Ansaldo[1], Emma Maggiolini[1], Tamara Ius[2], Miran Skrap[2], Davide Ricci[1] and Luciano Fadiga[1,3]*

[1] Robotics, Brain and Cognitive Sciences Department, Istituto Italiano di Tecnologia, Genoa, Italy
[2] Struttura Complessa di Neurochirurgia, Azienda Ospedaliero-Universitaria Santa Maria della Misericordia, Udine, Italy
[3] Section of Human Physiology, Department of Biomedical Sciences, University of Ferrara, Ferrara, Italy

Edited by:
Ulrich G. Hofmann, Albert-Ludwigs-University Freiburg, Germany

Reviewed by:
Anirban Dutta, Case Western Reserve University, USA
Luciano Lopes Furlanetti, Albert-Ludwigs University of Freiburg, Germany

***Correspondence:**
Luciano Fadiga, Robotics, Brain and Cognitive Sciences Department, Istituto Italiano di Tecnologia, Via Morego 30, Genoa, 16163, Italy
e-mail: luciano.fadiga@iit.it

Finding the most appropriate technology for building electrodes to be used for long term implants in humans is a challenging issue. What are the most appropriate technologies? How could one achieve robustness, stability, compatibility, efficacy, and versatility, for both recording and stimulation? There are no easy answers to these questions as even the most fundamental and apparently obvious factors to be taken into account, such as the necessary mechanical, electrical and biological properties, and their interplay, are under debate. We present here our approach along three fundamental parallel pathways: we reduced electrode invasiveness and size without impairing signal-to-noise ratio, we increased electrode active surface area by depositing nanostructured materials, and we protected the brain from direct contact with the electrode without compromising performance. Altogether, these results converge toward high-resolution ECoG arrays that are soft and adaptable to cortical folds, and have been proven to provide high spatial and temporal resolution. This method provides a piece of work which, in our view, makes several steps ahead in bringing such novel devices into clinical settings, opening new avenues in diagnostics of brain diseases, and neuroprosthetic applications.

Keywords: micro-electrocorticography (ECoG), Intracortical microelectrodes, carbon nanotubes, conductive polymers, hydrogel, neural recording, neural stimulation, brain-conformability

INTRODUCTION

The larger part of our understanding of brain neurophysiology derives from electrical signals experimentally recorded using different types of intracortical penetrating microelectrodes, i.e., multiple-insulated metal microwires (Musallam et al., 2007; Nicolelis and Lebedev, 2009; Marin and Fernández, 2010) or micromachined penetrating microelectrode arrays (Suner et al., 2005; Wise, 2005; Marin and Fernández, 2010) and electrocorticography (ECoG) electrodes (Leuthardt et al., 2004; Kellis et al., 2009; Ritaccio et al., 2011). However, long-term stability is still an issue as regards the clinical application of neural implants, and two parallel avenues of research are currently being explored with a view to resolving this problem. One is the ongoing commitment to improving today's intracortical penetrating microelectrodes, which, despite their superior neural recordings in term of accuracy, bandwidth, and resolution (Leuthardt et al., 2006, 2009), tend to induce acute and chronic inflammatory reactions due to the trauma of mechanical insertion and the tissue response to such a foreign body. Indeed, the latter causes the formation of a glial scar, which distances neurons from the recording sites and thereby impairs signal recording (Schwartz, 2004; Marin and Fernández, 2010). Simultaneously, there is also great effort being expended in the attempt to improve the quality of cortical recording up to a level that could provide sufficient information to decode, for example, motor cortical signals, through the use of very high resolution micro-ECoG arrays (Leuthardt et al., 2004, 2006; Kellis et al., 2009, 2010; Chao et al., 2010).

Although advances have been made, both approaches would greatly benefit from a key improvement, namely reducing the impedance of recording sites. Lowering the impedance is fundamental to enhance the signal recording quality, reduce the background noise, and, consequently, increase the signal-to-noise ratio. At the same time a lower impedance with no dimensional increase enables the injection of relatively large capacitive currents whilst minimizing electrode degradation due to Faradaic effects. Increasing the active surface area of electrodes through the deposition of high-surface-area materials, i.e., nanostructured coatings, has been shown to induce a dramatic drop in impedance (Cui and Martin, 2003; Abidian and Martin, 2008; Green et al., 2008; Keefer et al., 2008; Ferguson et al., 2009; Castagnola et al., 2010; Ansaldo et al., 2011; Baranauskas et al., 2011). This increases their signal-to-noise ratio while enabling electrode miniaturization, which reduces their invasiveness and minimizes tissue damage during insertion. It is expected that very low-impedance and tiny recording sites would also dramatically improve micro-ECoG array technologies, enhancing their sensitivity and spatial selectivity, thereby increasing the information content of the recorded signal. As a consequence, their inter-electrode distance could be reduced, enhancing the spatial resolution (Castagnola et al., 2013a,b).

Another actively pursued key research target is the development of soft, flexible, and conformable electrode substrates, which would reduce implant-related tissue stress. Indeed, the reciprocal movements of brain and skull during behavioral and metabolic processes can generate several negative effects when devices coupled to the bone are *in situ*. However, using a compliant material in penetrating micro-electrodes would help to minimize tissue damage arising from their micro-movements in brain tissue, thereby reducing long-term inflammation and glial scar formation (Rousche et al., 2001; Lee et al., 2004; Takeuchi et al., 2004). In the case of micro-ECoG arrays, the use of a conformable substrate would enable accommodation of both brain curvature and movement, keeping each electrode in the array in intimate contact with the cortical surface and improving the electrical coupling (Hollenberg et al., 2006; Leuthardt et al., 2009; Rubehn et al., 2009; Ritaccio et al., 2011; Khodagholy et al., 2011; Thongpang et al., 2011; Castagnola et al., 2013b). We set out to tackle all of these issues through the application of soft and high-surface-area material coatings to both intracortical and epicortical microelectrodes. We describe the use of a variety of such nanomaterial coatings, documenting their effects on impedance, charge transfer capability, signal-to-noise ratio, and signal recording quality of different types of miniaturized intracortical microelectrodes and very high-resolution micro-ECoG arrays. We also present a validated pragmatic approach to solving the biocompatibility issues and concerns raised by the use of nanomaterial-containing coatings, namely encapsulating nanocoated neural devices with a human fibrin hydrogel layer, which creates a mechanically stable barrier between the nanomaterials and the brain. Finally, we present our method of reducing the invasiveness and increasing the versatility of intracortical microelectrodes and micro-ECoG arrays, making them smaller, softer, and more flexible by exploiting a combination of nanocoatings and polymer-based circuits[1].

The results we present, in our opinion, provide a method which makes several steps ahead in bringing such novel devices into clinical settings, opening new avenues in diagnostics of brain diseases, and neuroprosthetic applications.

HIGH-SURFACE-AREA NANOCOATINGS

The impedance of electrodes is one of the main parameters influencing their suitability for both brain recording and stimulation. Assuming their metal surface is smooth and stable, the charge that can be exchanged with a saline solution, i.e., the current that can flow through it, is limited by the maximum voltage that can be applied without causing irreversible chemical reactions such as electrolysis. In the absence of Faradaic reactions, the metal interface will become charged, meaning that, practically speaking, the electrode must behave like a capacitor to prevent undesirable chemical reactions in the intracellular medium. One way to meet this requirement, which is particularly relevant for purely stimulating electrodes, is to introduce an active material that produces a controlled, reversible and rapid Faradaic reaction (pseudo-capacitive), for instance activated iridium oxide (Cogan et al., 2004; Gawad et al., 2009). A complementary approach, suitable for both stimulating and recording electrodes, would be to increase the electrode capacitance whilst containing its geometric size. This can be achieved, even when using electrochemically inert interfaces, by increasing the electrode surface area by augmenting its roughness/porosity. This, in turn, can be achieved by coating even commonly used metal electrodes with nanostructured high-surface-area (HSA) materials. Indeed, several HSA coatings made from a variety of nanostructured materials have been widely investigated as a means of enhancing the surface properties of traditional metal electrodes, decreasing their impedance, and increasing their charge transfer capability. These include platinum black (Robinson, 1968; Desai et al., 2010), various conductive polymers such as polypyrrole (PPy), polyaniline (PANI) and poly-[3,4 ethylenedioxythiophene] (PEDOT), (Cui et al., 2001; Cui and Martin, 2003; Yang et al., 2005; Ludwig et al., 2006; Kotov et al., 2009), and their carbon nanotube (CNT)-based nanocomposites (Keefer et al., 2008; Castagnola et al., 2009, 2013a,b; Ferguson et al., 2009; Jan et al., 2009; Lu et al., 2010; Ansaldo et al., 2011). As it would be preferable to record and stimulate using the same device, we set up a variety of CNT deposition methods, obtaining coatings to be tested in some of the most demanding electrode applications, i.e., intracortical and flexible epicortical neural recording and stimulation. By electrochemical deposition we were able to coat electrodes made from different metals with PEDOT-CNT, PPy-CNT, and Au-CNT nanostructured coatings. Using an *ad-hoc* process based on catalytic chemical vapor deposition (CVD), we synthetized CNTs directly on metal electrodes able to withstand high temperature (>600°C). It should be noted at this point that, although in the literature all CNT-containing composites (Keefer et al., 2008) are generally referred to as "CNT electrodes," only in few cases CNTs act as the ultimate electrochemical interface. In most instances, CNTs are mainly used to induce the surface nanostructuring, and, as they are encased in composites, the electrode-solution interface involves no graphitic carbon, but instead conductive polymers (CPs) or metals. In fact, similar results to these so-called "CNT electrodes" could be obtained by adding other additives, such as polyethylene glycol (PEG) or agar, to the deposition solutions, in place of CNTs, to promote HSA formation. However, CNTs are preferred because their high mechanical strength, good electrical properties, high specific area, and high aspect ratio confer composites with superior electrical conductivity and mechanical properties (Green et al., 2008; Gerwig et al., 2012). The main advantage in using electrochemical deposition for coating the electrode surface is that it can be carried out at room temperature, as opposed to *in situ* CNT synthesis, which requires high temperature. This means that it can be applied to a virtually unlimited variety of materials and devices. Conversely, when a direct interaction between CNTs and neural cells is allowed, it has been shown *in vitro* that the intimate contact achieved at this interface gives rise to an excellent electrical coupling (Mazzatenta et al., 2007; Shoval et al., 2009; Sorkin et al., 2009), hinting at a special affinity of exposed CNTs for neural tissue.

ELECTROPLATED HSA COATINGS

Deposition procedure

In the case of CP-CNT composites, polymer and CNT nanocomposites were co-electrodeposited from an aqueous suspension of 1 mg ml^{-1} multi-wall carboxylated CNTs (COOH-MWCNTs, NC 3151, <4% of -COOH functional groups,

[1] All animal experimental procedures were approved by the Italian Ministry of Health (Italian Law DL116/92) and were conducted in accordance with the guidelines established by the European Communities Council (Directive 2010/63/EU of September 22nd, 2010).

Nanocyl) containing 0.5 M of the corresponding monomer, 3,4-ethylenedioxythiophene (EDOT, Sigma-Aldrich) or pyrrole (Py, Sigma-Aldrich), and 0.4 wt% of poly(sodium 4-styrene sulfonate) (PSS, Sigma-Aldrich). COOH-MWCNTs were suspended in ultrapure water (Milli-Q, Millipore, USA) via horn sonication (6 s, 66% duty cycle pulses, 4 W ml^{-1}, for 30 min) while cooling in an ice bath. PSS and monomers were added to the suspension immediately afterwards, and the solution was kept deoxygenated by bubbling with nitrogen. The electrochemical deposition was carried out in an inert atmosphere in the potentiostatic mode. The polymerization potential was set to 0.55 V vs. Ag/AgCl reference electrode for PPy, and 0.8 V vs. Ag/AgCl reference electrode for PEDOT. For CP-agar coatings, the COOH-MWCNT suspension was replaced by 0.1 wt% agarose. PSS and monomer were added to the stirred solution before it jellified while cooling in an ice bath. Au-CNT nanocomposites were co-electrodeposited by applying monophasic voltage pulses (0.2–1.0 V, 240 s, duty cycle 50%), starting from a 10 mM potassium dicyanoaurate(I) (Sigma-Aldrich) aqueous solution containing 1.5 mg ml^{-1} of partially dispersed MWCNTs (NC 3100, Nanocyl) or 1.5 mg·ml^{-1} of partially dispersed SWCNTs (Cheaptubes). For Au-agar coating the CNTs were replaced by agarose (0.1 wt%).

Electroplated HSA coating benchmarking

We compared the electrochemical performance of different HSA coatings using identical planar 3.1 mm^2 gold and platinum electrodes as benchmarks. The electrochemical behavior of the microelectrodes was studied in a 0.9% sodium chloride (NaCl) aqueous solution, by both cyclic voltammetry (CV)—to quantify their capacitive charging—and electrochemical impedance spectroscopy (EIS)—to determine the electrical properties of the system over a large frequency range. During the CV tests, the working electrode potential was swept between 0.5 and −0.5 V or 0.6 and −1 V vs. Ag/AgCl, maintaining a scan rate of 100 mV/s. During the EIS measurements, a sine wave (10 mV RMS amplitude) was superimposed onto the open circuit potential while varying the frequency from 10^5 to 1 Hz.

All electrochemical depositions were carried out using a potentiostat/galvanostat (Parstat 2273, Princeton Applied Research), while a potentiostat/galvanostat/ZRA (Reference 600, Gamry Instruments, USA) was used for electrochemical characterization. The electrochemical cell was a three-electrode cell. A platinum wire was used as the counter electrode and an Ag/AgCl electrode was used as the reference electrode.

Figure 1A presents a comparison between the EIS spectra of identical planar platinum electrodes uncoated or coated with PPy-CNTs, PEDOT-CNTs, PEDOT-agar, Au-CNT, and Au-agar, respectively. In all cases the potentiostatic deposition of the CP composites was performed applying a charge density of 700 mC/cm^2. All nanocoatings tested resulted in a reduction in impedance across the entire frequency range (1–10^5 Hz). The impedance magnitude values at 100 Hz and 1 kHz are reported in **Table 1**, together with the corresponding total charge transfer capability (CTC_{tot}) values. The CTCs were calculated as the time-integral of an entire CV cycle between 0.5 and −0.5 V ($CTC_{tot}1$), or between 0.6 and −1 V ($CTC_{tot}2$). Typical CVs measured for differently coated electrodes are reported in **Figure 1B** (0.5 to −0.5 V range) and **Figure 1C** (0.6 to −1.0 V range for PPy-CNT- and

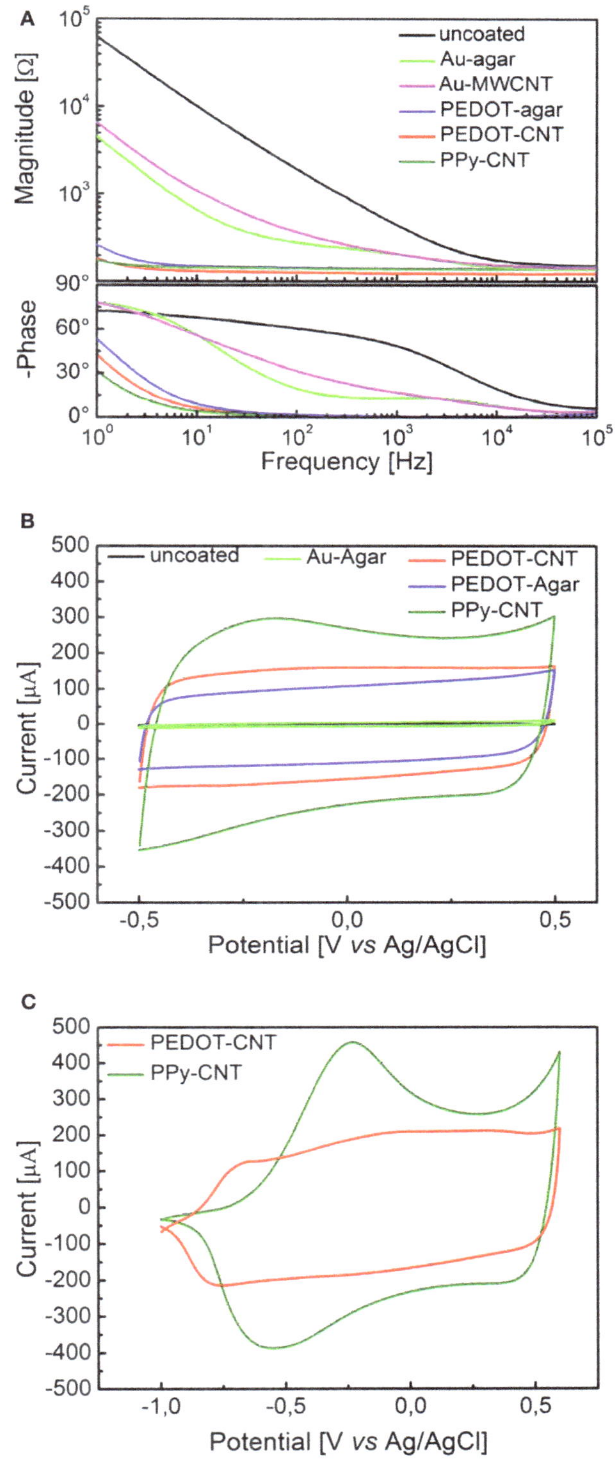

FIGURE 1 | (A) Impedance spectra of a 0.031 cm^2 Pt electrode, uncoated (black) and with electrodeposited Au-MWCNT (pink), Au-agar (green), PPy-CNT (dark green), PEDOT-agar (blue), or PEDOT-CNT (red). **(B)** Cyclic voltammograms between −0.5 and 0.5 V of a 0.031 cm^2 Pt electrode, uncoated (black), or with electrodeposited Au-agar (green), PPy-CNT (dark green), PEDOT-agar (blue), or PEDOT-CNT (red). **(C)**, Cyclic voltammograms between −1.0 and 0.6 V of a 0.031 cm^2 Pt electrode coated with PPy-CNT (dark green) and PEDOT-CNT (red).

Table 1 | Electrochemical characterization of HSA coatings.

	|Z|@ 100 Hz [Ω]	|Z|@ 1 kHz [Ω]	CTC_{tot}1[mC cm-2]	CTC_{tot}2[mC cm-2]
PEDOT-agar	142.6 ± 1.7	139.5 ± 1.6	149.7 ± 7.3	246.2 ± 4.9
PEDOT-CNT	127.6 ± 0.1	125.0 ± 0.2	92.3 ± 4.6	158.7 ± 8.2
PPy-CNT	138.7 ± 4.3	136.7 ± 4.1	67.7 ± 0.5	118.9 ± 4.8
Au-agar	291 ± 12	214.6 ± 8.3	3.1 ± 0.7	6.2 ± 0.5
Au-CNT	334 ± 50	192 ± 25	2.5 ± 0.3	4.6 ± 0.2
Uncoated	1915 ± 203	441 ± 7	0.5 ± 0.1	3.3 ± 0.2

PEDOT-CNT-coated electrodes). In both cases it can be observed that when the same charge density is applied during electrodeposition, the CTC_{tot} of the PPy-CNT coating is greater than that of the PEDOT-CNT coating, but that the peak potentials of the PEDOT composites are about 200 mV more negative than those of the PPy composite (**Figure 1C**), extending the PEDOT capacitive behavior over a wider potential window. Moreover, the PEDOT-CNT coating provided the lowest impedance at all frequencies above 2 Hz.

PROCEDURE FOR CHEMICAL VAPOR DEPOSITION OF CARBON NANOTUBES

In order to selectively synthetize CNTs on the metal tip of an electrode of arbitrary shape, we devised a nickel catalyst deposition method based on electrode electroplating, rather than relying on the more common physical deposition methods (such as dip-coating, spray-coating, evaporation, or sputtering). Nickel was electroplated from an aqueous solution containing 300 g l^{-1} nickel(II) sulfate hexahydrate ($NiSO_4 \cdot 6H_2O$, CAS 10101-97-0, *puriss.* p.a. Riedel-de Haën), 90 g l^{-1} nickel chloride hexaydrate ($NiCl_2$ 3 $6H_2O$, CAS 7791-20-0 *purum*, p.a.; >99.0% Fluka), and 45 mg l^{-1} boric acid (H_3BO_3, CAS 10043-35-3, *puriss.* p.a. Riedel-de Haën). Electrodeposition was performed in the potentiostatic mode at −0.9 V vs. an Ag/AgCl reference electrode. The depositions were carried out in an inert atmosphere at 45°C and pH 4. The amount of catalyst deposited onto the electrode was determined by controlling the charge passed during the deposition. The CVD process was performed in a quartz tube reactor, 120 cm long and 25 mm in diameter, passing through a Lenton PSC 12/--/600H split furnace. The catalyst was activated by flowing a forming gas (Ar 95 sccm, H_2, 5 sccm, ambient pressure) while heating the samples up to 650°C; the carbon feedstock was then introduced into the reaction chamber by bubbling the same gas mixture through a Drechsel washing bottle with glass filter disk, filled with absolute ethanol at room temperature. Reaction time was 15 min at 650°C.

APPLICATION OF NANOCOATINGS

INTRACORTICAL PLATFORM

Reduced impedance and increased charge transfer capability

In order to be able to compare all the previously described HSA coatings, including the CNTs directly synthetized on the electrode tip at high temperature, we selected as an intracortical electrode platform quartz glass insulated platinum/tungsten wires of 80 μm outer shank diameter and 20 μm metal core diameter (Thomas Recording, Giessen, Germany). We prepared and characterized identical electrodes coated with *in situ* synthetized CNTs (CVD-CNT) and with different electrochemically co-deposited composites, namely Au-CNT, Au-agar, PPy-CNT, PEDOT-CNT, and PEDOT-agar. The insulated wire was ground using a grinding machine (DIECKL-ST, Thomas Recording), thereby providing sharp tips with a typical geometric area of about 1000 μm^2 and an impedance magnitude ranging from 0.5 to 0.7 MΩ at 1 kHz. We used both of these single electrodes (**Figures 2A,B** reports optical and SEM images respectively) and 4-core quartz-platinum/tungsten microelectrodes (tetrodes) having similar electrical properties to perform direct comparisons of the coatings' performance in simultaneous neural recordings. The corresponding datasheet schematics from Thomas Recording are shown in **Figures 2C,D**. A SEM picture of the tetrode is shown in **Figure 2E**. Electrochemical characterizations of the typical uncoated (black), electroplated Au-CNT (green), PPy-CNT (red) and PEDOT-CNT (blue), and CNT-CVD coated (magenta) electrodes were performed using impedance spectroscopy (**Figure 3A**), and cyclic voltammetry between 0.6 and −1.0 V vs. Ag/AgCl (**Figure 3B**). The electrochemical performance reported here is related to "viable" electrodes, as defined in our previous work (Ansaldo et al., 2011), in which we emphasized that special attention must be paid when presenting "dramatic" changes in impedance and charge transfer capability in electrodes designed for intracortical neural recording and stimulation. Indeed, although electrode impedance could feasibly be lowered by many orders of magnitude by increasing the amount of material, thick coatings are usually mechanically unstable. Here we consider "viable" electrodes those capable of withstanding dura mater penetration, i.e., displaying no significant changes in appearance or electrochemical performance even after an acute intracortical recording session (Ansaldo et al., 2011). According to this definition, our viable CNT-CVD-coated electrodes typically had an impedance of 16.3 ± 4.8 kΩ at 1 kHz, with a 70.8 ± 1.1 mC·cm^2 CTC_{tot} (Castagnola et al., 2010; Ansaldo et al., 2011), a significant improvement with respect to the uncoated electrodes (typically 600 kΩ and 20 mC cm^{-2} CTC_{tot}). In the case of PPy-CNT and PEDOT-CNT coatings, viable electrodes were consistently produced by using charge densities of 0.6 C cm^{-2} during deposition. Impedance magnitude and CTC_{tot} were 5.7 ± 0.3 kΩ @1 kHz and 212.3 ± 23.9 mC cm^{-2}, respectively, for PPy-CNT-coated microelectrodes, and 4.5 ± 0.6 kΩ @1 kHz and 180.5 ± 40.2 mC cm^{-2} for PEDOT-CNT-coated microelectrodes. In the case of Au-CNT coatings, improvements were limited by the intrinsic behavior of gold, which produces nanorough lamellar surfaces rather that nanoporous ones. The best values obtained for viable electrodes were an impedance of 59.6 ± 11.2 kΩ@1 kHz and a

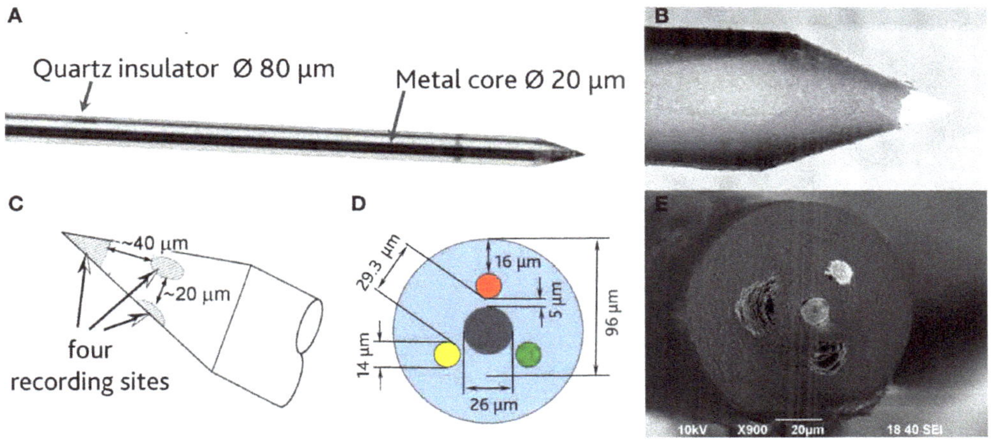

FIGURE 2 | (A) Optical image of a single sharp microelectrode. **(B)** Scanning electron micrograph of a single sharp microelectrode. **(C,D)** Schematic datasheet of a 4-core quartz-platinum/tungsten tetrode microelectrode (Thomas Recording, Giessen, Germany). **(E)** Tetrode scanning electron micrograph (s.e.m.).

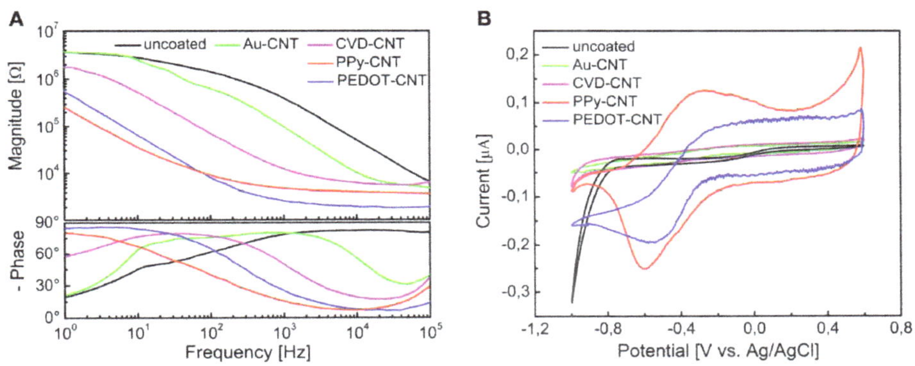

FIGURE 3 | (A) Impedance spectra of a single intracortical electrode, uncoated (black), or coated with Au-CNT (green) PPy-CNT (red), or PEDOT-CNT (blue), electrodeposited and CNT coated by direct growth with CVD. **(B)** Cyclic voltammograms of a single intracortical electrode, uncoated (black) or coated with Au-CNT (green), PPy-CNT (red) or PEDOT-CNT (blue), electrodeposited, and CNT coated by direct growth with CVD.

CTC_{tot} of 65.6 ± 13.6 mC cm^{-2} (Ansaldo et al., 2011). CTC_{tot} and $CTC_{tot}2$ were calculated as previously described. The reduction in impedance achieved depended on the coating, its nature and morphology, but all appeared to pave the way to a better signal-to-noise ratio in both single-neuron and multiunit recordings. The corresponding increase in CTC also makes these electrodes suitable for both recording and stimulation. The morphology of the different coatings can be appreciated by looking at the SEM pictures of grown CNT-CVD (**Figure 4A**), Au-CNT (**Figure 4B**), PPy-CNT (**Figure 4C**), and PEDOT-CNT (**Figure 4D**) electrodes. Nanorough lamellar coatings, similar to Au-CNT, can be also obtained by exploiting gold co-deposition in the presence of agarose gel (**Figures 5A,B**), or SWCNTs (**Figure 5C**).

To verify whether these coated microelectrodes are capable of stimulating the brain cortex, we estimated the charge injection limit for a set of typical electrodes, using cathodic-first charge-balanced biphasic symmetrical current pulses (Brummer et al., 1983; Cogan, 2008). The charge injection limit (Q_{inj}), defined as the maximum quantity of charge an electrode can inject before reaching the water electrolysis potential, was calculated as the time-integral of the current in the loading phase normalized by the geometric area of the uncoated microelectrode; water electrolysis potentials were determined experimentally via cyclic voltammetry. We used pulses having a total period of 2 ms and a cathodic duration of 500 µs (Ansaldo et al., 2011). To establish whether these electrodes could be used for long-term (chronic) neural stimulation and recording, we tested the stability of the different coatings under prolonged stimulation, and then compared the impedance of typical viable electrodes before and after applying a series of cathodic-first charge-balanced biphasic current pulses. The pulse duration was varied between 2 and 3 ms, the charge density between 0.4 and 1.6 mC cm^{-2}, and the cathodic pulse duration between 100 and 500 µs. The charge density applied was chosen according to the Q_{inj} for each material, namely 7 mC cm^{-2} for PPy-CNT microelectrodes, 4 mC cm^{-2} for CVD-CNT microelectrodes, and 0.8 mC cm^{-2} for Au-CNT microelectrodes. Even the relatively small Q_{inj} of Au-CNT electrodes is more than double that of the uncoated electrodes (0.2–0.4 mC cm^{-2}). As regards stability over time, CVD-CNT-coated electrodes were found to be stable, and could withstand a million 1.6 mC cm^{-2} pulses without

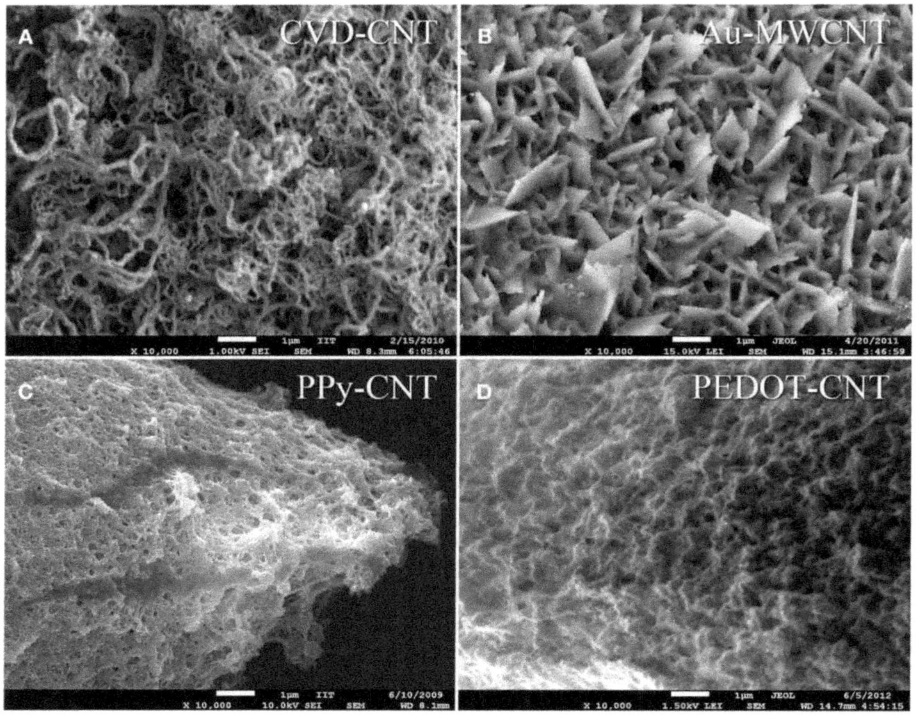

FIGURE 4 | Scanning electron micrograph of (A) as grown CNT-CVD coatings, (B) Au-MWCNT coating, (C) PPy-CNT coating, (D) PEDOT-CNT coating.

any degradation. PPy-CNT coatings rapidly degraded after a few thousand pulses at 1.6 mC cm^{-2}, while Au-CNT composite coatings were nearly as stable as CVD-CNTs, also being able to resist a million pulses, although their charge density had to be limited to 0.8 mC cm^{-2} in order to prevent Faradaic reactions (see Ansaldo et al., 2011). We can therefore conclude that CNTs selectively synthetized directly on the tip of neural microelectrodes by CVD are able to outperform the other so-called "CNT coatings" laid down by electrodeposition of CNT composites. Indeed, the CNT-CVD coating not only reduced microelectrode impedance, but was also able to withstand the repeated high-current pulses required for neural stimulation without degrading. This and its stability over time make it an excellent candidate for improving electrodes for use in chronic applications, especially when both neural recording and stimulation are required. Indeed, the only foreseeable limitation of CNT-CVD coatings resides in the high temperature (650°C) required for their deposition. Analysis of the PEDOT-CNT coating also yielded interesting results. In fact, it has already been reported in various studies that PEDOT may be a viable alternative to PPy for chronic, long-term implantations (Cui and Martin, 2003; Yang et al., 2005; Ludwig et al., 2006), as it is electrochemically more stable than PPy (Yamato et al., 1995). We measured a charge injection limit of 7 mC cm^{-2} on our PEDOT-CNT-coated microelectrodes. While this is identical to the charge on PPy-CNT-coated electrodes, PEDOT-CNT versions are able to withstand a million 1.6 mC cm^{-2}pulses without significant degradation, as demonstrated by the impedance spectra of a typical PEDOT-CNT coated electrode, reported in **Figure 6**. This suggests that PEDOT-CNT coatings are also excellent candidates for chronic applications, especially when both neural recording and stimulation have to be performed and a room-temperature deposition technique is required. Indeed, an initial validation of the suitability of these microelectrodes for *in vivo* use has already been obtained through acute intracortical recording sessions in rats (Ansaldo et al., 2011; Baranauskas et al., 2011).

CNT-composite coating improves multiunit signal-to-noise ratio of neural microelectrodes

Although it seems safe to assume that a low-impedance electrode has lower noise and is able to record larger signals, in fact the relationship between its resistivity and capacitance, and its ability to provide high-quality recordings are not straightforward. Indeed, the *in vivo* performance of an electrode is strongly influenced by many features of its surrounding environment (the brain), as well as the geometric area of the electrode (with respect to the size of the cells, i.e., the signal sources), and the presence of background biological activity, which remains too low to be properly detected, but contributes to the neural signal (the so-called biological noise) and therefore cannot be ignored. While the impedance reduction has a well-known impact on the Johnson-Nyquist noise (the thermal noise), any background signal that cannot be clearly isolated as neural activity will significantly contribute to total noise of a low-impedance electrode. Moreover, in the case of HSA-coated electrodes, the high specific capacitance, combined with the relatively high transversal resistivity of the coating, will significantly lower the speed of the signal on the electrode surface, meaning that the geometric size of the electrode can influence the frequency response at relatively low frequencies.

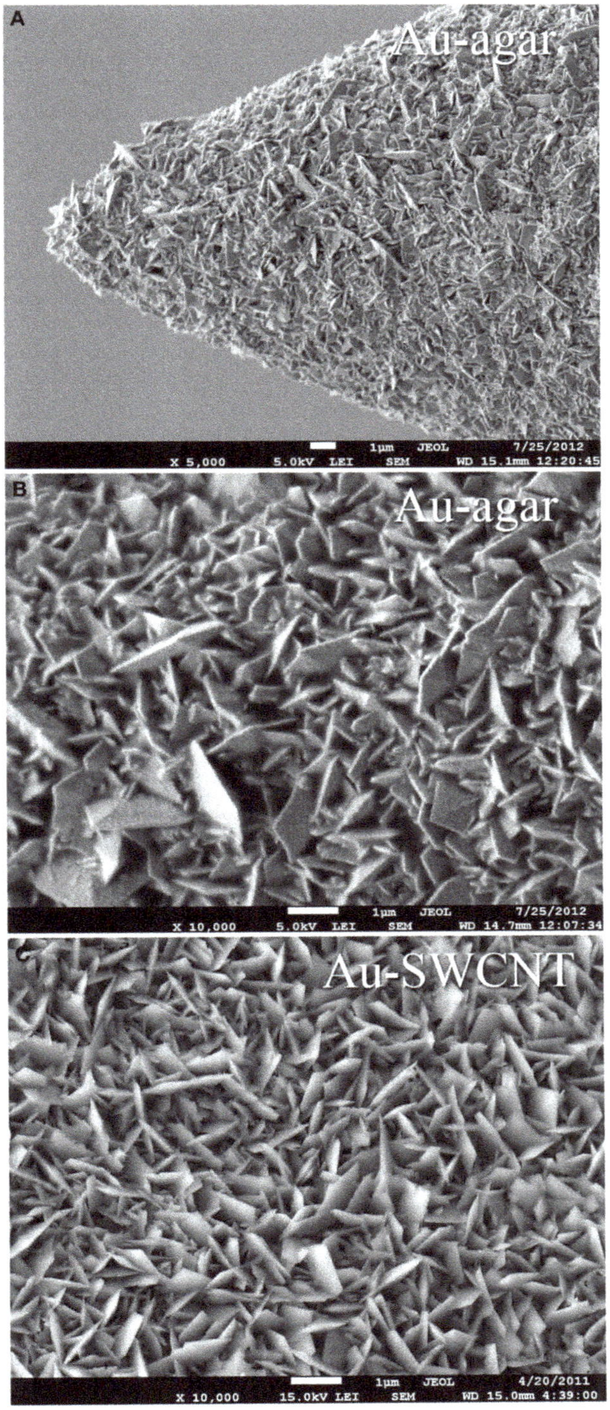

FIGURE 5 | Scanning electron micrograph of (A) a single tip Au-agar coated microelectrode, (B) Au-agar coating, (C) Au-SWCNT coating.

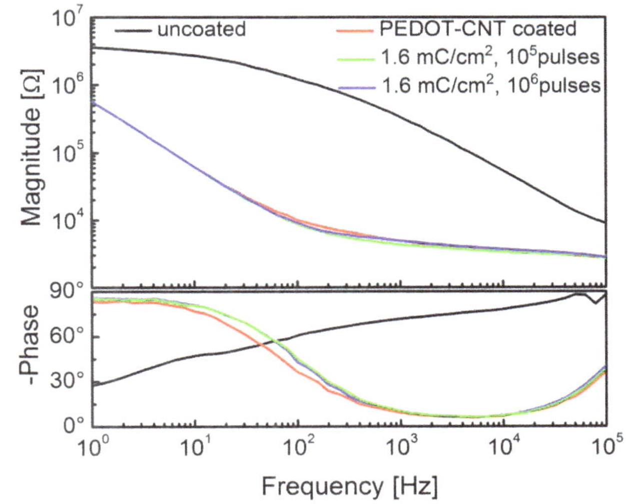

FIGURE 6 | Impedance spectra of a single intracortical electrode uncoated (black), and PEDOT-CNT-coated (red) and after stimulation experiments.

In order to investigate the effect of the very low impedance of CNT-based HSA coatings on signal acquisition, we devised a series of specific experiments using PPy-CNT coated electrodes to perform "acute" recording sessions on rats (Baranauskas et al., 2011). We studied in detail the impedance, the thermal, electronic and *in-vivo* noise, and the neural signals using ten single microelectrodes, PPy-CNT coated and uncoated, and two tetrodes, two of whose recording sites were coated with CNT-PPy while the other two remained untreated. This experiment enabled us to directly compare very closely positioned coated and uncoated electrodes during the same recording session.

As pointed out previously, during an *in vivo* recording session, neural signals are affected by several noise sources of both biological and non-biological origin. The non-biological sources include the electronic noise created by the amplifier, the thermal noise (Johnson-Nyquist), and the double-layer noise at the interface between the solution and microelectrode surface. The biological noise also includes additional thermal noise, created by the presence of brain tissue, and signals emitted by distant neurons. These neural signals are too small to be usefully distinguished, and therefore behave as noise for the majority of neural signal analyses (Harris et al., 2000; Quiroga et al., 2004; Ferguson et al., 2009). In the case of our electrodes, the non-biological noise contribution—including recording system noise, and filtering—was estimated by recording the noise signals from single microelectrodes immersed in a saline solution (NaCl 0.9%). In the case of PPy-CNT coated electrodes, we detected reduced noise over the entire useful frequency range (250–8000 Hz), and, in particular, in the range of frequencies corresponding to the multi-unit neural activity (MUA, ~150–1500 Hz). In the 250–8000 Hz frequency band, the overall noise measured was reduced by ~30%, from $5.9 \pm 0.2\,\mu V$ rms to $4.2 \pm 0.3\,\mu V$ rms. This difference was significant ($p < 0.015$; one-tailed t-test).

As discussed previously, the background noise is higher in the brain due to biological sources. Hence, in order to evaluate the biological noise contribution, we recorded from the deep layers of the primary somatosensory cortex (S1) in rats anaesthetized with Zoletil (30 mg/kg) and Xylazine (5 mg/kg). Indeed, under these conditions S1 switches between periods of high neural activity ("bursts") and periods of much lower activity ("pauses"). These periods of high and low activity are synchronized across large brain areas (>1 mm), and during the "pauses" the noise contribution of distant neuronal activity is minimal (Erchova et al., 2002), but during "bursts" it is possible to evaluate the background noise caused by the maximal activity of such neurons. In order to eliminate the effect of the presence of these burst spikes, the noise amplitude was estimated using a median value (Quiroga et al., 2004). We demonstrated that during "pauses," when the neuronal activity was low, the observed noise reduction ranged between 30 and 40%, comparable to data reported in the literature (Gabay et al., 2007; Keefer et al., 2008) though smaller than that of the saline test (55%). In contrast, during "bursts" the increased sensitivity provided by the PPy-CNT coating resulted in a larger contribution from distant neuronal activity, and a slight uptrend was observed from 11.2 ± 3.0 μV rms (uncoated) to 13.8 ± 4.0 μV rms (CNT-PPy, $p < 0.2$).

Moving on to the analysis of recorded neural signals, we estimated the amplitude for single spikes, local field potentials (LFP) and MUAs (Baranauskas et al., 2011). Tests were carried out using platinum/tungsten tetrodes featuring two PPy-CNT-coated and two uncoated recording sites. Although the average spike amplitudes of the two types of electrodes were similar (0.45 ± 0.03 mV vs. 0.40 ± 0.03 mV), the maximal spike amplitude was greater with the coated versions (increased from 0.52 ± 0.03 mV to 0.75 ± 0.04 mV). Moreover, more neuronal units were detected using the PPy-CNT coated electrodes (22 with respect to 16 units), as these were able to detect signals arising from more distant neurons in which smaller spikes dominate. This ability to detect a certain number of weaker signals may explain why the increase in maximal recorded amplitude was not accompanied by a similar improvement in average, further suggesting that average spike amplitude cannot be assumed as a reliable indicator of recording ability.

The contribution of MUA to the overall spectral power density (SPD) was estimated by subtracting the SPD of the signal recorded during "bursts" from the one recorded during "pauses." A significant increase in the SPD of the signals recorded using the PPy-CNT-coated electrode in the frequency range 200–1000 Hz was observed. Notably, analysis of the low frequency part of the spectrum (~1–250 Hz) recorded using PPy-CNT-coated microelectrodes revealed a marked reduction—of almost 3 orders of magnitude—in the 50 Hz interference (the frequency of the European electric power network), and total rejection of its higher harmonics. There are at least two reasons why this reduction in 50-Hz noise is particularly important from a neurophysiological standpoint. First, it reduces the risk of amplifier saturation during LFP recordings, and second the power line frequency of 50 Hz precisely matches the middle frequency of the so called "gamma range," which is thought to reflect a number of important brain functions (Gray et al., 1989; Fries et al., 2007). To sum up, we found that the most important improvements conferred by PPy-CNT coating of microelectrodes can be observed in the frequency range from 150 to 1500 Hz, which mainly corresponds to the multiunit signal and, partially, to the high-frequency end of LFPs. In this frequency range, the non-biological noise power is reduced by up to three-fold, while the neural signal power is increased by up to nine-fold. The combination of lower noise and stronger neural signal resulted in an approximately four-fold improvement in SNR in the middle of this frequency range. Our results also suggest that the coated microelectrodes offer considerable advantages for studying brain signals in the gamma frequency range, thanks to their greater electromagnetic noise rejection.

FLEXIBLE MICRO-ECoG ARRAYS

We developed a family of micro-electrocorticography (ECoG) arrays based on the commercially available flexible printed circuit (FPC) technology, tailoring the design according to the different neurophysiological experiments to be conducted. The choice of a well-established, reliable industrial process greatly reduced the time required to move from concept to prototype, and would likewise simplify production. We developed devices suitable for ECoG on both rats and primates (marmoset), as well as prototypes of devices suitable for the use on humans, having from 16 up to 128 recording sites with electrode diameters ranging from 75 up to 200 μm and an inter-electrode pitch from 300 up to 1.2 mm. Some examples are shown in **Figure 7**.

The FPCs consist of a double-sided copper circuit (9 μm thick) on a 25 μm polyimide film. After photo etching, the circuit is embedded in two polyimide coverlays (12.5 μm of polyimide plus 12.5 μm of pressure-sensitive acrylic adhesive) by cold lamination. The electrodes are then exposed by laser ablation, and passivated by a 1-μm thick layer of electroplated gold. The micro-ECoG devices were post-processed in our laboratory by electrochemical deposition of a nanostructured gold layer, which acts as an adhesion layer for PEDOT-CNT or PPy-CNT composites (Castagnola et al., 2013a,b). PEDOT-CNT or PPy-CNT nanocomposites were then co-deposited electrochemically onto the micro-ECoG recording sites to reduce their impedance and increase their charge transfer capabilities. SEM images showing the typical morphologies of these coatings when deposited on the micro-ECOG electrodes are shown in **Figure 8**.

Both the Au-CNT and Au-agar coatings present nanorough lamellar structures that reduce the electrode impedance by two-thirds with respect to the uncoated electrode (100 Hz, LFP central band), while the PEDOT-CNT and PPy-CNT composite coatings present a compact, sponge-like morphology, which provides a dramatic reduction in impedance of up to greater than 2 orders of magnitude over the whole frequency range of interest (1 Hz–1 kHz), and especially at 100 Hz. **Figure 9** reports the impedance spectra of 100 μm diameter ECoG array recording sites before and after Au-agar, PPy-CNT and PEDOT-CNT electrodeposition. The values shown were obtained by averaging the impedance spectra of 64 electrodes for each material studied. The impedance values (mean ± standard deviation) at 100 Hz were 774.5 ± 198.0 kΩ for the uncoated electrodes, 138.9 ± 24.9 kΩ for Au-CNTs, 5.0 ± 0.1 kΩ for PPy-CNTs, and 4.5 ± 0.2 kΩ for PEDOT-CNTs. It should be noted that our PEDOT-CNT-coated devices are fully compatible with sterilization in saturated water vapor at 122°C and 2 atm for 20 min, one of the most commonly used sterilization processes in hospitals, making them

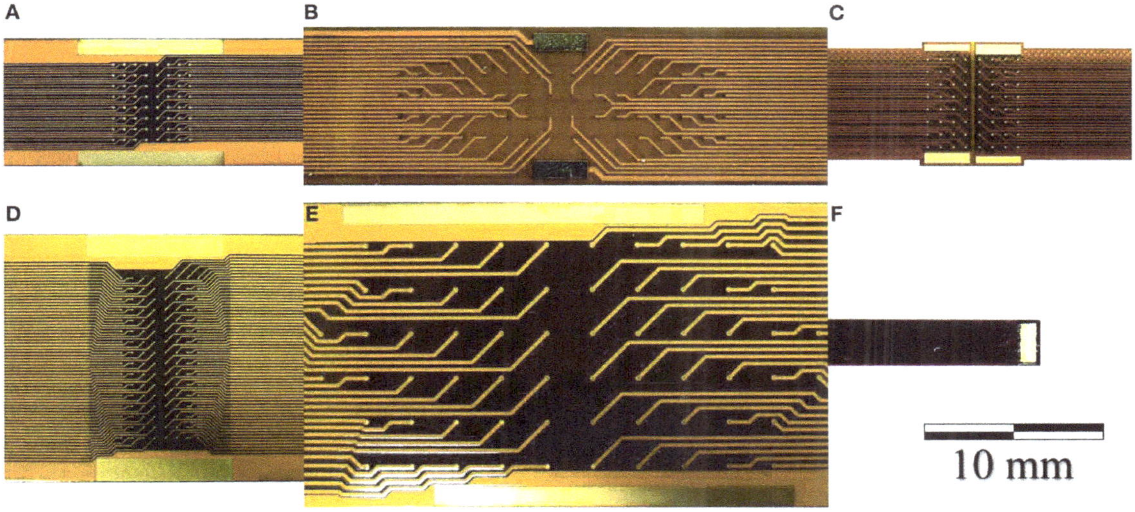

FIGURE 7 | Photographs of (A) a 64-electrode array with 4.2 × 4.2 mm total recording area and 140 μm diameter recording sites. (B) A 64-electrode array with 3.6 × 18.0 mm total recording area and 100 μm diameter recording sites; **(C)** A 64-electrode matrix with 5 × 5 mm total recording area, designed for the marmoset; **(D)** A 128-electrode array with 4.2 × 8.4 mm total recording area and 100 μm diameter recording sites; **(E)** A 64-electrode array with 12.5 × 27.5 mm total recording area and 200 μm diameter recording sites. **(F)** A 16-electrode array with 1.2 × 1.2 mm total recording area and 100 μm diameter recording sites.

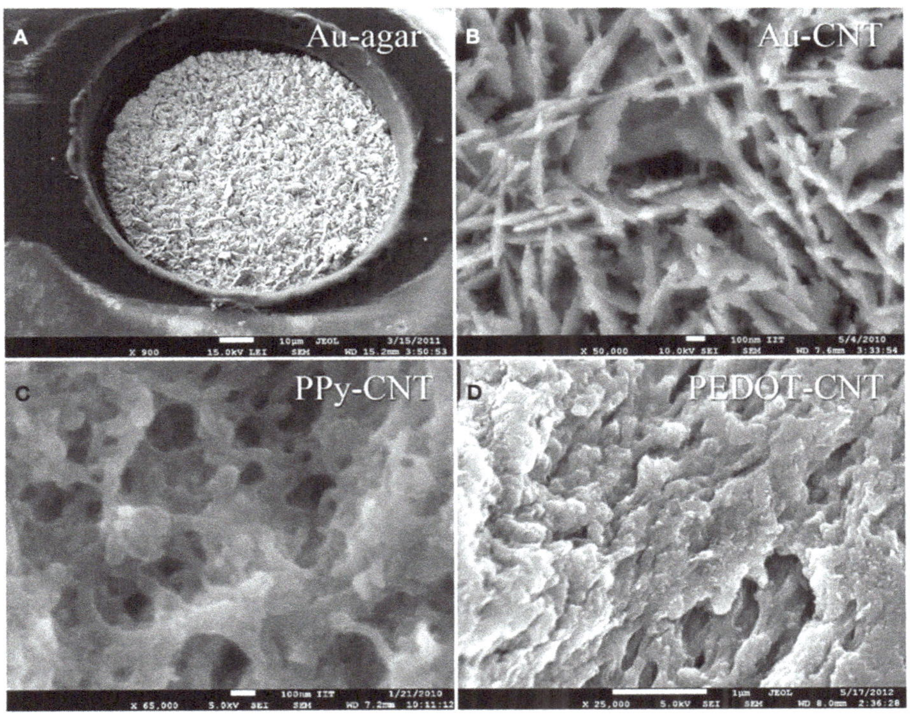

FIGURE 8 | s.e.m. images of: (A) a 100 μm Au-agar-coated recording site; (B) Au-CNT coating; **(C)** PPy-CNT coating; **(D)** PEDOT-CNT coating.

suitable candidates for clinical applications (see Castagnola et al., 2013a,b). In order to establish whether they are suitable for cortical stimulation, we investigated their ability to withstand a series of cathodic-first charge-balanced biphasic current pulses with a 2 ms pulse duration, 500 μs cathodic pulse duration, and 5.7 mC cm^{-2} charge density, measuring whether there was any change in the impedance spectra after each series. We chose to test PEDOT-CNT-coated micro-ECoG arrays alone, as we know from previous

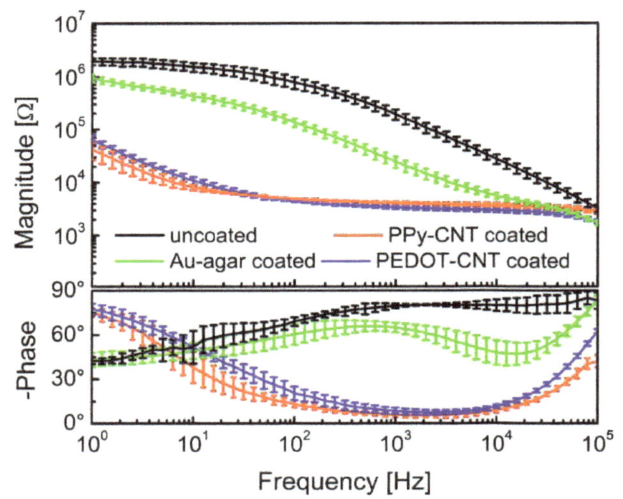

FIGURE 9 | Impedance spectra of 100-μm-diameter ECoG array recording sites (mean and standard deviation from 64 recording sites each) before (black) and after Au-agar (green), PPy-CNT (red) and PEDOT-CNT (blue) electrodeposition.

tests that PPy is not electrochemically stable under similar conditions. With our PEDOT-CNT arrays, impedance spectra did not change after four million pulses (data not shown), even when applying a ten times larger charge density, exhibiting the ability to handle the higher currents needed to stimulate neurons from the cortical surface. An example of somatosensory-evoked potentials (SEP) recorded using a 4 × 4 micro-ECoG array (inset) with a 1 × 1 mm total recording area, 100 μm diameter recording sites and 300 μm inter-electrode pitch coated with PEDOT-CNT is shown in **Figure 10**. The graphs show the response of each single electrode to the first 12-ms truncated Gaussian of a 9-Hz train of a rat multiwhisker deflections of 0.8 mm. The data are averaged from 20 repetitions of the stimulation pattern.

REDUCED INVASIVENESS AND INCREASED VERSATILITY THROUGH NANOCOATINGS AND POLYMER-BASED CIRCUITS: SMALLER AND SOFTER ELECTRODES

LOW-INVASIVE INTRACORTICAL MICROSPHERES

The insertion of any electrode into living brain tissue unavoidably results in a mechanical trauma that activates a cascade of events leading to a neural loss around the implant and its encapsulation in a high-impedance scar made of glial and immune cells, undermining the goal of maintaining long-term communication with neurons (Ward et al., 2009; Marin and Fernández, 2010). However, the physical properties of the whole device,—e.g., its size, shape and stiffness—can play a fundamental role in modulating the tissue reaction, and can be altered to reduce the insertion trauma and to aid accommodation of the large stiffness mismatch between the device and the nervous system tissue (Edell et al., 1992; Ward et al., 2009; Marin and Fernández, 2010). Aside from coating the electrodes with different biomolecules, anti-inflammatory compounds, hydrogels (Crompton et al., 2007; Zhong and Bellamkonda, 2007; Abidian and Martin, 2009), polymers (Ludwig et al., 2006; Leung et al., 2008; Grill et al., 2009) or carbon nanotubes (Lovat et al., 2005; Mazzatenta et al., 2007), another strategy is to modify the physical dimensions, and geometry of the neural probe (Stice et al., 2007; Ward et al., 2009).

Our approach was to minimize the physical size of the probe while maximizing the flexibility of the tether between the electrode and the connection to the external recording/stimulation system in order to be able to accommodate movements and motions of the brain with respect to the skull. As the smaller the size of the electrode, the greater the impedance, we endeavored to exploit the majority of the available surface of the probe, abandoning the standard shapes, which usually expose either flat or conical electrode surfaces. Instead we developed a process in which we created a conductive sphere (the electrode) that is much larger in diameter than the wire that connects it to the external recording chain. In fact, while the surface area of the electrode is crucial for recording and stimulation, even a very thin metallic wire used as connector will have a much lower impedance than that of the electrochemical interface. Another advantage of the spherical shape is that the electrode does not need a rigid stem, as it can be kept in position by the hydrostatic pressure of the brain.

To demonstrate this concept, we grew microspheres of fuzzy gold at the end of 12-μm polyimide-insulated Pt wires by electrochemical deposition, starting from a 10 mM potassium dicyanoaurate(I) agar gel (0.1 wt%), and applying monophasic voltage pulses (0.2–1.0 V, 240 s, duty cycle 50%). The temperature of the gel was kept at 45°C.

We characterized our microspheres both optically (**Figure 11A**) and electrochemically, measuring the size and impedance (**Figure 11B**) after 3, 6, 9, 12, and 13 h of electrodeposition. After the first 3 h, a huge reduction in impedance was observed, which can be linked to both the increased electrode size and the far greater surface area generated by the microstucturing. Over the following 10 h the impedance decreased by another order of magnitude, with a fairly linear trend in good accord with its increase in diameter. After 13 h we reached a diameter of 105 μm, and the corresponding impedance was less than 1 kΩ at 1 kHz. The impedance spectrum of a 105-μm diameter microsphere is shown in **Figure 11C**. An example of a signal trace recorded using a 100 μm diameter microsphere is shown in **Figure 11D**. The very thin Pt wire is extremely flexible and, once the microsphere is inserted, bends easily, reducing the mechanical stress on the surrounding tissue, while the sphere, as mentioned before, remains in place thanks to the hydrostatic pressure of the brain. The change in diameter of the microsphere can be better appreciated in **Figure 11E**.

ULTRA-FLEXIBLE AND BRAIN-CONFORMABLE micro-ECoG DEVICE WITH LOW-IMPEDANCE MICROELECTRODES

Although our flexible ECoG arrays were able to record brain activity in acute sessions, a long-term large-area implant comprising a high-resolution ECoG array would ideally require more flexible and brain-conformable devices that can accommodate brain curvature, compliantly covering neighboring gyri and crossing sulci while keeping the electrodes in intimate contact with the brain cortex. One way of attempting to meet this requirement is to reduce device thickness by developing appropriate technologies.

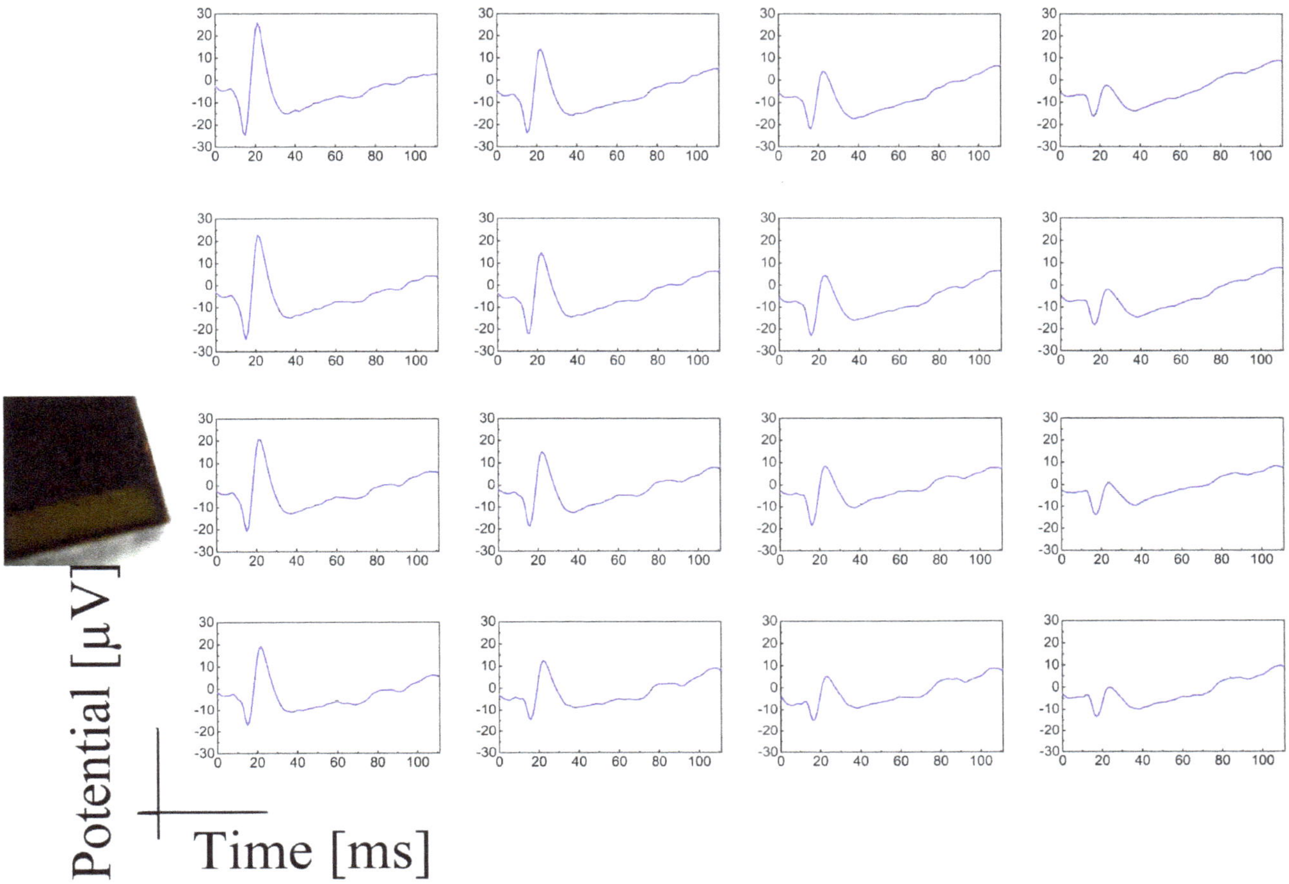

FIGURE 10 | SEP response of a 4 × 4 micro-ECoG array (inset) with a 1 × 1 mm total recording area, 100 μm diameter recording sites, and 300 μm inter-electrode pitch, coated with PEDOT-CNT to the first 12-ms truncated Gaussian of a 9-Hz train of rat multiwhisker deflections of 0.8° mm. The data are averaged on 20 repetitions of the stimulation pattern.

To this end we modified prototypes of gold-on-polyimide ultra-flexible micro-ECoG arrays. The fabrication procedure has been described elsewhere (Castagnola et al., 2013b), but relies on standard optical lithography. The ultra-flexible polyimide micro-ECoG arrays had a total thickness of approximately 8 μm. In spite of their thinness, these devices were mechanically quite robust, making their handling relatively unproblematic. We tested different layouts and electrode sizes (200 × 200 μm and 100 × 100 μm) suitable for different types of neurophysiological experiment. Some designs and details of the electrodes are reported in **Figure 12**.

We were able to selectively coat with PEDOT-CNT HSA composite both 100 × 100 μm and 200 × 200 μm electrodes, demonstrating that the absence of a well in the coverlay does not impair the possibility of obtaining spatially defined coatings, and we obtained reductions in impedance similar to those of our FCP ECoG arrays. Indeed, the impedance at 100 Hz was reduced from 1.6 ± 0.1 MΩ to 2.1 ± 0.7 kΩ with 100 × 100 μm electrodes and from 509.7 ± 177.5 to 0.63 ± 0.07 kΩ with 200 × 200 μm electrodes. The corresponding impedance spectra are shown in **Figure 13A**. Interestingly, the impedance decreased by up to four orders of magnitude in the 1–100 Hz frequency band (Castagnola et al., 2013b), where ECoG signals are typically recorded, with a significant downshift of the first frequency response pole. In order to validate the recording capability of our ultra-flexible micro-ECoGs, we tested our device *in vivo* by recording from the rat somatosensory cortex, using a stimulation protocol similar to the one described in section Flexible micro-ECoG arrays. An example of averaged SEP elicited using a 9-Hz train of truncated Gaussian 0.8-mm rat multiwhisker deflection (first 12 ms response) using PEDOT-coated 100 × 100 μm electrodes (average on 10 electrodes) is shown in **Figure 13B**, clearly demonstrating the ability of this device to record clear SEP responses.

BIOCOMPATIBILITY ISSUES AND FEAR OF NANOCOATINGS: A PRAGMATIC APPROACH AND PROOF OF CONCEPT

The toxicology of nanoparticles is hotly debated in scientific circles, and rather controversial results have been reported. However, experiments often document the *in vitro* or *in vivo* release of dispersed nanoparticles at very high concentrations, making it difficult to assess the real impact of nanomaterial-coated neural probes. Moreover, in the case of carbon nanotubes, a large

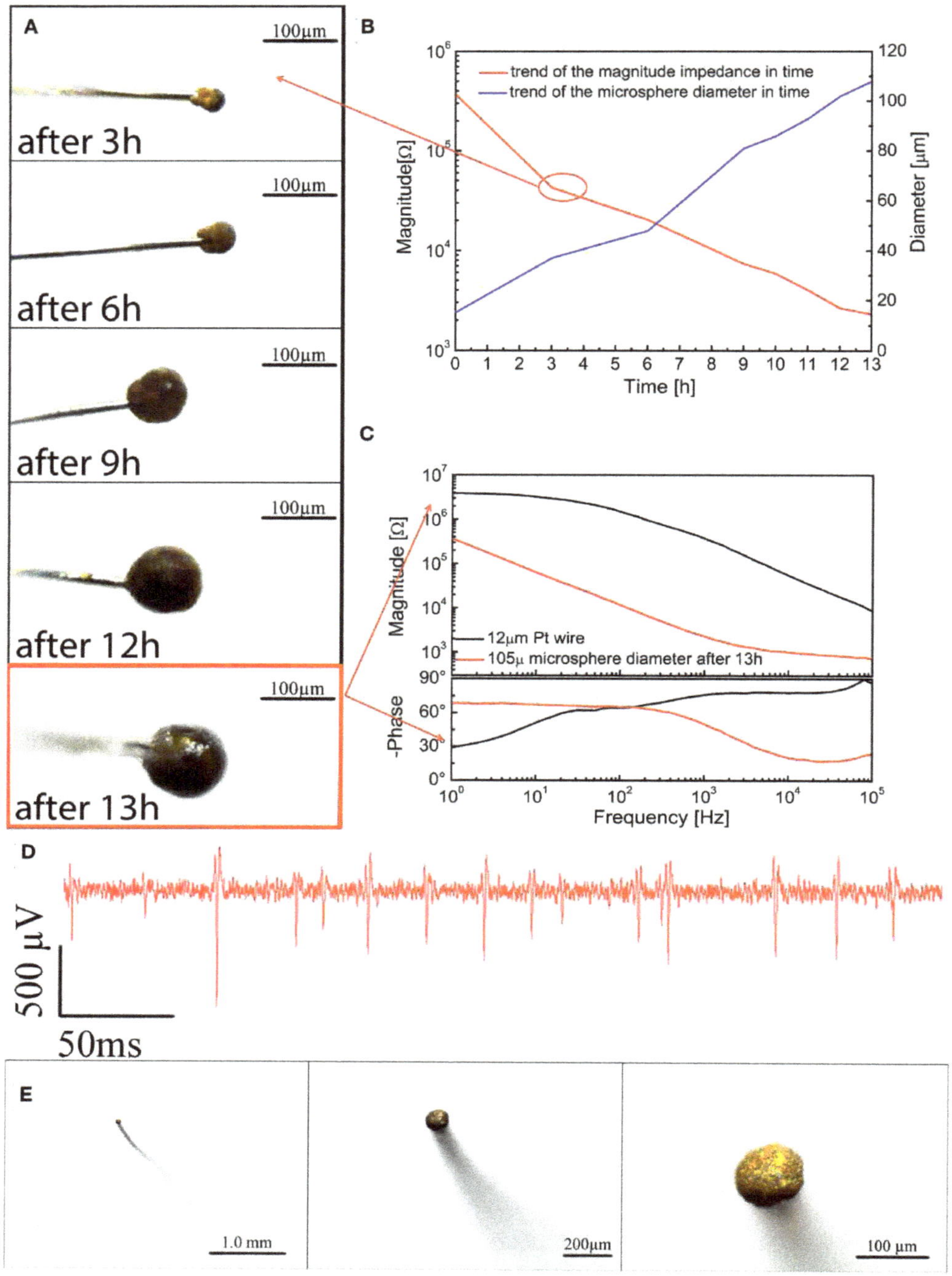

FIGURE 11 | (A) Optical images of the microspheres after 3, 6, 9, 12, and 13 h of electrodeposition; **(B)** impedance magnitude at 1 kHz and diameters of the microspheres after 3, 6, 9, 12, and 13 h of electrodeposition; **(C)** Impedance after 13 h of electrodeposition; **(D)** an example of spike activity recorded using a 100 μm microsphere; **(E)** from left to right different top view optical magnifications of a typical microsphere.

number of studies report effects that can easily be ascribed to the toxicity of the metal catalyst of unpurified CNTs.

One of the main sources of debate when dealing with nanoparticles, especially CNTs, lies in the fact that, as their properties are largely determined by their surface characteristics, any chemical functionalization will have a very strong influence on the way the particles are metabolized, and therefore any resulting tissue reaction. Some studies have demonstrated that specific types of CNTs can be biodegraded (Kagan et al., 2010; Bianco et al., 2011) even in the brain tissue, after internalization in the microglia (Nunes et al., 2012). The situation becomes even more complex if we consider that in many cases we are dealing with CNT composites, and

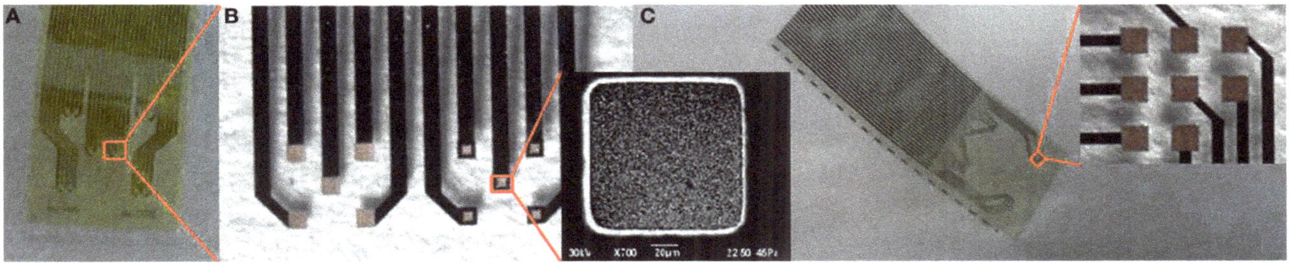

FIGURE 12 | (A) One possible ultraflexible micro-ECoG array layout. **(B)** Details of the two groups of five recording sites 200° × 200° μm and 100° × 100° μm in size, and a scanning electron micrograph of a 100 × 100 μm Au recording site (inset). **(C)** Other possible ultraflexible micro-ECoG array layouts and detail of a group of eight 200 × 200° μm recording sites (inset).

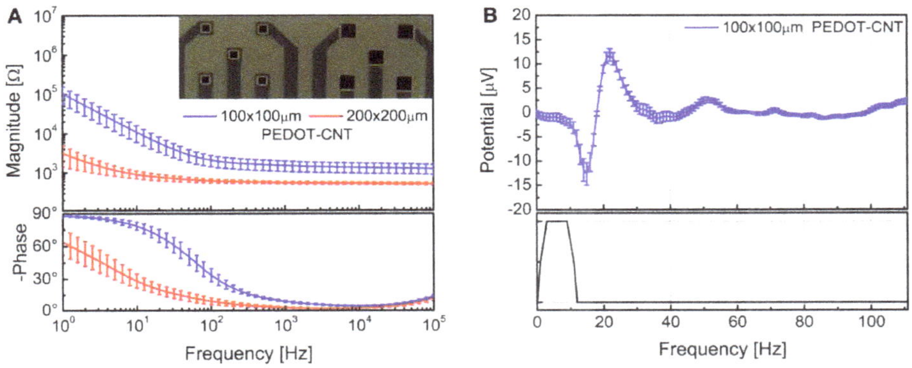

FIGURE 13 | (A) Impedance spectra of the 100 × 100 μm and 200 × 200 μm ultraflexible ECoG array recording sites (mean and standard deviation from 10 recording sites each) before and after PEDOT-CNT electrodeposition. **(B)** Averaged SEP elicited using a 9-Hz train of truncated Gaussian 0.8-mm rat multiwhisker deflection (first 12 ms response) using PEDOT-coated 100 × 100 μm electrodes (average on 10 electrodes).

not isolated particles. If the composite is stable, the surface interacting with the tissue can be considered as a macroscopic particle made of the matrix material, in which the CNTs are fully embedded and encapsulated. If one such composite (macro) particle is released, it may be degraded or not, depending on the material it is made of. If it were undegradable, it would, most probably, be encapsulated as a foreign body. If it were subject to particle degradation, the embedded CNTs would be released into the body in amounts that are vastly smaller than those used in current toxicological experimentation. This makes it very difficult to state whether or not there is a toxic effect at such low concentrations. In the case of nanocoated neural implants, addressing the toxicity of the HSA coating would itself take very long time, and it would be impossible to ascertain with absolute confidence that not one single tiny particle of nanocomposite detaches from the coating during the contact with the brain surface due to mechanical stress. For these reasons we proposed a completely different approach, namely to encapsulate the entire device with a coating that is transparent to ionic currents but, at the same time, protects the device from mechanical stress and prevents, in case of nanocoating failure, the release of particles into the brain tissue. To achieve this we used a hydrogel, specifically human fibrin, to encapsulate our HSA-coated neural micro-ECoG arrays, thereby creating a mechanically stable barrier that prevents direct exposure of the brain to nanomaterials, without, however, impairing their electrochemical and neural performance (Castagnola et al., 2013a,b).

We chose a commercially available two-component fibrin sealant that is approved for surgical purposes in both Europe and the United States (TISSEEL [fibrin sealant], Baxter, USA), and one that is commonly used in neurosurgical practice. We set out to develop a procedure compliant with the protocols approved by the competent medical surveillance agencies for the safe handling and use of fibrin in sterile operating theatres. We devised a process involving the sterilization of the HSA-coated micro-ECoG array before it is introduced to a sterile environment, the fibrin being applied to the device by the surgeon just before use (Castagnola et al., 2013a,b). To deposit the fibrin layer, the polyimide based FPC circuits were placed over an aluminium sample holder heated at 37°C. Meanwhile, the fibrin precursors, fibrinogen, and thrombin, were warmed up to the same temperature. The fibrinogen was spread over the electrodes with a spatula and, then, a large thrombin drop was placed over the whole fibrinogen-coated surface. After 5 min, a stable fibrin layer was formed and the micro–ECoG array was rinsed in ultrapure water to remove the residual thrombin solution.

A SEM image of a single recording/stimulation site after fibrin encapsulation is shown in **Figure 14A**, together with the

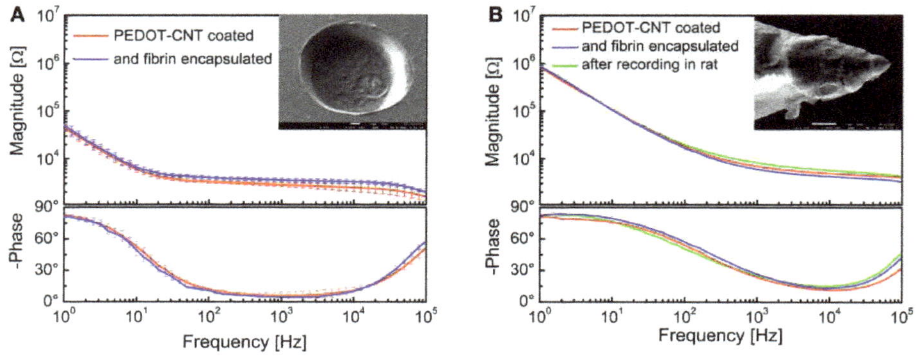

FIGURE 14 | Impedance spectra of (A) 140-μm-diameter ECoG array recording sites (mean and standard deviation from 64 recording sites each) coated with PEDOT-CNT composite, before and after fibrin encapsulation, and (B) intracortical PEDOT-CNT microelectrode before and after fibrin encapsulation and *in vivo* recording. s.e.m. images of a single recording/stimulation site encapsulated with fibrin are shown in the respective insets.

impedance spectra of a 140-μm diameter PEDOT-CNT-coated recording site ECoG array before and after fibrin encapsulation. We can observe that the fibrin encapsulation does not have any significant impact on the impedance spectra of PEDOT-CNT-coated microelectrodes (from 3.4 ± 0.2 kΩ to 3.9 ± 0.4 kΩ @ 100 Hz), confirming that the fibrin hydrogel acts as a good ionic conductor. These fibrin-encapsulated PEDOT-CNT-coated micro-ECoG arrays, being able to resist intense and prolonged current stimulation without the fibrin layer being affected by the current passage (Castagnola et al., 2013a,b) can therefore be considered suitable for cortical stimulation. Indeed, we used these devices *in vivo* to record SEPs from the rat somatosensory cortex, elicited through multiwhisker deflection using a protocol similar to the one reported above. We verified that after two 15-min-long epicortical recording sessions the fibrin coating was still in place, firmly adhering to the recording sites, and thereby effectively shielding the tissues from direct contact with the nanostructured coating. Furthermore, the microelectrode impedance did not change significantly, and the quality of the SEP recordings was not affected by the presence of the fibrin coating (Castagnola et al., 2013a,b).

After proving that the fibrin hydrogel is able to stay in place on the surface of micro-ECoG devices that are placed on the dura mater or cortex, we tested whether or not it can be used to encapsulate an intracortical electrode, and to withstand the mechanical stress generated by brain tissue penetration. To this end, we encapsulated our PEDOT-CNT-coated intracortical microelectrodes by a controlled two-stage dipping process, first into a vial containing fibrinogen, and then into a second vial containing thrombin. The impedance spectra of a PEDOT-CNT-coated electrode before and after fibrin encapsulation, and also after an *in vivo* intracortical recording session involving penetration of the rat brain tissue (including the dura mater), are shown in **Figure 14B**. A SEM picture of a microelectrode after fibrin encapsulation is shown in the inset. The fibrin encapsulation had no significant effect on the microelectrode impedance, which remained nearly identical, even after the intracortical recording. To check the persistence of the fibrin layer after the rat somatosensory cortex recording session, we stained it with methylene blue, which showed that the fibrin remained adherent to the HSA-coated tip. As previous experiments have shown us that fibrin tends to detach from uncoated, smooth electrodes, this experimental evidence suggests that there is an intimate adhesion between the fibrin layer and the rough HSA coating we applied to the tip (as previously hinted at by electrochemical measurements). In all probability, this adhesion is brought about by the hydrogel being trapped in the nanostructured microelectrode surface, preventing its slipping away.

As previously mentioned, we chose to test fibrin hydrogel due to its potentially ready transferral to human surgery applications. A particular advantage of fibrin hydrogel is that it can be autologous, i.e., obtained from the patient's own blood, thereby reducing to a minimum rejection risks, etc. However, while this approach appears feasible for acute use, unfortunately fibrin can be fully resorbed by the tissues within 2 weeks during *in vivo* implants (Schoeller et al., 2001; de Vries et al., 2002). Nevertheless, our results prove that it is possible to fully encapsulate recording and stimulation devices in hydrogel without impairing their performance, and suggests that it would be possible to extend the use of such a technique to chronic implants by replacing fibrin with an appropriate biocompatible non-resorbable hydrogel with similar physical properties. To this end, it may be advantageous to use synthetic hydrogels as they are better chemically defined, with respect to those composed of only natural materials, and it is possible to better control their polymerization, degradation, and biocompatibility (Aurand et al., 2012a,b). Among all, promising candidates are poly(2-hydroxyethyl methacrylate) (pHEMA) and polyurethane based hydrogels, that have a long-standing track record of successful biomedical applications and have been already tested in contact with the central and pheripheral nervous system (Woerly et al., 1998; Lukás et al., 2001; Dalton et al., 2002; Jhaveri et al., 2009; Rao et al., 2012). To be used for the encapsulation of nanocoated neural chronic implants, it is necessary to accurately fine-tune the hydrogel composition, the cross-linking molecules, and network mesh size, in order to achieve the desired properties in terms of semi-permeability, mechanical stiffness, degree of swelling, and resistance to degradation.

PERSPECTIVES FOR LONG TERM IMPLANTS

Despite the great efforts and expectations, at present electrodes for brain stimulation and recording are still far from the reliability, affordability, and long term stability necessary for a widespread clinical use in human cortical prosthesis. However, over the last 5 years, by careful selection of readymade technologies, we have been able to modify electrodes to make them smaller, more sensitive, more flexible, less invasive, and more reliable.

With a particular focus on electrodes for human use, we have shown that it is also possible to improve their recording capabilities in terms of sensitivity, signal-to-noise ratio, and electromagnetic interference rejection, by using a variety of HSA coatings based on nanomaterials. We have developed and systematically studied and compared a variety of HSA coatings—CVD-CNT, PPy-CNT, PEDOT-CNT, Au-CNT, Au-agar, PEDOT-agar—proving that such technologies enhance performance in both epicortical and intracortical recording and stimulation. We have also made these coatings mechanically stable and able to withstand penetration through the dura and the brain of an animal model (rat).

Despite the advantages of rigid microprobes, (Campbell et al., 1991; Rousche and Normann, 1992; Richter et al., 2013) particularly in ensuring a precise positioning of the electrodes during insertion into specific brain areas (Schjetnan and Luczak, 2011), they cannot yet provide reliable and stable long-term recordings. Indeed, even state-of-the-art rigid microelectrodes cause severe mechanical trauma during their insertion, resulting in a thick glial scar formation and a consequent loss of tissue-electrode coupling as time goes by (Turner et al., 1999; Polikov et al., 2005; Leach et al., 2010; Richter et al., 2013). That being said, (Krüger et al., 2010) did manage to achieve stable recordings for several years from electrodes experimentally implanted in monkeys thanks to the minimal invasiveness of their device at the cortical recording site. Although this proved the importance of minimizing the mechanical damage to the cortical area under investigation, their electrodes were inserted using a device that enables brain penetration through the white matter from a different area, making the technique very invasive and unsuitable for clinical applications. Hence many other studies have focused on the replacement of rigid with flexible electrodes, which it is hoped will reduce insertion trauma, being more similar mechanically to the soft brain tissue and thereby minimizing the stiffness mismatch between device and nervous system tissue (Rousche et al., 2001; Rubehn and Stieglitz, 2010; Richter et al., 2013). We too aimed to reduce the invasiveness of insertion, by minimizing the physical size of the probe without compromising its electrical impedance, and keeping the tether between the electrode and the external recording/stimulation system as flexible as possible to enable accommodation of brain movement and motions within the skull. We achieved a reduction in probe size by electrochemically growing a HSA gold sphere on the tip of a very thin wire (12 μm in diameter), envisioning the sphere as the ideal shape to be kept in position by the hydrostatic pressure of the brain. This technique also provided us with a very flexible tether, which is not involved in the long term positioning of the device. In a parallel approach, we aimed to overcome the issue of foreign-body response in intracortical implants, developing high-resolution micro-ECoG arrays with enhanced recording capabilities thanks to our HSA coatings. We developed a variety of flexible micro-ECoG arrays of HSA-coated electrodes, whose better signal quality make it feasible to further reduce electrode size and increase spatial resolution. We further improved our technology using novel ultrathin electrodes, which enable intimate contact with the surface of the brain, thereby enhancing the electrical coupling. Finally, we proved that it is possible to reliably encapsulate both intracortical and epicortical devices with a biocompatible hydrogel, which provides a mechanical barrier between the nanocomposite HSA materials, and the human body, without any loss of device performance.

Altogether, these results converge in a method that we believe represents several steps forward in terms of bringing such novel devices into clinical settings, opening new avenues for neurodiagnostics, and neuroprosthetic applications.

ACKNOWLEDGMENTS

We would like to thank Luca Maiolo, Marco Marrani, Antonio Minotti, Francesco Maita, Alessandro Pecora, and Guglielmo Fortunato for providing the ultra-flexible micro-ECoG devices. We would like to thank Gian Nicola Angotzi, Marianna Semprini, and Alessandro Vato for support during the use of the recording/stimulation set-up.

REFERENCES

Abidian, M. R., and Martin, D. C. (2008). Experimental and theoretical characterization of implantable neural microelectrodes modified with conducting polymer. *Biomaterials* 29, 1273–1283. doi: 10.1016/j.biomaterials.2007.11.022

Abidian, M. R., and Martin, D. C. (2009). Multifunctional nanobiomaterials for neural interfaces. *Adv. Funct. Mater.* 19, 573–585. doi: 10.1002/adfm.200801473

Ansaldo, A., Castagnola, E., Maggiolini, E., Fadiga, L., and Ricci, D. (2011). Superior electrochemical performance of carbon nanotubes directly grown on sharp microelectrodes. *ACS Nano* 5, 2206–2214. doi: 10.1021/nn103445d

Aurand, E. R., Lampe, K. J., and Bjugstad, K. B. (2012a). Defining and designing polymers and hydrogels for neural tissue engineering. *Neurosci. Res.* 72, 199–213. doi: 10.1016/j.neures.2011.12.005

Aurand, E. R., Wagner, J., Lanning, C., and Bjugstad, K. B. (2012b). Building biocompatible hydrogels for tissue engineering of the brain and spinal cord. *J. Funct. Biomater.* 3, 839–863. doi:10.3390/jfb3040839

Baranauskas, G., Maggiolini, E., Castagnola, E., Ansaldo, A., Mazzoni, A., Angotzi, G. N., et al. (2011). Carbon nanotube composite coating of neural microelectrodes preferentially improves the multiunit signal-to-noise ratio. *J. Neural Eng.* 8:66013. doi: 10.1088/1741-2560/8/6/066013

Bianco, A., Kostarelos, K., and Prato, M. (2011). Making carbon nanotubes biocompatible and biodegradable. *Chem. Commun.* 47, 10182–10188. doi: 10.1039/c1cc13011k

Brummer, S. B., Robblee, L. S., Hambrecht, T., and Hambrecht, F. T. (1983). Criteria for selecting electrodes for electrical stimulation: theoretical and practical considerations. *Ann. N. Y. Acad. Sci.* 405, 159–171. doi: 10.1111/j.1749-6632.1983.tb31628.x

Campbell, P. K., Jones, K. E., Huber, R. J., Horch, K. W., and Normann, R. A. (1991). A silicon based three dimensional neural interface: manufacturing processes for an intracortical electrode array. *IEEE Trans. Biomed. Eng.* 38, 758–768. doi: 10.1109/10.83588

Castagnola, E., Ansaldo, A., Fadiga, L., and Ricci, D. (2010). Chemical vapour deposited carbon nanotube coated microelectrodes for intracortical neural recording. *Phys. Status Solidi (B)* 247, 2703–2707. doi: 10.1002/pssb.201000217

Castagnola, E., Ansaldo, A., Maggiolini, E., Angotzi, G. N., Skrap, M., Ricci, D., et al. (2013a). Biologically compatible neural interface to safely couple nanocoated electrodes to the surface of the brain, *ACS Nano* 5, 3887–3895. doi: 10.1021/nn305164c

Castagnola, E., Biso, M., and Ricci, D. (2009). Improvement of polypyrrole and carbon nanotube co-deposition techniques for high charge-transfer electrodes. *Phys. Status Solidi (B)* 246, 2469–2472. doi: 10.1002/pssb.200982283

Castagnola, E., Maiolo, L., Maggiolini, E., Minotti, A., Marrani, M., Maita, F., et al. (2013b). "Ultra-flexible and brain-conformable microelectrocorticography device with low impedance PEDOT-carbon nanotube coated microelectrodes," in *Proceeding of the 6th International IEEE/EMBS Conference on Neural Engineering* (San Diego, CA), 927–930. doi: 10.1109/NER.2013.6696087

Chao, Z. C., Nagasaka, Y., and Fujii, N. (2010). Long-term asynchronous decoding of arm motion using electrocorticographic signals in monkeys. *Front. Neuroeng.* 3:3. doi: 10.3389/fneng.2010.00003

Cogan, S. F. (2008). Neural stimulation and recording electrodes. *Annu. Rev. Biomed. Eng.* 10, 275–309. doi: 10.1146/annurev.bioeng.10.061807.160518

Cogan, S. F., Plante, T. D., and Ehrlich, J. (2004). Sputtered iridium oxide films (SIROFs) for low-impedance neural stimulation and recording electrodes. *Conf. Proc. IEEE Eng. Med. Biol. Soc.* 6, 4153–4156. doi: 10.1109/IEMBS.2004.1404158

Crompton, K. E., Goud, J. D., Bellamkonda, R. V., Gengenbach, T. R., Finkelstein, D. I., Horne, M. K., et al. (2007). Polylysine-functionalised thermoresponsive chitosan hydrogel for neural tissue engineering. *Biomaterials* 28, 441–449. doi: 10.1016/j.biomaterials.2006.08.044

Cui, X., Lee, V. A., Raphael, Y., Wiler, J. A., Hetke, J. F., Anderson, D. J., et al. (2001). Surface modification of neural recording electrodes with conducting polymer/biomolecule blends. *J. Biomed. Mater. Res.* 56, 261–272. doi: 10.1002/1097-4636(200108)56:2%3C261::AID-JBM1094%3E3.0.CO;2-I

Cui, X., and Martin, D. C. (2003). Electrochemical deposition and characterization of poly(3,4-ethylenedioxythiophene) on neural microelectrode arrays. *Sens. Actuators B Chem.* 89, 92–102. doi: 10.1016/S0925-4005(02)00448-3

Dalton, P. D., Flynn, L., and Shoichet, M. S. (2002). Manufacture of poly(2-hydroxyethyl methacrylate-co-methyl methacrylate) hydrogel tubes for use as nerve guidance channels. *Biomaterials* 23, 3843–3851. doi: 10.1089/neu.2009.0948

Desai, S. A., Rolston, J. D., Guo, L., and Potter, S. M. (2010). Improving impedance of implantable microwire multi-electrode arrays by ultrasonic electroplating of durable platinum black. *Front. Neuroeng.* 3:5. doi: 10.3389/fneng.2010.00005

de Vries, J., Menovsky, T., van Gulik, S., and Wesseling, P. (2002). Histological effects of fibrin glue on nervous tissue. *Surg. Neurol.* 57, 415–422. doi: 10.1016/S0090-3019(02)00736-X

Edell, D. J., Van Toi, V., McNeil, V. M., and Clark, L. D. (1992). Factors influencing the biocompatibility of insertable silicon microshafts in cerebral cortex. *IEEE Trans. Biomed. Eng.* 39, 635–643. doi: 10.1109/10.141202

Erchova, I. A., Lebedev, M. A., and Diamond, M. E. (2002). Somatosensory cortical neuronal population activity across states of anaesthesia. *Eur. J. Neurosci.* 15, 744–752. doi: 10.1046/j.0953-816x.2002.01898.x

Ferguson, J. E., Boldt, C., and Redish, A. D. (2009). Creating low-impedance tetrodes by electroplating with additives. *Sens. Actuators A Phys.* 156, 388–393. doi: 10.1016/j.sna.2009.10.001

Fries, P., Nikolic, D., and Singer, W. (2007). The gamma cycle. *Trends Neurosci.* 30, 309–316. doi: 10.1016/j.tins.2007.05.005

Gabay, T., Ben-David, M., Kalifa, I., Sorkin, R., Abrams, Z. R., Ben-Jacob, E., et al. (2007). Electro-chemical and biological properties of carbon nanotube based multi-electrode arrays. *Nanotechnology* 18:035201. doi: 10.1088/0957-4484/18/3/035201

Gawad, S., Giugliano, M., Heuschkel, M., Wessling, B., Markram, H., Schnakenberg, U., et al. (2009). Substrate arrays of iridium oxide microelectrodes for *in vitro* neuronal interfacing. *Front. Neuroeng.* 2:1. doi: 10.3389/neuro.16.001.2009

Gerwig, R., Fuchsberger, K., Schroeppel, B., Link, G. S., Heusel, G., Kraushaar, U., et al. (2012). PEDOT-CNT composite microelectrodes for recording and electrostimulation applications: fabrication, morphology, and electrical properties. *Front. Neuroeng.* 5:8. doi: 10.3389/fneng.2012.00008

Gray, C. M., Konig, P., Engel, A. K., and Singer,W. (1989). Oscillatory responses in cat visual cortex exhibit inter-columnar synchronization which reflects global stimulus properties. *Nature* 338, 334–337. doi: 10.1038/338334a0

Green, R. A., Williams, C. M., Lovell, N. H., and Poole-Warren, L. A. (2008). Novel neural interface for implant electrodes: improving electroactivity of polypyrrole through MWNT incorporation. *J. Mater. Sci. Mater. Med.* 19, 1625–1629. doi: 10.1007/s10856-008-3376-7

Grill, W. M., Norman, S. E., and Bellamkonda, R. V. (2009). Implanted neural interfaces: biochallenges and engineered solutions. *Annu. Rev. Biomed. Eng.* 11, 1–24. doi: 10.1146/annurev-bioeng-061008-124927

Harris, K. D., Henze, D. A, Csicsvari, J., Hirase, H., and Buzsáki, G. (2000). Accuracy of tetrode spike separation as determined by simultaneous intracellular and extracellular measurements. *J. Neurophysiol.* 84, 401–414.

Hollenberg, B. A., Richards, C. D., Richards, R., Bahr, D. F., and Rector, D. M. (2006). A MEMS fabricated flexible electrode array for recording surface field potentials. *J. Neurosci. Methods* 153, 147–153. doi: 10.1016/j.jneumeth.2005.10.016

Jan, E., Hendricks, J. L., Husaini, V., Richardson-Burns, S. M., Sereno, A., Martin, D. C., et al. (2009). Layered carbon nanotube-polyelectrolyte electrodes outperform traditional neural interface materials. *Nano Lett.* 9, 4012–4018. doi: 10.1021/nl902187z

Jhaveri, S. J., Hynd, M. R., Dowell-Mesfin, N., Turner, J. N., Shain, W., and Ober, C. K. (2009). Release of nerve growth factor from HEMA hydrogel-coated substrates and its effect on the differentiation of neural cells. *Biomacromolecules* 10, 174–183. doi: 10.1021/bm801101e

Kagan, V. E., Konduru, N. V., Feng, W., Allen, B. L., Conroy, J., Volkov, Y., et al. (2010). Carbon nanotubes degraded by neutrophil myeloperoxidase induce less pulmonary inflammation. *Nat. Nanotech.* 5, 354–359. doi: 10.1038/nnano.2010.44

Keefer, E. W., Botterman, B. R., Romero, M. I., Rossi, A. F., and Gross, G. W. (2008). Carbon nanotube coating improves neuronal recordings. *Nat. Nanotech.* 3, 434–439. doi: 10.1038/nnano.2008.174

Kellis, S., Miller, K., Thomson, K., Brown, R., House, P., and Greger, B. (2010). Decoding spoken words using local field potentials recorded from the cortical surface. *J. Neural Eng.* 7:56007. doi: 10.1088/1741-2560/7/5/056007

Kellis, S. S., House, P. A., Thomson, K. E., Brown, R., and Greger, B. (2009). Human neocortical electrical activity recorded on nonpenetrating microwire arrays: applicability for neuroprostheses. *Neurosurg. Focus* 27:E9. doi: 10.3171/2009.4.FOCUS0974

Khodagholy, D., Doublet, T., Gurfinkel, M., Quilichini, P., Ismailova, E., Leleux, P., et al. (2011). Highly conformable conducting polymer electrodes for *in vivo* recordings. *Adv. Mater.* 23, H268–H272. doi: 10.1002/adma.201102378

Kotov, N. A., Winter, J. O., Clements, I. P., Jan, E., Timko, B. P., Campidelli, S., et al. (2009). Nanomaterials for neural interfaces. *Adv. Mater.* 21, 3970–4004. doi: 10.1002/adma.200801984

Krüger, J., Caruana, F., Dalla Volta, R., and Rizzolatti, G. (2010). Seven years of recording from monkey cortex with a chronically implanted multiple microelectrode. *Front. Neuroeng.* 3:6. doi: 10.3389/fneng.2010.00006

Leach, J. B., Achyuta, A. K., and Murthy, S. K. (2010). Bridging the divide between neuroprosthetic design, tissue engineering and neurobiology. *Front. Neuroeng.* 2:18. doi: 10.3389/neuro.16.018.2009

Lee, K.-K., He, J., Singh, A., Massia, S., Ehteshami, G., Kim, B., et al. (2004). Polyimide-based intracortical neural implant with improved structural stiffness. *J. Micromech. Microeng.* 14, 32–37. doi: 10.1088/0960-1317/14/1/305

Leung, B. K., Biran, R., Underwood, C. J., and Tresco, P. A. (2008). Characterization of microglial attachment and cytokine release on biomaterials of differing surface chemistry. *Biomaterials* 29, 3289–3297. doi: 10.1016/j.biomaterials.2008.03.045

Leuthardt, E. C., Freudenberg, Z., Bundy, D., and Roland, J. (2009). Microscale recording from human motor cortex: implications for minimally invasive electrocorticographic brain-computer interfaces. *Neurosurg. Focus* 27:E10. doi: 10.3171/2009.4.FOCUS0980

Leuthardt, E. C., Schalk, G., Moran, D., and Ojemann, J. G. (2006). The emerging world of motor neuroprosthetics: a neurosurgical perspective. *Neurosurgery* 59, 1–14. doi: 10.1227/01.NEU.0000221506.06947.AC

Leuthardt, E. C., Schalk, G., Wolpaw, J. R., Ojemann, J. G., and Moran, D. W. (2004). A brain-computer interface using electrocorticographic signals in humans. *J. Neural Eng.* 1, 63–71. doi: 10.1088/1741-2560/1/2/001

Lovat, V., Pantarotto, D., Lagostena, L., Cacciari, B., Grandolfo, M., Righi, M., et al. (2005). Carbon nanotube substrates boost neuronal electrical signaling. *Nano Lett.* 5, 1107–1110. doi: 10.1021/nl050637m

Ludwig, K. A., Uram, J. D., Yang, J., Martin, D. C., and Kipke, D. R. (2006). Chronic neural recordings using silicon microelectrode arrays electrochemically deposited with a poly(3,4-ethylenedioxythiophene) (PEDOT) film. *J. Neural Eng.* 3, 59–70. doi: 10.1088/1741-2560/3/1/007

Lukás, J., Smetana, K., Petrovický, P., Palecková, V., Vacik, J., Dvoránková, B., et al. (2001). Biological properties of copolymer of 2-hydroxyethyl methacrylate with sulfopropyl methacrylate. *J. Mater. Sci. Mater. Med.* 12, 639–646. doi: 10.1023/A:1011297828955

Lu, Y., Li, T., Zhao, X., Li, M., Cao, Y., Yang, H., et al. (2010). Electrodeposited polypyrrole/carbon nanotubes composite films electrodes for neural interfaces. *Biomaterials* 31, 5169–5181. doi: 10.1016/j.biomaterials.2010.03.022

Marin, C., and Fernández, E. (2010). Biocompatibility of intracortical microelectrodes: current status and future prospects. *Front. Neuroeng.* 3:8. doi: 10.3389/fneng.2010.00008

Mazzatenta, A., Giugliano, M., Campidelli, S., Gambazzi, L., Businaro, L., Markram, H., et al. (2007). Interfacing neurons with carbon nanotubes: electrical signal transfer and synaptic stimulation in cultured brain circuits. *J. Neurosci.* 27, 6931–6936. doi: 10.1523/JNEUROSCI.1051-07.2007

Musallam, S., Bak, M. J., Troyk, P. R., and Andersen, R. A. (2007). A floating metal microelectrode array for chronic implantation. *J. Neurosci. Meth.* 160, 122–127. doi: 10.1016/j.jneumeth.2006.09.005

Nicolelis, M. A. L., and Lebedev, M. A. (2009). Principles of neural ensemble physiology underlying the operation of brain-machine interfaces. *Nat. Rev. Neurosci.* 10, 530–540. doi: 10.1038/nrn2653

Nunes, A., Bussy, C., Gherardini, L., Meneghetti, M., Herrero, M. A., Bianco, A., et al. (2012). *In vivo* degradation of functionalized carbon nanotubes after stereotactic administration in the brain cortex. *Nanomedicine* 7, 1485–1494. doi: 10.2217/nnm.12.33

Polikov, V. S., Tresco, P. A., and Reichert, W. M. (2005). Response of brain tissue to chronically implanted neural electrodes. *J. Neurosci. Methods.* 148, 1–18. doi: 10.1016/j.jneumeth.2005.08.015

Quiroga, R. Q., Nadasdy, Z., and Ben-Shaul, Y. (2004). Unsupervised spike detection and sorting with wavelets and superparamagnetic clustering. *Neural Comput.* 16, 1661–1687. doi: 10.1162/089976604774201631

Rao, L., Zhou, H., Li, T., Li, C., and Duan, Y. Y. (2012). Polyethylene glycol-containing polyurethane hydrogel coatings for improving the biocompatibility of neural electrodes. *Acta Biomaterialia* 8, 2233–2242. doi: 10.1016/j.actbio.2012.03.001

Richter, A., Xie, Y., Schumacher, A., Löffler, S., Kirch, R. D., Al-Hasani, J., et al. (2013). A simple implantation method for flexible, multisite microelectrodes into rat brains. *Front. Neuroeng.* 6:6. doi: 10.3389/fneng.2013.00006

Ritaccio, A., Boatman-Reich, D., Brunner, P., Cervenka, M. C., Cole, A. J., Crone, N., et al. (2011). Proceedings of the second international workshop on advances in electrocorticography. *Epilepsy Behav.* 22, 641–650. doi: 10.1016/j.yebeh.2011.09.028

Robinson, D. A. (1968). The electrical properties of metal microelectrodes. *Proc. IEEE* 56, 1065–1071. doi: 10.1109/PROC.1968.6458

Rousche, P. J., and Normann, R. A. (1992). A method for pneumatically inserting an array of penetrating electrodes into cortical tissue. *Ann. Biomed. Eng.* 20, 413–422. doi: 10.1007/BF02368133

Rousche, P. J., Pellinen, D. S., Pivin, D. P., Williams, J. C., Vetter, R. J., and Kipke, D. R. (2001). Flexible polyimide-based intracortical electrode arrays with bioactive capability. *IEEE Trans. Biomed. Eng.* 48, 361–371. doi: 10.1109/10.914800

Rubehn, B., Bosman, C., Oostenveld, R., Fries, P., and Stieglitz, T. (2009). A MEMS-based flexible multichannel ECoG-electrode array. *J. Neural Eng.* 6:036003. doi: 10.1088/1741-2560/6/3/036003

Rubehn, B., and Stieglitz, T. (2010). *In vitro* evaluation of the long-term stability of polyimide as a material for neural implants. *Biomaterials* 31, 3449–3458. doi: 10.1016/j.biomaterials.2010.01.053

Schjetnan, A. G., and Luczak, A. (2011). Recording large-scale neuronal ensembles with silicon probes in the anesthetized rat. *J. Vis. Exp.* 56:e3282. doi: 10.3791/3282

Schoeller, T., Lille, S., Wechselberger, G., Otto, A., Mowlawi, A., and Piza-Katzer, H. (2001). Histomorphologic and volumetric analysis of implanted autologouspreadipocyte cultures suspended in fibrin glue: a potential new source for tissue augmentation. *Aesthetic Plast. Surg.* 25, 57–63. doi: 10.1007/s002660010096

Schwartz, A. B. (2004). Cortical neural prosthetics. *Annu. Rev. Neurosci.* 27, 487–507. doi: 10.1146/annurev.neuro.27.070203.144233

Shoval, A., Adams, C., David-Pur, M., Shein, M., Hanein, Y., and Sernagor, E. (2009). Carbon nanotube electrodes for effective interfacing with retinal tissue. *Front. Neuroeng.* 2:4. doi: 10.3389/neuro.16.004.2009

Sorkin, R., Greenbaum, A., David-Pur, M., Anava, S., Ayali, A., Ben-Jacob, E., et al. (2009). Process entanglement as a neuronal anchorage mechanism to rough surfaces. *Nanotechnology* 20:015101. doi: 10.1088/0957-4484/20/1/015101

Stice, P., Gilletti, A., Panitch, A., and Muthuswamy, J. (2007). Thin microelectrodes reduce GFAP expression in the implant site in rodent somatosensory cortex. *J. Neural Eng.* 4, 42–53. doi: 10.1088/1741-2560/4/2/005

Suner, S., Fellows, M. R., Vargas-Irwin, C., Nakata, G. K., and Donoghue, J. P. (2005). Reliability of signals from a chronically implanted, silicon-based electrode array in non-human primate primary motor cortex. *IEEE Trans. Neural Syst. Rehabil. Eng.* 13, 524–541. doi: 10.1109/TNSRE.2005.857687

Takeuchi, S., Suzuki, T., Mabuchi, K., and Fujita, H. (2004). 3D flexible multichannel neural probe array. *J. Micromech. Microeng.* 14, 104–107. doi: 10.1088/0960-1317/14/1/014

Thongpang, S., Richner, T. J., Brodnick, S. K., Schendel, A., Kim, J., Wilson, J. A., et al. (2011). A micro-electrocorticography platform and deployment strategies for chronic BCI applications. *Clin. EEG Neurosci.* 42, 259–265. doi: 10.1177/155005941104200412

Turner, J. N., Shain, W., Szarowski, D. H., Andersen, M., Martins, S., Isaacson, M., et al. (1999). Cerebral astrocyte response to micromachined silicon implants. *Exp. Neurol.* 156, 33–49. doi: 10.1006/exnr.1998.6983

Ward, M. P., Rajdev, P., Ellison, C., and Irazoqui, P. P. (2009).Toward a comparison of microelectrodes for acute and chronic recordings. *Brain Res.* 1282, 183–200. doi: 10.1016/j.brainres.2009.05.052

Wise, K. D. (2005). Silicon microsystems for neuroscience and neural prostheses. *IEEE Eng. Med. Biol. Mag.* 24, 22–29. doi: 10.1109/MEMB.2005.1511497

Woerly, S., Pinet, E., De Robertis, L., Bousmina, M., Laroche, G., Roitback, T. et al. (1998). Heterogeneous PHPMA hydrogels for tissue repair and axonal regeneration in the injured spinal cord. *J. Biomater. Sci. Polym. Ed.* 9, 681–711. doi: 10.1163/156856298X00091

Yamato, H., Ohwa, M., and Wernet, W. (1995). Stability of polypyrrole and poly (3, 4 _ ethylenedioxythiophene) for biosensor application. *J. Electroanal. Chem.* 397, 163–170. doi: 10.1016/0022-0728(95)04156-8

Yang, J., Kim, D. H., Hendricks, J. L., Leach, M., Northey, R., and Martin, D. C. (2005). Ordered surfactant-templated poly(3,4-ethylenedioxythiophene) (PEDOT) conducting polymer on microfabricated neural probes. *Acta Biomater.* 1, 125–136. doi: 10.1016/j.actbio.2004.09.006

Zhong, Y., and Bellamkonda, R. V. (2007). Dexamethasone-coated neural probes elicit attenuated inflammatory response and neuronal loss compared to uncoated neural probes. *Brain Res.* 1148, 15–27. doi: 10.1016/j.brainres.2007.02.024

17

Calibrating Doppler imaging of preterm intracerebral circulation using a microvessel flow phantom

Fleur A. Camfferman[1], Ginette M. Ecury-Goossen[2], Jhuresy E. La Roche[2], Nico de Jong[3,4], Willem van 't Leven[3], Hendrik J. Vos[3,4], Martin D. Verweij[4], Kazem Nasserinejad[5], Filip Cools[1], Paul Govaert[1,2] and Jeroen Dudink[2,6]*

[1] Department of Neonatology, Universitair Ziekenhuis Brussel, Vrije Universiteit Brussel, Brussels, Belgium
[2] Department of Neonatology, Erasmus Medical Centre, Rotterdam, Netherlands
[3] Department of Biomedical Engineering, Erasmus Medical Centre, Rotterdam, Netherlands
[4] Department of Imaging Physics, Delft University of Technology, Delft, Netherlands
[5] Department of Biostatistics, Erasmus Medical Centre, Rotterdam, Netherlands
[6] Department of Radiology, Erasmus Medical Centre, Rotterdam, Netherlands

Edited by:
Silvia Comani, Università degli Studi G. D'Annunzio, Italy

Reviewed by:
Narendra Reddy Dereddy, Maria Fareri Children's Hospital at Westchester Medical Center, USA
Gordon Niall Stevenson, National Health Service, UK

Correspondence:
Jeroen Dudink, Erasmus Medical Center, Sophia Children's Hospital, Dr. Molewaterplein 60, Rotterdam 3015 GJ, Netherlands
e-mail: j.dudink@erasmusmc.nl

Introduction: Preterm infants are born during critical stages of brain development, in which the adaptive capacity of the fetus to extra-uterine environment is limited. Inadequate brain perfusion has been directly linked to preterm brain damage. Advanced high-frequency ultrasound probes and processing algorithms allow visualization of microvessels and depiction of regional variation. To assess whether visualization and flow velocity estimates of preterm cerebral perfusion using Doppler techniques are accurate, we conducted an *in vitro* experiment using a microvessel flow phantom.

Materials and Methods: An in-house developed flow phantom containing two microvessels (inner diameter 200 and 700 μm) with attached syringe pumps, filled with blood-mimicking fluid, was used to generate non-pulsatile perfusion of variable flow. Measurements were performed using an Esaote MyLab70 scanner.

Results: Microvessel mimicking catheters with velocities as low as 1 cm/s were adequately visualized with a linear ultrasound probe. With a convex probe, velocities <2 cm/s could not be depicted. Within settings, velocity and diameter measurements were highly reproducible [intra-class correlation 0.997 (95% CI 0.996–0.998) and 0.914 (0.864–0.946)]. Overall, mean velocity was overestimated up to threefold, especially in high velocity ranges. Significant differences were seen in velocity measurements when using steer angle correction and in vessel diameter estimation ($p < 0.05$).

Conclusion: Visualization of microvessel-size catheters mimicking small brain vessels is feasible. Reproducible velocity and diameter results can be obtained, although important overestimation of the values is observed. Before velocity estimates of microcirculation can find its use in clinical practice, calibration of the ultrasound machine for any specific Doppler purpose is essential. The ultimate goal is to develop a sonographic tool that can be used for objective study of regional perfusion in routine practice.

Keywords: preterm brain, cerebral circulation, cerebral perfusion, microcirculation, flow phantom, calibration, cerebral blood flow, Doppler

INTRODUCTION

Central to normal human brain development and function is maintenance of adequate blood flow and oxygenation. This requires complex regulatory mechanisms, which at the early stages of human development exist in a vulnerable equilibrium and are notoriously difficult to monitor. Severe neonatal conditions, such as prematurity, birth trauma, infections, and congenital malformations, often compromise brain perfusion during this critical period of brain development and will grow into an avalanche of neurodevelopmental problems, including cognitive deficits, motor disability, and psychiatric diseases (Sherlock et al., 2005; Volpe, 2009) with ensuing lifelong burdens for the growing individuals and their families, and a major socio-economic impact for the health care system and the whole of society (Petrou et al., 2001).

Brain injury as a complication of preterm birth is directly or indirectly linked to low brain perfusion and oxygenation (Meek et al., 1999; Kissack et al., 2004). Although little is known about the ability of the preterm to regulate cerebral blood flow (CBF) in

Abbreviations: BMF, blood-mimicking fluid; CBF, cerebral blood flow; CD, color Doppler; ICC, intra-class correlation; ICV, internal cerebral vein; NIRS, near-infrared spectroscopy; PD, power Doppler; PI, pulsatility index; PRC, processing; PRF, pulse repetition frequency; PRS, persistence; PW, pulsed wave; PWD, pulsed wave Doppler; RI, resistance index.

response to changes in perfusion pressure, there is some evidence that the autoregulatory range is limited compared with that of adults and absent in sick infants (Greisen, 2005). Muscular walls are even absent in fragile medullary channels of the preterm brain, suggesting that some functional tools for autoregulation are not present yet (Kuban and Gilles, 1985). Consequently, extremes of systemic perfusion are transmitted unaltered to brain tissue. It is still a challenge to study neonatal organ and brain–blood perfusion systematically. A reliable, objective, repeatable, safe, and bedside method to characterize neonatal blood perfusion is needed.

Alternative methods to approximate blood flow, like blood pressure, diuresis, heart rate, and limb oxygen saturation are extensively used, but are notoriously poor surrogates of neonatal brain perfusion. Standard techniques for adult brain studies are undesirable or very difficult to apply in the neonate. CBF measured with radioactive Xenon or jugular occlusion plethysmography are disruptive to the infant and cannot be repeated frequently. MRI perfusion scans (such as arterial spin labeling) are not suited for (repeated) monitoring and require transport of often critically ill and clinically unstable infants to the radiology ward (Liem and Greisen, 2010). Now, tissue oxygen delivery can be studied using optical near-infrared spectroscopy (NIRS), a bedside and safe technique, which allows continuous monitoring. However, NIRS is not quantitative and only provides indirect information about blood flow in regions that cannot be precisely pinpointed. Although trends in CBF may be inferred from changes in cerebral oxygenation and/or blood volume, NIRS does not allow a direct measure of CBF (van Bel et al., 2008; Marin and Moore, 2011).

EEG monitoring, like NIRS, is a safe and bedside neuro monitoring tool, which gained renewed interest of clinicians and researchers because of improved hardware and software in recent years. However, changes in EEG signal reflect large neuronal electrophysiological changes in a late and often irreversible stage of brain injury evolution (Hellström-Westas, 2006).

Brain ultrasound is a widely used non-invasive and bedside tool for evaluation of neonatal brain anatomy and detection of brain injury. Color Doppler (CD) has already found a limited application in the analysis of patent ductus arteriosus and birth asphyxia. Indices like pulsatility index and resistance index have been developed and used as proxies for flow (Pezzati et al., 2002; Basu et al., 2014). Recent advances in ultrasound technique have made visualization of small diameter vessels (microcirculation) possible (Macé et al., 2011). Yet, conventional pulsed wave Doppler (PWD) is regularly used for absolute flow velocity measurements. Triplex mode imaging is used in current daily practice, in which flow information is overlaid to an anatomical B-mode image, and absolute flow velocities are measured in the PW Doppler panel (WHO, 2011). Flow information is visualized either in CD or power Doppler (PD). In CD, the color indicates average velocity in the vessel, which is sensitive to the angle of the vessel. In PD, the color indicates the total amount of Doppler energy in the echo from the vessel, which is not sensitive to the angle. The general effect is that PD should be able to detect lower flow velocities and smaller vessels, at the cost of loss of quantitative velocity information. Moreover, the additional method of directional PD gives the PD, but estimates the direction of the flow and colors it subsequently.

Although there is no general consensus on the definition of "microcirculation" in the preterm brain, it is often defined as arteriolar and venular flow. Extrapolating from descriptions of vessel anatomy in fetuses, the diameter of microvessels visualized with Doppler in cerebral white matter of a preterm infant between 24 and 30 weeks is expected to be between 50 and 100 μm (Kuban and Gilles, 1985; Anstrom et al., 2004). The large arteries of the circle of Willis of 24-week-old fetuses have diameters around 400–500 μm (Vasovic et al., 2007). High-frequency linear probes permit visualization of vessels with a diameter below 200 μm. Therefore, visualization of the brain microcirculation of the preterm infant is feasible, making this a potential tool for *in vivo*, safe, bedside, repeatable measurement of CBF. Still, one of the challenges of ultrasound is that the vessel caliber cannot be accurately measured, so that flow cannot be estimated (Kehrer et al., 2003, 2005).

Models using a flow phantom and advanced (power) Doppler technique may be of use to objectively quantify regional flow variation. To mimic preterm brain tissue, this model should depict very small vessel sizes (about 200 μm) and very low flow (<2 cm/s).

As far as we know, no studies are reported to assess the accuracy of current PW, CD, and directional PD techniques in the visualization of microperfusion. Our aim was to evaluate if velocity measurements of microvessels are reproducible and accurate using sensitive modern ultrasound techniques. The second aim was to determine which Doppler technique (color versus PD, type of probe) is best used to visualize these small vessels. To this purpose, we set up an *in vitro* experiment using a microvessel flow phantom designed to mimic preterm cerebral perfusion. We hypothesized that current ultrasound technique is sufficiently accurate to estimate flow in preterm brain microvessels.

MATERIALS AND METHODS

MICROVESSEL FLOW PHANTOM

The flow phantom (**Figure 1**) consisted of an acrylic container filled with agar-based tissue-mimicking material, built according

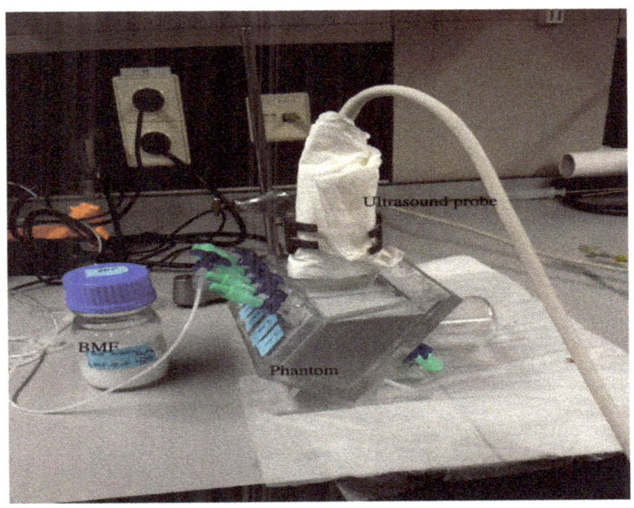

FIGURE 1 | The test setting. Flow phantom with a fixed ultrasound probe. BMF, blood-mimicking fluid.

to Teirlinck et al. (1998). The tissue-mimicking material contained two vessels made of polyethylene terephthalate glycol-modified (Paradigm Optics, Vancouver, WA, USA) with an inner diameter of 200 μm each, and three silicone vessels (ERIKS bv, Alkmaar, the Netherlands) with an inner diameter of 700, 1000, and 2000 μm respectively. The blood-mimicking fluid (BMF) used to run through the vessels was based on the recipe by Ramnarine et al. (1998). However, our BMF contains half the amount of dextran and glycerol compared to the original recipe. This reduces the viscosity of the fluid, which is necessary to prevent blockage of the small vessels used in this study.

We intended to simulate the internal cerebral veins (ICV) and intracerebral medullary veins of very preterm infants using this microvessel flow phantom. Based on measurements performed in daily clinical practice, the distance from the anterior fontanel to the ICV is 2.5–5 cm, and intracerebral medullary veins are located at a depth of 2 cm. Blood flow velocity in the ICV is about 5 cm/s and in medullary veins this lies around 1 cm/s (Pfannschmidt and Jorch, 1989; Deeg and Lode, 2005). ICV diameter is estimated to be 500 μm in these neonates, while the diameter of the intracerebral medullary veins is around 100 μm (Kuban and Gilles, 1985). Since capillaries for the flow phantom with a diameter of 100 and 500 μm were not available, we used the 200 and 700 μm vessels for this study.

TEST SETTING

To generate steady flow through the capillaries, we used a calibrated syringe pump (Harvard Apparatus Pump 11 Elite, Instech Laboratories, Plymouth Meeting, USA) to infuse BMF at velocities ranging from 1 to 10 cm/s. This pump can produce regular flows as low as 1.28 pL/min. To calibrate the syringe pump, we calculated expected BMF volume based on pump speed and duration of the experiment and compared this with the volume of BMF collected at the flow phantom outlet. Recording time was started at the first drop.

For each vessel size, flow settings (microliter per second) were calculated according to the following equation:

$$Q = \left(V_{\text{avg}} \times \pi r^2\right) \times 10^9 \tag{1}$$

Q is flow in microliter per second, V_{avg} is average velocity in meter per second, and r is the radius of the vessel in meter.

Measurements were obtained using an Esaote system (Mylab 70, Genova, Italy) with a linear (Esaote LA 435 Linear Array Ultrasound Probe, 6.0–18.0 MHz) and convex probe (Esaote CA123 Convex Array Ultrasound Probe, 3.3–9.0 MHz). A standard ultrasound preset was used, identical to the preset used for imaging in daily clinical practice. This standard preset was optimized for neonatal preterm microvessel visualization prior to a large local prospective cohort study. The aim of that study was to explore the feasibility of CD for monitoring of cerebral perfusion in very preterm infants at the level of microvessels (unpublished data of Raets et al. – Preterm cerebral microcirculation assessed with color Doppler: a pilot study). According to Ten Cate et al. (2013), the Esaote Ultrasound machine, as used in this experiment, proved to be more suitable for microcirculation imaging in comparison to the other ultrasound brands. This is most probably mainly caused by fundamental differences in processing the Doppler signal or internal settings inaccessible to users. Settings used in this study are summarized in **Table 1**. For the linear probe, settings included a transmit frequency of 7.7 MHz in flow visualization and 5.9 MHz in PW Doppler, a gain of 50%, and an imaging depth of 30 mm. For the convex probe, settings included a transmit frequency of 5 MHz in flow visualization and 6.3 MHz in PW Doppler, a gain of 54%, and imaging depth of 76 mm. Thermal and mechanical indices were always kept below 1.0.

The syringe pump was set to generate non-pulsatile perfusion of predefined volumes for each of the vessels (see above). Using the convex and linear probes, peak flow velocity and diameter of the capillaries were measured at 2 cm depth. Detection and diameter sizing measurements were performed using CD and directional PD. To obtain diameter measurements, a Doppler image was frozen, and diameter was estimated using a manual caliber measurement. Velocity measurements were performed in the PW Doppler panel by manually putting a marker at the extreme bound of the PW profile. Since the flow was non-pulsatile, this extreme bound was persistent over the entire measurement period (1 or more seconds) and easily identifiable. When enabled, the steering angle was aligned parallel to the capillary. The velocity measurements were repeated three times at each predefined velocity. In order to minimize bias, a single observer obtained the measurements in the presence of a second observer.

In order to prevent motion artifacts, the probes were fixed using a tripod. With set flow velocities of 5 cm/s and above, a pulsatile flow pattern was witnessed. This disturbance vanished when using a 10 mL low friction glass syringe (GASTIGHT #1010, Hamilton Company, Bonaduz, Switzerland) or a 60 mL plastic syringe instead of a 10 mL plastic syringe. Therefore, for all set flow velocities of 5 cm/s and more we used the glass syringe.

Table 1 | Ultrasound settings used in this study.

Doppler mode	Probe	Frequency (MHz)	Gain (%)	PRF (kHz)	PRS	PRC	Wall filter
PWD	Linear	5.9	53–60	0.5–10	–	6	100 Hz
	Convex	6.3	50–56	0.75–2	–	6	65 Hz
CD	Linear	7.7	50	0.37	16	M/2	1
	Convex	5	64	1.5	16	H/2	2
Directional PD	Linear	7.7	50	1–2.5	3, 4	M/2, H/2	2, 3
	Convex	5	64	1–2	3, 4, 6	L/2, M/2	2, 4

PWD, pulsed wave Doppler; CD, color Doppler mode; PD, power Doppler; PRF, pulse repetition frequency; PRS, persistence; PRC, processing.

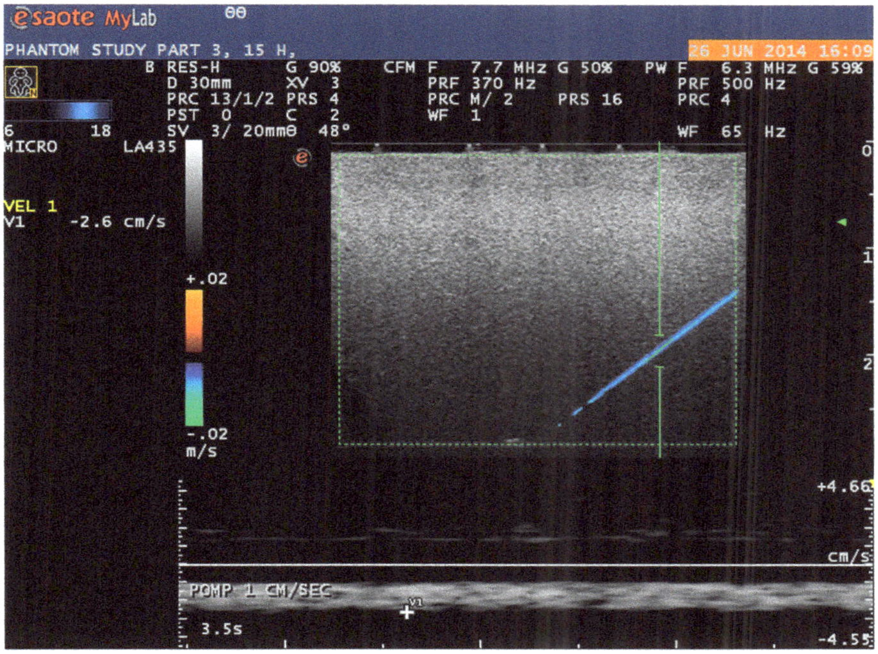

FIGURE 2 | Ultrasound image of phantom microvessel. Ultrasound image showing a 200 μm flow phantom catheter as depicted by a linear probe in color Doppler mode.

STATISTICAL ANALYSIS

To assess the reproducibility of the velocity measurements and whether velocity measured with the ultrasound corresponded with the actual set velocity, one-way random intra-class correlation (ICC) coefficient was computed with single measures. Based on bootstrap sampling, the 95% confidence interval for ICC coefficient was calculated. To compare the measured diameter with the actual diameter of the capillaries, we used the Student's one sample t-test. Statistically significant was assumed if two-sided p value was <0.05. All statistical analyses were performed in R (version 3.1.1; R Foundation for Statistical Computing, Vienna, Austria – http://www.R-project.org).

RESULTS

VELOCITY MEASUREMENTS

Microvessels mimicking catheters with a size of 200 and 700 μm with BMF velocities as low as 1 cm/s were adequately visualized using a linear probe (**Figure 2**). With a convex probe, however, velocities below 2 cm/s in the 700 μm vessel and below 3 cm/s in the 200 μm vessel could not be depicted.

Measurements of velocity and diameter proved to be highly reproducible, with an overall ICC coefficient of 0.997 (95% CI 0.996–0.998) and 0.914 (0.864–0.946), respectively.

As shown in **Table 2**, in all different settings, ICC coefficient of three consecutive velocity measurements stayed above 0.9 with a variation coefficient below 1.0, except for velocities measured in the 200 μm vessel with the convex probe.

Differences between true (pump) velocity and the peak measured Doppler velocity are shown in **Figure 3**. Overall, PWD

Table 2 | Reproducibility of velocity measurements.

Vessel diameter (μm)	Doppler mode	Probe	Steer angle correction	ICC (95% CI)	
200	Color	Linear	–	0.998 (0.991–1.000)	
			+	0.999 (0.996–0.999)	
		Convex	–	0.985 (0.643–0.989)	a
			+	0.991 (0.673–0.995)	a
	Power	Linear	–	0.997 (0.991–00.998)	
			+	0.997 (0.988–0.999)	
		Convex	–	0.915 (0.357–0.945)	a
			+	0.992 (0.702–0.998)	a
700	Color	Linear	–	0.999 (0.996–1.000)	
			+	0.999 (0.976–1.000)	
		Convex	–	0.986 (0.964–0.998)	b
			+	0.999 (0.992–1.000)	b
	Power	Linear	–	0.995 (0.933–0.997)	
			+	0.999 (0.996–0.999)	
		Convex	–	0.997 (0.991–0.999)	b
			+	0.999 (0.993–0.999)	b

Reproducibility of consecutive velocity measurements as showed by ICC (intra-class correlation) coefficients. Color, color Doppler; power, power Doppler; v, velocity.

[a] *No visualization if $v \leq 2$ cm/s.*

[b] *No visualization if $v = 1$ cm/s.*

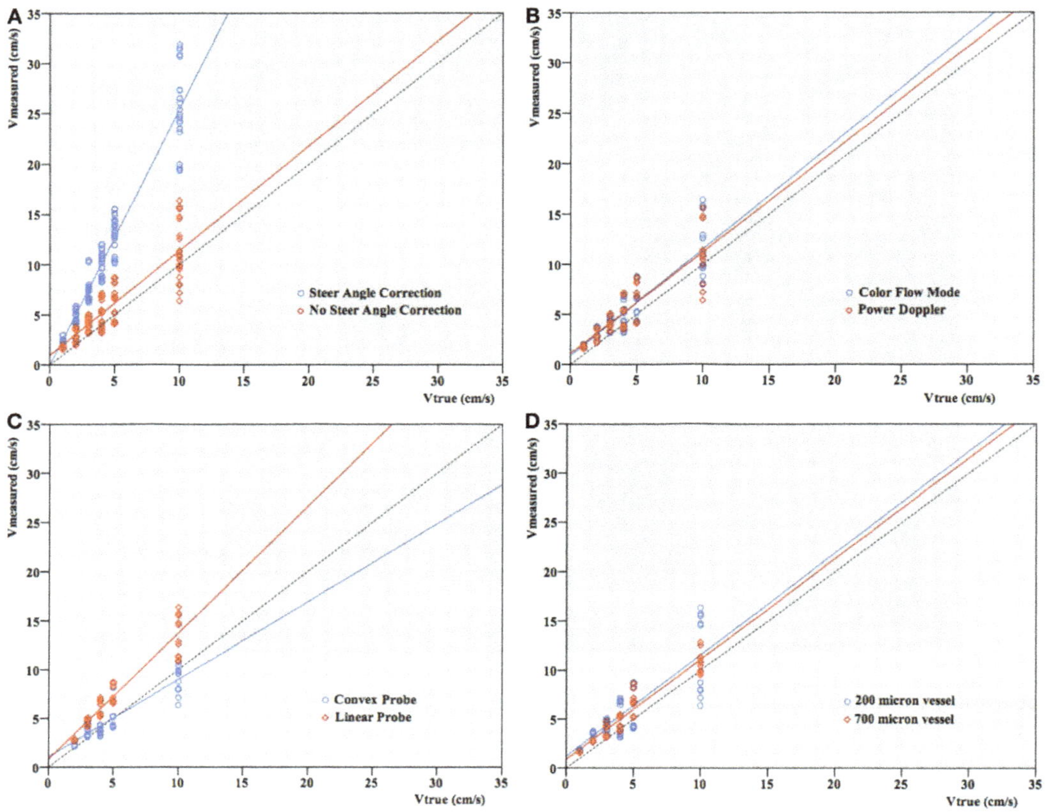

FIGURE 3 | Pump velocity versus measured Doppler velocity. Relation between true velocity (centimeter per second) and velocity measured (centimeter per second) in different settings: **(A)** with or without steer angle correction, **(B)** color Doppler versus power Doppler, **(C)** convex versus linear probe, **(D)** vessel size. Since applying steer angle correction leads to significant ($p < 0.001$) overestimation of velocity, velocities in **(B–D)** are without applying steer angle correction. The dotted line represents the line of equality.

overestimated velocity with a 1.1- to 3.5-fold overestimation. This is independent of the flow visualization method in the triplex mode, as expected (**Figure 3B**). If velocity increased, spreading of the velocities measured in the different settings seemed to be more pronounced. However, this appeared to depend almost uniquely on the highly significant differences that were seen in velocity measurements with versus without steer angle correction ($p < 0.001$). When leaving out the steer angle velocity estimates, correlation between true velocities and measured velocity ameliorated.

Overall, ICC coefficient between average velocity measured by Doppler and the true velocity was 0.352 (0.269–0.442). As shown in a Bland–Altman plot (**Figure 4**), overall agreement between true velocity (Velocity pump) and velocity estimated by Doppler was poor. However, results suggest consistent overestimation.

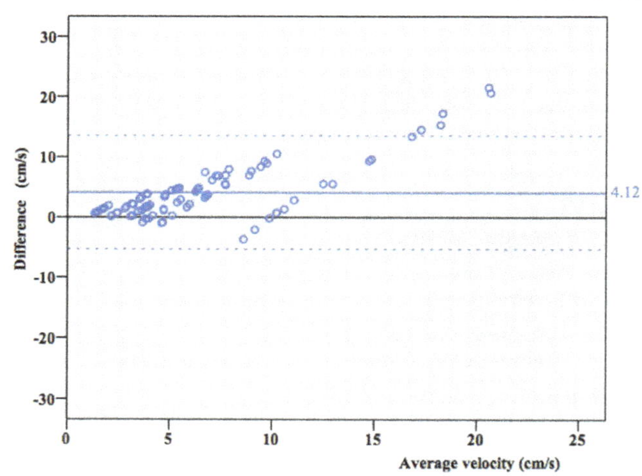

FIGURE 4 | Agreement between true velocity and Doppler velocity. Bland–Altman plot of agreement between true velocity (V_{true}) and velocity estimated by Doppler measurements ($V_{measured}$). The mean difference is 4.12 cm/s (95% CI 3.10–5.15 cm/s), dotted lines represent ± 2 SD borders.

DIAMETER MEASUREMENTS

Student's t-test for vessel size showed significant differences in diameter estimation (p-values <0.001 and 0.005, respectively). As shown in **Figure 5**, vessel size was mostly overestimated by ultrasound.

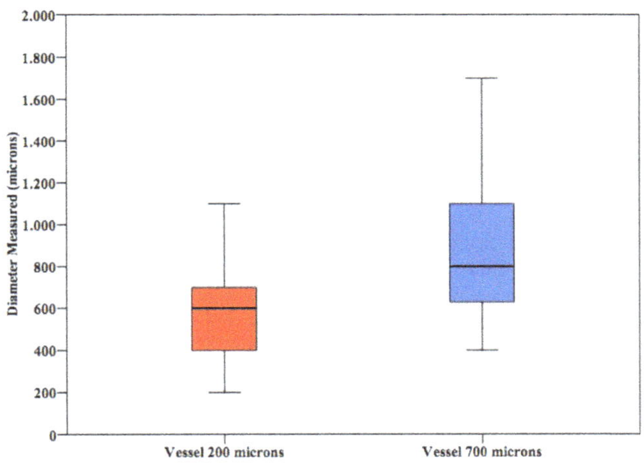

FIGURE 5 | Vessel diameter. Vessel diameter measured (±SD) for the 200 μm vessel and the 700 μm vessel. Note the significant overestimation.

DISCUSSION

In this flow phantom study, we found that Doppler ultrasound imaging is able to visualize microvessel-size catheters with low flow, mimicking cerebral microcirculation. Within the different settings, reproducible velocity and diameter results can be obtained. Our overall results showed that vessel diameter and velocity are overestimated when measured by Doppler ultrasound. This corresponds with results of previous phantom studies (Goertz et al., 2000; Raine-Fenning et al., 2008a; Schulten-Wijman et al., 2008; Xu et al., 2008). However, these studies were designed mainly to determine optimal machine settings and minimal detectable flow. To our best knowledge, this is the first *in vitro* experiment to calibrate for neonatal brain microcirculation.

Overestimation of flow velocity was observed in our study with convex as well as linear ultrasound probes. Previous publications (Guo et al., 1995; Teirlinck et al., 1998; Schulten-Wijman et al., 2008) described a similar phenomenon. Several aspects of Doppler technique and processing of the signals may contribute to this overshooting, as detailed below.

First, it might be explained by sampling inaccuracy. The flow can be assumed parabolic in the low-Reynolds number regime asserted in our measurements. In such a flow, the peak velocity is two times higher than the average flow as predicted by Eq. 1. Moreover, we manually picked the maximum Doppler velocity in the PW panel, as in current clinical practice, not the average velocity. The effect of the flow profile on such Doppler-based velocity estimation is complex, but tends to overestimate the mean velocity (Ricci et al., 2014).

A second explanation might be the way that raw ultrasound data are filtered and processed within the ultrasound machine to produce an image. Most ultrasound machines consider the mean propagation speed c in tissue to be 1540 cm/s and use this value to calculate many values, of which velocity is 1 (Zagzebski, 1996; Gill, 2012). If the true propagation speed is higher than 1540 cm/s, this may lead to overestimation of predicted velocity. Exact propagation speed of preterm brain tissue is unknown and additionally depends on several other factors, like temperature and hydration status (Kremkau et al., 1981). Also, in the process of filtering background scatter, some information might be lost or adapted, all according to the software used. At present, we are not familiar with the manufacturer's confidential post-processing algorithms to create an image from raw data. Especially, when desiring to depict smaller vessels and lower flow velocities, insight in these methods and cooperation with the manufacturer in the development of new software might be of importance.

Third, overshooting might be explained by insonation angle. Since both velocity and direction of blood flow determine Doppler shift, which is the main principle of Doppler ultrasound, insonation angle is an important determinant in calculating velocity. To make velocity quantification error as small as possible, the Doppler angle must be kept as small as possible (Zagzebski, 1996). Current study was performed in a flow phantom with an insonation angle of about 60°, which is considered the maximal insonation angle in clinical practice but still gives an important velocity estimation error. Additionally, increasing insonation angle worsens several Doppler artifacts, such as an intrinsic spectral broadening, which leads to a systematic overestimation in velocity measurements (Gill, 2012).

Pulsed wave Doppler and CD ultrasound depend on the time shift of pulsed wave echoes to calculate velocity and direction. In PD, on the other hand, the color displayed is determined by the Doppler signal power rather than the effective time shift. In theory, this makes PD more sensitive for visualization of low flow velocity (Murphy and Rubin, 1997; Martinoli et al., 1998). Yet, our study shows that both directional PD and CD are able to detect flow velocities down to 1 cm/s with the linear array, which would indicate applicability of both methods in the current framework of preterm intracerebral circulation imaging. The measured velocities with PD were independent of the CD or PD visualization method, which is expected because of the independent nature of data acquisition and processing between PW Doppler and the visualization method.

As expected, applying the steer angle artificially corrects for the angle between flow direction and ultrasound beam. Since the measured Doppler value is divided by the cosine of the angle that the sonographer sets, it should always result in larger apparent velocities in the image (Szabo, 2013). This is consistent with our findings.

Considering the specific characteristics of the linear and convex ultrasound probes and their use in clinical practice, we expected the linear probe to be more suitable for microcirculation imaging. Indeed, lower flow velocities were visualized using the linear probe in the 200 μm vessel compared to the convex probe. As seen in **Figure 3**, velocities were mainly overestimated by the linear probe while the convex probe underestimated them. Apart from that, results show no obvious superiority for this probe and its specific settings, with reference to the diameter and blood flow velocity of the microvessels.

Since B-mode ultrasound is insufficiently accurate in estimating the diameter of microvessels, we tried to approach true diameter using CD and PD. Reproducible results were obtained; however, overestimation was equally observed as in the velocity measurements. This inaccuracy in measuring diameter is a known problem of Doppler technique. Due to the relatively long transmit pulses in Doppler, axial accuracy of CD systems is rather low, resulting in the encoding of the color sometimes beyond the true flow field (Guo et al., 1995).

Additionally, when adjusting instrument parameters, for instance, increasing the gain, overestimation of vessel diameter is more likely (Browne et al., 2004; Raine-Fenning et al., 2008b). Mitchell (1990) stated that a jet area depicted by color imaging is likely to be more dependent on instrument parameters than on vascular anatomy or physiological characteristics. However, current understanding of ultrasound technique and new *in vitro* models like this microcirculation flow model might give the opportunity to calibrate machine settings for measurement of diameter and true blood flow in near future. In a small spinoff pilot study, ultrasound settings were adjusted according to flow phantom measurements allowing accurate caliber visualization during Doppler imaging, showing the feasibility of this technique.

In conclusion, Doppler ultrasound might be an additional diagnostic tool for quantification of neonatal brain blood flow. This study shows that, before starting to use velocity estimates in patients, calibration of the ultrasound machine for that purpose is needed. The ultimate goal of this type of research is to develop a sonographic tool that can be used for objectively studying regional (3D) perfusion in routine practice.

AUTHOR CONTRIBUTIONS

Fleur A. Camfferman has written the manuscript and created figures. Ginette M. Ecury-Goossen has performed the analysis and has written the manuscript. Jhuresy E. La Roche has performed the analysis. Hendrik J. Vos provided technical support and has written the manuscript. Nico de Jong, Willem Van 'T Leven, and Martin D. Verweij provided technical support and contributed to the manuscript. Kazem Nasserinejad analyzed the data and contributed to the manuscript. Filip Cools contributed to the manuscript and the figures. Paul Govaert and Jeroen Dudink have written the manuscript, designed the experiments, and provided expert consultation. Additionally, Jeroen Dudink provided senior supervision.

REFERENCES

Anstrom, J. A., Brown, W. R., Moody, D. M., Thore, C. R., Challa, V. R., and Block, S. M. (2004). Subependymal veins in premature neonates: implications for hemorrhage. *Pediatr. Neurol.* 30, 46–53. doi:10.1016/S0887-8994(03)00404-1

Basu, S., Dewangan, S., Barman, S., Shukla, R. C., and Kumar, A. (2014). Postnatal changes in cerebral blood flow velocity in term intra-uterine growth-restricted neonates. *Paediatr. Int. Child Health* 34, 189–193. doi:10.1179/2046905514Y.0000000124

Browne, J. E., Watson, A. J., Hoskins, P. R., and Elliott, A. T. (2004). Validation of a sensitivity performance index test protocol and evaluation of colour Doppler sensitivity for a range of ultrasound scanners. *Ultrasound Med. Biol.* 30, 1475–1483. doi:10.1016/j.ultrasmedbio.2004.09.005

Deeg, K. H., and Lode, H. M. (2005). Trans-fontanellar Doppler sonography of the intracranial veins in infants – part I – normal values. *Ultraschall Med.* 26, 507–517. doi:10.1055/s-2005-858881

Gill, R. (2012). *The Physics and Technology of Diagnostic Ultrasound.* Sydney: High Frequency Publishing.

Goertz, D. E., Christopher, D. A., Yu, J. L., Kerbel, R. S., Burns, P. N., and Foster, F. S. (2000). High-frequency color flow imaging of the microcirculation. *Ultrasound Med. Biol.* 26, 63–71. doi:10.1016/S0301-5629(99)00101-5

Greisen, G. (2005). Autoregulation of cerebral blood flow in newborn babies. *Early Hum. Dev.* 81, 423–428. doi:10.1016/j.earlhumdev.2005.03.005

Guo, Z., Moreau, M., Rickey, D. W., Picot, P. A., and Fenster, A. (1995). Quantitative investigation of in vitro flow using three-dimensional colour Doppler ultrasound. *Ultrasound Med. Biol.* 21, 807–816. doi:10.1016/0301-5629(95)00007-E

Hellström-Westas, L. (2006). Continuous electroencephalography monitoring of the preterm infant. *Clin. Perinatol.* 33, 633–647. doi:10.1016/j.clp.2006.06.003

Kehrer, M., Blumenstock, G., Ehehalt, S., Goelz, R., Poets, C., and Schöning, M. (2005). Development of cerebral blood flow volume in preterm neonates during the first two weeks of life. *Pediatr. Res.* 58, 927–930. doi:10.1203/01.PDR.0000182579.52820.C3

Kehrer, M., Krägeloh-Mann, I., Goelz, R., and Schöning, M. (2003). The development of cerebral perfusion in healthy preterm and term neonates. *Neuropediatrics* 34, 281–286. doi:10.1055/s-2003-44663

Kissack, C. M., Garr, R., Wardle, S. P., and Weindling, A. M. (2004). Postnatal changes in cerebral oxygen extraction in the preterm infant are associated with intraventricular hemorrhage and hemorrhagic parenchymal infarction but not periventricular leukomalacia. *Pediatr. Res.* 56, 111–116. doi:10.1203/01.PDR.0000128984.03461.42

Kremkau, F. W., Barnes, R. W., and McGraw, C. P. (1981). Ultrasonic attenuation and propagation speed in normal human brain. *J. Acoust. Soc. Am.* 70, 29–38. doi:10.1121/1.386578

Kuban, K. C. K., and Gilles, F. H. (1985). Human telencephalic angiogenesis. *Ann. Neurol.* 17, 539–548. doi:10.1002/ana.410170603

Liem, K. D., and Greisen, G. (2010). Monitoring of cerebral haemodynamics in newborn infants. *Early Hum. Dev.* 86, 155–158. doi:10.1016/j.earlhumdev.2010.01.029

Macé, E., Montaldo, G., Cohen, I., Baulac, M., Fink, M., and Tanter, M. (2011). Functional ultrasound imaging of the brain. *Nat. Methods* 8, 662–664. doi:10.1038/nmeth.1641

Marin, T., and Moore, J. (2011). Understanding near-infrared spectroscopy. *Adv. Neonatal Care* 11, 382–388. doi:10.1097/ANC.0b013e3182337ebb

Martinoli, C., Derchi, L. E., Rizzatto, G., and Solbiati, L. (1998). Power Doppler sonography: general principles, clinical applications, and future prospects. *Eur. Radiol.* 8, 1224–1235. doi:10.1007/s003300050540

Meek, J. H., Tyszczuk, L., Elwell, C. E., and Wyatt, J. S. (1999). Low cerebral blood flow is a risk factor for severe intraventricular haemorrhage. *Arch. Dis. Child. Fetal Neonatal Ed.* 81, F15–F18. doi:10.1136/fn.81.1.F15

Mitchell, D. G. (1990). Color Doppler imaging: principles, limitations, and artifacts. *Radiology* 177, 1–10. doi:10.1148/radiology.177.1.2204956

Murphy, K. J., and Rubin, J. M. (1997). Power Doppler: it's a good thing. *Semin. Ultrasound CT MR* 18, 13–21. doi:10.1016/S0887-2171(97)90034-2

Petrou, S., Sach, T., and Davidson, L. (2001). The long-term costs of preterm birth and low birth weight: results of a systematic review. *Child Care Health Dev.* 27, 97–115. doi:10.1046/j.1365-2214.2001.00203.x

Pezzati, M., Dani, C., Biadaioli, R., Filippi, L., Biagiotti, R., Giani, T., et al. (2002). Early postnatal Doppler assessment of cerebral blood flow velocity in healthy preterm and term infants. *Dev. Med. Child Neurol.* 44, 745–752. doi:10.1017/S0012162201002870

Pfannschmidt, J., and Jorch, G. (1989). Transfontanelle pulsed Doppler measurement of blood flow velocity in the internal jugular vein, straight sinus, and internal cerebral vein in preterm and term neonates. *Ultrasound Med. Biol.* 15, 9–12. doi:10.1016/0301-5629(89)90126-9

Raine-Fenning, N. J., Nordin, N. M., Ramnarine, K. V., Campbell, B. K., Clewes, J. S., Perkins, A., et al. (2008a). Determining the relationship between three-dimensional power Doppler data and true blood flow characteristics: an in-vitro flow phantom experiment. *Ultrasound Obstet. Gynecol.* 32, 540–550. doi:10.1002/uog.6110

Raine-Fenning, N. J., Nordin, N. M., Ramnarine, K. V., Campbell, B. K., Clewes, J. S., Perkins, A., et al. (2008b). Evaluation of the effect of machine settings on quantitative three-dimensional power Doppler angiography: an in-vitro flow phantom experiment. *Ultrasound Obstet. Gynecol.* 32, 551–559. doi:10.1002/uog.6138

Ramnarine, K. V., Nassiri, D. K., Hoskins, P. R., and Lubbers, J. (1998). Validation of a new blood-mimicking fluid for use in Doppler flow test objects. *Ultrasound Med. Biol.* 24, 451–459. doi:10.1016/S0301-5629(97)00277-9

Ricci, S., Matera, R., and Tortoli, P. (2014). An improved Doppler model for obtaining accurate maximum blood velocities. *Ultrasonics* 54, 2006–2014. doi:10.1016/j.ultras.2014.05.012

Schulten-Wijman, M. J., Struijk, P. C., Brezinka, C., De Jong, N., and Steegers, E. A. (2008). Evaluation of volume vascularization index and flow index: a phantom study. *Ultrasound Obstet. Gynecol.* 32, 560–564. doi:10.1002/uog.6112

Sherlock, R. L., Anderson, P. J., Doyle, L. W., and Victorian Infant Collaborative Study G. (2005). Neurodevelopmental sequelae of intraventricular haemorrhage at 8 years of age in a regional cohort of ELBW/very preterm infants. *Early Hum. Dev.* 81, 909–916. doi:10.1016/j.earlhumdev.2005.07.007

Szabo, T. L. (2013). *Diagnostic Ultrasound Imaging: Inside Out*, 2 Edn. Oxford: Academic Press.

Teirlinck, C. J. P. M., Bezemer, R. A., Kollmann, C., Lubbers, J., Hoskins, P. R., Fish, P., et al. (1998). Development of an example flow test object and comparison of five of these test objects, constructed in various laboratories. *Ultrasonics* 36, 653–660. doi:10.1016/S0041-624X(97)00150-9

Ten Cate, D. F., Luime, J. J., van der Ven, M., Hazes, J. M., Kooiman, K., de Jong, N., et al. (2013). Very different performance of the power Doppler modalities of several ultrasound machines ascertained by a microvessel flow phantom. *Arthritis Res. Ther.* 15, R162. doi:10.1186/ar4345

van Bel, F., Lemmers, P. M., and Naulaers, G. (2008). Monitoring neonatal regional cerebral oxygen saturation in clinical practice: value and pitfalls. *Neonatology* 94, 237–244. doi:10.1159/000151642

Vasovic, L. P., Jovanovic, I. D., Ugrenovic, S. Z., and Andelkovic, Z. P. (2007). The posterior part of the human cerebral arterial circle (CAC): arterial caliber from gestational weeks 13 to 24. *J. Anat.* 211, 612–619. doi:10.1111/j.1469-7580.2007.00806.x

Volpe, J. J. (2009). Brain injury in premature infants: a complex amalgam of destructive and developmental disturbances. *Lancet Neurol.* 8, 110–124. doi:10.1016/S1474-4422(08)70294-1

World Health Organization. (2011). *Manual of Diagnostic Ultrasound.* eds H. Lutz and E Buscarini (Geneva: WHO).

Xu, X., Sun, L., Cannata, J. M., Yen, J. T., and Shung, K. K. (2008). High-frequency ultrasound Doppler system for biomedical applications with a 30-MHz linear array. *Ultrasound Med. Biol.* 34, 638–646. doi:10.1016/j.ultrasmedbio.2007.09.012

Zagzebski, J. A. (1996). *Essentials of Ultrasound Physics*, 1st Edn. Philadelphia: Mosby.

18

The relationship between eye movement and vision develops before birth

Veronika Schöpf[1]*, Thomas Schlegl[2], Andras Jakab[2], Gregor Kasprian[1], Ramona Woitek[1], Daniela Prayer[1] and Georg Langs[2,3]*

[1] *Division of Neuro- and Musculoskeletal Radiology, Department of Biomedical Imaging and Image-guided Therapy, Medical University of Vienna, Vienna, Austria*
[2] *Computational Imaging Research Laboratory, Department of Biomedical Imaging and Image-guided Therapy, Medical University of Vienna, Vienna, Austria*
[3] *Computer Science and Artificial Intelligence Lab, Massachusetts Institute of Technology, Cambridge, MA, USA*

Edited by:
Silvia Comani, Università degli Studi "G. d'Annunzio," Italy

Reviewed by:
Christos Papadelis, Boston Children's Hospital – Harvard Medical School, USA
Xiaobing Li, Nanjing Medical University Suzhou Hospital, China

Correspondence:
Georg Langs, Computational Imaging Research Laboratory, Department of Biomedical Imaging and Image-guided Therapy, Medical University of Vienna, Währinger Gürtel 18-20, 1090 Vienna, Austria
e-mail: georg.langs@meduniwien.ac.at;
Veronika Schöpf, Division of Neuro- and Musculoskeletal Radiology, Department of Biomedical Imaging and Image-guided Therapy, Medical University of Vienna, Währinger Gürtel 18-20, 1090 Vienna, Austria
e-mail: veronika.schoepf@meduniwien.ac.at

While the visuomotor system is known to develop rapidly after birth, studies have observed spontaneous activity in vertebrates in visually excitable cortical areas already before extrinsic stimuli are present. Resting state networks and fetal eye movements were observed independently *in utero*, but no functional brain activity coupled with visual stimuli could be detected using fetal fMRI. This study closes this gap and links *in utero* eye movement with corresponding functional networks. BOLD resting-state fMRI data were acquired from seven singleton fetuses between gestational weeks 30–36 with normal brain development. During the scan time, fetal eye movements were detected and tracked in the functional MRI data. We show that already *in utero* spontaneous fetal eye movements are linked to simultaneous networks in visual- and frontal cerebral areas. In our small but in terms of gestational age homogenous sample, evidence across the population suggests that the preparation of the human visuomotor system links visual and motor areas already prior to birth.

Keywords: functional connectivity, development, eye movement, ICA, *in utero* fMRI

INTRODUCTION

Postnatal sensory development is critical (Lewis and Maurer, 2005), as external stimuli shape the cortical architecture and its initial genetic roadmap (Bengoetxea et al., 2012). The nervous structures responsible for initial stimulus processing and evidence from animal studies suggest that already before the onset of vision, genetic factors, and spontaneous activity form the basis for subsequent topographic refinement of functional networks driven by experience. Vaidya and Gordon (2013) suggested that both genetic and experience-dependent maturational processes shape intrinsic connectivity networks.

Spontaneous neuronal activity is suspected to affect initial organization necessary for subsequent formation of more mature networks (Katz and Shatz, 1996). Recently, spontaneous retinal activity was described in mice *in vivo*, but the extent to which corresponding structured information is transmitted through the sensory system is still unknown (Ackman et al., 2012). Comparable activity has not yet been observed in humans. While substantial work exists on postnatal visual development in children, little is known about the events during the prenatal stimulus scarce period, when intrinsic activity is expected to dominate. Responses to visual stimuli were reported from as early as the 28th gestational week using neural electromagnetic activity measures acquired with magnetic resonance encephalography (MEG; Eswaran et al., 2004). *In utero* resting state networks (Schöpf et al., 2012; Thomason et al., 2013), and fetal eye movements (Birnholz, 1981; Woitek et al., 2013) were observed independently, but no visual stimulus response could be located in fetal functional magnetic resonance imaging (fMRI; Fulford et al., 2003). It is well established that resting-state fMRI is a powerful tool to study the organization of functional brain networks (Rosazza et al., 2012). The analysis of fMRI is not trivial and often requires data driven algorithms, such as independent component analysis [e.g., Schöpf et al. (2010a,b)]. The emergence of the visuomotor system is particularly informative regarding the precursory period of post-natal vision. It involves the relationship of intrinsic and extrinsic components suspected to shape the subsequent development of perception. The interaction of active eye movements and vision remains central in adult perception. In this work we investigated the relationship between eye movements and functional activity *in utero*, to identify the corresponding functional networks present before birth.

Even-though the questions where functional visual activity occurs *in utero*, and how primary visual areas do respond to extrinsic stimuli are not yet answered, voxel based morphometry studies in congenitally blind subjects hint at brain areas that change due to the processing of extrinsic stimuli. While congenitally blind subjects exhibit lower cortical volume in both frontal areas (BA 44, 45) and visual areas (BA 17, 18; Ptito et al., 2008), compared to a control population, functional connectivity between frontal areas (parts of BA 44, 45, and 47) and occipital areas is stronger in early blind (Liu et al., 2007). This suggests an ambiguous relationship between associated intrinsic and extrinsic processing systems (Golland et al., 2007). It might indicate that an initial abundance in connectivity between such areas as those implicated for language and visual processing is pruned after vision onset. While this then results in a clearer separation between the two systems, the network as a whole is relevant during initial organization of functional architecture.

Here we use data driven methodology to first show that there exists a link between spontaneous eye movements and functional networks in the occipital brain regions associated with vision. Furthermore, we detected stable functional networks involving both occipital and frontal regions.

MATERIALS AND METHODS

SUBJECTS

Seven singleton fetuses between gestational weeks (GW) 30–36 [mean: 32.86 (SD 1.81); mean age of mothers at MRI: 32.29 years (3.99 SD)] with no pathological brain development were scanned after informed consent was obtained from the mothers. The ethics committee of the Medical University of Vienna approved the study.

IMAGE ACQUISITION

Magnetic resonance imaging was performed on a 1.5 T unit (Philips Medical Systems, Best, The Netherlands) using a SENSE (sensitivity encoding) cardiac coil with five elements. The pregnant women were examined in supine position, and neither contrast agents nor sedatives were administered. Measurements were performed using single-shot gradient-recalled echo-planar imaging (EPI). Fifteen axial slices with slice thickness of 3 mm were acquired with a matrix size of 144 × 144, FOV of 250 × 250 mm and TE/TR of 50/1000 ms and a flip angle of 90°. Axial slices were positioned perpendicular to the fetal brainstem. Two experienced neuroradiologists (GK and DP) evaluated the MR images.

TRACKING OF EYE MOVEMENTS RELATIVE TO HEAD AXIS

We tracked the movements of both fetal eyes computationally based on the fMRI data (see **Figure 1**). First, we identified the MR slice that contained the eyes, and then pixels were classified by means of a random forest classifier (Breiman, 2001) to assign each pixel a probability of being part of an eye. Based on this probability map, eye center locations were estimated, and the segmentation of the eye was refined by mathematical morphology operations. The lens was detected along the eye border, and the view direction was calculated as the direction from eye center to the lens center. The head axis was defined as the symmetry axis between the two eyes. Relative eye angles were calculated as the difference between each eye angle (left and right) and the head central axis. Eye positions and relative eye angles were calculated for each frame in the MRI sequence resulting in a sequence of relative angles for the both eyes for each fMRI frame (see **Figure 2**).

Based on the eye tracking sequences we create regressors and event indicators defined as explanatory variables that reflect the onset of eye movement. Eye movement events are defined as the time points when the eye movement is initiated. We obtain these points by marking peaks of the derivative of the absolute value of the first derivative of the relative eye angles. These are time points when the change of relative eye angle accelerates. We discard peaks below a value of 1.4, and used the time points of the remaining peaks as event-indicators. For each eye this vector is then convolved with a standard hemodynamic response function corresponding to the TR of the fMRI sequence to obtain the final explanatory vector for each eye.

$$e :\leftrightarrow (d(|d(\alpha_1)/dt|)/dt > t) \vee (d(|d(\alpha_2)/dt|)/dt > t)$$

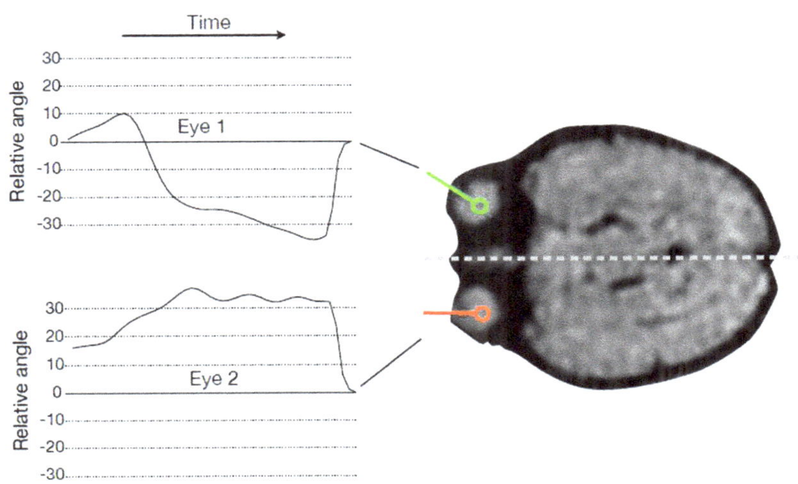

FIGURE 1 | Tracking eye movements over time. For every time point in the fMRI sequence, the angle of gaze direction relative to head orientation was recorded for every subject and both eyes.

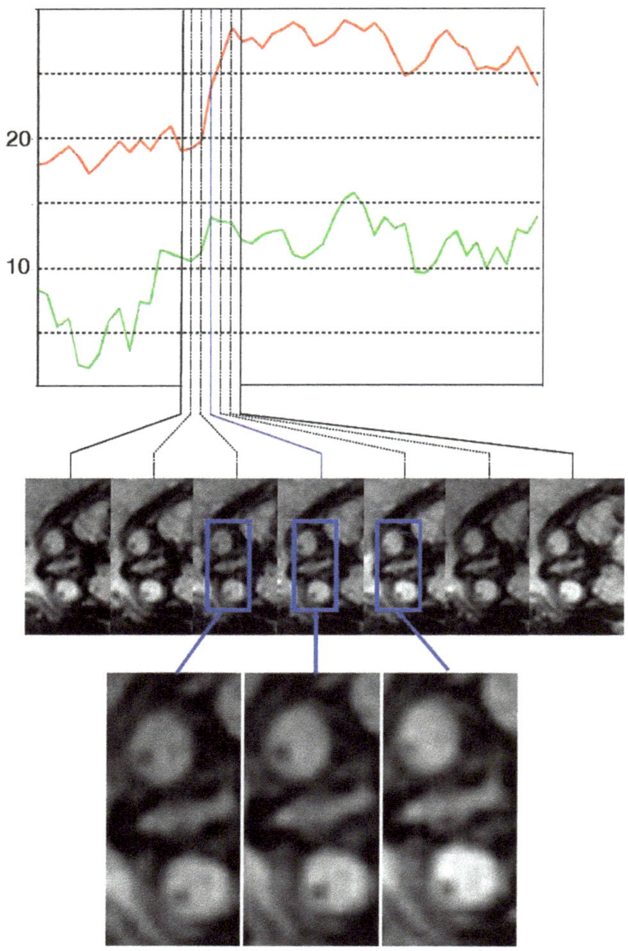

FIGURE 2 | An example of an eye movement sequence. The top plot shows the measures eye angles relative to the head axis (red for eye 1 and green for eye 2). The images below show the imaging data depicting the eyes at the corresponding time points. The eye movements are in the range of 5–7° in this sequence, and therefore qualitative analysis by a reader is difficult.

Description of main movement regressor: eye movement onset left/right jointly.

MOTION CORRECTION AND REGISTRATION

Image preprocessing was performed with FSL (FMRIB's Software Library, www.fmrib.ox.ac.uk/fsl) including motion correction as implemented in MCFLIRT version 5.5 (Oakes et al., 2005).

NUISANCE REGRESSORS

To lessen the confounding effects of non-neural signal fluctuations, we used a GLM based procedure to orthogonalize the fMRI signal to nuisance signals. Typically, such signals are originating from fetal head or maternal respiratory motion, and physiological noise, such as cardiac effects. We utilized the CompCor approach (Behzadi et al., 2007) which uses anatomical priors and principal component analysis to define non-neural signal. Fetal specific atlases were used to derive the CSF and WM compartments. We used CompCor regressors from an eroeded white matter mask, and from a region surrounding the cortical surface, including the CSF and the skull. For each region average signal and the most dominant six principal components were used as regressors. Furthermore derived nuisance regressors from the head and eye tracking information: (1,2) head position, (3,4) change of head position (x,y), (5) head angle, (6) change of head angle. The measurements from head tracking were convolved with a Gaussian filter, with SD 2.

ANALYSIS

Single subject independent component analysis was performed using probabilistic ICA as implemented in Multivariate Exploratory Linear Decomposition Optimized into Independent Components (MELODIC) version 3.10, a part of FSL (FMRIB's Software Library, www.fmrib.ox.ac.uk/fsl), using FastICA (Beckmann and Smith, 2004). The number of sources was estimated from the data by maximizing the Laplacian approximation to the Bayesian evidence of the model order (Minka, 2000; Beckmann and Smith, 2004). For the optimization of the non-Gaussian sources, contrast function, and convergence thresholds, as suggested by Hyvärinen et al. (2001), were used. Estimated component maps were divided by the SD of the residual noise and thresholded by fitting a mixture model to the intensity values histogram (Beckmann and Smith, 2004). Cross correlation coefficients of the derived independent components with all eye movement parameters were calculated.

RESULTS

To investigate if the networks active at movement onsets are stable, and can be detected from the data regardless of the eye movement, we performed ICA on the fMRI data. On average 13 independent components were estimated per subject (SD 4.03). Correlation of single-subject component time courses with the eye movement regressor was calculated. The independent component with maximum correlation coefficients for each subjects were evaluated [mean correlation coefficient: 0.33 (SD 0.07)]. The networks showing the highest correlation with fetal eye movement (see **Figure 3**) include association related areas as the angular gyrus, the inferior parietal gyrus, the superior frontal gyrus, as well as a primary visual area the medial occipital gyrus and motion associated function.

DISCUSSION

The present results indicate a relationship between fetal eye movements and activation in visual brain areas, motor areas, and orbitofrontal areas *in utero*. The observed functional networks correlating to visuomotor activity may offer a new perspective of the time period in which the orbitofrontal prepares for extrinsic sensory processing. The presence and relationship of the reported functional networks between visual and frontal areas in fetuses may prepare the developing brain for the processing of visual patterns as a precursor for the subsequent postnatal stimulus driven development of visual perception. Although observations are

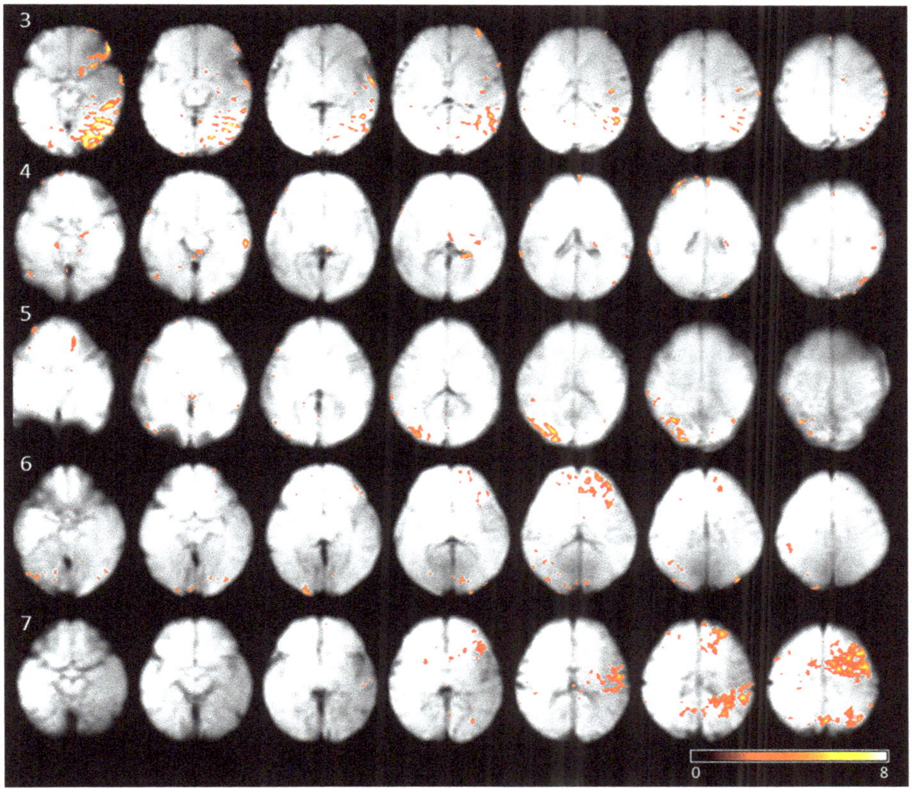

FIGURE 3 | Results of subjects 3–7 of the independent components with the maximum correlation coefficients with the eye movement on-set regressor derived from eye tracking. Maps are overlaid on individual mean EPIs.

based on a limited number of subjects, the results were consistent across the population.

FETAL EYE MOVEMENTS

Previous work on *in utero* fMRI provides insight in the developing brain ranging from stimulus processing (Schöpf et al., 2011) to intrinsic resting-state activity (Schöpf et al., 2012; Thomason et al., 2013). The observation of brain networks *in utero* suffers from the uncertainty of the status of the fetus at rest or asleep, which cannot be controlled. According to the categorization of fetal behavioral states from Romanini and Rizzo (1995), periods of "quiet sleep" or "quiet awake" can only be differentiated upon fetal eye movement. Four fetal eye movement patterns were initially characterized based on early ultrasound observations (Birnholz, 1981): Type I eye movements were described as single, transient deviations consisting of a bulb deviation, and a slower return back to the resting position, single but prolonged eye movements as Type II, complex sequences of eye movements to different directions without periodicity as Type III, and repetitive nystagmoid eye movements as Type IV. Additionally splitting of Type I eye movements into Type Ia (fast deviation, slower reposition) and Type Ib (fast deviation, equally fast reposition) was based on eye movement observation during MRI measurements (Woitek et al., 2013). It has already been shown that MRI sequences provide a valuable tool for visualizing and categorizing fetal eye movements (Brémond-Gignac et al., 1997; Woitek et al., 2013). While this method was initially developed to serve as an indicator for ocular development and as an indirect biomarker to detect malformations affecting the brainstem, our study investigates for the first time the networks responsible for the processing of eye movement *in utero*, enabling the purest form of a natural self induced stimulus, eye movement.

FUNCTIONAL SENSORI MOTOR NETWORKS *IN UTERO*

We did not observe activations in the frontal eye field, which is known to be related to saccadic eye movements. As saccades are very fast (20–400 ms), we do not expect them to be correlated with the MRI tracked motion events due to the limited temporal resolution of the MRI eye tracking.

Slow pursuit or gazing movements (looking at directions intentionally or following a moving object) are controlled with involvement of deep-parieto-occipital cortex. Although we cannot confirm on intentional focusing *in utero,* we do see parietal–occipital activity in four out of seven cases. It is known from studies on macaques that the parieto-occipital cortex shows activation during self-generated eye movements (Law et al., 1998) and plays a crucial role in encoding extrapersonal visual space (Galletti et al., 1995). As we did not provide the fetus with visual stimuli, the activation we observed in the parietal–occipital area might hint at the generator of intrinsic eye movements in human fetuses.

There is only little motor activity and little involvement of the supplementary motor cortex or the typical frontal eye field (see below). These results are in line with findings in macaques reporting on fetal eye motion mainly governed by brainstem and midbrain processes. They suggest supratentorial control of eye motion gaining functional importance during brain development.

The networks we observed in fetuses differ from those known in the adult brain, and do not include a number of regions typically associated with eye movements in adults. Instead, they include areas identified with extrinsic stimulus processing (V1 in subjects 3,4,5,6) and motor control (subjects 3,4,6,7). So far no visual stimulus fMRI response activity *in utero* could be located (Fulford et al., 2003).

THE FETAL- VERSUS THE ADULT BRAIN

Most experiments investigating sensory systems *in utero*, as for example visual and auditory systems, were constituted based on block length and stimulus sequences of adult paradigm settings, which might be a poor fit for fetal function and could explain the non-detection of activity patterns in, e.g., the primary sensory areas [for a review see Schöpf et al. (2011)]. The lack of previous localizations in primary sensory areas as a response to sensory stimuli strongly indicates that conventional fMRI paradigms used in adult settings do not capture the fetal brain settings. In light of (Dehorter et al., 2012) proposition that the developing brain is not a small adult brain but that the voltage- and transmitter-gated currents act like network driven patterns following a developmental sequence, the present results point to endogenous activity in the developing cortex as modulating the formation of functional units in the sensorimotor system. Instead of linking primary sensory activity to external stimuli, they evidence a link to spontaneous eye motion as part of the sensorimotor system. The function of these early patterns is to enable heterogeneous neurons to fire and wire together and prepare for subsequent stimulus driven development rather than to code specific modalities at this point.

Colonnese et al. (2010) already observed the change of functional units and a switch to mature visual response shortly before delivery in humans based on recordings from the visual cortex of preterm human infants. They proposed a "bursting" period of visual responsiveness during which weak retinal information is amplified by endogenous network oscillations, which in turn enable a primitive form of vision. Colonnese et al. (2010) concluded that an intrinsic program that is able to switch cortical responses in anticipation of patterned vision operates early visual developmental processing.

LIMITATIONS

A constraining factor of the presented work is the limited sample size. According to this issue results are based on a single subject level analysis. As the sample was very homogenous with regard to gestational age this setting was chosen specifically to abstain from technical nuisance introduction emerging from registration to a template, which could influence the quality of single eye movement trackings. On the other hand, this homogeneity of developmental age does not allow for the analysis of eye movement related networks across gestational development, which will be of interest in future investigation. Furthermore, an important open question regarding our understanding of the hemodynamic developmental trajectory across *in utero* development, could be addressed by model driven data analysis.

ACKNOWLEDGMENTS

This work was supported by the Austrian National Bank Anniversary Fund (FETALMORPHO) to Gregor Kasprian, the EU FP7 projects KHRESMOI and VISCERAL to Georg Langs, the Austrian Science Fund (P23205-B09) to Veronika Schöpf. Andras Jakab is supported by the European Union FP7 Marie Curie IEF Research grant FABRIC – "exploring the Formation and Adaptation of the Brain Connectome," grant no. 2012-PIEF-GA-33003.

REFERENCES

Ackman, J. B., Burbridge, T. J., and Crair, M. C. (2012). Retinal waves coordinate patterned activity throughout the developing visual system. *Nature* 490, 219–225. doi: 10.1038/nature11529

Beckmann, C. F., and Smith, S. M. (2004). Probabilistic independent component analysis for functional magnetic resonance imaging. *IEEE Trans. Med. Imaging* 23, 137–152. doi: 10.1109/TMI.2003.822821

Behzadi, Y., Restom, K., Liau, J., and Liu, T. T. (2007). A component based noise correction method (CompCor) for BOLD and perfusion based fMRI. *Neuroimage* 37, 90–101. doi: 10.1016/j.neuroimage.2007.04.042

Bengoetxea, H., Ortuzar, N., Bulnes, S., Rico-Barrio, I., Lafuente, J. V., and Argandoña, E. G. (2012). Enriched and deprived sensory experience induces structural changes and rewires connectivity during the postnatal development of the brain. *Neural Plast.* 2012, 305693. doi: 10.1155/2012/305693

Birnholz, J. C. (1981). The development of human fetal eye movement patterns. *Science* 213, 679–681. doi: 10.1126/science.7256272

Breiman, L. (2001). Random forests. *Mach. Learn.* 45, 5–32. doi: 10.1023/A:1010933404324

Brémond-Gignac, D. S., Benali, K., Deplus, S., Cussenot, O., Ferkdadji, L., Elmaleh, M., et al. (1997). In utero eyeball development study by magnetic resonance imaging. *Surg. Radiol. Anat.* 19, 319–322. doi: 10.1007/BF01637602

Colonnese, M. T., Kaminska, A., Minlebaev, M., Milh, M., Bloem, B., Lescure, S., et al. (2010). A conserved switch in sensory processing prepares developing neocortex for vision. *Neuron* 67, 480–498. doi: 10.1016/j.neuron.2010.07.015

Dehorter, N., Vinay, L., Hammond, C., and Ben-Ari, Y. (2012). Timing of developmental sequences in different brain structures: physiological and pathological implications. *Eur. J. Neurosci.* 35, 1846–1856. doi: 10.1111/j.1460-9568.2012.08152.x

Eswaran, H., Lowery, C. L., Wilson, J. D., Murphy, P., and Preissl, H. (2004). Functional development of the visual system in human fetus using magnetoencephalography. *Exp. Neurol.* 190(Suppl.), S52–S58. doi: 10.1016/j.expneurol.2004.04.007

Fulford, J., Vadeyar, S. H., Dodampahala, S. H., Moore, R. J., Young, P., Baker, P. N., et al. (2003). Fetal brain activity in response to a visual stimulus. *Hum. Brain Mapp.* 20, 239–245. doi: 10.1002/hbm.10139

Galletti, C., Battaglini, P. P., and Fattori, P. (1995). Eye position influence on the parieto-occipital area PO (V6) of the macaque monkey. *Eur. J. Neurosci.* 7, 2486–2501. doi: 10.1111/j.1460-9568.1995.tb01047.x

Golland, Y., Bentin, S., Gelbard, H., Benjamini, Y., Heller, R., Nir, Y., et al. (2007). Extrinsic and intrinsic systems in the posterior cortex of the human brain revealed during natural sensory stimulation. *Cereb. Cortex* 17, 766–777. doi: 10.1093/cercor/bhk030

Hyvärinen, A., Karhunen, J., and Oja, E. (2001). *Independent Component Analysis.* Toronto, ON: John Wiley & Sons.

Katz, L. C., and Shatz, C. J. (1996). Synaptic activity and the construction of cortical circuits. *Science* 274, 1133–1138. doi: 10.1126/science.274.5290.1133

Law, I., Svarer, C., Rostrup, E., and Paulson, O. B. (1998). Parieto-occipital cortex activation during self-generated eye movements in the dark. *Brain* 121 1, 2189–2200. doi: 10.1093/brain/121.11.2189

Lewis, T. L., and Maurer, D. (2005). Multiple sensitive periods in human visual development: evidence from visually deprived children. *Dev. Psychobiol.* 46, 163–183. doi: 10.1002/dev.20055

Liu, Y., Yu, C., Liang, M., Li, J., Tian, L., Zhou, Y., et al. (2007). Whole brain functional connectivity in the early blind. *Brain* 130, 2085–2096. doi: 10.1093/brain/awm121

Minka, T. (2000). *Automatic Choice of Dimensionality for PCA*. Technical Report 514. Cambridge, MA: MIT Media Lab Vision and Modeling Group.

Oakes, T. R., Johnstone, T., Ores Walsh, K. S., Greischar, L. L., Alexander, A. L., Fox, A. S., et al. (2005). Comparison of fMRI motion correction software tools. *Neuroimage* 28, 529–543. doi: 10.1016/j.neuroimage.2005.05.058

Ptito, M., Schneider, F. C. G., Paulson, O. B., and Kupers, R. (2008). Alterations of the visual pathways in congenital blindness. *Exp. Brain Res.* 187, 41–49. doi: 10.1007/s00221-008-1273-4

Romanini, C., and Rizzo, G. (1995). Fetal behaviour in normal and compromised fetuses. An overview. *Early Hum. Dev.* 43, 117–131. doi: 10.1016/0378-3782(95)01667-8

Rosazza, C., Minati, L., Ghielmetti, F., Mandelli, M. L., and Bruzzone, M. G. (2012). Functional connectivity during resting-state functional MR imaging: study of the correspondence between independent component analysis and region-of-interest-based methods. *AJNR Am. J. Neuroradiol.* 33, 180–187. doi: 10.3174/ajnr.A2733

Schöpf, V., Kasess, C. H., Lanzenberger, R., Fischmeister, F., Windischberger, C., and Moser, E. (2010a). Fully exploratory network ICA (FENICA) on resting-state fMRI data. *J. Neurosci. Methods* 192, 207–213. doi: 10.1016/j.jneumeth.2010.07.028

Schöpf, V., Windischberger, C., Kasess, C., Lanzenberger, R., and Moser, E. (2010b). Group ICA of resting-state data: a comparison. *MAGMA* 23, 317–325. doi: 10.1007/s10334-010-0212-0

Schöpf, V., Kasprian, G., Brugger, P., and Prayer, D. (2012). Watching the fetal brain at "rest". *Int. J. Dev. Neurosci.* 30, 11–17. doi: 10.1016/j.ijdevneu.2011.10.006

Schöpf, V., Kasprian, G., and Prayer, D. (2011). Functional imaging in the fetus. *Top. Magn. Reson. Imaging* 22, 113–118. doi: 10.1097/RMR.0b013e3182699283

Thomason, M. E., Dassanayake, M. T., Shen, S., Katkuri, Y., Alexis, M., Anderson, A. L., et al. (2013). Cross-hemispheric functional connectivity in the human fetal brain. *Sci. Transl. Med.* 5, 173ra24. doi: 10.1126/scitranslmed.3004978

Vaidya, C. J., and Gordon, E. M. (2013). Phenotypic variability in resting-state functional connectivity: current status. *Brain Connect.* 3, 99–120. doi: 10.1089/brain.2012.0110

Woitek, R., Kasprian, G., Lindner, C., Stuhr, F., Weber, M., Schöpf, V., et al. (2013). Fetal eye movements on magnetic resonance imaging. *PLoS ONE* 8:e77439. doi: 10.1371/journal.pone.0077439

19

Beyond cell replacement: unresolved roles of NG2-expressing progenitors

Enrica Boda* and Annalisa Buffo

Department of Neuroscience Rita Levi-Montalcini, Neuroscience Institute Cavalieri Ottolenghi, University of Turin, Turin, Italy

Edited by:
Luca Bonfanti, University of Turin, Italy

Reviewed by:
Hans Georg Kuhn, University of Gothenburg, Sweden
Akiko Nishiyama, University of Connecticut, USA

****Correspondence:***
Enrica Boda, Department of Neuroscience Rita Levi-Montalcini, Neuroscience Institute Cavalieri Ottolenghi, University of Turin, Regione Gonzole 10, Orbassano 10043 (Turin), Italy
e-mail: enrica.boda@unito.it

NG2-expressing parenchymal precursors (NG2+p) serve as primary source of myelinating oligodendrocytes in both the developing and adult Central Nervous System (CNS). However, their abundance, limited differentiation potential at adult stages along with stereotypic reaction to injury independent of the extent of myelin loss suggest that NG2+p exert functions additional to myelin production. In support of this view, NG2+p express a complex battery of molecules known to exert neuromodulatory and neuroprotective functions. Further, they establish intimate physical associations with the other CNS cell types, receive functional synaptic contacts and possess ion channels apt to constantly sense the electrical activity of surrounding neurons. These latter features could endow NG2+p with the capability to affect neuronal functions with potential homeostatic outcomes. Here we summarize and discuss current evidence favoring the view that NG2+p can participate in circuit formation, modulate neuronal activity and survival in the healthy and injured CNS, and propose perspectives for studies that may complete our understanding of NG2+p roles in physiology and pathology.

Keywords: buffering, depolarization, myelin, neuroprotection, neuromodulation

INTRODUCTION

During Central Nervous System (CNS) ontogenesis, myelinating oligodendrocytes originate from highly ramified neural precursors expressing the platelet-derived growth factor alpha receptor (PDGFRa) and the NG2 chondroitin sulfate proteoglycan (Zhu et al., 2008a,b). These precursors persist in the adult CNS parenchyma, where constitute the main proliferative cell type and make up about 5% of all CNS cells (Dawson et al., 2003). At adult stages, they can engage into maturation to sustain a certain degree of basal myelin turnover and plasticity (Wang and Young, 2013; Young et al., 2013) and are rapidly mobilized to replace oligodendrocytes in demyelination (Redwine and Armstrong, 1998; Zawadzka et al., 2010). Herein we will refer to these cells as NG2-expressing precursors (NG2+p), although NG2 is also expressed by pericytes of the vasculature (Stallcup, 2002) and reported in astrocyte subsets (Matthias et al., 2003).

Currently, the only unequivocally established functions of NG2+p are to regenerate themselves and produce oligodendrocytes in the healthy, diseased and aged CNS (Zhu et al., 2008a,b; Kang et al., 2010; Tripathi et al., 2010; Young et al., 2013). However, the persistence of a large pool of quiescent (i.e., neither engaged in proliferation nor maturation) NG2+p with limited differentiation potential at adult ages has suggested that these cells do not only represent a transitional stage along the oligodendroglial lineage, but rather a novel type of glia endowed with specific properties and functions (Nishiyama et al., 2002). Consistently, NG2+p appear uniformly distributed in the gray and white matter and provide a stereotypic reaction to injury independently of the extent of myelin loss, suggesting that they may play roles additional to myelin production. Along this line, it has been proposed that NG2+p may be multipotent progenitors endowed with the ability to generate astrocytes and neurons in defined conditions. However, to date consensus is established only for the generation of astrocyte subsets at perinatal stages (Rivers et al., 2008; Zhu et al., 2008a,b; Huang et al., 2014). Here we will overview and discuss features potentially related to surveillance, neuromodulation and neuroprotection that still render NG2+p very enigmatic and prompt further investigations on this type of glia.

NG2+p ANATOMICAL RELATIONSHIP WITH CNS CELLS AND PARACRINE INTERACTIONS

In both human and rodent CNS, NG2+p appear distributed rather homogeneously in gray and white matter areas, with no correlation between their density and that of myelin (Butt et al., 2005; Staugaitis and Trapp, 2009). NG2+p processes extend tridimensionally to cover non-overlapping fields that are likely maintained by homotypic repulsive mechanisms (Hughes et al., 2013). Accordingly, in the intact tissue contacts among NG2+p processes are rarely observed (Hughes et al., 2013) and, despite some NG2+p express connexin 32 (Melanson-Drapeau et al., 2003), cells are never coupled via gap-junctions (Wallraff et al., 2004; Butt et al., 2005). Thus, at variance with astrocytes, NG2+p do not function as a syncythium, but are rather individual functional units. However, they partly couple to mature oligodendrocytes, indicating some privileged communication with other elements in the lineage (Maglione et al., 2010).

Confocal and electron microscopy analyses showed that NG2+p establish intimate anatomical and functional contacts with other CNS cells. NG2+p processes form multiple contacts with dendrites and axons, and NG2+p arborizations intertwine amongst and can encapsulate neuronal somata (Wigley and Butt,

2009; see also **Figures 1A,A′**) in ways suggestive of their participation in perineuronal nets (Butt et al., 2005). Electron microscopy further revealed that NG2+p processes make contacts with the axonal membrane at the paranodes and nodes of Ranvier (Butt et al., 1999), and interdigitate between pre- and post-synaptic neuronal elements (Ong and Levine, 1999). Contacts with axons include also functional neuron-to-NG2+p synapses (see below). Of note, tight NG2+p-neuron associations exist also in the CNS of adult non-mammalian vertebrates (i.e., zebrafish; März et al., 2010), in line with a fundamental mechanism of communication conserved through species.

Intimate physical interactions also occur with astrocytes. Both cell types often contact the same neurons/axonal terminals (Wigley and Butt, 2009) but NG2+p never ensheat neuronal synapses as astrocytes do. Interestingly, areas of immediate apposition in NG2+p and astrocyte processes are sites of communication, where astrocyte-derived signals induce Ca^{2+} transients in NG2+p (Hamilton et al., 2010). At those sites synaptophysin-positive clusters indicative of secretory vesicle accumulation were observed in NG2+p, pointing to potential secretory spots (Wigley and Butt, 2009). NG2+p also make direct contacts with microglia (Nishiyama et al., 1997), pericytes and myelin (Butt et al., 2005). Hence, NG2+p connect to distinct cell types and functionally-relevant cellular domains, suggesting that they may actively sense and integrate information from diverse sources. An additional level of integration occurs through paracrine signals produced by neighboring cells including neurons, astrocytes and microglia, and influences NG2+p during developmental myelination and in pathology (see Clemente et al., 2013 for review). Is the output of this integration (see below) limited to the regulation of NG2+p differentiation or survival? It is surprising that NG2+p are generally considered only as a sink and not as a source of signals. Hence, if and how NG2+p affect surrounding cells remains essentially unknown.

PRIVILEGED CONTACTS WITH NEURONS

What makes NG2+p unique amongst other glial cells is their connection with neurons through synapses that sense neuronal activity at the quantal level with high temporal and spatial resolution. These contacts emerge in parallel with neuronal synaptogenesis and appear ubiquitary, being present in all regions examined so far (cerebellar and cerebral cortex, Lin et al., 2005; Kukley et al., 2008; Ge et al., 2009; Tanaka et al., 2009; Vélez-Fort et al., 2010; hippocampus, Lin and Bergles, 2004; Mangin et al., 2008; brain stem, Müller et al., 2009; white matter tracts, Kukley et al., 2007; Ziskin et al., 2007; Káradóttir et al., 2008; De Biase et al., 2010; Etxeberria et al., 2010). Synapses include glutamatergic and Gamma-Aminobutyric Acid (GABA)-ergic inputs, and both produce depolarizations. Full functionality of these contacts *in vivo* is attested by recordings of evoked, spontaneous, and miniature currents both in physiology and during remyelination (Etxeberria et al., 2010; Vélez-Fort et al., 2010). Glutamatergic contacts are lost as NG2+p progress in differentiation (De Biase et al., 2010; Kukley et al., 2010), in line with a role in the regulation of the cell cycle or of functions specific of the progenitor stage. Notably, glutamatergic inputs increase in frequency and amplitude in NG2+p cells during CNS maturation (Mangin et al., 2008), whereas in the cerebral cortex GABAergic signaling shifts from activation of synaptic receptors to indirect activation of extrasynaptic channels through spillover (Vélez-Fort et al., 2010; Balia et al., 2013; Passlick et al., 2013).

Glutamate- and GABA-induced depolarizations in NG2+p are overall modest in amplitude with the notable exception of cerebellar climbing fiber inputs that induce relevant potential variations (Lin et al., 2005). Thus, to affect the cell physiology, a number of convergent inputs from diverse synapses likely require be integrated. Transduction of synaptic signal may also rely on calcium-mediated mechanisms such as calcium entry though permeable α-amino-3-hydroxy-5-methyl-4-isoxazolepropionic acid

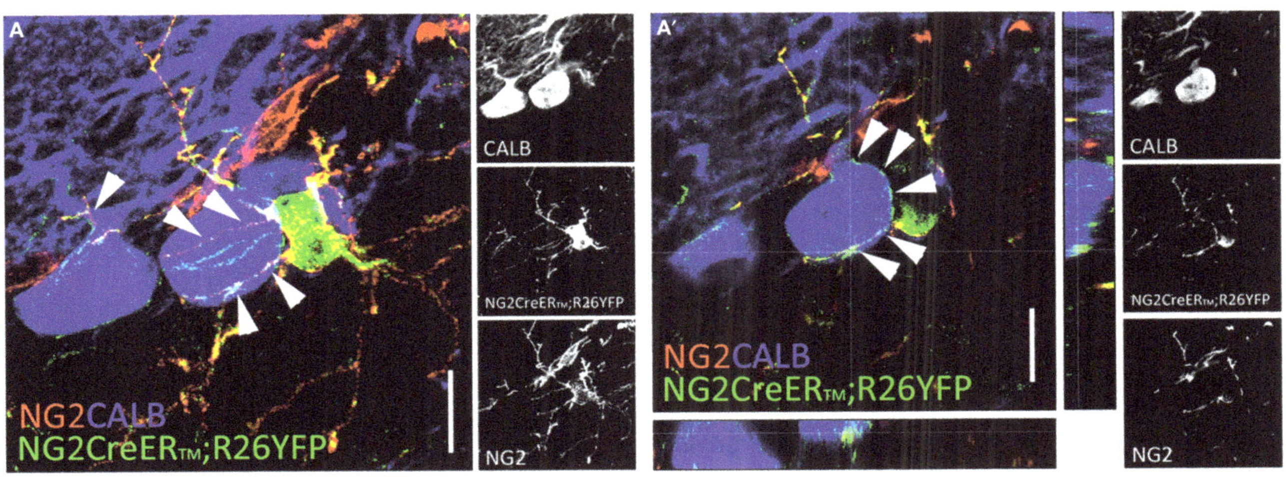

FIGURE 1 | NG2+p distribution in the adult cerebellum. (A,A′) Two weeks after tamoxifen induction, multiprocessed cells identified by NG2 (red), and YFP (green) expression appear closely associated to calbindin+ (blue) Purkinje cells in adult NG2CreER™; R26YFP mouse cerebellum. NG2+p arborizations envelop Purkinje cell somata and dendrites [arrowheads in **(A,A′)**]. **(A)** Confocal stack comprising 20 optical section 1 mm thick. **(A′)** Single confocal plane. Scale bars: 10 μm.

(AMPA) or N-methyl-D-aspartate (NMDA) receptors, and activation of voltage dependent conductances that provide signal amplification and can trigger calcium transients from intracellular stores. Notably, in the hippocampus neuron-to-NG2+p synapses undergo activity-dependent modifications analogous to long term potentiation (LTP) at excitatory synapses (Ge et al., 2006), showing that these contacts possess the machinery to sustain plastic changes. Moreover, glutamate or GABA evoked signals can be integrated intracellularly with responses to other mediators such as adenosine triphosphate (ATP), which, upon release by both axons and astrocytes, triggers calcium currents through P2Y and P2X receptors (Hamilton et al., 2010). Yet, depolarizations and calcium transients are mostly described as very local events that take place at the cell processes, where synapses are mostly found, and could therefore influence spatially restricted functions such as local protein synthesis, motility, or secretion (see also above, Kirby et al., 2006; Tanaka et al., 2009; Haberlandt et al., 2011; Wake et al., 2011; Hughes et al., 2013).

What is the functional significance of neuronal inputs? Since NG2+p do not appear able to transmit electrical signals to other cells, information derived from neuronal activity is likely to instruct functions specific to these progenitors. Several reports showed that neurotransmitters can affect proliferation and migration of NG2+p *in vitro* (Luyt et al., 2007; Gallo et al., 2008; Tong et al., 2009). Other studies related alterations in circuit activities at adult ages (including motor activity, sleep-wake cycles, experimental spreading depression, or enriched environment) to modulation of NG2+p proliferation and maturation (Ehninger et al., 2011; Simon et al., 2011; Tamura et al., 2012; Bellesi et al., 2013). However, these findings, which appeared somewhat contradictory, only established a rather aspecific link between neuronal activity and NG2+p behaviors. In a recent report Mangin et al. (2012) addressed this issue more directly and found that sensory stimuli from the whisker pad regulate NG2+p number and distribution in the neonatal barrel cortex by negatively affecting cell proliferation. These data are in keeping with an inhibitory role of glutamatergic inputs on NG2 cell amplification and suggest that different inputs levels would result in proliferation-mediated accumulation of NG2+p at sites of relatively low electric activity. Such accumulations could then specifically predispose cells to start myelination (Mangin et al., 2012), as the achievement of a critical density is one of the key factors for myelin formation (Rosenberg et al., 2008). Electrical activity itself could likely further support the progression of postmitotic progenitors along the lineage, as it has long been known to be a myelination promoter (Demerens et al., 1996; Stevens et al., 2002; Lundgaard et al., 2013). Thus, the response of NG2+p to neuronal activity appears crucial to regulate their number and engagement in myelination during development, thereby contributing to structure the CNS architecture. Similarly, it could underlie myelin refinements related to learning and memory during adulthood. Yet, how these findings apply to the adult CNS and whether the large abundance of NG2+p present at adult stages is exclusively required to sustain the low grade of myelin turnover so far detected and/or experience-related circuit modulations remain to be assessed. Indeed, the occurrence of myelin remodeling appears rather low in the adult CNS (Zatorre et al., 2012; Young et al., 2013) and at least in the gray matter the overall rate of NG2+p proliferation does not differ in myelin rich vs. myelin low territories (our unpublished observations) thus showing to be unrelated to myelin turnover. Further, exploiting the high metabolic charge of electric activity solely to tonically limit NG2+p proliferation appears poorly efficient, particularly in light of data showing that homotypic density cues play a major role in the regulation of NG2+p proliferation at adult stages (Hughes et al., 2013). Moreover, the observation that an important part of NG2+ clones in the gray matter do not generate oligodendrocytes in the adult brain (Levison et al., 1999; Zhu et al., 2011) raises the question as to whether NG2+p responses to neuronal inputs may include functions other than proliferation control or lineage progression.

NG2+p FUNCTIONS BEYOND MYELINATION?

Recently discovered features of NG2+p point to additional neuromodulatory and neuroprotective actions of this population. Some of these traits appear specifically related to the particular capability of NG2+p to sense and respond to electrical activity. Others, including the expression of growth factors, morphogens, cytokines, chemokines, and extracellular matrix (ECM) components, can instead be viewed as properties inherent in the progenitor nature of these cells, and may well correspond to the reparative bystander actions that germinal neural progenitors exert either *in situ* or upon grafting in the lesioned CNS (Martino and Pluchino, 2006; Butti et al., 2012).

Of note, evidence that NG2+p express synaptophysin suggests they may be capable of regulated secretion and bidirectional communication with astrocytes and neurons (Wigley and Butt, 2009). Of relevance in this context, Maldonado et al. (2013) have shown that during postnatal maturation NG2+p become progressively more sensitive to extracellular potassium increases generated by action potentials thanks to upregulation of Kir4.1 inward rectifying potassium channels. These channels mediate inward currents in conditions of high potassium and constitute one of the mechanisms through which astrocytes perform potassium buffering in the extracellular space, which is a requisite for correct neuronal transmission and excitability. In adult NG2+p, besides contributing to set the resting membrane potential, these channels may help with removing high extracellular potassium and regulating neuronal functions at sites of close appositions to neurons (see above) (Maldonado et al., 2013). This could be a NG2+p specific mechanisms occurring upon single neuron firing, which may remain undetected by astrocytes (Maldonado et al., 2013).

NG2+p are also known to express several ECM components such as tenascins, versicans, neurocans, phosphacan, hyaluronan and even hyaluronan, and proteoglycan link protein 1 (HPLN1), which act as synaptic stabilizers by anchoring the neurotransmitter receptors to the cytoskeleton and contribute to perineuronal nets formation (Butt et al., 2005; Sim et al., 2009; see also Sim and Goldman, 2013). Given the intimate association of NG2 processes with neuronal pre- and post-synaptic elements and that neighboring pairs of NG2+p and neurons receive synaptic contacts from the same neurons (Bergles et al., 2000; Lin et al., 2005; Mangin et al., 2008), it can be hypothesized that NG2+p monitor neuron-neuron synapses and, depending on synchronization levels, act on synaptic stabilization and network organization by modifying the perisynaptic microenvironment. Interestingly, human NG2+p also show enriched levels of thrombospondin 2 (Sim et al., 2006), which is known as a synaptogenic cue released by immature astrocytes (Christopherson et al., 2005). Seminal studies demonstrating the role of astroglia in synaptic strengthening and formation also attributed a relevant effect to cells of the oligodendroglial lineage (Pfrieger and Barres, 1997). However, these data should be re-considered in light of the need to clarify the purity of cells and actual maturation stages. Yet, in line with an early function in circuit formation, acute deletion of cycling oligodendroglial cells have been reported to induce rapid changes in the expression of molecules involved in synaptic plasticity, axon growth and guidance in the cerebellum at birth, indicative of fast activation of remodeling mechanisms (Doretto et al., 2011). Previous experiments at later developmental stages have shown that myelin formation shapes cerebellar connections by removing exuberant collateral branches of Purkinje neurons (Gianola et al., 2003). These results suggest that cycling NG2+p participate in shaping cerebellar circuits well before myelination starts.

Neuroprotective mechanisms have been also proposed to be activated in NG2+ cells upon lesion. NG2+p provide a stereotyped response to injury, unrelated to the extent of myelin loss and of their own damage, which includes a precocious activation of proliferation and hypertrophy and is mediated by inflammatory and danger related signals (Levine et al., 2001; Nielsen et al., 2006). The sensitivity of these cells to changes in nerve conduction and neurotransmission could also influence NG2+p reactivity. Tanaka et al. (2009) reported that GABA-receptor mediated excitation in NG2+p after ischemic stroke increases brain-derived neurotrophic factor (BDNF) production, which was instead blocked by inhibition of GABA-mediated depolarization. The authors further hypothesize that NG2+p-derived BDNF participate in post-stroke reparative mechanisms. Given the well-known actions of BDNF in promoting synaptic transmission, plasticity, and growth (Lu et al., 2013), these speculations could be extended to include modulatory actions of neuronal functions in physiological conditions. Along this line, reactive NG2+p responding to depolarizing waves induced by experimental cortical spreading depression were reported to upregulate the peptide galanin and proposed to release it to receptor positive cortical neurons with the purpose of limiting excitotoxic damage (Shen et al., 2003). In a recent *in vitro* study Sypecka and Sarnowska (2013) provided first evidence in support of a pro-survival action of NG2+p on the injured nervous tissue. In co-cultures of primary NG2+p with organotypic hippocampal slices subjected to oxygen-glucose deprivation, the authors observed a significant rescue of neuronal viability and identify BDNF, interleukin-10, stem cell factor (SCF) as agents through which NG2+p perform immunomodulatory and protective functions in their experimental setting. Accordingly, NG2+p derived from human embryonic stem cells express transforming growth factor (TGF) β2, a potent inhibitor of inflammation, midkine, and activine A, two neurosupportive factors that are highly upregulated early after injury (Munz et al., 2001; Zhang et al., 2006; Yoshida et al., 2014). NG2+p cells could therefore share the capability of mature oligodendrocytes to produce neurotrophic factors, influence adjacent cells (Wilkins et al., 2001; Dai et al., 2003) and especially neurons in physiology and conditions of cell stress (Lee et al., 2012; Frühbeis et al., 2013). Further, in amyloidosis models it has been reported that NG2+p internalize and degrade β-amyloid1-42 by autophagy (Li et al., 2013). Thus, together with astrocytes and microglia, NG2+ glia could also participate in the clearance of amyloid as part of their reactive response (Boda et al., 2011; Behrendt et al., 2013).

The potential reparative and supportive actions may be specifically triggered by NG2+p reactivity or be already present in resting conditions and become amplified as a consequence of the NG2+p widespread cytogenic response to damage. However, these considerations remain speculative, because a detailed and comprehensive examination of NG2+p changes upon lesion is not available. What is instead better assessed is the contribution of NG2+p to scar formation and the inhibitory role of chondroitin sulfate proteoglycans—including NG2—in axon remodeling and regrowth of transected axons (Galtrey and Fawcett, 2007), recently accompanied by evidence for conduction blockade exerted by NG2 at nodes of Ranvier after spinal cord transection (Petrosyan et al., 2013). While these inhibitory effects are mostly seen as detrimental for circuit rewiring, they could be part of a mechanism necessary to contain excitoxicity and damage extension, as formerly shown for astrocytes (Buffo et al., 2010). Further, actions restricting plasticity may be compensated by an increment in the availability of prosurvival factors determined by both NG2+p reactivity and proliferation.

CONCLUDING REMARKS

Intense research over the last decades has revealed key insights into NG2+p physiopathology related to myelinogenesis. Nevertheless, fundamental aspects of NG2+p biology remain undetermined. For example, while NG2+p are known to respond to signals produced by neurons, astrocytes, and microglia, whether this communication is reciprocal and how it occurs is substantially neglected. NG2+p-derived signaling may include morphogenic, neuromodulatory, and neuroprotective factors whose elucidation may also have therapeutic implications for the implementation of the endogenous reparative potential of injured CNS. *In vivo* approaches aimed at selectively and timely ablating NG2+p in the CNS, together with the identification of active paracrine/juxtacrine factors produced by NG2+p, will be highly instrumental to address these issues, especially to understand how much it is crucial to maintain such a high number of cells to sustain myelin turnover and plasticity in the adult CNS and whether any relevant alteration in neuronal functions occurs in the absence of NG2+p in the intact or injured CNS.

ACKNOWLEDGMENTS

The work of Enrica Boda and Annalisa Buffo is supported by the Italian Ministry for University and Research (MIUR, PRIN 20107MSMA4, Annalisa Buffo). Enrica Boda is supported by a postdoctoral fellowship of the Giuseppe Levi Foundation, Accademia Nazionale dei Lincei, Rome, Italy. We thank Elena Frola and Giulia Pregno for the courtesy of the pictures in **Figure 1**.

REFERENCES

Balia, M., Vélez-Fort, M., Passlick, S., Schäfer, C., Audinat, E., Steinhäuser, C., et al. (2013). Postnatal down-regulation of the GABAA Receptor γ2 subunit in neocortical NG2 cells accompanies synaptic-to-extrasynaptic switch in the GABAergic transmission mode. *Cereb. Cortex*. doi: 10.1093/cercor/bht309. [Epub ahead of print].

Behrendt, G., Baer, K., Buffo, A., Curtis, M. A., Faull, R. L., Rees, M. I., et al. (2013). Dynamic changes in myelin aberrations and oligodendrocyte generation in chronic amyloidosis in mice and men. *Glia* 61, 273–286. doi: 10.1002/glia.22432

Bellesi, M., Pfister-Genskow, M., Maret, S., Keles, S., Tononi, G., and Cirelli, C. (2013). Effects of sleep and wake on oligodendrocytes and their precursors. *J. Neurosci.* 33, 14288–14300. doi: 10.1523/JNEUROSCI.5102-12.2013

Bergles, D. E., Roberts, J. D., Somogyi, P., and Jahr, C. E. (2000). Glutamatergic synapses on oligodendrocyte precursor cells in the hippocampus. *Nature.* 405, 187–191. doi: 10.1038/35012083

Boda, E., Viganò, F., Rosa, P., Fumagalli, M., Labat-Gest, V., Tempia, F., et al. (2011). The GPR17 receptor in NG2 expressing cells: focus on *in vivo* cell maturation and participation in acute trauma and chronic damage. *Glia* 59, 1958–1973. doi: 10.1002/glia.21237

Buffo, A., Rolando, C., and Ceruti, S. (2010). Astrocytes in the damaged brain: molecular and cellular insights into their reactive response and healing potential. *Biochem. Pharmacol.* 79, 77–89. doi: 10.1016/j.bcp.2009.09.014

Butt, A. M., Duncan, A., Hornby, M. F., Kirvell, S. L., Hunter, A., Levine, J. M., et al. (1999) Cells expressing the NG2 antigen contact nodes of Ranvier in adult CNS white matter. *Glia* 26, 84–91.

Butt, A. M., Hamilton, N., Hubbard, P., Pugh, M., and Ibrahim, M. (2005). Synantocytes: the fifth element. *J. Anat.* 207, 695–706. doi: 10.1111/j.1469-7580.2005.00458.x

Butti, E., Bacigaluppi, M., Rossi, S., Cambiaghi, M., Bari, M., Cebrian Silla, A., et al. (2012). Subventricular zone neural progenitors protect striatal neurons from glutamatergic excitotoxicity. *Brain* 135, 3320–3335. doi: 10.1093/brain/aws194

Christopherson, K. S., Ullian, E. M., Stokes, C. C., Mullowney, C. E., Hell, J. W., Agah, A., et al. (2005). Thrombospondins are astrocyte-secreted proteins that promote CNS synaptogenesis. *Cell* 120, 421–433. doi: 10.1016/j.cell.2004.12.020

Clemente, D., Ortega, M. C., Melero-Jerez, C., and de Castro, F. (2013). The effect of glia-glia interactions on oligodendrocyte precursor cell biology during development and in demyelinating diseases. *Front. Cell. Neurosci.* 7:268. doi: 10.3389/fncel.2013.00268

Dai, X., Lercher, L. D., Clinton, P. M., Du, Y., Livingston, D. L., Vieira, C., et al. (2003). The trophic role of oligodendrocytes in the basal forebrain. *J. Neurosci.* 23, 5846–5853.

Dawson, M. R., Polito, A., Levine, J. M., and Reynolds, R. (2003). NG2-expressing glial progenitor cells: an abundant and widespread population of cycling cells in the adult rat CNS. *Mol. Cell. Neurosci.* 24, 476–488. doi: 10.1016/S1044-7431(03)00210-0

De Biase, L. M., Nishiyama, A., and Bergles, D. E. (2010). Excitability and synaptic communication within the oligodendrocyte lineage. *J. Neurosci.* 30, 3600–3611. doi: 10.1523/JNEUROSCI.6000-09.2010

Demerens, C., Stankoff, B., Logak, M., Anglade, P., Allinquant, B., Couraud, F., et al. (1996). Induction of myelination in the central nervous system by electrical activity. *Proc. Natl. Acad. Sci. U.S.A.* 93, 9887–9892. doi: 10.1073/pnas.93.18.9887

Doretto, S., Malerba, M., Ramos, M., Ikrar, T., Kinoshita, C., De Mei, C., et al. (2011). Oligodendrocytes as regulators of neuronal networks during early postnatal development. *PLoS ONE* 6:e19849. doi: 10.1371/journal.pone.0019849

Ehninger, D., Wang, L. P., Klempin, F., Römer, B., Kettenmann, H., and Kempermann, G. (2011). Enriched environment and physical activity reduce microglia and influence the fate of NG2 cells in the amygdala of adult mice. *Cell Tissue Res.* 345, 69–86. doi: 10.1007/s00441-011-1200-z

Etxeberria, A., Mangin, J. M., Aguirre, A., and Gallo V. (2010). Adult-born SVZ progenitors receive transient synapses during remyelination in corpus callosum. *Nat. Neurosci.* 13, 287–289. doi: 10.1038/nn.2500

Frühbeis, C., Fröhlich, D., Kuo, W. P., Amphornrat, J., Thilemann, S., Saab, A. S., et al. (2013). Neurotransmitter-triggered transfer of exosomes mediates oligodendrocyte-neuron communication. *PLoS Biol.* 11:e1001604. doi: 10.1371/journal.pbio.1001604

Gallo, V., Mangin, J. M., Kukley, M., and Dietrich, D. (2008) Synapses on NG2-expressing progenitors in the brain: multiple functions? *J. Physiol.* 586, 3767–3781. doi: 10.1113/jphysiol.2008.158436

Galtrey, C. M., and Fawcett, J. W. (2007). The role of chondroitin sulfate proteoglycans in regeneration and plasticity in the central nervous system. *Brain Res. Rev.* 54, 1–18. doi: 10.1016/j.brainresrev.2006.09.006

Ge, W. P., Yang, X. J., Zhang, Z., Wang, H. K., Shen, W., Deng, Q. D., et al. (2006). Long-term potentiation of neuron-glia synapses mediated by Ca2+-permeable AMPA receptors. *Science* 312, 1533–1537. doi: 10.1126/science.1124669

Ge, W. P., Zhou, W., Luo, Q., Jan, L. Y., and Jan, Y. N. (2009). Dividing glial cells maintain differentiated properties including complex morphology and functional synapses. *Proc. Natl. Acad. Sci. U.S.A.* 106, 328–333. doi: 10.1073/pnas.0811353106

Gianola, S., Savio, T., Schwab, M. E., and Rossi, F. (2003). Cell-autonomous mechanisms and myelin-associated factors contribute to the development of Purkinje axon intracortical plexus in the rat cerebellum. *J. Neurosci.* 23, 4613–4624.

Haberlandt, C., Derouiche, A., Wyczynski, A., Haseleu, J., Pohle, J., Karram, K., et al. (2011). Gray matter NG2 cells display multiple Ca2+-signaling pathways and highly motile processes. *PLoS ONE* 6:e17575. doi: 10.1371/journal.pone.0017575

Hamilton, N., Vayro, S., Wigley, R., and Butt, A. M. (2010). Axons and astrocytes release ATP and glutamate to evoke calcium signals in NG2-glia. *Glia* 58, 66–79. doi: 10.1002/glia.20902

Huang, W., Zhao, N., Bai, X., Karram, K., Trotter, J., Goebbels, S., et al. (2014) Novel NG2-CreERT2 knock-in mice demonstrate heterogeneous differentiation potential of NG2 glia during development. *Glia* 62, 896–913. doi: 10.1002/glia.22648

Hughes, E. G., Kang, S. H., Fukaya, M., and Bergles, D. E. (2013). Oligodendrocyte progenitors balance growth with self-repulsion to achieve homeostasis in the adult brain. *Nat. Neurosci.* 16, 668–676. doi: 10.1038/nn.3390

Kang, S. H., Fukaya, M., Yang, J. K., Rothstein, J. D., and Bergles, D. E. (2010). NG2+ CNS glial progenitors remain committed to the oligodendrocyte lineage in postnatal life and following neurodegeneration. *Neuron* 68, 668–681. doi: 10.1016/j.neuron.2010.09.009

Káradóttir, R., Hamilton, N. B., Bakiri, Y., and Attwell, D. (2008). Spiking and nonspiking classes of oligodendrocyte precursor glia in CNS white matter. *Nat. Neurosci.* 11, 450–456. doi: 10.1038/nn2060

Kirby, B. B., Takada, N., Latimer, A. J., Shin, J., Carney, T. J., Kelsh, R. N., et al. (2006). *In vivo* time-lapse imaging shows dynamic oligodendrocyte progenitor behavior during zebrafish development. *Nat. Neurosci.* 9, 1506–1511. doi: 10.1038/nn1803

Kukley, M., Capetillo-Zarate, E., and Dietrich, D. (2007). Vesicular glutamate release from axons in white matter. *Nat. Neurosci.* 10, 311–320. doi: 10.1038/nn1850

Kukley, M., Kiladze, M., Tognatta, R., Hans, M., Swandulla, D., Schramm, J., et al. (2008). Glial cells are born with synapses. *FASEB J.* 22, 2957–2969. doi: 10.1096/fj.07-090985

Kukley, M., Nishiyama, A., and Dietrich, D. (2010). The fate of synaptic input to NG2 glial cells: neurons specifically downregulate transmitter release onto differentiating oligodendroglial cells. *J. Neurosci.* 30, 8320–8331. doi: 10.1523/JNEUROSCI.0854-10.2010

Lee, Y., Morrison, B. M., Li, Y., Lengacher, S., Farah, M. H., Hoffman, P. N., et al. (2012). Oligodendroglia metabolically support axons and contribute to neurodegeneration. *Nature* 487, 443–448. doi: 10.1038/nature11314

Levine, J. M., Reynolds, R., and Fawcett, J. W. (2001). The oligodendrocyte precursor cell in health and disease. *Trends Neurosci.* 24, 39–47. doi: 10.1016/S0166-2236(00)01691-X

Levison, S. W., Young, G. M., and Goldman, JE. (1999). Cycling cells in the adult rat neocortex preferentially generate oligodendroglia. *J. Neurosci. Res.* 57, 435–446.

Li, W., Tang, Y., Fan, Z., Meng, Y., Yang, G., Luo, J., et al. (2013). Autophagy is involved in oligodendroglial precursor-mediated clearance of amyloid peptide. *Mol. Neurodegener.* 8, 27. doi: 10.1186/1750-1326-8-27

Lin, S. C., and Bergles, D. E. (2004). Synaptic signaling between GABAergic interneurons and oligodendrocyte precursor cells in the hippocampus. *Nat Neurosci.* 7, 24–32. doi: 10.1038/nn1162

Lin, S. C., Huck, J. H., Roberts, J. D., Macklin, W. B., Somogyi, P., and Bergles D. E. (2005). Climbing fiber innervation of NG2-expressing glia in the mammalian cerebellum. *Neuron* 46, 773–785. doi: 10.1016/j.neuron.2005.04.025

Lu, B., Nagappan, G., Guan, X., Nathan, P. J., and Wren, P. (2013). BDNF-based synaptic repair as a disease-modifying strategy for neurodegenerative diseases. *Nat. Rev. Neurosci.* 14, 401–416. doi: 10.1038/nrn3505

Lundgaard, I., Luzhynskaya, A., Stockley, J. H., Wang, Z., Evans, K. A., Swire, M., et al. (2013). Neuregulin and BDNF induce a switch to NMDA receptor-dependent myelination by oligodendrocytes. *PLoS Biol.* 11:e1001743. doi: 10.1371/journal.pbio.1001743

Luyt, K., Slade, T. P., Dorward, J. J., Durant, C. F., Wu, Y., Shigemoto, R., et al. (2007). Developing oligodendrocytes express functional GABA(B) receptors that stimulate cell proliferation and migration. *J. Neurochem.* 100, 822–840. doi: 10.1111/j.1471-4159.2006.04255.x

Maglione, M., Tress, O., Haas, B., Karram, K., Trotter, J., Willecke, K., et al. (2010). Oligodendrocytes in mouse corpus callosum are coupled via gap junction channels formed by connexin47 and connexin32. *Glia* 58, 1104–1117. doi: 10.1002/glia.20991

Maldonado, P. P., Vélez-Fort. M., Levavasseur, F., and Angulo, M. C. (2013). Oligodendrocyte precursor cells are accurate sensors of local K+ in mature gray matter. *J. Neurosci.* 33, 2432–2442. doi: 10.1523/JNEUROSCI.1961-12.2013

Mangin, J. M., Kunze, A., Chittajallu, R., and Gallo, V. (2008). Satellite NG2 progenitor cells share common glutamatergic inputs with associated interneurons in the mouse dentate gyrus. *J. Neurosci.* 28, 7610–7623. doi: 10.1523/JNEUROSCI.1355-08.2008

Mangin, J. M., Li, P., Scafidi, J., and Gallo, V. (2012). Experience-dependent regulation of NG2 progenitors in the developing barrel cortex. *Nat. Neurosci.* 15, 1192–1194. doi: 10.1038/nn.3190

Martino, G., and Pluchino, S. (2006). The therapeutic potential of neural stem cells. *Nat. Rev. Neurosci.* 7, 395–406. doi: 10.1038/nrn1908

März, M., Schmidt, R., Rastegar, S., and Strähle, U. (2010) Expression of the transcription factor Olig2 in proliferating cells in the adult zebrafish telencephalon. *Dev. Dyn.* 239, 3336–3349. doi: 10.1002/dvdy.22455

Matthias, K., Kirchhoff, F., Seifert, G., Hüttmann, K., Matyash, M., Kettenmann, H., et al. (2003). Segregated expression of AMPA-type glutamate receptors and glutamate transporters defines distinct astrocyte populations in the mouse hippocampus. *J. Neurosci.* 23, 1750–1758.

Melanson-Drapeau, L., Beyko, S., Davé, S., Hebb, A. L., Franks, D. J., Sellitto, C., et al. (2003) Oligodendrocyte progenitor enrichment in the connexin32 null-mutant mouse. *J. Neurosci.* 23, 1759–1768.

Müller, J., Reyes-Haro, D., Pivneva, T., Nolte, C., Schaette, R., Lübke, J., et al. (2009). The principal neurons of the medial nucleus of the trapezoid body and NG2(+) glial cells receive coordinated excitatory synaptic input. *J. Gen. Physiol.*134, 115–127. doi: 10.1085/jgp.200910194

Munz, B., Tretter, Y. P., Hertel, M., Engelhardt, F., Alzheimer, C., and Werner, S. (2001). The roles of activins in repair processes of the skin and the brain. *Mol. Cell. Endocrinol.* 180, 169–177. doi: 10.1016/S0303-7207(01)00514-7

Nielsen, H. H., Ladeby, R., Drøjdahl, N., Peterson, A. C., and Finsen, B. (2006). Axonal degeneration stimulates the formation of NG2+ cells and oligodendrocytes in the mouse. *Glia* 54, 105–115. doi: 10.1002/glia.20357

Nishiyama, A., Watanabe, M., Yang, Z., and Bu J. (2002) Identity, distribution, and development of polydendrocytes: NG2-expressing glial cells. *J. Neurocytol.* 31, 437–455. doi: 10.1023/A:1025783412651

Nishiyama, A., Yu, M., Drazba, J. A., and Tuohy, V. K. (1997). Normal and reactive NG2+ glial cells are distinct from resting and activated microglia. *J. Neurosci. Res.*48, 299–312.

Ong, W. Y., and Levine, J. M. (1999) A light and electron microscopic study of NG2 chondroitin sulfate proteoglycan-positive oligodendrocyte precursor cells in the normal and kainate-lesioned rat hippocampus. *Neuroscience* 92, 83–95. doi: 10.1016/S0306-4522(98)00751-9

Passlick, S., Grauer, M., Schäfer, C., Jabs, R., Seifert, G., and Steinhäuser, C. (2013). Expression of the γ2-subunit distinguishes synaptic and extrasynaptic GABA(A) receptors in NG2 cells of the hippocampus. *J. Neurosci.* 33, 12030–12040. doi: 10.1523/JNEUROSCI.5562-12.2013

Petrosyan, H. A., Hunanyan, A. S., Alessi, V., Schnell, L., Levine, J., and Arvanian, V. L. (2013). Neutralization of inhibitory molecule NG2 improves synaptic transmission, retrograde transport, and locomotor function after spinal cord injury in adult rats. *J. Neurosci.* 33, 4032–4043. doi: 10.1523/JNEUROSCI.4702-12.2013

Pfrieger, F. W., and Barres, B. A. (1997). Synaptic efficacy enhanced by glial cells *in vitro*. *Science* 277, 1684–1687. doi: 10.1126/science.277.5332.1684

Redwine, J. M., and Armstrong, R. C. (1998). *In vivo* proliferation of oligodendrocyte progenitors expressing PDGFalphaR during early remyelination. *J. Neurobiol.* 37, 413–428.

Rivers, L. E., Young, K. M., Rizzi, M., Jamen, F., Psachoulia, K., Wade, A., et al. (2008). PDGFRA/NG2 glia generate myelinating oligodendrocytes and piriform projection neurons in adult mice. *Nat. Neurosci.* 11, 1392–1401. doi: 10.1038/nn.2220

Rosenberg, S. S., Kelland, E. E., Tokar, E., De la Torre, A. R., and Chan, J. R. (2008). The geometric and spatial constraints of the microenvironment induce oligodendrocyte differentiation. *Proc. Natl. Acad. Sci. U.S.A.* 105, 14662–14667. doi: 10.1073/pnas.0805640105

Shen, P. J., Larm, J. A., and Gundlach, A. L. (2003). Expression and plasticity of galanin systems in cortical neurons, oligodendrocyte progenitors and proliferative zones in normal brain and after spreading depression. *Eur. J. Neurosci.* 18, 1362–1376. doi: 10.1046/j.1460-9568.2003.02860.x

Sim, F. J., and Goldman, S. A. (2013). "Gene expression patterns of oligodendrocyte progenitor cells and oligodendroglia," in *Neuroglia*, eds E. Kettenmann and B. Ransom (Oxford: Oxford University Press), 358–373.

Sim, F. J., Lang, J. K., Waldau, B., Roy, N. S., Schwartz, T. E., Pilcher, W. H., et al. (2006). Complementary patterns of gene expression by human oligodendrocyte progenitors and their environment predict determinants of progenitor maintenance and differentiation. *Ann. Neurol.* 59, 763–779. doi: 10.1002/ana.20812

Sim, F. J., Windrem, M. S., and Goldman, S. A. (2009). Fate determination of adult human glial progenitor cells. *Neuron Glia Biol.* 5, 45–55. doi: 10.1017/S1740925X09990317

Simon, C., Götz, M., and Dimou, L. (2011). Progenitors in the adult cerebral cortex: cell cycle properties and regulation by physiological stimuli and injury. *Glia* 59, 869–881. doi: 10.1002/glia.21156

Stallcup, W. B. (2002) The NG2 proteoglycan: past insights and future prospects. *J. Neurocytol.* 31, 423–435. doi: 10.1023/A:1025731428581

Staugaitis, S. M., and Trapp, B. D. (2009) NG2-positive glia in the human central nervous system. *Neuron Glia Biol.* 5, 35–44. doi: 10.1017/S1740925X09990342

Stevens, B., Porta, S., Haak, L. L., Gallo, V., and Fields, R. D. (2002). Adenosine: a neuron-glial transmitter promoting myelination in the CNS in response to action potentials. *Neuron* 36, 855–868. doi: 10.1016/S0896-6273(02)01067-X

Sypecka, J., and Sarnowska, A. (2013). The neuroprotective effect exerted by oligodendroglial progenitors on ischemically impaired hippocampal cells. *Mol. Neurobiol.* 49, 685–701. doi: 10.1007/s12035-013-8549-9

Tamura, Y., Eguchi, A., Jin, G., Sami, M. M., and Kataoka, Y. (2012). Cortical spreading depression shifts cell fate determination of progenitor cells in the adult cortex. *J. Cereb. Blood Flow Metab.* 32, 1879–1887. doi: 10.1038/jcbfm.2012.98

Tanaka, Y., Tozuka, Y., Takata, T., Shimazu, N., Matsumura, N., Ohta, A., et al. (2009). Excitatory GABAergic activation of cortical dividing glial cells. *Cereb. Cortex* 19, 2181–2195. doi: 10.1093/cercor/bhn238

Tong, X. P., Li, X. Y., Zhou, B., Shen, W., Zhang, Z. J., Xu, T. L., et al. (2009). Ca(2+) signaling evoked by activation of Na(+) channels and Na(+)/Ca(2+) exchangers is required for GABA-induced NG2 cell migration. *J. Cell Biol.* 186, 113–128. doi: 10.1083/jcb.200811071

Tripathi, R. B., Rivers, L. E., Young, K. M., Jamen, F., and Richardson, W. D. (2010). NG2 glia generate new oligodendrocytes but few astrocytes in a murine experimental autoimmune encephalomyelitis model of demyelinating disease. *J. Neurosci.* 30, 16383–16390. doi: 10.1523/JNEUROSCI.3411-10.2010

Vélez-Fort, M., Maldonado, P. P., Butt, A. M., Audinat, E., and Angulo, M. C. (2010). Postnatal switch from synaptic to extrasynaptic transmission between interneurons and NG2 cells. *J. Neurosci.* 30, 6921–6929. doi: 10.1523/JNEUROSCI.0238-10.2010

Wake, H., Lee, P. R., and Fields, R. D. (2011). Control of local protein synthesis and initial events in myelination by action potentials. *Science* 333, 1647–1651. doi: 10.1126/science.1206998

Wallraff, A., Odermatt, B., Willecke, K., and Steinhäuser, C. (2004) Distinct types of astroglial cells in the hippocampus differ in gap junction coupling. *Glia* 48, 36–43. doi: 10.1002/glia.20040

Wang, S., and Young, K. M. (2013). White matter plasticity in adulthood. *Neuroscience*. doi: 10.1016/j.neuroscience.2013.10.018. [Epub ahead of print].

Wigley, R., and Butt, A. M. (2009) Integration of NG2-glia (synantocytes) into the neuroglial network. *Neuron Glia Biol.* 5, 21–28. doi: 10.1017/S1740925X09990329

Wilkins, A., Chandran, S., and Compston, A. (2001). A role for oligodendrocyte-derived IGF-1 in trophic support of cortical neurons. *Glia* 36, 48–57. doi: 10.1002/glia.1094

Yoshida, Y., Sakakima, H., Matsuda, F., and Ikutomo, M. (2014). Midkine in repair of the injured nervous system. *Br. J. Pharmacol.* 171, 924–930. doi: 10.1111/bph.12497

Young, K. M., Psachoulia, K., Tripathi, R. B., Dunn, S. J., Cossell, L., Attwell, D., et al. (2013). Oligodendrocyte dynamics in the healthy adult CNS: evidence for myelin remodeling. *Neuron* 77, 873–885. doi: 10.1016/j.neuron.2013.01.006

Zatorre, R. J., Fields, R. D., and Johansen-Berg, H. (2012). Plasticity in gray and white: neuroimaging changes in brain structure during learning. *Nat. Neurosci.* 15, 528–536. doi: 10.1038/nn.3045

Zawadzka, M., Rivers, L. E., Fancy, S. P., Zhao, C., Tripathi, R., Jamen., F., et al. (2010). CNS-resident glial progenitor/stem cells produce Schwann cells as well as oligodendrocytes during repair of CNS demyelination. *Cell Stem Cell* 6, 578–590. doi: 10.1016/j.stem.2010.04.002

Zhang, Y. W., Denham, J., and Thies, R. S. (2006). Oligodendrocyte progenitor cells derived from human embryonic stem cells express neurotrophic factors. *Stem Cells Dev.* 15, 943–952. doi: 10.1089/scd.2006.15.943

Zhu, X., Bergles, D. E., and Nishiyama, A. (2008a). NG2 cells generate both oligodendrocytes and gray matter astrocytes. *Development* 135, 145–157. doi: 10.1242/dev.004895

Zhu, X., Hill, R. A., Dietrich, D., Komitova, M., Suzuki, R., and Nishiyama, A. (2011). Age-dependent fate and lineage restriction of single NG2 cells. *Development* 138, 745–753. doi: 10.1242/dev.047951

Zhu, X., Hill, R. A., and Nishiyama, A. (2008b). NG2 cells generate oligodendrocytes and gray matter astrocytes in the spinal cord. *Neuron Glia Biol.* 4, 19–26. doi: 10.1017/S1740925X09000015

Ziskin, J. L., Nishiyama, A., Rubio, M., Fukaya, M., and Bergles, D. E. (2007). Vesicular release of glutamate from unmyelinated axons in white matter. *Nat. Neurosci.* 10, 321–330. doi: 10.1042/AN20110001

20

Stress and traumatic brain injury: a behavioral, proteomics, and histological study

Sook-Kyung C. Kwon[1†], Erzsebet Kovesdi[1†], Andrea B. Gyorgy[1], Daniel Wingo[1], Alaa Kamnaksh[1], John Walker[1], Joseph B. Long[2] and Denes V. Agoston[1]*

[1] Department of Anatomy, Physiology and Genetics, School of Medicine, Uniformed Services University, Bethesda, MD, USA
[2] Division of Military Casualty Research, Walter Reed Army Institute of Research, Silver Spring, MD, USA

Edited by:
Marten Risling, Karolinska Institutet, Sweden

Reviewed by:
Linda Noble, University of California at San Francisco, USA
Robert Vink, University of Adelaide, Australia

***Correspondence:**
Denes V. Agoston, Department of Anatomy, Physiology and Genetics, School of Medicine, Uniformed Services University, 4301 Jones Bridge Road, Bethesda, MD 20814, USA.
e-mail: vagoston@usuhs.edu

[†]Sook-Kyung C. Kwon and Erzsebet Kovesdi have contributed equally.

Psychological stress and traumatic brain injury (TBI) can both result in lasting neurobehavioral abnormalities. Post-traumatic stress disorder and blast induced TBI (bTBI) have become the most significant health issues in current military conflicts. Importantly, military bTBI virtually never occurs without stress. In this experiment, we assessed anxiety and spatial memory of rats at different time points after repeated exposure to stress alone or in combination with a single mild blast. At 2 months after injury or sham we analyzed the serum, prefrontal cortex (PFC), and hippocampus (HC) of all animals by proteomics and immunohistochemistry. Stressed sham animals showed an early increase in anxiety but no memory impairment at any measured time point. They had elevated levels of serum corticosterone (CORT) and hippocampal IL-6 but no other cellular or protein changes. Stressed injured animals had increased anxiety that returned to normal at 2 months and significant spatial memory impairment that lasted up to 2 months. They had elevated serum levels of CORT, CK-BB, NF-H, NSE, GFAP, and VEGF. Moreover, all of the measured protein markers were elevated in the HC and the PFC; rats had an increased number of TUNEL-positive cells in the HC and elevated GFAP and Iba1 immunoreactivity in the HC and the PFC. Our findings suggest that exposure to repeated stress alone causes a transient increase in anxiety and no significant memory impairment or cellular and molecular changes. In contrast, repeated stress and blast results in lasting behavioral, molecular, and cellular abnormalities characterized by memory impairment, neuronal and glial cell loss, inflammation, and gliosis. These findings may have implications in the development of diagnostic and therapeutic measures for conditions caused by stress or a combination of stress and bTBI.

Keywords: stress, blast traumatic brain injury, anxiety, memory, gliosis, inflammation, neurogenesis

INTRODUCTION

Traumatic brain injury (TBI) is one of the leading causes of death and chronic disability worldwide (Bruns and Hauser, 2003; Tagliaferri et al., 2006). Blast induced TBI (bTBI) caused by explosive devices is especially frequent in recent conflicts in Iraq and in Afghanistan (Warden and French, 2005; Taber et al., 2006; Warden, 2006). Epidemiological studies have shown that mild bTBI (mbTBI) can result in chronic neurobehavioral changes such as increased anxiety and memory impairment (Ryan and Warden, 2003; Okie, 2005). Importantly, virtually no bTBI occurs on the battlefield without the exposure to psychological stress. Exposure to stress alone (i.e., traumatic and/or life-threatening events) without physical injury can lead to a chronic condition called post-traumatic stress disorder (PTSD) in some but not all affected individuals (Breslau and Kessler, 2001). PTSD is especially frequent among soldiers; about 14% of soldiers suffer from PTSD-like symptoms compared to 4% of the US adult population (Keane et al., 2006; Richardson et al., 2010).

Although bTBI shares some of the clinical features of the closed head and the penetrating TBIs, bTBI appears to be a fundamentally different form of neurotrauma (Ling et al., 2009). Several factors are responsible for the uniqueness of bTBI; explosive blast rapidly dissipates very high levels of energy in the form of supersonic pressure waves (Mayorga, 1997; Okie, 2005). Within the brain parenchyma, the high-energy high-velocity blast waves can cause substantial damage to blood vessels, neuronal and glial cell bodies and their processes (Kaur et al., 1997; Cernak et al., 2001). Clinical hallmarks of severe bTBI include an unusually early onset (hours after injury) and rapid development of diffuse malignant cerebral edema, and delayed (10–14 days post-injury) vasoconstriction (Armonda et al., 2006; Ling et al., 2009; Ling and Ecklund, 2011). Given that blast almost always affects the whole body, subclinical thoracic or abdominal injuries can also contribute to the pathophysiology of bTBI (Cernak et al., 2010). It has been thought that the secondary injury process in bTBI includes vascular changes, neuroinflammation, and gliosis (Kaur et al., 1997; Mayorga, 1997; Cernak et al., 2001; Taber et al., 2006).

Exposure to mild blast poses especially difficult challenges. Even though there are no life-threatening injuries in mbTBI and soldiers do not lose consciousness, 6–9 months later many soldiers develop neurobehavioral abnormalities that include memory impairment, anxiety, and mood disorders (Belanger et al., 2007; Brenner et al., 2009). These symptoms indicate damage to the hippocampus (HC) and the prefrontal cortex (PFC), brain structures that are also indicated as the neuroanatomical substrates of PTSD (Jaffee and Meyer, 2009). Stress is a constant factor on the battlefield

(Warden et al., 1997; Brenner et al., 2009); soldiers are repeatedly exposed to various life-threatening situations and to the visual and audible cues of blasts without necessarily suffering from any visible physical injury.

In order to better understand the long-term consequences of stress with and without the exposure to blast, we used a rodent model of stress and mbTBI and assessed the behavior of animals at various time points after sham or injury and analyzed their sera and brains for cellular and molecular changes. Due to our experimental setup, we were unable to determine the effect of blast injury alone. During our pilot studies we learned that handling and transporting animals (associated with the exposure to blast) resulted in a significant amount of stress as indicated by substantially elevated serum CORT levels of animals.

MATERIALS AND METHODS

ANIMALS, HOUSING CONDITIONS, AND EXPERIMENTAL SCHEDULE

Sprague-Dawley male rats (245–265 g; Charles River Laboratories, Wilmington, MA, USA) were housed in cages with free access to food and water in a reverse 12/12 h light/dark cycle. The experimental schedule is depicted in **Figure 1**. After 7 days of acclimation and handling in our animal facility, control animals (C) were housed two per cage; stressed sham injured (SS) and stressed injured animals (SI) were housed individually. All animals were handled according to protocol approved by the Institutional Animal Care and Use Committee (IACUC) at the Uniformed Services University of the Health Sciences. All behavioral tests were conducted during animals' dark cycle.

INJURY

On the day of the exposure, animals in the SS and SI groups were transported from USU (Bethesda, MD, USA) to Walter Reed Army Institute of Research (Silver Spring, MD, USA) for injury. Blast TBI was generated using a compression-driven shock tube as described earlier (Long et al., 2009). Before injury, rats in the SI group were anesthetized with 4% isoflurane (Forane, Baxter Healthcare Corporation, Deerfield, IL, USA), placed in an animal holder in a transverse prone position and then transferred to the shock tube where they were exposed to whole body blast overpressure (20.6 ± 3 psi). Immediately after exposure, the duration of apnea was measured and rats were moved back to their home cages. Animals in the SS group received the same amount of anesthesia and underwent the same procedure but were not exposed to blast overpressure. However, SS as well as SI animals were exposed to the sounds of the blast, which is likely an additional stressor. Following exposures (or sham), animals were transported back to USU.

CHRONIC STRESS

Rats in the SI and SS groups were exposed to a combination of predator and unpredictable stressors for 1 week prior to and 1 week after the first behavioral testing session (**Figure 1**). Unpredictable stress is a face-valid model of human stress that has been shown to reliably elevate stress hormone levels in rodents (Fride et al., 1986; Weinstock et al., 1992).

A combination of fox urine and unpredictable stress (Campbell et al., 2003) was performed with modifications (Berger and Grunberg, in preparation). Rats were exposed to fox urine for 10 min/day (Red fox urine, Buck Stop Lure Company, Stanton, MI, USA) as a predator stress, and loud noises and sudden cage movements at irregular times as an unpredictable stressor. During the stress routine, rats were moved to the animal facility's procedure room. Each rat was transferred to a clean empty cage with a cotton ball containing 15 ml of fox urine; each day the position of the cotton ball was changed. Within the 10 min stress period, rats were exposed to loud noises and irregular cage movement. After stress, the rats were immediately moved back to their home cages and transferred back to the animal housing room. Control rats were neither transferred to the procedure room nor exposed to any of the stressors.

SCHEDULE OF BEHAVIORAL TESTS

Before chronic stress and injury all animals underwent a baseline open field (OF) measurement (**Figure 1**). Horizontal activity results were used to create three groups with no statistical significance among them. After the first stress phase and blast (or sham) injury, rats underwent a series of behavioral evaluations. In each behavioral session OF was conducted first to ascertain whether animals had any motor problems, which can confound other behavioral tests. One day after OF, elevated plus maze (EPM) was performed to measure anxiety levels. Barnes maze (BM) was performed last to measure spatial learning and memory. The three behavioral assessments were performed on separate days starting at 24 h, 1, and 2 months after injury (**Figure 1**).

Open field

The OF test is an indicator of potential motor deficits but can also reflect fluctuations in anxiety levels based on changes in exploratory behavior (Heath and Vink, 1999). Several studies have shown this test to reliably measure anxiety and depression in rodents (von Horsten et al., 1998) including after TBI (Vink et al., 2003). OF tests were performed using Omnitech Electronics' Digiscan infrared photocell system (test box model RXYZCM, Omnitech Electronics, Columbus, OH; Elliott and Grunberg, 2005). The OF system is a

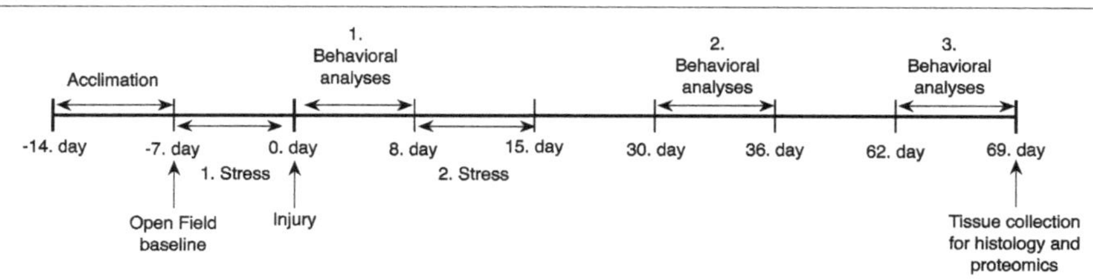

FIGURE 1 | Outline of the experimental schedule.

40 × 40 × 30 ($L \times W \times H$) cm clear Plexiglas arena with a perforated lid. During the 60 min testing period, we measured horizontal activity (locomotor activity), time spent in the margins (anxiety), and in the center. Data were automatically gathered and transmitted to a computer via an Omnitech Model DCM-BBU analyzer.

Elevated plus maze

The EPM is a widely used, ethologically relevant test that assesses anxiety states in rodents (Carobrez and Bertoglio, 2005; Salzberg et al., 2007; Walf and Frye, 2007). The maze is an elevated structure (1 m above ground) consisting of four intersecting arms. The arms of the maze are 50 cm long and 10 cm wide; the closed arms have walls on three sides that are 40 cm high while the open arms have none. The lighting in the middle of the maze was set at 90 lux. On testing days rats were placed one by one in the center of the maze facing one of the open arms; each animal was allowed to explore freely for 5 min while its movement was video-tracked. Total distance traveled, number of entries made, and time spent (duration) in each arm was recorded using ANY-maze 4.2 Software (Stoelting Company, Wood Dale, IL, USA).

Barnes maze

Barnes maze was used to assess spatial learning and memory (Barnes, 1979; Maegele et al., 2005; Doll et al., 2009). BM represents a widely used, validated, and less stressful alternative to the commonly used water maze test (Harrison et al., 2009). The maze is a circular platform (1.2 m in diameter) with 18 evenly spaced holes around the periphery. One of the holes is the entrance to a darkened escape box that is not visible from the surface of the board. Each rat was tested twice per day for six consecutive days to find the escape box (only day 1 of the first BM session had three trials). In each trial, latency to locate and enter the escape box was measured (ANY-maze 4.2 Software, Stoelting Company, Wood Dale, IL, USA).

During the first (teaching) trial of the first BM session, all animals were trained to locate the escape chamber. Each animal was placed in the escape box and covered for 30 s. The escape box was then removed with the animal inside and moved to the center of the maze. The rat was removed from the box and allowed to explore the maze for a few seconds, after which the rat was returned to its home cage. No latency times were recorded for the teaching trials. The escape box and the maze were cleaned with 30% ethanol solution between each trial. In the second trial the same rat was placed under a start box in the center of the maze for 30 s; the start box was then removed and the rat was allowed to explore freely to find the escape chamber. Training sessions ended after the animal had entered the escape box or when a pre-determined time (240 s) had elapsed. If the animal had not found the escape box during the given time period, it was placed in the escape box for 1 min at the end of the trial.

TISSUE COLLECTION AND PROCESSING

On day 67 post-injury (or sham; **Figure 1**) all animals were deeply anesthetized with isoflurane until a tail pinch produced no reflex movement. Anesthesia was maintained using a mask/nose cone attached to the anesthetic vaporizer, and blood was collected (1.5 ml) from a tail vein. For proteomics and ELISA assays, rats were decapitated under deep anesthesia. Brains were immediately removed and placed on ice. The PFC and HC were dissected, frozen, and stored at −80°C. For histology, rats were transcardially perfused with cold phosphate-buffered saline (PBS) followed by 4% buffered paraformaldehyde solution under deep isoflurane anesthesia. Following overnight post-fixation in 4% buffered paraformaldehyde solution brains were consecutively immersed in cold 15 and 30% sucrose solutions in 1× PBS for cryoprotection and then frozen on dry ice. Frozen brains were sectioned coronally at a 20-μm thickness using a cryostat (Cryocut 1800; Leica Microsystems, Bannockburn, IL, USA) and sections were kept at −80°C until use.

PROTEOMICS

Preparation of samples

Sample preparation, printing, scanning, and data analysis were performed as described later in detail (Gyorgy et al., 2010). Flash-frozen tissues were briefly pulverized in liquid nitrogen; 200 mg of the frozen powder was transferred into 1 ml of T-per lysis buffer (Thermo Fisher, Waltham, MA, USA) with protease and phosphatase inhibitors (Thermo Fisher) and then sonicated. Samples were centrifuged for 15 min at 4°C; the supernatants were aliquoted and stored at −80°C. Protein concentrations were measured by using a BCA assay (Thermo Fisher). Blood samples were promptly centrifuged after removal at 10,000×*g* for 15 min at 4°C; the supernatants were aliquoted, flash-frozen, and stored at −80°C. Tissue samples were diluted in print buffer (10% glycerol, 0.05% SDS, 50 mM DTT in 1× TBS) to a final protein concentration of 1 mg/ml, while serum samples were diluted 1:10. Samples were then subjected to an 11-point serial 1:2 dilution and transferred into Genetix 384-well plates (X7022, Fisher Scientific, Pittsburgh, PA, USA) as described (Gyorgy et al., 2010). Plates were transferred into an Aushon 2470 Arrayer (Aushon Biosystems, Billerica, MA, USA) and samples were printed on ONCYTE Avid (tissue samples) or ONCYTE Nova (serum samples) single-pad nitrocellulose coated glass slides (Grace Bio-Labs, Bend, OR, USA).

Printing parameters

The Aushon Arrayer was programmed to use 16 pins (4 × 4 pattern). Each sample was printed in 12 dilutions (12 rows) and in triplicate (3 columns), resulting in a block of 3 × 12 dots per sample. The Spot Diameter was set to 250 nm with a spacing of 500 nm between dots on the *x*-axis and 375 nm on the *y*-axis. Wash time was set at 2 s without delays. The printer was programmed for a single deposition per dot for printing serum and tissue extracts.

Immunochemical detection

Primary antibodies were diluted to 10× the optimal Western analysis concentration in antibody incubation buffer (0.1% bovine serum albumin (BSA), protease inhibitors (EDTA-free Halt protease and phosphatase inhibitor cocktail, Thermo Fisher, Waltham, MA, USA; 1× TBS, 0.5% Tween 20) as described (Gyorgy et al., 2010). Primary antibodies were used in the following dilutions: VEGF 1:100 (Abcam ab-53465), s100b 1:50 (Abcam ab-41548), GFAP 1:500 (Abcam ab-7260), Tau-protein 1:20 (Santa Cruz sc-1995), CK-BB 1:20 (Santa Cruz sc-15157), NSE 1: 100 (Abcam, Cat# ab53025), NF-H 1:20 (Sigma N4142). Slides were incubated with the primary antibody solution overnight at 4°C covered by a cover slip (Nunc* mSeries LifterSlips, Fisher Scientific, Pittsburg, PA).

The following day slides were washed and then incubated with an Alexa Fluor® 635 goat anti-mouse (Cat# A-31574), goat anti-rabbit (Cat# A-31576), or rabbit anti-goat IgG (H + L; Cat# A-21086) secondary antibodies from Invitrogen at 1:6000 dilution in antibody incubation buffer for 1 h at room temperature (RT). After washing and drying, the fluorescent signals were measured in a Scan Array Express HT microarray scanner (Perkin Elmer, Waltham, MA, USA) using a 633 nm wavelength laser and a 647 nm filter. Data from the scanned images were imported into a Microsoft Excel-based bioinformatics program developed in house for analysis (Gyorgy et al., 2010).

Data analysis and bioinformatics

The program calculates total net intensity after local background subtraction for each spot. The intensity data from the dilution series of each sample are then plotted against dilution on a log–log graph. The linear regression of the log–log data was calculated after the removal of flagged data, which include signal to noise ratios of less than 2, spot intensities in the saturation range or noise range, or high variability between duplicate spots (>10–15%). The total amount of antigen is determined by the *y*-axis intercept (Gyorgy et al., 2010).

CORTICOSTERONE ASSAY

Serum corticosterone (CORT) levels were measured using Cayman's Corticosterone EIA Kit according to the manufacturer's instructions (Cayman Chemical, Ann Arbor, MI, USA). Each sample was diluted 1:500 and measured in triplicate.

IL-6 AND INFγ ASSAYS

INFγ and IL-6 levels were measured from brain tissues using the rat Interferon gamma ELISA and the Rat IL-6 ELISA kits (both are from Thermo Fisher, Waltham, MA, USA). The IL-6 ELISA kit required a 1:5 dilution using the supplied dilution buffer in order to avoid saturation in the wells. After the dilution of brain samples, the assay was performed according to the manufacturer's instructions.

HISTOLOGY

Immunohistochemistry

Every first and tenth coronal section containing either the PFC, the dorsal HC (DHC), or the ventral HC (VHC) were mounted on positively charged glass slides with two sections per slide. Three slides per animal, containing sections with identical *z*-axes, were selected per brain region for each immunostaining. Slides containing the frozen sections were equilibrated at RT and hydrated with 1× PBS for 30 min. Antigen retrieval was performed by incubating the sections in 10 mM citrate buffer (pH 6.0) at 80°C for 30 min followed by cooling down to RT. After rehydration with 1× PBS, sections were permeabilized with 0.5% Triton X-100 in PBS for 1 h and blocked in 1× PBS containing 5% normal goat serum (NGS), 5% BSA, 0.1% sodium azide, and 0.5% Triton X-100 for 1 h. The same solution minus NGS was used to dilute primary antibodies. The following primary antibodies were used: mouse anti-GFAP (Millipore, Temecula, CA, USA; 1:400) rabbit anti-doublecortin (DCX; Cell Signaling Technology, Beverly, MA, USA; 1:1000), and goat anti-Iba1 (Abcam, Cambridge, MA, USA; 1:1000). Sections were incubated with the primary antibodies overnight at 4°C. After washing with 1× PBS, they were incubated with appropriate secondary antibodies (Alexa Fluor 555 goat anti-mouse IgG, 488 goat anti-rabbit IgG, or 488 donkey anti-goat IgG (Invitrogen, Carlsbad, CA) was applied for 1 h at RT 1:100), Hoechst 33342 (Molecular Probes, Eugene, OR, USA) at 1 μg/ml was applied for 2 min, sections washed and coverslipped using anti-fading media (Vectashield, Vector Laboratories, Burlingame, CA, USA).

TUNEL assay

Apoptotic cell death marked by DNA fragmentation was determined using a TUNEL *in situ* cell death detection kit, POD (Roche, Indianapolis, IN, USA) according to the manufacturer's instructions. Sections were hydrated with PBS and endogenous peroxidase activity was quenched by 3% H_2O_2 in methanol for 10 min at RT. Sections were permeabilized by 0.1 M sodium citrate buffer (pH 6.0) at 70°C for 30 min followed by PBST for 30 min at RT. TUNEL reaction was performed for 1 h at 37°C and the signal was converted using converter-POD. TUNEL-positive cells were visualized by DAB substrate. Dark brown TUNEL-positive cells were counted from four sections per animal.

Histological data acquisition

Histological sections were visualized in an Olympus IX-71 microscope using the appropriate filters and images were collected using a SPOT digital camera (Diagnostic Instruments Inc., Sterling Heights, MI, USA). The collected images were colored using TIFFany Caffeine Software.

STATISTICAL ANALYSIS AND COMPARISON OF DATA

Behavioral test results were analyzed with ANOVA and Tukey *post hoc* tests. Differences with a *p*-value of <0.05 were considered significant. Statistical analyses were performed using GraphPad InStat software. Proteomics and ELISA results were analyzed with Student's *t*-test. Data are reported as the average ± standard error of the mean. Proteomics data results were followed up with a one-way ANOVA. For each of our numerical measurements, we determined statistical significance among experimental groups by ($p < 0.05$ depicted by one star; $p < 0.01$ by two and $p < 0.001$ by three).

RESULTS

BEHAVIORAL EFFECTS

Locomotor activity

Twenty-four hours after exposure to blast (or sham), rats in the SI group showed a decrease in horizontal activity compared to rats in the SS and C groups (**Figure 2A**) but the difference was statistically insignificant. Animals in the SI group spent significantly more time in the periphery and significantly less time in the center (**Figures 2B,C**) compared to C and SS animals. SS animals showed no significant difference compared to C animals.

At 1 and 2 months after injury (or sham), we found no significant differences in any of the measured parameters between animals in all experimental groups (**Figures 2A–C**).

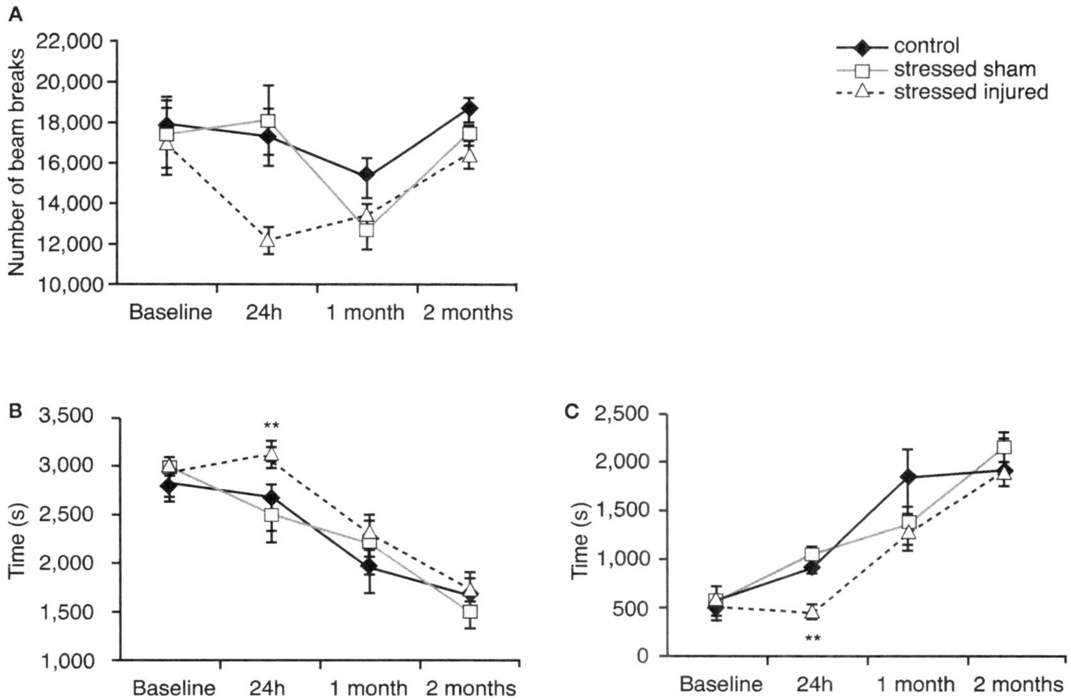

FIGURE 2 | Locomotor activity of animals in the various experimental groups. Open field was used to assess **(A)** horizontal activity (number of beam breaks), **(B)** time spent in the peripheral zone (seconds) and **(C)** time spent in the central zone (seconds). $^{**}p < 0.01$ SI compared to C rats. Data are presented in mean ± SEM. (C: $n = 4$; SS: $n = 6$; and SI: $n = 6$).

Anxiety

Forty-eight hours after blast (or sham) injury, we found that SI rats traveled significantly shorter distances than C animals (**Figure 3A**). Animals in the SS group also traveled shorter distances but the differences were not statistically significant. Animals in both SS and SI groups spent significantly less time in the open arms and more time in the closed arms (**Figures 3B,C**).

At 1 month both SS and SI groups traveled shorter distances compared to C animals (**Figure 3A**). Among the stressed groups only SI animals exhibited raised anxiety by spending less time in the open arms and more time in the closed arms (**Figures 3B,C**). Animals in the SS group did not show significant differences in the time spent in the open arms vs. closed arms compared to the controls.

Two months after blast or sham injury, all animals performed similarly with no significant differences in total distance traveled or time spent in the open and the closed arms.

Spatial learning and memory

During the first BM session, performed between days 3 and 8 post-blast (or sham; see **Figure 1** for schedule) we observed significant differences in the performance of animals on the last testing day only (day 8). SS rats needed significantly more time to find the escape box compared to C rats. SI rats spent less time finding the escape box than SS rats, but more time compared to C rats; the difference was not statistically significant (**Figure 4A**).

During the second BM session, performed between days 32 and 36 post-blast (or sham), we found no difference in the latency times of animals in the SS and the C groups. However, SI animals required significantly longer times to find the escape box on day 33 through 36 (**Figure 4B**).

The last BM session was performed between days 64 and 69 post-injury (or sham). Again, the performance of SS animals was not statistically different from animal in the control group (**Figure 4C**). In contrast, SI rats performed very poorly in the BM on day 64. These animals had increased latency times similar to those measured during the first BM session (**Figures 4C,D**) showing significant memory problems on days 65 and 68, indicating lasting memory impairment caused by blast.

EFFECTS ON PROTEIN MARKERS

Serum changes

At the end of the last behavioral session (69 days post-injury or sham), we obtained serum from each animal and compared NF-H, CK-BB, GFAP, VEGF, and NSE levels across all experimental groups. We found that serum levels of all protein markers listed above were significantly elevated at this late time point in SI animals (**Figure 5**). As expected, serum CORT levels were significantly elevated in both SS and SI groups. However, the difference in serum CORT levels between the two groups was statistically insignificant.

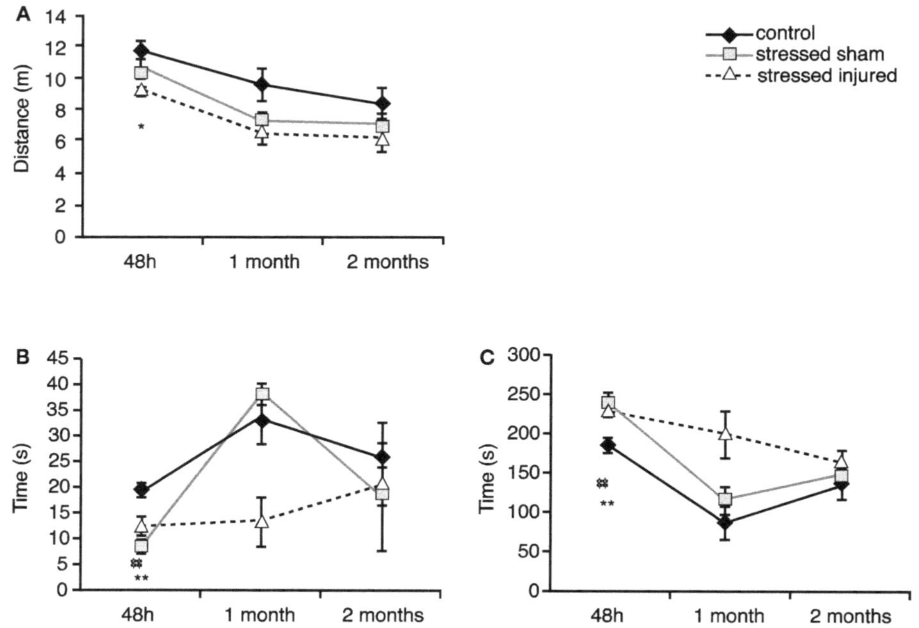

FIGURE 3 | Anxiety of animals in the various experimental groups. Elevated plus maze was used to assess **(A)** total distance traveled (meter), **(B)** time spent in the open arms (seconds) and **(C)** time spent in the closed arms (seconds). $*p < 0.05$ and $**p < 0.01$ SI compared to C rats, $^{##}p < 0.01$ SS to C rats. Data are presented in mean ± SEM. (C: $n = 4$; SS: $n = 6$; and SI: $n = 6$).

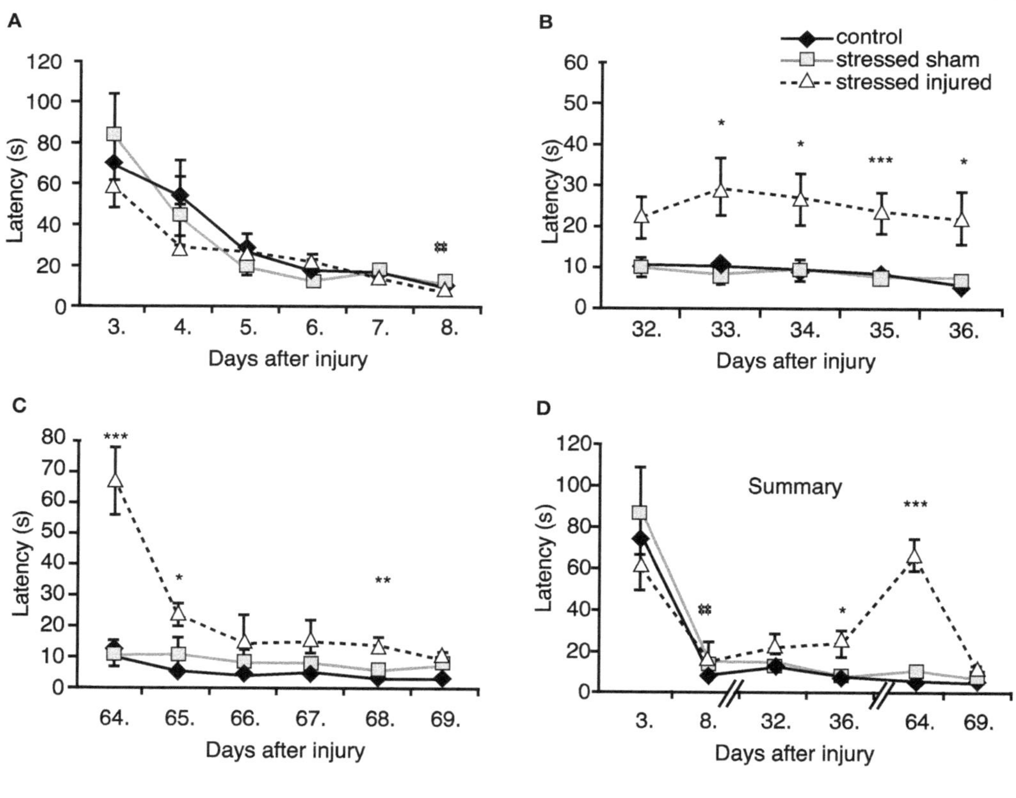

FIGURE 4 | Spatial learning and memory of animals in the various experimental groups. Barnes maze was used to determine latencies to find the escape box **(A)** 3–8 days post-injury, **(B)** 32–36 days post-injury, **(C)** 64–69 days post-injury. **(D)** Summarized time-line of latencies of the three sets of Barnes maze test. $*p < 0.05$, $**p < 0.01$, and $***p < 0.01$ SI compared to C rats, $^{##}p < 0.01$ SS to C rats. Data are presented in mean ± SEM (C: $n = 4$; SS: $n = 6$; and SI: $n = 6$).

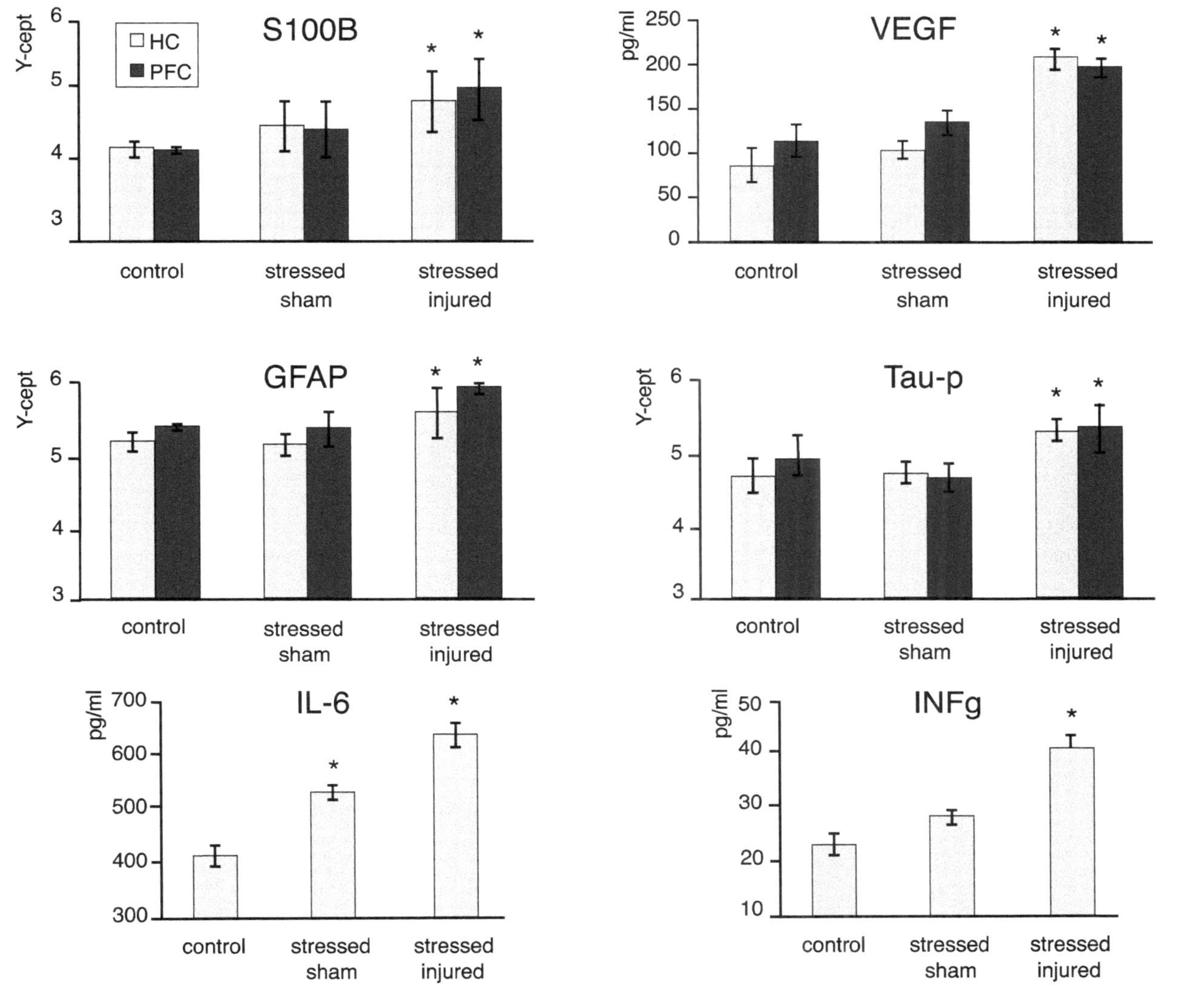

FIGURE 5 | Protein markers in the PFC and the HC of animals in the various experimental groups. Tissue extracts were prepared from dissected PFC and HC regions of C, SS, and SI rat brains. The tissue levels of the selected marker proteins were assayed using either RPPM or ELISA. The *y*-axis intercept (Y-cept) and pg/ml (IL-6 and IFNg) indicate the measured protein levels. *$p < 0.05$, **$p < 0.01$ compared to C rats, error bars are ± SEM. (C: $n = 2$; SS: $n = 3$; and SI: $n = 3$).

Changes in the brain

At the end of the last behavioral session we analyzed changes in the expression of S100β, VEGF, GFAP, Tau-protein, IL-6, and INFγ in the PFC and the HC of all animals. We found significantly elevated levels of all markers (except IL-6) in the PFC and the HC of SI animals only (**Figure 6**). Interestingly, we found that IL-6 levels were significantly increased in the HC of SS animals while no such effect of stress alone was seen on hippocampal INFγ levels.

CELLULAR CHANGES

Astrogliosis

To identify the cellular changes underlying the observed behavioral abnormalities, we analyzed the HC and the PFC for GFAP expression at 2 months post-blast (or sham). Consistent with our proteomics data, we found that exposure to stress alone (SS) had no observable effect on GFAP expression in the PFC or the HC (**Figure 7**). However, in SI animals we detected a noticeable increase in GFAP immunoreactivity in the PFC and the VHC.

Importantly, an increase in GFAP+ cells displaying a stellar morphology characteristic of reactive astrocytes was observed in the PFC and the VHC of SI animals (**Figure 7C**, and insert).

Inflammation

Similar to the gliotic response above, exposure to stress alone had no significant effect on Iba1 immunoreactivity in the PFC or the HC (**Figure 8**). While increased Iba1 immunoreactivity was observed in the SI group, there was a noticeable increase in Iba1 immunoreactivity (albeit to a lesser degree) in the PFC of SS animals. No significant differences were observed in Iba1 immunoreactivity in the DHC of any of the experimental groups.

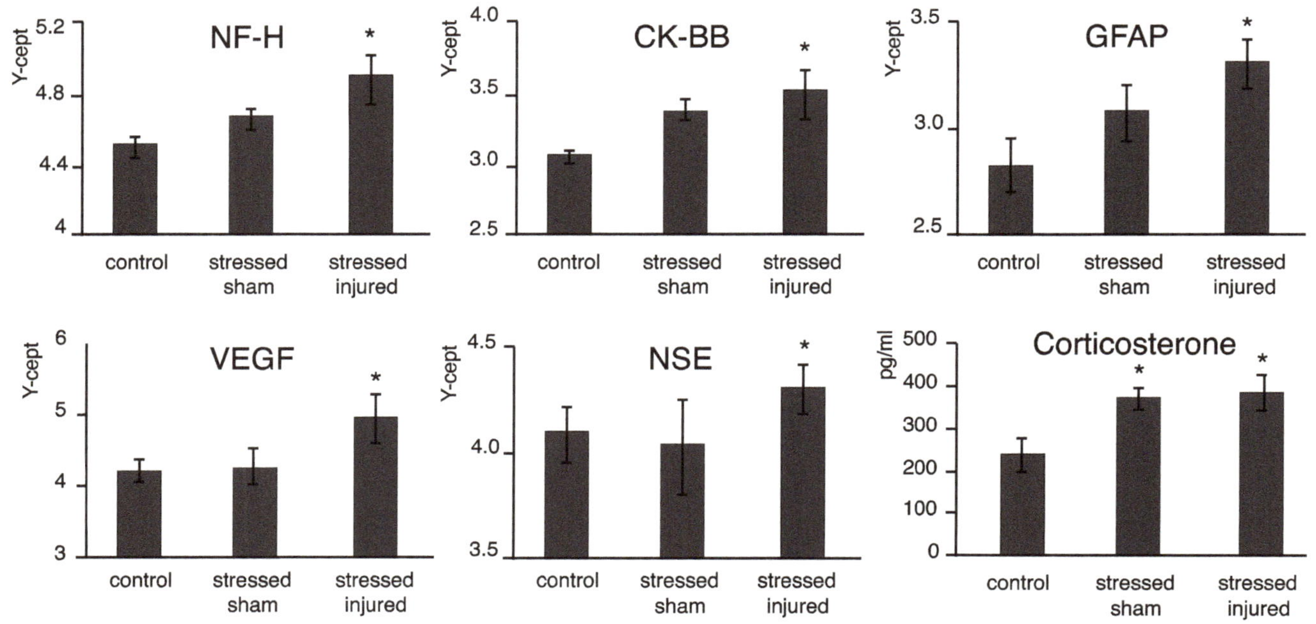

FIGURE 6 | Serum markers of animals in the various experimental groups. Blood was drawn and sera were prepared from the C, SS, and SI rats. The levels of the selected marker proteins were assayed using either RPPM or ELISA, and corticosterone levels were assayed using ELISA. The *y*-axis intercept (Y-cept) and pg/ml (corticosterone) indicate the measured protein levels. $*p < 0.05$, $**p < 0.01$ compared to C rats, error bars are ± SEM (C: $n = 4$; SS: $n = 6$; and SI: $n = 6$).

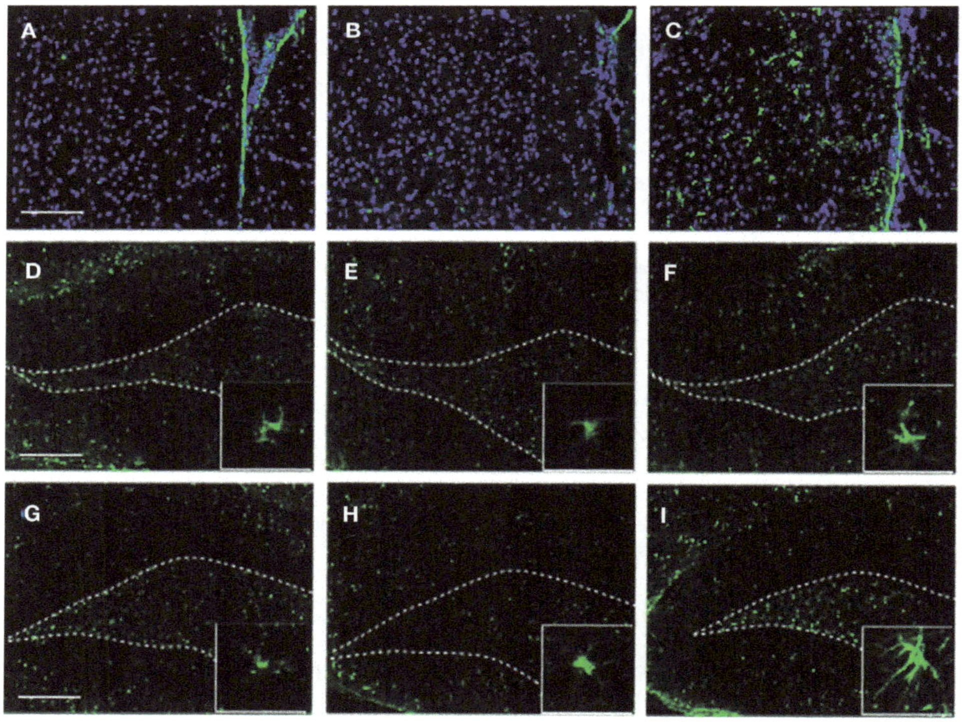

FIGURE 7 | GFAP immunoreactivity in selected brain regions of animals in the various experimental groups. Frozen coronal sections containing the PFC, DHC, and VHC were cut and processed for immunohistochemistry using a GFAP antibody. Sections were stained with Hoechst 33342 to mark cellular nuclei. PFC of **(A)** C, **(B)** SS, and **(C)** SI rats; DHC of **(D)** C, **(E)** SS, and **(F)** SI rats; VHC of **(G)** C, **(H)** SS, and **(I)** SI rats. Inlays display morphological extension of stellar-like processes in VHC of SI rats. White-dotted line outlines DG layer of hippocampus.

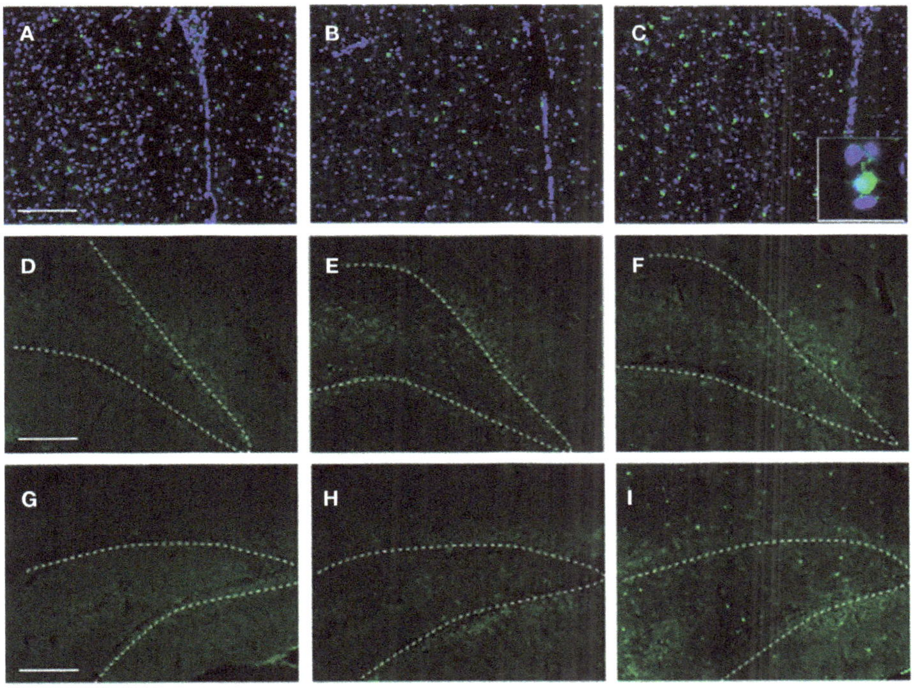

FIGURE 8 | Iba1 immunoreactivity in selected brain regions of animals in the various experimental groups. Frozen coronal sections containing the PFC, DHC, and VHC were cut and processed for immunohistochemistry using an Iba1 antibody. Sections were stained with Hoechst 33342 to mark cellular nuclei. PFC of **(A)** C, **(B)** SS, and **(C)** SI rats; DHC of **(D)** C, **(E)** SS, and **(F)** SI rats; VHC of **(G)** C, **(H)** SS, and **(I)** SI rats. White-dotted line outlines DG layer of hippocampus.

Apoptotic cell death

TUNEL histology was used to determine the extent of apoptotic cell death in the PFC, VHC, and DHC across all experimental groups. The number of TUNEL-positive cells was significantly increased in the hilus of the VHC and the DHC of the SI group (**Figure 9**). Interestingly, there was no increase in the number of TUNEL-positive cells in the PFC of animals in any of the experimental groups (**Figure A1** in Appendix). The exposure to stress alone resulted in no increase in the number of TUNEL-positive cells in any of the SS brain regions investigated.

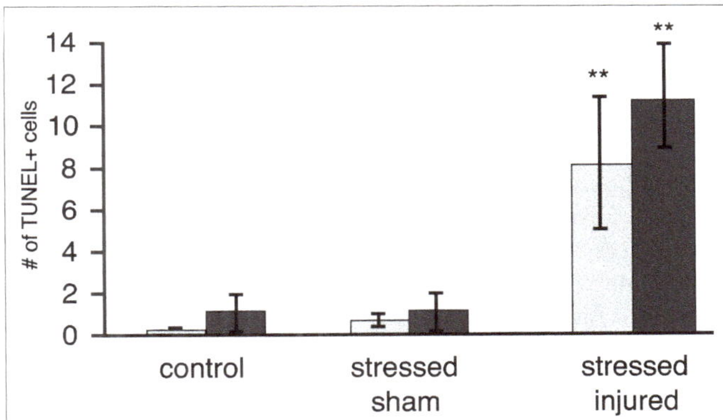

FIGURE 9 | TUNEL-positive cells in selected brain regions of animals in the various experimental groups. Frozen coronal sections containing the hilus of the DHC and VHC of C, SS, and SI rats were cut and processed for TUNEL histology. The number of TUNEL-positive cells were counted and expressed as positive cells per unit area ± SEM. *$p < 0.05$ and **$p < 0.01$ compared to C rats.

Neurogenesis

To gain insight into the potential effects of stress (with or without injury) on hippocampal *de novo* neurogenesis, we performed DCX immunohistochemistry. We observed a noticeable increase in DCX expression in the VHC of SI animals; DCX immunoreactive cells displayed specific morphologies with elaborate processes reaching well into the DG (**Figure 10F** and insert). Stress alone caused an apparent increase in DCX positive cells in the VHC compared to the controls (**Figure 10**). However, the DCX+ cells in SS animals lacked the elaborate processes seen in SI animals.

DISCUSSION

The main finding of this study is that repeated stress alone caused a transient increase in anxiety and no major cellular and molecular abnormalities, while the exposure to stress and a single mild blast resulted in a transient (but longer lasting) increase in anxiety and chronic memory impairment. These behavioral changes are associated with neuroinflammation, vascular changes, and neuronal and glial cell loss.

Repetitive stress alone resulted in an early (48 h) increase in anxiety that dissipated at later time points. Our finding is consistent with previous studies where the exposure of rats to a fear-provoking environment resulted in a short-term increase in anxiety

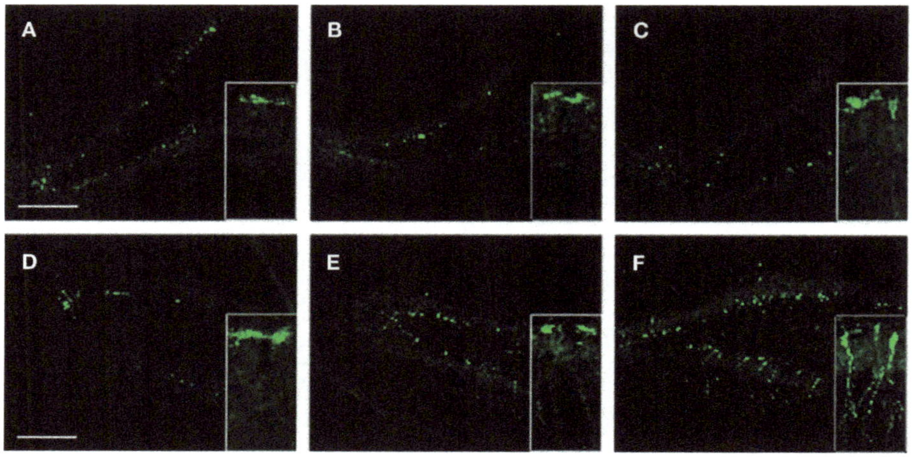

FIGURE 10 | DCX immunoreactivity in selected brain regions of animals in the various experimental groups. Frozen coronal sections containing the PFC, DHC, and VHC were cut. Immunohistochemistry was performed using a DCX antibody. Sections were stained with Hoechst 33342 to mark cellular nuclei. DHC of **(A)** C, **(B)** SS, and **(C)** SI rats; VHC of **(D)** C, **(E)** SS, and **(F)** SI rats. Inlays show the finer details of the cell bodies and processes of DCX cells within the DG of the VHC.

(Pynoos et al., 1996). Other studies also reported increased anxiety that lasted up to 7 days after daily exposure to predator odor (Adamec and Shallow, 1993; Cohen et al., 1996, 2000, 2003; Adamec et al., 1997, 1999). On the other hand, exposure of stressed animals to blast appears to prolong the period of increased anxiety, as these animals had elevated anxiety levels up to 1 month after injury. Importantly, anxiety levels of even these animals returned to normal at 2 months post-injury (or sham).

These findings suggest that the long-term effects of stress and injury can dissipate. However, epidemiological studies show that traumatic event(s) or repeated stress can result in PTSD, a chronic condition (Woon et al., 2010), although not all individuals exposed to traumatic events develop PTSD (Gross and Hen, 2004; Yehuda and LeDoux, 2007). The neuroanatomical substrates mediating symptom formation in PTSD include the medial PFC, amygdala, and HC (Bremner, 2007; Liberzon and Sripada, 2008). Within the HC, the VHC is predominantly involved in mediating anxiety-related functions while the DHC is involved in learning and memory-associated functions (Henke, 1990; Moser et al., 1995). *In vivo* imaging studies have found correlation between hippocampal volume and susceptibility to PTSD development (Karl et al., 2006). A recent meta-analytic study concluded that hippocampal volume reduction is associated with the exposure to trauma independent of PTSD diagnosis, but additional hippocampal reduction is associated with the development of PTSD compared to the trauma-exposed group without PTSD (Woon et al., 2010). A recent comprehensive *in vivo* imaging study showed that the volume of CA3/DG fields of the HC was significantly reduced in veterans with combat-related PTSD (Wang et al., 2010).

Both genetic and epigenetic factors are suspected in individuals' susceptibility to developing PTSD. These include an abnormal serotonin system and an altered response to CORT (Gross and Hen, 2004). Stress can alter the function of the hypothalamus–pituitary–adrenal axis (HPA), which in turn leads to abnormally elevated levels of CORT (Yehuda, 2006). Chronically elevated levels of CORT, as we observed, can adversely affect the architecture of the HC. However, a recent study found that chronically elevated CORT levels did not reduce cell number but caused a pronounced loss of synapses, suggesting that volume measures can substantially underestimate the effects of CORT on hippocampal structure and importantly on function (Tata et al., 2006; Tata and Anderson, 2010).

The HC, specifically the DHC, is also a critical neuroanatomical substrate of learning and memory (Henke, 1990; Moser and Humpel, 2005); elevated CORT levels can adversely affect memory (Bannerman et al., 2004). Although we found that CORT levels remained elevated even after 2 months in both SS and SI groups, we found that SS animals did not display memory deficits. Previous studies showed that following daily (foot-shock) stress for 14 days, CORT levels were elevated during the first 7 days post-stress, but returned to control levels by day 14 (Kant et al., 1987). However, there have been no studies to our knowledge that measure the long-term (e.g., 2 months) effects of stress on CORT levels.

In contrast to the transient increase in anxiety, we found that memory impairment was both specific to blast injury and also appeared to be a "chronic" condition. In BM, the performance of SS animals was not significantly different from C animals at any given time point, except on day 8 post-injury. Previous behavioral paradigms, in which rats were exposed to another form of predator stress (Diamond et al., 2006) have indicated that stress can have different effects on memory formation and consolidation depending on the time of exposure. Importantly, our data showed that memory impairment was at its highest at 2 months post-injury. These findings suggest that blast injury predominantly affects the DHC as evidenced by impaired spatial memory.

We found an increased number of TUNEL-positive cells in the hilus of the HC but not in the PFC of animals in the SI group at 2 months post-injury. This apparent lasting apoptotic processes after TBI is quite unusual. The limited information available indicates that in other models of TBI apoptotic activity returned to control levels 2 months after injury (Luo et al., 2002). There were no significant differences in the number of TUNEL-positive cells of animals that were exposed to chronic stress only. As discussed above, SS animals had elevated serum CORT levels but showed no increase in the number of TUNEL-positive cells in their HC or PFC. These findings suggest that in addition to elevated CORT levels, other factors like inflammation may be required to sustain the increase in apoptotic cell death.

Our immunohistochemical data showed an increase in Iba1 immunoreactivity in the PFC as well as the HC of SI animals. Within the HC of SI animals, Iba1 immunoreactivity appeared to be higher in the VHC than in the DHC. However, we also found that exposure to stress alone resulted in an increase in hippocampal IL-6 (but not INFγ) levels 2 month after injury (or sham). IL-6 and INFγ are inflammatory cytokines produced by activated microglia and astroglia and are involved in mediating various responses to injury (Morganti-Kossmann et al., 2001, 2002; Nimmo et al., 2004). Depending on the cellular and molecular context, IL-6 can be neurotoxic or can act as a neuroprotectant (Toulmond et al., 1992).

IL-6 can act as a potent inhibitor of *de novo* hippocampal neurogenesis; one of several innate regenerative processes triggered by TBI (Vallieres et al., 2002). After a latency period following TBI, the rate of *de novo* hippocampal neurogenesis increases (Dash et al., 2001; Chirumamilla et al., 2002; Lee and Agoston, 2010). Newborn neurons, marked by DCX expression, migrate from the SGL to the granule cell layer (GCL) where many of the surviving neurons differentiate into granule cells (Altman and Das, 1965; Cameron et al., 1993). We found an apparent increase in DCX positive cells at 2 months after injury in the VHC but not in the DHC of SI rats. Additionally, these cells showed elaborate processes extending well into the DG. Animals in the SS group also showed an increase in DCX immunoreactivity in the VHC but the cells lacked the elaborate processes observed in SI rats. These findings suggest an increase in *de novo* neurogenesis in the VHC in response to stress, but particularly to the combination of stress and blast. This may indicate that increased *de novo* neurogenesis in the VHC is partly responsible for the normalization of anxiety observed at 2 months.

The apparent increase in DCX+ cells in the VHC of SI animals contradict what the Iba1 immunohistochemistry and the IL-6 ELISA data would imply. In addition to chronically elevated CORT levels, elevated hippocampal IL-6 levels and the presence of Iba1+ cells in the HC would imply a decrease or repression in neurogenetic activity as neuroinflammation and elevated CORT levels are known inhibitors of hippocampal *de novo* neurogenesis (Cameron and Gould, 1994; Yu et al., 2004; Montaron et al., 2006); with males showing a greater vulnerability to elevated CORT (Brummelte and Galea, 2010). However, the regulation of *de novo* hippocampal neurogenesis is rather complex; large numbers of molecules are involved and the exact nature of the regulatory process is currently not fully understood (Kempermann and Gage, 2000; Kempermann, 2002). Even though it has been accepted that an increase in DCX+ cells indicates increased *de novo* neurogenesis, DCX is only transiently expressed by *de novo* neurons. Thus, a more detailed BrdU/Prox1 double immunohistochemical and stereological quantification of the histology results is required to determine changes in *de novo* neurogenesis after stress and blast.

One of the positive regulators of *de novo* neurogenesis is VEGF; we and others have found that VEGF is significantly upregulated in various forms of TBI (Jin et al., 2002; Lee and Agoston, 2010) increased VEGF level promotes survival of *de novo* hippocampal neurons by blocking apoptotic cell death (Lee and Agoston, 2010). Consistent with the previous observation, we found that injury and stress, but not stress alone, increases VEGF levels in the HC and also in the PFC. Consistent with the previous observation, we found that injury and stress, but not stress alone, increases VEGF levels in the HC and also in the PFC. Previous studies have demonstrated that an increase in VEGF concentration can also increase vascular permeability as indicated by the breach of the BBB (Dvorak et al., 1995). Interestingly, a recent clinical study has shown that increased serum level of VEGF is indicative of good outcome after ischemic stroke (Sobrino et al., 2009).

We found increased serum levels of several neuronal and glia-specific proteins including NF-H, NSE, CK-BB, and GFAP 2 months post-injury. These molecules have previously been used to assess the extent and the outcome of TBI (Berger, 2006; Korfias et al., 2009). For example, NF-H has been used as a biomarker of neuronal loss and BBB damage and predicting outcome (Anderson et al., 2008). That serum levels of these proteins remain elevated at 2 month after injury suggest ongoing neuronal and glial cell loss as well as a chronically increased BBB permeability in which elevated levels of VEGF may play a role (Ay et al., 2008; Gerstner et al., 2009).

We also found significantly elevated levels of S100β and GFAP in the HC and in the PFC of SI animals. Elevated tissue levels of S100β may indicate astroglial proliferation and overall glial response to injury (Kleindienst et al., 2005). Elevated expression of GFAP by astrocytes, combined with morphological changes (reactive astrogliosis), is a hallmark of CNS neurotrauma (Eng and Ghirnikar, 1994; Fitch and Silver, 2008). We found that the VHC and the DHC appear to have differential expression of stellar GFAP astroglia following exposure to stress only and to the combination stress and injury. The role of increased GFAP immunoreactivity and stellar astroglia in CNS injury is complex. Astrocytic responses can lead to either reparative or detrimental outcomes depending on the type and time after injury (Eng and Ghirnikar, 1994; Fitch and Silver, 2008). However, increasing evidence also indicates a protective role of astrogliosis in reducing the toxic effects of extracellular glutamate and enabling barrier reconstruction after TBI (Buffo et al., 2010). In light of our behavioral findings, showing normalized anxiety levels of SI animals at 2 months post-injury, we speculate that the apparent increase in GFAP positive cells in the VHC may contribute to reparative pathomechanisms and the restoration of normal anxiety levels. Chronic stress has been shown to significantly reduce both the number and somal volume of astroglia in the HC (Czeh et al., 2006). Interestingly, we did see a differential effect of stress alone and stress and injury in the DHC and VHC. While the VHC displayed an apparent increase in GFAP+ cells with stellar processes, the same was not observed in the DHC and memory impairment remained significant 2 months post-injury. A possible explanation for the lasting memory deficits occurring in SI animals is that stress may selectively impair the restorative and/or regenerative action of reactive astrocytes in the DHC. While compelling, the results obtained require further exploration.

In summary, we found that when stressed animals are exposed to a single mild blast overpressure, there are lasting behavioral, molecular, and cellular abnormalities characterized by memory impairment, neuronal and glial cell losses, inflammation, and gliosis. In contrast, stress alone resulted only in a transient increase in anxiety, no memory deficit and no detectable tissue damage. If our findings are independently verified, the potential ramifications can be significant in developing tools to assess the severity and to predict the outcome of psychological and physical traumas.

ACKNOWLEDGMENTS

We thank the Neurotrauma Team (WRAIR) for their technical help during the exposures; Ms. Cara Olsen (USU) for her help in statistical analysis; Drs. Grunberg and Wu (USU) for their input in designing and interpreting the behavioral experiments. The work was supported by CDMRP, grant# W81XWH-08-2-0176.

REFERENCES

Adamec, R. E., Burton, P., Shallow, T., and Budgell, J. (1999). NMDA receptors mediate lasting increases in anxiety like behavior produced by the stress of predator exposure - implications for anxiety associated with posttraumatic stress disorder. *Physiol. Behav.* 65, 723–737.

Adamec, R. E., and Shallow, T. (1993). Lasting effects on rodent anxiety of a single exposure to a cat. *Physiol. Behav.* 54, 101–109.

Adamec, R. E., Shallow, T., and Budgell, J. (1997). Blockade of CCK(B) but not CCK(A) receptors before and after the stress of predator exposure prevents lastingincreasesinanxiety-likebehav- ior:implications foranxietyassociated with posttraumatic stress disorder. *Behav. Neurosci.* 111, 435–449.

Altman, J., and Das, G. D. (1965). Autoradiographic and histological evidence of postnatal hippocampal neurogenesis in rats. *J. Comp. Neurol.* 124, 319–335.

Anderson, K. J., Scheff, S.W., Miller, K. M., Roberts, K. N., Gilmer, L. K., Yang, C., and Shaw, G. (2008). The phospho- rylated axonal form of the neuro- filament subunit NF-H (pNF-H) as a blood biomarker of traumatic brain injury. *J. Neurotrauma* 25, 1079–1085. Armonda, R. A., Bell, R. S., Vo, A. H., Ling, G., Degraba, T. J., Crandall, B., Ecklund, J., and Campbell, W. W. (2006). Wartime traumatic cerebral vasospasm: recent review of combat casualties. *Neurosurgery* 59, 1215–1225; discussion 1225.

Ay, I., Francis, J. W., and Brown, R. H. Jr. (2008). VEGFincreasesblood–brain barrier permeability to Evans blue dye and tetanus toxin fragment C but not adeno-associated virus in ALS mice. *Brain Res.* 1234, 198–205.

Bannerman, D. M., Rawlins, J. N., Mchugh, S. B., Deacon, R. M., Yee, B. K., Bast, T., Zhang, W. N., Pothuizen, H. H., and Feldon, J. (2004). Regional dissociations within the hippocam- pus - memory and anxiety. *Neurosci. Biobehav. Rev.* 28, 273–283.

Barnes,C.A.(1979).Memorydeficitsasso- ciated with senescence: a neurophysiologicalandbehavioralstudyintherat. *J. Comp. Physiol. Psychol.* 93, 74–104. Belanger, H. G., Vanderploeg, R. D.,

Curtiss, G., and Warden, D. L. (2007). Recent neuroimaging techniques in mild traumatic brain injury. *J. Neuropsychiatry Clin.Neurosci.*19,5–20. Berger, R. P. (2006). The use of serum biomarkers to predict outcome after traumatic brain injury in adults and children. *J. Head Trauma Rehabil.* 21, 315–333.

Bremner,J.D.(2007).Functionalneuroim- aginginpost-traumaticstressdisorder. *Expert Rev. Neurother.* 7, 393–405.

Brenner, L. A., Vanderploeg, R. D., and Terrio, H. (2009). Assessment and diagnosis of mild traumatic brain injury, posttraumatic stress disorder, and other polytrauma conditions: burden of adversity hypothesis. *Rehabil. Psychol.* 54, 239–246.

Breslau, N., and Kessler, R. C. (2001). The stressor criterion in DSM-IV post-traumatic stress disorder: an empiri- cal investigation. *Biol. Psychiatry* 50, 699–704.

Brummelte, S., and Galea, L. A. (2010). Chronic high corticosterone reduces neurogenesis in the dentate gyrus of adult male and female rats. *Neuroscience* 168, 680–690.

Bruns, J., and Hauser, W. A. (2003). The epidemiology of traumatic brain injury: areview.*Epilepsia* 44(Suppl.),2. Buffo, A., Rolando, C., and Ceruti, S. (2010). Astrocytes in the damaged brain: molecular and cellular insights into their reactive response and heal- ingpotential. *Biochem. Pharmacol.* 79, 77–89.

Cameron, H. A., and Gould, E. (1994). Adult neurogenesis is regulated by adrenal steroids in the dentate gyrus. *Neuroscience* 61, 203–209.

Cameron, H. A., Woolley, C. S., Mcewen, B. S., and Gould, E. (1993). Differentiation of newly born neurons and glia in the dentate gyrus of the adult rat. *Neuroscience* 56, 337–344.

Campbell, T., Lin, S., Devries, C., and Lambert, K. (2003). Coping strate- gies in male and female rats exposed to multiple stressors. *Physiol. Behav.* 78, 495–504.

Carobrez, A. P., and Bertoglio, L. J. (2005). Ethological and temporal analyses of anxiety-like behavior: the elevated plus-mazemodel 20 yearson.*Neurosci. Biobehav. Rev.* 29, 1193–1205.

Cernak, I., Merkle, A. C., Koliatsos, V. E., Bilik, J. M., Luong, Q. T., Mahota, T. M., Xu, L., Slack, N., Windle, D., and Ahmed, F. A. (2010). The pathobiol- ogy of blast injuries and blast-induced neurotrauma as identified using a new experimental model of injury in mice. *Neurobiol. Dis.* 41, 538–551.

Cernak, I., Wang, Z., Jiang, J., Bian, X., and Savic, J. (2001). Ultrastructural and functional characteristics of blast injury-induced neurotrauma. *J. Trauma.* 50, 695–706.

Chirumamilla, S., Sun, D., Bullock, M. R., and Colello, R. J. (2002). Traumatic brain injury induced cell proliferation intheadultmammaliancentralnervous system. *J. Neurotrauma* 19, 693–703.

Cohen, H., Benjamin, J., Kaplan, Z., and Kotler, M. (2000). Administration of high-dose ketoconazole, an inhibitor of steroid synthesis, preventspposttraumaticanxietyin an animal model. *Eur. Neuropsychopharmacol.* 10, 429–435.

Cohen, H., Friedberg, S., Michael, M., Kotler, M., and Zeev, K. (1996). Interaction of CCK-4 induced anxiety and post-cat exposure anxiety in rats. *Depress. Anxiety* 4, 144–145.

Cohen, H., Zohar, J., and Matar, M. (2003). The relevance of differential response to trauma in an animal model of posttraumatic stress disorder. *Biol. Psychiatry* 53, 463–473.

Czeh, B., Simon, M., Schmelting, B., Hiemke, C., and Fuchs, E. (2006). Astroglial plasticity in the hippocam- pus is affected by chronic psychoso- cial stress and concomitant fluoxetine treatment. *Neuropsychopharmacology* 31, 1616–1626.

Dash, P. K., Mach, S. A., and Moore, A. N. (2001). Enhanced neurogenesis in the rodent hippocampus following traumaticbraininjury. *J. Neurosci. Res.* 63, 313–319.

Diamond, D. M., Campbell, A. M., Park, C. R., Woodson, J. C., Conrad, C. D., Bachstetter, A. D., and Mervis, R. F. (2006). Influence of predator stress on the consolidation versus retrieval of long-term spatial memory and hip- pocampal spinogenesis. *Hippocampus* 16, 571–576.

Doll, H., Truebel, H., Kipfmueller, F., Schaefer, U., Neugebauer, E. A., Wirth, S., and Maegele, M. (2009). Pharyngeal selective brain cooling improves neurofunctional and neurocognitive out- comeafterfluidpercussionbraininjury in rats. *J. Neurotrauma* 26, 235–242.

Dvorak, H. F., Brown, L. F., Detmar, M., and Dvorak, A. M. (1995). Vascular permeability factor/vascular endothe- lial growth factor, microvascular hyperpermeability, and angiogenesis. *Am. J. Pathol.* 146, 1029–1039.

Elliott, B. M., and Grunberg, N. E. (2005). Effects of social and physical enrich- ment on open field activity differ in maleandfemaleSprague-Dawleyrats. *Behav. Brain Res.* 165, 187–196.

Eng, L. F., and Ghirnikar, R. S. (1994). GFAP and astrogliosis. *Brain Pathol.* 4, 229–237.

Fitch, M. T., and Silver, J. (2008). CNSinjury, glialscars,andinflammation:inhibitory extracellularmatricesandregeneration failure. *Exp. Neurol.* 209, 294–301.

Fride, E., Dan, Y., Feldon, J., Halevy, G., and Weinstock, M. (1986). Effects of prenatal stress on vulnerability to stress in prepubertal and adult rats. *Physiol. Behav.* 37, 681–687.

Gerstner, E. R., Duda, D. G., Di Tomaso, E., Ryg, P. A., Loeffler, J. S., Sorensen, A. G., Ivy, P., Jain, R. K., and Batchelor, T. T. (2009). VEGF inhibitors in the treatment of cerebral edema in patients with brain cancer. *Nat. Rev. Clin. Oncol.* 6, 229–236.

Gross, C., and Hen, R. (2004). Geneticand environmental factors interact to influenceanxiety. *Neurotox. Res.* 6, 493–501.

Gyorgy, A. B., Walker, J., Wingo, D., Eidelman, O., Pollard, H. B., Molnar, A., and Agoston, D. V. (2010). Reverse phase protein microarray technology in traumatic brain injury. *J. Neurosci. Methods.* 192, 96–101.

Harrison, F. E., Hosseini, A. H., and Mcdonald, M. P. (2009). Endogenous anxiety and stress responses in water mazeand Barnesmazespatialmemory tasks. *Behav. Brain Res.* 198, 247–251. Heath, D. L., and Vink, R. (1999). Optimization of magnesium therapy after severe diffuse axonal brain injury in rats. *J. Pharmacol. Exp. Ther.* 288, 1311–1316.

Henke, P.G. (1990). Hippocampal pathway to the amygdala and stress ulcer development. *Brain Res. Bull.* 25, 691–695.

Jaffee, M. S., and Meyer, K. S. (2009). A brief overview of traumatic brain injury

(TBI) and post-traumatic stress disorder (PTSD) within the Department of Defense. *Clin. Neuropsychol.* 23, 1291–1298.

Jin, K., Zhu, Y., Sun, Y., Mao, X. O., Xie, L., and Greenberg, D. A. (2002). Vascular endothelial growth factor (VEGF) stimulates neurogenesis in vitro and invivo. *Proc.Natl.Acad.Sci.U.S.A.* 99, 11946–11950.

Kant, G. J., Leu, J. R., Anderson, S. M., and Mougey, E. H. (1987). Effects of chronic stress on plasma corticoster- one, ACTH and prolactin. *Physiol. Behav.* 40, 775–779.

Karl, A., Schaefer, M., Malta, L. S., Dorfel, D., Rohleder, N., and Werner, A. (2006). A meta-analysis of structural brainabnormalitiesin PTSD. *Neurosci. Biobehav. Rev.* 30, 1004–1031.

Kaur, C., Singh, J., Lim, M. K., Ng, B. L., Yap, E. P., and Ling, E. A. (1997). Ultrastructural changes of macroglial cells in theratbrainfollowinganexpo- sure to a non-penetrative blast. *Ann. Acad.Med.Singap.* 26, 27–29.

Keane, T. M., Marshall, A. D., and Taft, C. T. (2006). Posttraumatic stress disorder: etiology, epidemiology, and treatment outcome. *Annu. Rev. Clin. Psychol.* 2, 161–197.

Kempermann, G. (2002). Regulation of adult hippocampal neurogenesis – implicationsfornoveltheoriesof major depression. *BipolarDisord.* 4, 17–33.

Kempermann, G., and Gage, F. H.(2000). Neurogenesis in the adult hippocampus. *Novartis Found. Symp.* 231, 220–235; discussion 235–241, 302–226.

Kleindienst,A.,Mcginn,M.J.,Harvey,H.B.,Colello, R. J., Hamm, R. J., and Bullock, M. R. (2005). Enhanced hippocampal neurogenesisbyintraventricularS100B infusion is associated with improved cognitiverecoveryaftertraumaticbrain injury. *J. Neurotrauma* 22, 645–655.

Korfias,S.,Papadimitriou,A.,Stranjalis,G., Bakoula, C., Daskalakis, G., Antsaklis, A., and Sakas, D. E.(2009). Serum biochemicalmarkersofbrain injury. *Mini Rev. Med. Chem.* 9, 227–234.

Lee, C., and Agoston, D.V. (2010).Vascular endothelial growth factor is involved in mediating increased de novo hippocampal neurogenesis in response to traumaticbraininjury. *J. Neurotrauma* 27, 541–553.

Liberzon, I., and Sripada, C. S.(2008). The functional neuroanatomy of PTSD: a critical review. *Prog. Brain Res.* 167, 151–169.

Ling, G., Bandak, F., Armonda, R., Grant, G., and Ecklund, J. (2009). Explosive blast neurotrauma. *J. Neurotrauma* 26, 815–825.

Ling, G. S., and Ecklund, J. M. (2011). Traumatic brain injury in modern war. *Curr.Opin.Anaesthesiol.* doi: 10.1097/ACO.0b013e32834458da. [Epub ahead of print].

Long, J. B., Bentley, T. L., Wessner, K. A., Cerone, C., Sweeney, S., and Bauman, R. A.(2009). Blast overpressure in rats: recreating a battlefield injury in the laboratory. *J.Neurotrauma* 26, 827–840.

Luo, C., Jiang, J., Lu, Y., and Zhu, C. (2002). Spatialandtemporalprofileofapoptosis following lateral fluid percussion brain injury. *Chin. J. Traumatol.* 5, 24–27.

Maegele, M., Lippert-Gruener, M., EsterBode, T., Sauerland, S., Schafer, U., Molcany, M., Lefering, R., Bouillon, B., Neiss, W. F., Angelov, D. N., Klug, N., Mcintosh, T. K., and Neugebauer, E. A. (2005). Reversal of neuromo- tor and cognitive dysfunction in an enrichedenvironmentcombinedwith multimodal early onset stimulation after traumatic brain injury in rats. *J. Neurotrauma* 22, 772–782.

Mayorga, M. A. (1997). The pathology of primary blast overpressure injury. *Toxicology* 121, 17–28.

Montaron, M. F., Drapeau, E., Dupret, D., Kitchener, P., Aurousseau, C., Le Moal, M., Piazza, P. V., and Abrous, D. N. (2006). Lifelong corticosterone level determines age-related decline in neurogenesisandmemory. *Neurobiol. Aging* 27, 645–654.

Morganti-Kossmann, M. C., Rancan, M., Otto,V. I., Stahel, P. F., and Kossmann, T. (2001). Role of cerebral inflamma- tion after traumatic brain injury: a revisited concept. *Shock* 16, 165–177.

Morganti-Kossmann, M. C., Rancan, M., Stahel, P. F., and Kossmann, T. (2002). Inflammatory response in acutetraumaticbraininjury: adouble- edged sword. *Curr. Opin. Crit. Care* 8, 101–105.

Moser, K. V., and Humpel, C. (2005). Vascular endothelial growth factor counteracts NMDA-induced cell death of adult cholinergic neurons in rat basal nucleus of Meynert. *Brain Res.Bull.* 65, 125–131.

Moser, M. B., Moser, E. I., Forrest, E., Andersen, P., and Morris, R. G.(1995). Spatial learning with a minislab in the dorsalhippocampus. *Proc. Natl.Acad. Sci. U.S.A.* 92, 9697–9701.

Nimmo, A. J., Cernak, I., Heath, D. L., Hu, X., Bennett, C. J., and Vink, R. (2004). Neurogenicinflammationisassociated with development of edema and functionaldeficitsfollowingtraumaticbrain injuryinrats. *Neuropeptides* 38, 40–47.

Okie, S. (2005). Traumatic brain injury in thewarzone. *N. Engl. J. Med.* 352, 2043–2047.

Pynoos, R. S., Ritzmann, R. F., Steinberg, A. M., Goenjian, A., and Prisecaru, I. (1996). A behavioral animal model of posttraumatic stress disorder featuring repeated exposure to situ- ational reminders. *Biol. Psychiatry* 39, 129–134.

Richardson,L.K.,Frueh,B.C.,andAcierno, R. (2010). Prevalence estimates of combat-related post-traumatic stress disorder: critical review. *Aust. N. Z. J. Psychiatry* 44, 4–19.

Ryan, L. M., and Warden, D. L. (2003). Post concussion syndrome. *Int. Rev. Psychiatry* 15, 310–316.

Salzberg, M., Kumar, G., Supit, L., Jones, N. C., Morris, M. J., Rees, S., and O'brien, T. J. (2007). Early postnatal stress confers enduring vulnerability to limbic epileptogenesis. *Epilepsia* 48, 2079–2085.

Sobrino, T.,Arias, S., Rodriguez-Gonzalez, R., Brea, D., Silva, Y., De La Ossa, N. P., Agulla, J., Blanco, M., Pumar, J. M., Serena, J., Davalos, A., and Castillo, J. (2009). High serum levels of growth factors are associated with good outcome in intracerebral hemor- rhage. *J. Cereb. BloodFlowMetab.* 29, 1968–1974.

Taber, K. H., Warden, D. L., and Hurley, R. A. (2006). Blast-related traumatic brain injury: what is known? *J. NeuropsychiatryClin.Neurosci.* 18, 141–145.

Tagliaferri, F., Compagnone, C., Korsic, M., Servadei, F., and Kraus, J. (2006).A systematic review of brain injury epi- demiology in Europe. *Acta Neurochir. (Wien)* 148, 255–268.

Tata, D. A., and Anderson, B. J. (2010). The effects of chronic glucocorticoid exposure on dendritic length, synapse numbers and glial volume in animal models: implications for hippocam- pal volume reductions in depression. *Physiol. Behav.* 99, 186–193.

Tata, D.A., Marciano,V.A., and Anderson, B. J. (2006). Synapse loss from chroni- cally elevated glucocorticoids: rela- tionship to neuropil volume and cell number in hippocampal area CA3. *J. Comp. Neurol.* 498, 363–374.

Toulmond, S., Vige, X., Fage, D., and Benavides, J. (1992). Local infusion of interleukin-6 attenuates the neurotoxic effects of NMDA on rat striatal cholinergic neurons. *Neurosci. Lett.* 144, 49–52.

Vallieres, L., Campbell, I. L., Gage, F. H., and Sawchenko, P. E. (2002). Reduced hippocampal neurogenesis in adult transgenic mice with chronic astro- cytic production of interleukin-6. *J. Neurosci.* 22, 486–492.

Vink, R., O'Connor, C. A., Nimmo, A. J., and Heath, D. L. (2003). Magnesium attenuates persistent functional defi- cits following diffuse traumatic brain injury in rats. *Neurosci. Lett.* 336, 41–44.

von Horsten, S., Exton, M. S., Voge, J., Schult, M., Nagel, E., Schmidt, R. E., Westermann, J., and Schedlowski, M. (1998). Cyclosporine A affects open field behavior in DA rats. *Pharmacol. Biochem. Behav.* 60, 71–76.

Walf,A.A., and Frye, C.A.(2007). The use of the elevated plus maze as an assay of anxiety-related behavior in rodents. *Nat. Protoc.* 2, 322–328.

Wang, Z., Neylan, T. C., Mueller, S. G., Lenoci,M.,Truran,D.,Marmar,C. R., Weiner, M. W., and Schuff, N. (2010). Magnetic resonance imaging of hip- pocampal subfields in posttraumatic stress disorder. *Arch. Gen. Psychiatry* 67, 296–303.

Warden, D. (2006). Military TBI during the Iraq and Afghanistan wars. *J. Head Trauma Rehabil.* 21, 398–402.

Warden, D. L., and French, L. (2005). Traumatic brain injury in the war zone. *N.Engl.J.Med.* 353, 633–634.

Warden,D.L.,Labbate,L.A.,Salazar,A.M., Nelson, R., Sheley, E., Staudenmeier, J., and Martin, E. (1997). Posttraumatic stress disorder in patients with trau- matic brain injury and amnesia for the event? *J. Neuropsychiatry Clin. Neurosci.* 9, 18–22.

Weinstock, M., Matlina, E., Maor, G. I., Rosen, H., and Mcewen, B. S. (1992). Prenatal stress selectively alters the reactivity of the hypothalamic-pitu- itary adrenal system in the female rat. *Brain Res.* 595, 195–200.

Woon, F. L., Sood, S., and Hedges, D. W. (2010). Hippocampal volume deficits associated with exposure to psycho- logical trauma and posttraumatic stress disorder in adults: a meta-anal- ysis. *Prog. Neuropsychopharmacol. Biol. Psychiatry* 34, 1181–1188.

Yehuda,R.(2006).Advances inunderstand- ingneuroendocrinealterationsin PTSD andtheirtherapeuticimplications. *Ann. N. Y.Acad. Sci.* 1071, 137–166.

Yehuda, R., and LeDoux, J. (2007). Response variation following trauma: a translational neuroscience approach to understanding PTSD. *Neuron* 56, 19–32.

Yu, I. T., Lee, S. H., Lee, Y. S., and Son, H. (2004). Differential effects of corticosteroneanddexamethasoneonhippoc ampal neurogenesis in vitro. *Biochem. Biophys. Res. Commun.* 317, 484–490..

APPENDIX

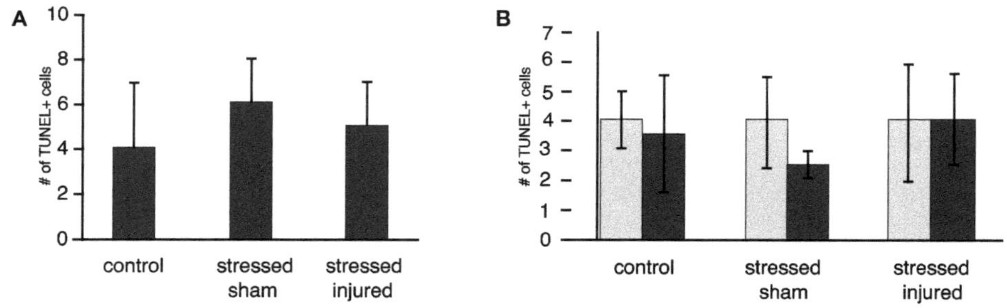

FIGURE A1 | TUNEL-positive cells in selected brain regions of animals in the various experimental groups. Frozen coronal sections containing the **(A)** PFC and **(B)** DG of the DHC and VHC of C, SS, and SI rats were counted and expressed as positive cells per unit area ± SEM. *$p < 0.05$ and **$p < 0.01$ compared to C rats.

21

Frontal lobe neurology and the creative mind

Leonardo C. de Souza[1], Henrique C. Guimarães[1], Antônio L. Teixeira[1], Paulo Caramelli[1], Richard Levy[2,3,4,5,6], Bruno Dubois[2,3,4,5,7] and Emmanuelle Volle[2,3,4,5]*

[1] Neuropsychiatric Branch, Neurology Division, University Hospital, Universidade Federal de Minas Gerais, Belo Horizonte, Brazil
[2] Inserm, U 1127, ICM Frontlab, Paris, France
[3] CNRS, UMR 7225, ICM Frontlab, Paris, France
[4] Sorbonne Universités, UPMC Univ Paris 06, UMR S 1127, Paris, France
[5] Institut du Cerveau et de la Moelle épinière, ICM Frontlab, Paris, France
[6] AP-HP, Hôpital Saint-Antoine, Service de Neurologie, Paris, France
[7] AP-HP, Hôpital de la Salpêtrière, Neurology Department, Institut de la Mémoire et de la Maladie d'Alzheimer, Paris, France

Edited by:
Anna Abraham, Kuwait University, Kuwait

Reviewed by:
Hugues Duffau, Montpellier University Medical Center and INSERM U1051, France
Dahlia Zaidel, University of California, USA

***Correspondence:**
Emmanuelle Volle, ICM Research Center, Hôpital Pitié Salpêtrière, 47, bd de l'hôpital, 75013 Paris, France
e-mail: emmavolle@gmail.com

Concepts from cognitive neuroscience strongly suggest that the prefrontal cortex (PFC) plays a crucial role in the cognitive functions necessary for creative thinking. Functional imaging studies have repeatedly demonstrated the involvement of PFC in creativity tasks. Patient studies have demonstrated that frontal damage due to focal lesions or neurodegenerative diseases are associated with impairments in various creativity tasks. However, against all odds, a series of clinical observations has reported the facilitation of artistic production in patients with neurodegenerative diseases affecting PFC, such as frontotemporal dementia (FTD). An exacerbation of creativity in frontal diseases would challenge neuroimaging findings in controls and patients, as well as the theoretical role of prefrontal functions in creativity processes. To explore this paradox, we reported the history of a FTD patient who exhibited the emergence of visual artistic productions during the course of the disease. The patient produced a large amount of drawings, which have been evaluated by a group of professional artists who were blind to the diagnosis. We also reviewed the published clinical cases reporting a change in the artistic abilities in patients with neurological diseases. We attempted to reconcile these clinical observations to previous experimental findings by addressing several questions raised by our review. For instance, to what extent can the cognitive, conative, and affective changes following frontal damage explain changes in artistic abilities? Does artistic exacerbation truly reflect increased creative capacities? These considerations could help to clarify the place of creativity—as it has been defined and explored by cognitive neuroscience—in artistic creation and may provide leads for future lesion studies.

Keywords: creativity, prefrontal cortex, frontotemporal dementia, artistic, divergent thinking

Beyond its cultural, aesthetic or artistic aspects, creativity can be defined from a neuroscientific perspective as "the ability to produce a work that is both original (new, unusual, novel, unexpected) and valuable (useful, good, adaptive, appropriate)" (Sternberg and Lubart, 1999; Dietrich, 2004). Creative thinking usually involves the ability to break with conventional well-established ideas and to develop alternative behaviors in new and unexpected situations. In this sense, creativity may be considered to be a particular form of adaptation or problem solving (Runco, 2004; Sternberg, 2006). In this theoretical view, creativity relies on fundamental cognitive processes such as working memory, attention, planning, cognitive flexibility, mentalizing, and abstract thinking (Carlsson et al., 2000; Dietrich, 2004; Bogousslavsky, 2005; Changeux, 2005). These functions depend largely on the integrity of the prefrontal cortex (PFC), a brain region that is essential for behavioral adaptation and highly integrated mental functions. Functional neuroimaging data in healthy subjects also show that the PFC plays an important role in the cognitive processes involved in creativity (Gonen-Yaacovi et al., 2013). Therefore, both cognitive theories and neuroimaging data suggest that the integrity of the PFC is essential for creative thinking, and that neurological diseases that damage PFC regions (or their connections) would affect cognitive creativity processes. Some experimental studies have indeed demonstrated the impairment of creativity after prefrontal damage (Rankin et al., 2007; de Souza et al., 2010; Shamay-Tsoory et al., 2011; Abraham et al., 2012).

However, in contrast with these theories and experiments, a series of clinical observations reports the facilitation of artistic abilities in some patients with neurodegenerative disease affecting the frontal lobes, raising the question of a possible increased creativity following frontal damage (Palmiero et al., 2012; Schott, 2012; Gretton and ffytche, 2014). An exacerbation of creativity in neurological diseases affecting the frontal lobes would question the role of the PFC in creativity.

Herein, we propose that cognitive aspects of creativity depend on the integrity of PFC subregions and we hypothesize that some of these contradictory data may be reconciled by considering the repercussion of frontal symptoms into the patients' production, by taking into account affective and conative aspects of creativity, and by comparing the artistic and neuroscientific perspectives of creativity. This discussion will be illustrated using a clinical case of artistic production during the course of the behavioral variant frontotemporal dementia (bvFTD).

PREFRONTAL FUNCTIONS AND CREATIVITY

The PFC is highly developed in humans and plays a crucial role in elaborating and controlling voluntary and goal-directed behaviors, expanding behavior far beyond the sole repertoire of automatic and reflexive actions. The PFC enables adaptive behavior according to one's own objectives and to the context while taking into account past experiences and needs (Goldman-Rakic, 1995; Shallice and Burgess, 1996; Fuster et al., 2000; Miller and Cohen, 2001; Levy and Volle, 2009; Volle et al., 2013). This central role in adaptive behavior is supported by intense connections between the PFC and other brain regions (Dubois et al., 1995; Mesulam, 1998). The strong connective properties of this region suggest that the PFC is involved in integrating or combining different types of information according to the task goal. The PFC is connected with the sensory systems involved in perception, enabling access to information about the current environment. The PFC receives information about past events and knowledge though connections to long-term memory circuits. The PFC is also part of the limbic system and receives information on the individual needs, emotions, and motivations (Schoenbaum et al., 2009; Fellows, 2013) to guide decisions. The PFC interacts with motor systems that program, perform and monitor the plan of actions (Catani and Thiebaut de Schotten, 2012; Yeterian et al., 2012; Cole et al., 2013; Rojkova et al., under revision). Thus, the PFC can be considered to be a convergence hub that enables the integration of different types of information and the formation of mental representations of both the external and inner worlds (Ramnani and Owen, 2004; Reynolds et al., 2006; Nee et al., 2013) that can guide more sophisticated patterns of behavior.

Furthermore, the connections between the PFC and other brain regions are usually reciprocal, enabling the PFC to exert control over other brain systems, in addition to receiving information. For instance, control signals over the action system may inhibit actions that would not be suitable in a given context, and control over perceptual systems enables the selection of relevant information in the environment (Picton et al., 2007; Levy and Wagner, 2011; Volle et al., 2012). The supervisory role of the PFC also allows the selection and the voluntary retrieval of information in memory (Martin and Cheng, 2006; Thompson-Schill and Botvinick, 2006; Badre and Wagner, 2007; Strenziok et al., 2013). Several recent models describe a hierarchical postero-anterior organization of the control functions that are exerted by PFC in which an increased control requirement for behavioral adaptation recruits more anterior PFC subregions (Koechlin et al., 2003; Koechlin and Hyafil, 2007; Azuar et al., 2014). Other models also describe a posteroanterior PFC gradient in the abstraction degree of the mental representations that can be formed; more anterior regions support more abstract thinking (Christoff et al., 2001, 2009; Badre and Wagner, 2007; Volle et al., 2010).

Overall, the PFC enables the formation and control of mental representations according to an internal goal by selecting information from the environment or from memory, by forming or selecting rules, and by resisting spontaneous prepotent responses (Levy and Volle, 2009). These prefrontal properties are assumed to support creativity as well as complex human abilities such as planning, reasoning, problem solving, abstract thinking (Carlsson et al., 2000; Godefroy, 2003; Dietrich, 2004; Bogousslavsky, 2005; Changeux, 2005; Burgess et al., 2009; Levy and Volle, 2009). In other words, our knowledge of PFC structure and functions supports the assumption that the PFC is essential for cognitive processes that underlie creative thinking. Experimental studies using creativity tasks in healthy participants and in patients confirm this hypothesis.

EXPERIMENTAL STUDIES ON THE NEURAL CORRELATES OF CREATIVITY

FUNCTIONAL NEUROIMAGING APPROACH: A ROLE FOR THE FPC IN CREATIVITY

Functional imaging studies have attempted to explore the cerebral bases of creativity processes using various experimental tasks (see Arden et al., 2010; Dietrich and Kanso, 2010; Jung, 2013 for reviews). Some studies relied on ecological tasks attempting to imitate creativity in real life, but most of them employed tasks drawn from theoretical cognitive models. Studies with a more ecological approach used tasks such as story writing (Bechtereva et al., 2004; Howard-Jones et al., 2005; Shah et al., 2013), object design (Kowatari et al., 2009; Ellamil et al., 2012), or music improvisation (Bengtsson et al., 2007; Berkowitz and Ansari, 2008; Limb and Braun, 2008; de Manzano and Ullen, 2012).

Among the studies based on theory-based creativity tasks, the most frequent framework used to examine the brain correlates of creativity was the divergent thinking approach (Runco and Acar, 2012). Divergent thinking tests typically require generating the maximal number of new or unusual responses. One of the classical divergent thinking tasks is the *Alternate Uses task*, which assesses the ability to produce many alternative uses of a common object such as a brick.

Another approach, which was proposed by Mednick (Mednick, 1962; Mednick et al., 1964), considers that creativity results from "the forming of associative elements into new combinations, which either meet specified requirements or are in some way useful. The more mutually remote the elements of the new combination, the more creative the process or solution." One experimental task to test this hypothesis is to present three unrelated words without obvious connections between them (e.g., stain, glass, and red), and to ask the subject to find a fourth word that is related to each of these words (e.g., wine) (Jung-Beeman et al., 2004; Kounios et al., 2006). This task has been mainly used to investigate the phenomenon of "insight" or "Aha!" or "Eureka" (Kounios et al., 2006). "Aha" describes a subjective experience that occurs when solving a problem for which the solution suddenly comes to mind without effort or difficulty and is associated with a feeling of pleasure and confidence (Luo et al., 2004; Aziz-Zadeh et al., 2009; Qiu et al., 2010; Tian et al., 2011). This "Aha" experience is the cornerstone of another approach in creativity studies, that of problem solving with insight. Problems that raise an insight phenomenon include statements with strong implicit constraints that guide the search for a solution in the incorrect direction. The solution to these problems requires breaking these constraints and implicit associations and opening the search space to more possibilities. According to the classical model from Wallas (Kozbelt, 2011), this element is part of a creative process that follows four stages. Insight follows a preparation and an incubation phases and is followed by a verification phase. For many authors, the creative process is not this linear but instead alternates between phases of idea generation, evaluation, and the selection of ideas (Changeux, 2005; Simonton, 2010; Ward and Kolomyts, 2010; Ellamil et al., 2012).

A recent coordinate-based meta-analysis (Gonen-Yaacovi et al., 2013) using GingerALE free software (Eickhoff et al., 2012; http:www.brainmap.org/ale/) reviewed the published data regarding the investigation of the neural basis of creative thinking in functional neuroimaging studies. This study included 34 articles reporting 44 different experiments that employed the different creative paradigms aforementioned, i.e., divergent thinking tasks (Seger et al., 2000; Howard-Jones et al., 2005; Asari et al., 2008; Fink et al., 2009, 2010; Chrysikou and Thompson-Schill, 2011; Abraham et al., 2012; Ellamil et al., 2012; Kröger et al., 2012; Rutter et al., 2012) combination tasks and problem solving (Jung-Beeman et al., 2004; Luo et al., 2004; Geake and Hansen, 2005; Vartanian and Goel, 2005; Kounios et al., 2006; Mashal et al., 2007; Siebörger et al., 2007; Aziz-Zadeh et al., 2009; Qiu et al., 2010; Tian et al., 2011; Aziz-Zadeh et al., 2012; Cardillo et al., 2012; Green et al., 2012; Huang et al., 2013), as well as ecological tasks attempting to capture real life creativity instead of hypothesized cognitive processes (Bechtereva et al., 2004; Howard-Jones et al., 2005; Bengtsson et al., 2007; Berkowitz and Ansari, 2008; Limb and Braun, 2008; Kowatari et al., 2009; Ellamil et al., 2012; de Manzano and Ullen, 2012; Shah et al., 2013).

Despite the diversity of tasks used in these studies, the results showed a common set of brain regions as the neural basis of creative thinking, including multiple areas within the PFC and regions involved in semantic memory (the temporo-parietal region and posterior temporal and antero-lateral temporal cortex).

Additionally, this meta-analysis showed that distinct prefrontal subregions support distinct cognitive creativity processing. More specifically, tasks based on divergent thinking (to imagine alternative uses of objects or new designs) and those requiring the combination of information (to compose a sentence with unrelated words or to combine different figures to produce a new one, e.g.) were associated with both common and distinct prefrontal areas. Caudal lateral PFC was involved in both task categories, while more anterior PFC areas appear to be more task-oriented. For instance, within the frontal pole, the lateral part was more related to combination tasks, while its medial portion was engaged in divergent thinking tasks.

Together, these findings underlie the importance of PFC in creativity and suggest that different processes involved in creative thinking rely on distinct subregions within the PFC, in particular along the posterior-anterior axis and the medial-lateral axis. If PFC subregions are involved in creativity tasks, as suggested by functional imaging, one expects that damage to these areas would provoke impairment in the same tasks.

EXPERIMENTAL PATIENT STUDIES: DECREASED CREATIVITY AFTER PREFRONTAL DAMAGE

Whether PFC regions are critical to creativity has been explored in very few patient studies. Creative thinking has been studied in patients with focal brain lesions (Shamay-Tsoory et al., 2011; Abraham et al., 2012) and in one of the most frequent causes of frontal damage: frontotemporal dementia (FTD) (Rankin et al., 2007; de Souza et al., 2010). FTD is a neurodegenerative disease and the second most common cause of dementia in patients under 65 years of age. FTD encompasses three different clinical syndromes: the behavioral variant (bvFTD) and the language variants, i.e., progressive non-fluent aphasia and semantic dementia (SD).

de Souza et al. (2010) investigated creativity in patients with bvFTD, using a standardized test of divergent thinking, the Torrance Test of Creative Thinking (TTCT; Torrance, 2004). The TTCT includes both verbal and figurative tasks. TTCT establishes objective criteria to measure creative production, by scoring three main aspects: (1) the fluency, i.e., the total number of responses, (2) the flexibility, i.e., the number of different categories to which the responses belong, and (3) originality, which is the number of new responses, here considered as responses that are statistically infrequent. Fluency and flexibility are usually defined as executive functions and are classically assessed in neuropsychological testing. The results from de Souza and colleagues showed that bvFTD patients performed worse than controls (a normal and a pathological control group) in all dimensions of the TTCT (fluency, flexibility, and originality) for both figurative and verbal tasks. bvFTD patients had also impaired performance in frontal functions such as flexibility, inhibition, abstraction and planning. These findings are consistent with previous data demonstrating that bvFTD patients have impairments in the production of new ideas either in an ecological task of artistic drawing or on the TTCT (Rankin et al., 2007). This study also showed that behavioral disorders such as perseverations and behavioral disinhibition (often sexual) could partly account for the "originality" of frontal patients in their responses in TTCT. In other words, some of the production features may be considered to be manifestations of the behavioral disorders that characterize bvFTD; these were not observed in the control subjects.

In this study, brain correlates of creative abilities were also explored in bvFTD patients, and perfusion in prefrontal regions measured using SPECT correlated with creativity performance at the TTCT (de Souza et al., 2010). More interestingly, there was a clear concordance among the regions reported in this study and those observed in functional neuroimaging studies in healthy subjects (Gonen-Yaacovi et al., 2013), in particular in the left inferior frontal gyrus [BA 47], the left posterior inferior and middle temporal gyri [BA 37], the left inferior parietal lobule [BA39/40], and the left precuneus [BA 23].

Focal prefrontal lesions also impact creative thinking, as demonstrated by two recent lesion studies that examined the consequences of focal brain damage (such as stroke) on creative performance (Shamay-Tsoory et al., 2011; Abraham et al., 2012). Shamay-Tsoory et al. (2011) compared patients' performance on the TTCT according to distinct lesion locations: frontal pole, posterior part of the PFC, or outside the PFC. The results showed that damage to the frontal pole was specifically associated with a deficit at the TTCT. More especially, the originality criterion was the most compromised, and patients with damage to the frontal pole were less original in their response than other patients. Abraham et al. (2012) used several creativity tests in patients with various lesion locations and showed that patients with lateral frontal damage were impaired in both fluency and originality aspects of divergent thinking tasks.

Taken together, these data supports the critical role of PFC in creative thinking. From a cognitive perspective, cerebral findings from patient studies agree with functional neuroimaging results (Carlsson et al., 2000; Seger et al., 2000; Bechtereva et al., 2004; Jung-Beeman et al., 2004; Goel and Vartanian, 2005; Howard-Jones et al., 2005; Asari et al., 2008; Aziz-Zadeh et al., 2009; Fink et al., 2009, 2010; Kowatari et al., 2009). These findings are also consistent with studies that used SPECT (Chavez-Eakle et al., 2007), voxel-based morphometry (Jung et al., 2010b; Takeuchi et al., 2010a; Gansler et al., 2011), and diffusion tensor imaging (Jung et al., 2010a; Takeuchi et al., 2010b).

However, against all odds, a series of medical observations have reported the facilitation of artistic abilities in patients with damage to the frontal lobes (Palmiero et al., 2012; Schott, 2012).

CLINICAL OBSERVATIONS OF CREATIVITY IN NEUROLOGICAL PATIENTS

The description of patients developing artistic abilities raises the question of enhanced creativity following frontal damage, which would challenge the neuroimaging findings in controls and patients and the theoretical role of prefrontal functions in creativity processing. To better understand the relationships between frontal damage, frontal functions, artistic ability, and creativity, we performed a mini-review of published articles reporting changes in artistic production by neurological patients.

A MINI-REVIEW OF MEDICAL REPORTS ON CREATIVITY

We actively searched the *PubMed database* for previous medical reports of changes in artistic skills in neurological patients. Unlike experimental studies on creativity that were usually based on various experimental tasks using objective measures and more instructed tasks, these clinical reports were based on a subjective evaluation of spontaneous patients' productions in the artistic domain. We used the following key-words terms: "dementia, frontotemporal+dementia, Alzheimer's+disease, semantic+dementia, or stroke" AND "creativity, artistry, or artist." We looked for articles published until March 2014. We also included articles cited in previous reviews on creativity in patients (Palmiero et al., 2012; Schott, 2012; Gretton and ffytche, 2014). We did not include Parkinson disease, as artistic facilitation in this condition may most likely relate to the dopa medication rather than to the brain damage itself (Lhommee et al., 2014). The papers found throughout this research were evaluated for relevance and duplicate cases were excluded.

We found 35 relevant papers reporting the degradation, emergence, preservation or improvement of creative expression in 53 patients after the onset of different neurological diseases (see **Table 1**): 19 patients with temporal variant FTD (semantic dementia), 10 patients with behavioral variant FTD, eight patients with Alzheimer's disease, four patients with primary progressive non-fluent aphasia, and 12 patients with various neurological diseases (Espinel, 1996; Miller et al., 1998, 2000; Crutch et al., 2001; Thomas-Anterion et al., 2002, 2010; Kleiner-Fisman et al., 2003; Mell et al., 2003; Mendez and Perryman, 2003; Annoni et al., 2005; Fornazzari, 2005; Lythgoe et al., 2005; Serrano et al., 2005; Chatterjee et al., 2006; Drago et al., 2006a,b; Budrys et al., 2007; Finney and Heilman, 2007; Midorikawa et al., 2008; Seeley et al., 2008; Liu et al., 2009; Thomas-Anterion, 2009; Chakravarty, 2011; Chatterjee et al., 2011; van Buren et al., 2013; Galarza et al., 2014; Takahata et al., 2014). All reported patients with temporal FTD ($n = 19$) presented the emergence ($n = 11$), increase ($n = 2$), or preservation ($n = 6$) of creative production but no degradation of artistic abilities (Miller et al., 1996, 1998; Edwards-Lee et al., 1997; Drago et al., 2006b; Wu et al., 2013). Most case reports on behavioral variant FTD ($n = 10$) noted the emergence ($n = 4$), increase ($n = 4$), or preservation ($n = 1$) of artistic abilities (Miller et al., 1998; Thomas-Anterion et al., 2002; Mendez and Perryman, 2003; Serrano et al., 2005; Liu et al., 2009; Thomas-Anterion, 2009). The effects of Alzheimer's disease on artistic production were more heterogeneous, with observations of both increase (Fornazzari, 2005; Chakravarty, 2011) and degradation (Cummings and Zarit, 1987; Crutch et al., 2001; Serrano et al., 2005; van Buren et al., 2013). Other neurological degenerative diseases or strokes of various locations were associated with heterogeneous profiles (Annoni et al., 2005; Lythgoe et al., 2005; Thomas-Anterion et al., 2010; Takahata et al., 2014). The cognitive, behavioral, and artistic changes reported in the reviewed studies are synthetized in **Table 2**.

This non-systematic review highlights that some FTD patients develop enhanced artistic abilities and suggests that the relations between FTD, frontal functions, artistic abilities and creativity are unclear, as discussed below. We first would like to illustrate the paradoxical relationship between frontal symptoms and creativity by reporting the clinical observation of a patient who developed artistic abilities during the course of bvFTD. This is a new clinical case (unpublished original data) that will be discussed in conjunction with the other reviewed findings.

CLINICAL VIGNETTE

Mrs. YCFZ (case number 963564), a retired dentist secretary aged 83 years, was evaluated in October 2010 in the Cognitive and Behavioral Neurology Unit of the Clinics Hospital from the Federal University of Minas Gerais (Belo Horizonte, Brazil). She was referred to the unit for the evaluation of behavioral and cognitive symptoms that had been evolving for approximately 2 years. Her preceding medical history was unremarkable, except for systemic hypertension, which was well controlled.

The family reported that the patient demonstrated striking behavioral changes. She was progressively uninterested in previously appreciated household chores, and she narrowed her usual cooking repertoire, abandoning the preparation of traditional dishes from her native country, El Salvador. Increased appetite manifested as a troublesome binge eating cookies. Additionally, the patient became progressively less concerned with personal grooming. The patient developed a new stereotyped and fixed routine. For example, she started to eat one banana every day at

Table 1 | Synthesis of published articles reporting changes in artistic creativity in neurological patients.

Author and year	Diagnosis	Neuroimaging data	Change in abilities	Previous interest in Art?	Art domain	Neuropsychological data
Miller et al., 1998, 2000 (Pt 3)	Frontal FTD	SPECT: bifrontal and temporal hypoperfusion (right > left)	E	Occasionally produced novels (not a professional)	Photo	MMSE = 26/30 Preserved language and constructions Impaired executive tests (WCST, Stroop, TMT) Behavioral disinhibition and compulsions
Thomas-Anterion et al., 2002 and Thomas-Anterion, 2009	Frontal FTD	CT scan: frontotemporal atrophy SPECT: frontal hypoperfusion	E	No	Drawing	Language and memory impairment Impaired executive tests Emotional difficulties Apathy Stereotypies
Mendez and Perryman, 2003 (Pt 1)	Frontal FTD	MRI: frontotemporalatrophy PET-FDG: Bifrontal and right temporal hypometabolism	I	Yes (professional graphic artist)	Drawing	MMSE = 22/30 Preserved language, face processing and visuospatial tests Decreased verbal fluency Concrete interpretation of proverbs Compulsions and hoarding Poor insight
Mendez and Perryman, 2003 (Pt 2)	Frontal FTD	MRI: normal SPECT: Bifrontal and right temporal hypoperfusion	I	Yes (professional photographer and graphic designer)	Drawing	MMSE = 23/30 Preserved visuospatial and face processing tests Decreased verbal fluency, executive functions and memory Difficulties with proverbs Inappropriate social behaviors and compulsions Loss of insight
Mendez and Perryman, 2003 (Pt 3)	Frontal FTD	MRI: frontotemporal atrophy SPECT: Frontal and right anterior temporal hypoperfusion	I	Occasionally caricatures (not a professional)	Drawing	MMSE 20/30 Preserved visuospatial and face processing tests Decreased verbal fluency and memory Difficulties with similarities and proverbs Poor insight Compulsions Disinhibited behaviors, impulsivity
Mendez and Perryman, 2003 (Pt 4)	Frontal FTD	MRI: frontotemporal atrophy SPECT: Bifrontal and bitemporal hypoperfusion	P	Yes (professional artist)	Not specified	MMSE 23/30 Preserved visuospatial and face processing tests Decreased verbal fluency Good proverb interpretation Disinhibition of personal behavior Compulsive behaviors
Serrano et al., 2005 (Pt 3)	Frontal FTD	MRI: normal SPECT: Left fronto-temporoparietal hypoperfusion	I	Yes (painter)	Painting	Impaired language skills Impaired executive tests (TMT, spans) Preserved performance on similarity test Compulsive behaviors

(Continued)

Table 1 | Continued

Author and year	Diagnosis	Neuroimaging data	Change in abilities	Previous interest in Art?	Art domain	Neuropsychological data
Liu et al., 2009	Frontal FTD (a)	MRI: atrophy in bilateral anterior and left lateral frontal regions.	E	No	Painting Sculpture	MMSE 28/30 Preserved visuospatial skills Impaired executive tests Abstraction difficulties Lack of emotion, empathy and insight Impaired verbal memory and semantic Antisocial and compulsive behaviors Paintings contain sexual disinhibition Obsessions about art and dots and stripes
Thomas-Anterion, 2009 (Pt 2)	Frontal FTD	No imaging data	E	No	Drawing Poetry	No neuropsychological data Obsession about art
Budrys et al., 2007	Frontal FTD (b)	MRI: bilateral frontotemporal atrophy	D	Yes (professional artist)	Painting	MMSE 25/30 Aphasia and amnesia Difficulties on abstract reasoning Verbal and writing perseverations
Edwards-Lee et al., 1997 (Pt LTLV 1) and Miller et al., 2000	Temporal FTD	MRI: bitemporal atrophy, SPECT: Bitemporal hypoperfusion	P	Yes (pianist)	Music	MMSE = 1/30 Preserved attentional and visuospatial skills Impaired executive tests (Stroop, TMT) Compulsive behaviors
Edwards-Lee et al., 1997 (Pt LTLV 3) and Miller et al., 2000	Temporal FTD	MRI: left temporal lobe atrophy SPECT: Left temporal hypoperfusion	P	Yes	"Artistic skills"	MMSE 26/30 Preserved visuospatial skills Semantic anomia Memory impairment
Edwards-Lee et al., 1997 (Pt LTLV 5) and Miller et al., 2000	Temporal FTD	MRI: generalized atrophy SPECT: Bitemporal hypoperfusion	E	No	Painting	MMSE = 15/30 Preserved visuospatial skills Executive tests markedly impaired (TMT, Stroop, verbal fluency) Anomic aphasia and impaired memory
Miller et al., 1998 and 2000	Temporal FTD (c)	SPECT: bitemporal (Left > right) and mild left frontal hypoperfusion	E	No	Painting drawing	MMSE = 16/30 Preserved visuospatial skills Letter fluency = 2 Perseverations on executive tests Disinhibition and compulsive behavior
Miller et al., 1998	Temporal FTD	No imaging data	E	No	Painting	No neuropsychological data Disinhibition in language.
Miller et al., 1998 and 2000	Temporal FTD	MRI: bifrontal and left temporal atrophy SPECT: Left frontal and bitemporal hypoperfusion	I	Yes	Sculpture	MMSE = 9/30 Mild deficit in visuospatial tests Decreased verbal fluency Impaired memory and naming Disinhibition and compulsive behavior

(Continued)

Table 1 | Continued

Author and year	Diagnosis	Neuroimaging data	Change in abilities	Previous interest in Art?	Art domain	Neuropsychological data
Miller et al., 1998 and 1998 (also in Miller et al., 1996 and Edwards-Lee et al., 1997 Patient RTLV 4)	Temporal FTD	MRI: bitemporal atrophy SPECT: Bilateral temporal hypoperfusion	E	No	Painting	MMSE = 15/30 Fluent verbal output, with semantic anomia Letter fluency = 2 Disinhibition and compulsive behavior
Midorikawa et al., 2008 (Pt 1)	Temporal FTD	MRI: left temporal atrophy	E	No	Painting	Language deficits (semantic deficits) Abnormal behaviors (intrusiveness, repetitive actions)
Midorikawa et al., 2008 (Pt 2)	Temporal FTD	MRI: left temporal atrophy	E	No	Painting	Language deficits (semantic deficits)
Miller et al., 2000 (Pt 1)	Temporal FTD	SPECT: bitemporal, left greater than right, hypoperfusion with frontal sparing	P	Yes (previous inventor)	Inventor	MMSE = 21/30 Boston naming test: 1/60 Normal on Rey Complex Figure Disinhibited behavior
Miller et al., 2000 (Pt 2)	Temporal FTD	MRI: focal left temporal atrophy SPECT: bitemporal, left greater than right, hypoperfusion with frontal sparing	P	Yes (previous bridge)	Bridge	MMSE = 25/30 Normal on Wisconsin Card Sort Test Normal visual reproduction abilities Intact social skills
Miller et al., 2000 (Pt 3)	Temporal FTD	SPECT: bitemporal hypoperfusion with frontal sparing	P	Yes (previous inventor)	Inventor	MMSE = 22/30 Boston naming test: 16/60 Apathy
Miller et al., 2000 (Pt 4)	Temporal FTD	SPECT: bitemporal, left greater than right, hypoperfusion with frontal sparing	E	No	Music	MMSE = 17/30 Boston naming test: 4/60 Normal visual reproduction abilities Personality changes (childlike, euphoric) Compulsive behavior
Miller et al., 2000 (Pt 5)	Temporal FTD	SPECT: moderate left temporal and mild left frontal hypoperfusion	E	No	Music	MMSE = 25/30 Decreased verbal output
Miller et al., 2000 (Pt 6)	Temporal FTD	Positron emission tomography showed left anterior hypometabolism	P	Yes (music)	Music	MMSE = 15/30 Fluent speech with perseverations
Drago et al., 2006a	Temporal FTD	MRI: anterior bitemporal atrophy	I	Yes (visual artist)	Painting	Preserved visuospatial skills Language deficits Behavioral disorders (more impulsive and belligerent)
Wu et al., 2013 (Pt 1)	Temporal FTD	MRI: bilateral (left greater than right) anterior temporal atrophy extending to hippocampal and orbitofrontal regions	E	No	Verbal (poetry)	MMSE 26/30 Normal performance on visual memory and visuospatial function Impairment in verbal memory Preserved executive function Disinhibition

(Continued)

Table 1 | Continued

Author and year	Diagnosis	Neuroimaging data	Change in abilities	Previous interest in Art?	Art domain	Neuropsychological data
Wu et al., 2013 (Pt 2)	Temporal FTD	MRI: atrophy in (left greater than right) anterior temporal lobe atrophy	E	No	Verbal (rhyming)	MMSE 30/30 Marked anomia, with intact comprehension and repetition Impairment in executive functions and in visual memory Preserved short-term verbal memory
Wu et al., 2013 (Pt 3)	Temporal FTD	MRI: marked atrophy in the anterior temporal lobes and amygdala, right greater than left, with moderate atrophy of the orbitofrontal cortex, right anterior insula, and right parahippocampus	E	No	Verbal (writer)	MMSE 28/30 Poor performance on tasks of semantic knowledge, executive function and famous face recognition Disinhibition
Mell et al., 2003	PPA (Non-Fluent)	MRI: bifrontal atrophy and mild temporal atrophy	I	Yes (art teacher)	Painting	Preserved visuospatial skills Non-fluent and effortful language Impaired executive tests
Serrano et al., 2005 (Pt 2)	PPA (Non-Fluent)	CT scan: diffuse cortical atrophy with left predominance	P	Yes (painter)	Painting	Preserved visuospatial skills Language deficits
Finney and Heilman, 2007	PPA (Non-Fluent)	MRI: focal atrophy of the left anterior temporal lobe and left insula	D	Yes (painter)	Painting	MMSE 25/30 Boston naming test 47/60 Categorical letter fluency 8 Preserved visuospatial skills
Seeley et al., 2008	PPA (d)	MRI: predominantly left inferolateral frontal atrophy SPECT: Predominantly left frontal hypoperfusion	I	Yes	Visual Art	MMSE = 20/30 Deficits limited to language and executive functions (span; fluency; TMT); Perseverations
Espinel, 1996	Mixed Alzheimer's disease	No imaging data	I	Yes (professional artist)	Painting	No neuropsychological data
Cummings and Zarit, 1987	Alzheimer's disease	No imaging data	D	Yes (professional artist)	Painting	MMSE: varies from 21 to 10 over 2.5 years Boston naming test: varies from 28 to 19 over 2.5 years FAS: varies from 7 to 0 over 2.5 years
Crutch et al., 2001 (and van Buren et al., 2013, Pt 1)	Alzheimer's disease	MRI: generalized brain atrophy	D	Yes (professional artist)	Painting Drawing	MMSE 22/30 WAIS 94 Calculation 0/24 Impaired visuospatial abilities Impaired verbal memory
Maurer and Prvulovic, 2004	Alzheimer's disease	No imaging data	D	Yes (professional artist)	Painting Drawing	Severe visuoconstructive deficits Prosopagnosia Gestural apraxia

(Continued)

Table 1 | Continued

Author and year	Diagnosis	Neuroimaging data	Change in abilities	Previous interest in Art?	Art domain	Neuropsychological data
Fornazzari, 2005	Alzheimer's disease	MRI: large arachnoid cyst SPECT: Bilateral temporo-parietal hypoperfusion	P	Yes (painter)	Painting	MMSE 26/30 Preserved visuospatial abilities Deficits in episodic memory, language, gestural praxis and executive functions
Serrano et al., 2005 (Pt 1)	Alzheimer's disease	CT scan: diffuse cortical atrophy	D	Yes (painter)	Painting	MMSE = 22/30 Impaired visuospatial skills Impaired executive tests (similarities, TMT) and memory
Chakravarty, 2011	Alzheimer's disease	CT scan: Diffuse cortical atrophy	E	No	Painting	MMSE = 16/30 CDR = 3
van Buren et al., 2013 (Pt 2)	Alzheimer's disease	No imaging data	D	No	Painting	Short term memory loss and emotional dysregulation Memory impairment
Kleiner-Fisman et al., 2003	Corticobasal degeneration	MRI: right-predominant atrophy PET-FDG: marked hypoperfusion on right hemisphere and left frontal region	D	Yes (professional illustrator)	Graphic Arts	Severely impaired visuo-spatial skills, spatial neglect Deficits on attention, initiation, memory and executive functions Poor insight Personality changes, irritability Apathy
Sahlas, 2003	Lewy Body Dementia	No imaging data	D	Yes (professional artist)	Painting Writing	No neuropsychological data but reports of deterioration of visuospatial functions
Drago et al., 2006a	Lewy Body Dementia	No imaging data	D	Yes (visual artist)	Painting	MMSE = 6/30 Poor orientation and apraxic gaze
Annoni et al., 2005 (Pt 1)	Stroke	MRI: left occipital region (V1 and V2)	I	Yes (professional painter)	Painting	MMSE = 29/30 Normal neuropsychological exam Emotional dysfunction Increased impulsiveness
Annoni et al., 2005 (Pt 2)	Stroke	MRI: left paramedian thalamus infarct	I	Yes (professional painter)	Painting	MMSE = 28/30 Normal neuropsychological exam Mild emotional dyscontrol Moderate tendency to perseveration in phonological and figural fluency No compulsive behaviors
Chatterjee et al., 2011 (Pt 1)	Stroke	No imaging data (left hemisphere stroke)	Change	Yes (professional painter)	Painting	No neuropsychological data
Chatterjee et al., 2011 (Pt 2)	Stroke	No imaging data (left hemisphere stroke)	Change	Yes (professional painter)	Painting	No neuropsychological data
Chatterjee et al., 2011 (Pt 3)	Stroke	No imaging data (right hemisphere stroke)	Change	Yes (professional painter)	Painting	No neuropsychological data but reports left spatial neglect

(Continued)

Table 1 | Continued

Author and year	Diagnosis	Neuroimaging data	Change in abilities	Previous interest in Art?	Art domain	Neuropsychological data
Takahata et al., 2014	Stroke	CT and MRI: infarction in the left prefrontal region	I	Yes	Painting	MMSE = 26/30 Preserved visuospatial abilities Deficits in episodic memory and executive functions Behavioral perseverations No impulsiveness and no compulsiveness.
Thomas-Anterion, 2009 (Pt 3)	Stroke	MRI: left posterior insula and parietal operculum infarct	E	No	Painting	Normal neuropsychological exam Compulsive art production with specific colors
Lythgoe et al., 2005	Subarachnoid hemorrhage	CT: no focal injury	E	No	Painting Poetry Sculpture	Almost normal, except difficulties in switching and inhibition control Patient obsessed with art
Galarza et al., 2014	Intracerebral hemorrhage associated to a cerebral arteriovenous malformation	MRI: extensive damage of left temporal lobe due to lobectomy.	Change	Yes	Music	Low performance in confrontation naming tests. Impairment on episodic memory tests for verbal modality, but not for visual modality. Preserved emotion recognition, except for fear.

This table synthesizes the published medical reports of changes in artistic skills in neurological patients. Abbreviations: CT, Computerized tomography; D, Degradation of artistic abilities; E, Emergence of artistic abilities; FTD, Frontotemporal dementia; I, Increase of artistic abilities; MMSE, Mini-Mental State Examination; P, Preservation of preceding artistic abilities; PET-FDG, Fluorodeoxyglucose positron emission tomography; PPA, Primary Progressive Aphasia; Pt, Patient; SPECT, Brain perfusion scintigraphy; TMT, Trail Making Test; WCST, Wisconsin Card Sorting Test. (a) Frontal FTD associated to ALS in a patient with previous bipolar disorder; (b) Frontal FTD due to Neuronal Intermediate Filament Inclusion Disease; (c) Temporal FTD associated to ALS; (d) Primary Progressive Aphasia due to corticobasal degeneration.

10 o'clock precisely. She also presented with repetitive and ritualistic behaviors such as compulsive writing, obsessions regarding time schedules and compulsive handbag checking. In this context, the patient started to produce drawings in a compulsive manner. Mrs. YCFZ also had memory complaints, but behavioral disorders remained the most impaired domain throughout the course of the illness. Basic activities of daily living were globally preserved, although she needed assistance for some instrumental activities such as financial operations.

The standard neurological examination was normal, without eye movement disorders or extrapyramidal signs. Formal neuropsychological evaluation (November 2010—**Table 3**) showed an impairment in global cognitive efficiency both on the Mini-Mental State Exam (MMSE: 16/30; Folstein et al., 1975) and on the Mattis Dementia Rating Scale (103/144; Porto et al., 2003). Executive tasks such as DRS initiation/perseveration subscale, FAS letter fluency and digit span were altered. There was a marked episodic memory deficit, which was characterized by low performance on both learning and delayed recall tasks from the Rey Auditory Verbal Learning Test (Malloy-Diniz et al., 2007) and in the DRS memory subscale. There was a moderate impairment in the naming task (9/15; Bertolucci et al., 2001). The visual abilities assessed using the Visual Object and Space Perception Battery (Warrington and James, 1991; Quental et al., 2013) were preserved (number location and cube analysis). The patient had no deficit on gesture execution, and no signs of Balint or Gertsmann syndromes. Brain computed tomography scanning in 2009 showed a remarkable atrophy in temporopolar regions bilaterally and a mild frontal polar atrophy (**Figure 1**). Brain MRI performed 2 years later showed no signs of cerebrovascular disease and confirmed the same regional atrophy pattern with additional diffuse brain shrinkage. On clinical follow-up after 36 months, the global cognitive efficiency assessed using MMSE remained stable (see **Table 4**), although language and functional abilities deteriorated, as assessed using the Functional Activities Questionnaire (Pfeffer et al., 1982). The diagnosis of probable bvFTD was retained on a clinical basis.

The patient was never notably interested in art. However, during the course of her disease, she began to draw compulsively on a daily basis (**Figure 2**). We sought to systematically analyze her drawing production using independent tools for this assessment. For this purpose, we used the consensual assessment technique (CAT; Amabile, 1982) to measure the global creativity of each drawing combined with a questionnaire adapted from Drago and colleagues (Drago et al., 2006a). The criteria assessed in this questionnaire included "Aesthetics": How beautiful is the painting? "Closure": How complete is the painting? "Abstraction": How abstractive is the painting? "Obsessions/Repetition": How obsessive/repetitive is the painting? "Evocative Impact": How strongly does the painting induce feelings or thoughts? "Novelty": How

Table 2 | Synthesis of cognitive, behavioral and artistic changes in previous published cases of patients listed in Table 1 and in our patient.

Pathology	Bv-FTLD	Temp-FTLD	nfPPA-FTLD	Alzheimer's disease	Other
Number of patients	11	19	4	8	12
Artistic emergence	5	11	0	1	2
Artistic increase (or preservation)	4 (1)	2 (6)	2 (1)	1 (1)	4 (3)
Artistic degradation	1	0	1	5	3
Artistic domain = visual	10	8	4	8	11
Intact visuospatial abilities	7 out of 7 reported	9 out of 10 reported	3	The degradation of artistic skills was associated with impaired visuospatial abilities in 6 cases out of 8 reported	
Positive behavioral symptoms reported					
Perseverations	3	2	1	–	1
Disinhibition	5	7	–	–	2
Compulsions obsessions	9	5	–	–	2
Negative dysexecutive symptoms reported					
1 or several deficits	10 out of 10 reported	7 out of 9 reported	3	3	3
Abstraction difficulties	5 out of 8 reported	–	–	1	–

This table summarizes the patterns of artistic changes (emergence, increase/preservation, or degradation of artistic abilities) and behavioral and neuropsychological findings in previously reported neurological patients. Neuropsychological deficits and behavioral disorders may be underreported due to the absence of specific mention in the original papers. "out of x reported" means the number of patients for which this given cognitive or behavioral aspect was assessed and reported in the article. We did not include Parkinson's disease because changes in creativity in these patients may be linked with dopamine rather than neurodegeneration. Bv-FTD, Behavioral variant of fronto-temporal lobar degeneration; temp-FTD, temporal variant of fronto-temporal lobar degeneration or semantic dementia; PPA-FTD, non-fluent primary progressive aphasia form of fronto-temporal lobar degeneration; Other, Corticobasal degeneration, Lewy body dementia, stroke, subarachnoid hemorrhage and cerebral arteriovenous malformation.

Table 3 | Neuropsychological assessment of the patient YCFZ (November 2010).

Test	Patient score	Standard deviation
MATTIS TOTAL SCORE (/144)	**103**	**−9.47**
MATTIS–Attention (/37)	33	−1.83
MATTIS–Initiation (/37)	19	−4.26
MATTIS–Construction (/6)	6	
MATTIS–Concepts (/39)	37	
MATTIS–Memory (/25)	8	−2.59
Verbal SPAN (DIRECT–INDIRECT)	**4–3**	
Rey auditory verbal learning test		
Immediate recall list A	18	−6.1
Delayed recall list A	0	−2.6
Recognition test list A	3	−4.3
NAMING (BOSTON–CERAD) (/15)	**9**	
FAS–Total	19	−9.9
Letter F	7	
Letter A	6	
Letter S	6	
VISUAL OBJECT AND SPACE PERCEPTION		
Number location (/20)	20	Cut-off: 9*
Cube analysis (/20)	20	Cut-off: 9§

**This cut-off distinguished controls from patients with early Alzheimer's disease with 63% sensitivity and 74% specificity (Quental et al., 2013).*

§This cut-off distinguished controls from patients with early Alzheimer's disease with 75% sensitivity and 68% specificity (Quental et al., 2013).

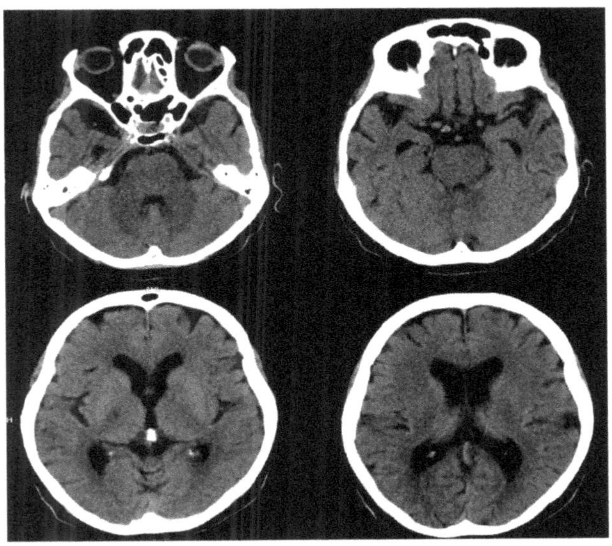

FIGURE 1 | Brain computed tomography scan performed in 2009 showing marked atrophy in bilateral temporopolar and frontal regions.

original or new is the painting? "Representation": How well is the subject of the painting rendered? "Technique": How much skill does the painting demonstrate?

We selected 20 drawings from May 2010 to September 2013 and asked 12 independent professional visual artists from Brazil (5 men, 7 women, aged from 31 to 70 years old, 5 of which

Table 4 | Longitudinal cognitive assessment of Mrs YCFZ, from November 2010–September 2013.

	November 2010	January 2011	May 2011	February 2012	June 2012	September 2012	November 2012	February 2013	September 2013
Time orientation (/5)	2	1	1	1	0	1	1	0	0
Spatial orientation (/5)	4	4	3	4	3	2	3	3	3
Registration (/3)	2	3	3	3	3	3	3	3	3
Mental calculation (/5)	0	1	1	0	1	1	0	0	2
Recall (/3)	0	0	0	0	0	0	1	0	0
Language (/8)	7	8	8	8	8	8	8	8	8
Copy (/1)	1	1	1	0	1	0	0	1	1
MMSE (/30)	**16**	**18**	**17**	**16**	**16**	**15**	**16**	**15**	**17**
Animal Fluency (Cut-off: 13)	9	7	5	5	6	NA	6	8	7
Functional Activities Questionnaire (0–30)	23	NA	NA	29	26	29	30	28	30

The table presents the MMSE total scores (in bold) and subscores for time and spatial orientation, registration of three words, mental calculation, recall of three words, language and copy of pentagons. Data for Animal Fluency and for the Functional Activities Questionnaire–FAQ (Pfeffer et al., 1982) for Activities of Daily Living are also presented. A cut-off point higher than 9 in the FAQ indicates impaired function and cognitive impairment. (NA, Not available).

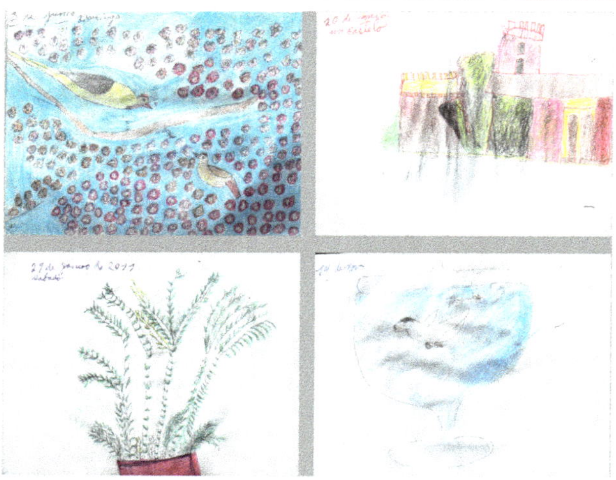

FIGURE 2 | Drawings with higher and lower CAT scores. Left panel: drawings with the highest global scores (8.5 for the upper drawing, range 4–10; 7.4 for the lower drawing, range 3–10). **Right panel:** drawings with the lowest global scores (5.8 for the upper drawing, range 4–10; 6.0 for the lower drawing, range 2–10).

were professors at Fine Art universities, most of which had formal artistic training in Fine Arts) to judge the drawings according to global creativity and the criteria explored in the questionnaire. The experts were also encouraged to make free comments. This expert group was blind to the clinical condition of the patient, and no information on her artistic status or training was given.

The results of this evaluation are presented in **Table 5**. The mean global creativity score across experts and drawings was 6.6, but varied markedly depending on the expert, ranging from 3.2 to 9.6. Scores for each criterion also showed a considerable heterogeneity between the experts ranging from 0 to 10 for each drawing. This heterogeneity suggests that the 12 scorers, all experts in the domain of visual arts, had a different conception of what creativity and its related features should be.

CAT does not give an absolute assessment of creativity but provides relative scores enabling the comparison between different productions or different groups of participants. Therefore, we attempted to evaluate the evolving profile of the patient's drawings across time periods. First, we pooled drawings performed each year from 2010 to 2013 and looked at scores across the years (**Figure 3**). We observed an increase in scores from the first drawings (2010) to the last drawings (2013) in all of the evaluated aspects. Then, we statistically compared two periods: an early (drawings from 2010 and 2011; $n = 8$) and a late period (those from 2012 and 2013; $n = 12$) using a non-parametric Wilcoxon signed rank test. An increase in creativity scores was statistically significant for abstraction ($Z = -2.756$, $p = 0.006$), obsession ($Z = -2.045$, $p = 0.041$) and novelty ($Z = -2.312$, $p = 0.021$) subscores (**Figure 3**).

In their free comments, expert artists mentioned that most of the drawings were beautiful and creative, drawn with care, and found the compositions interesting or original. They insisted on the "naïve" character of the drawings, frequently describing them as simple and infantile ("these drawings are similar to those from my daughter of 6 years of age," translated general comment from expert 1). The experts agreed on the representational rather than abstract nature of the productions. Repetitions, obsessions, or stereotypies were diversely interpreted. Many experts highlighted the repetitive and obsessive character of the drawings, but they often found them useful for the composition, the expression, or the rhythm of the picture, and gave low obsession scores for this reason. There was a large variability in the scores for repetitions and obsessions (minimal 0, maximal 9.1, with a mean of 5.2). The drawings were often described as expressive and containing negative emotions ("sinister paranoid atmosphere," translated from expert 8 about drawing 19), but harmony was also evoked for some of them. Other comments highlighted bizarre or interesting compositions or strange/poor color choices.

Overall, the quantitative and qualitative creativity assessments showed great heterogeneity, especially in the general creativity of the drawings, the role of repetitions in the composition, or the emotional content. The disparity of judgment between

Table 5 | CAT assessment of the drawings from patient YCFZ (2010–2013).

	Global Score	Aesthetics	Closure	Abstraction	Obsessions/ repetitions	Evocative impact	Novelty	Representation	Technique
Artist 1	4.8	4.4	5.7	4.1	4.1	3.8	3.6	4.7	3.3
Artist 2	3.2	0.3	9.2	1.5	8.5	0.3	0.9	3.0	0.0
Artist 3	3.2	0.3	9.2	1.5	8.5	0.3	0.9	3.0	0.0
Artist 4	9.4	9.1	9.4	9.1	9.1	9.8	9.3	9.8	9.6
Artist 5	6.6	4.6	4.4	1.5	3.4	4.0	2.1	3.9	3.6
Artist 6	9.6	9.5	10.0	0.0	0.0	8.7	10.0	9.8	10.0
Artist 7	9.3	8.9	9.2	1.3	5.3	8.2	8.4	8.7	8.8
Artist 8	3.2	3.0	3.1	3.3	4.6	3.6	3.2	3.0	2.9
Artist 9	7.0	5.6	7.7	3.9	4.5	6.2	6.5	7.5	6.5
Artist 10	7.9	7.2	8.5	7.5	3.7	7.6	7.8	7.3	6.5
Artist 11	6.8	5.7	8.4	1.7	5.4	6.1	3.8	7.4	5.6
Artist 12	8.5	8.2	9.3	5.1	4.9	6.8	7.8	9.5	8.7
Mean	**6.6**	**5.6**	**7.8**	**3.3**	**5.2**	**5.4**	**5.3**	**6.4**	**5.4**
SD	**2.5**	**3.2**	**2.2**	**2.7**	**2.5**	**3.1**	**3.3**	**2.8**	**3.5**
Min	**3.2**	**0.3**	**3.1**	**0.0**	**0.0**	**0.3**	**0.9**	**3.0**	**0.0**
Max	**9.6**	**9.5**	**10.0**	**9.1**	**9.1**	**9.8**	**10.0**	**9.8**	**10.0**

The professional artists scored (from 0 to 10) each of the drawings for global creativity and according to the following criteria (adapted from Drago et al., 2006a): Aesthetics: How beautiful is the painting? Closure: How complete is the painting? Abstraction: How abstractive is the painting? Obsessions/Repetition: How obsessive/repetitive is the painting? Evocative Impact: How strongly does the painting induce feelings or thoughts? Novelty: How original or new is the painting? Representation: How well is the subject of the painting rendered? Technique: How much skill does the painting demonstrate? Mean scores attributed by each judge to the 20 assessed drawings are provided together with standard deviation, minimum and maximum values (in bold).

the professional artists with academic training for most indicates that personal subjectivity strongly influenced the scoring. Despite a large inter-judge variability, an improvement of the patient's artistic skills was considered during a 3-year evolution period, especially for the abstraction, novelty, and repetition criteria, while language and autonomy declined. This suggests that the artistic creative capacity of the patient did not parallel her cognitive deterioration.

This observation is consistent with the potential emergence of an artistic inclination during the evolution of bvFTD, as previously reported, and highlights the interference between cognitive and behavioral frontal symptoms and creative production.

DISCUSSION: WHAT DO ARTISTIC PATIENTS TELL US ABOUT CREATIVITY?

The difference between controlled patient studies and medical reports of creativity following frontal damage raises interesting questions regarding the mental components of creative thinking, their measurements, and their neural bases. Experimental approaches of creativity have demonstrated that various PFC regions are critical to creative capacity. Conversely, some frontal patients exhibit new or significant artistic productions despite their frontal dysfunctions, as was the case for the reported patient. Can this be explained? Does this mean that their creative capacities increased?

CLINICAL CONSIDERATIONS FOR PATIENTS WITH NEW OR SIGNIFICANT ARTISTIC PRODUCTION

Artistic facilitation is a rare phenomenon in neurological patients. The link between artistic production and neurological diseases appears to be anecdotal, especially when the high incidence of strokes and neurodegenerative diseases are considered. SD (FTD with temporal prominent atrophy) is the most frequent diagnosis associated with increased creative production (**Table 2**). In contrast with controlled studies that included unselected patients with neurodegenerative diseases, case reports point to particular patients who are especially concerned with making art. To our knowledge, no such exceptional patient with artistic facilitation has been explored using theory-based creativity tests. So it cannot be ruled out that controlled studies with unselected patients may miss some exceptional patients.

Because artistic facilitation has been observed in diseases as different as temporal and frontal variants of FTD, Alzheimer's disease, or stroke affecting distinct brain regions, clinical reports do not argue for a specific neuroanatomical or neuropsychological pattern associated with enhanced artistic production. For instance, it has been proposed that the emergence of artistic talent in FTD patients results from the release of the inhibition exerted by anterior regions over the posterior regions involved in visuospatial processing (Kapur, 1996; Mendez, 2004; Seeley et al., 2008). This theory may not explain the improved or preserved creative output in patients with predominant posterior injury (Annoni et al., 2005; Fornazzari, 2005) or in patients with no frontal dysfunction (Schrag and Trimble, 2001; Thomas-Anterion et al., 2010). Nevertheless, it is remarkable that most positive changes of artistic abilities concerned visual arts (41 cases out of 54 reviewed, including the current case report) when most patients had preserved visuospatial skills each time this was reported. In the related cases of creative production associated with either bvFTD or SD, degeneration mostly affected the left temporal and/or frontal regions, which may explain the predominance of visual arts in the patients' production being more related to the visuospatial functions of the right hemisphere. However, Wu and colleagues (Wu et al., 2013) recently reported two SD patients in whom the emergence of artistic activities in the verbal domain was associated with a predominantly left atrophy. Additionally, this left-right hypothesis is not in agreement with functional imaging data, as the meta-analysis from Gonen-Yaacovi and colleagues demonstrated a left dominance of activation in both verbal and visual tasks. Unfortunately, most of the published clinical reports do not provide extensive or detailed neuropsychological and anatomical data, which would enable a better characterization of the relationship between frontal or visuospatial alterations and creative output.

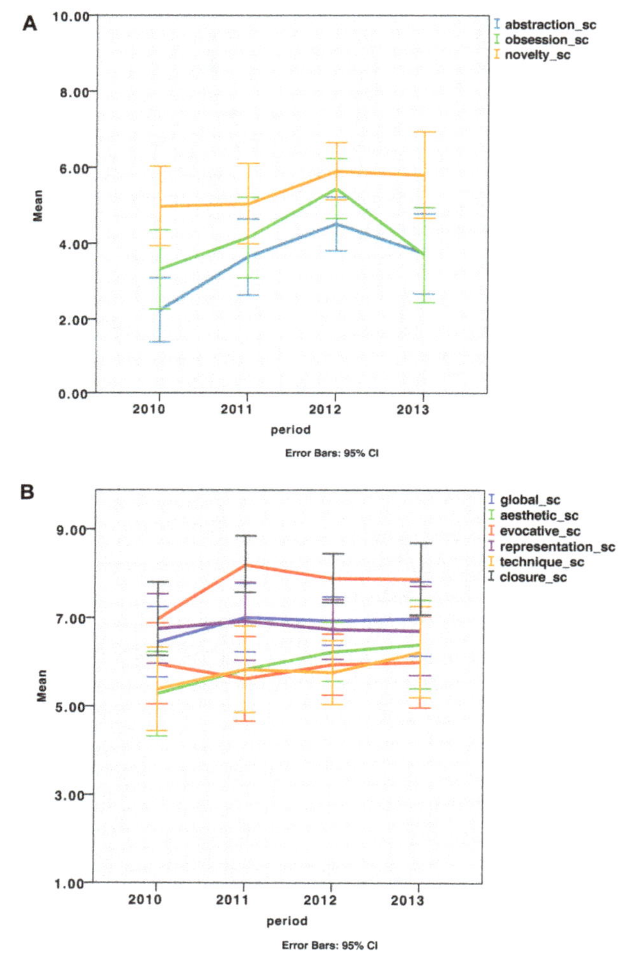

FIGURE 3 | Scores of the drawings across a 36-month period. (A) Subscores with a significant improvement between the first (2010–2011) and the second period (2012–2013) of the drawings. Significant increases were observed for the abstraction, obsession and novelty subscores. **(B)** The global score and several subscores did not show a significant improvement between the first and the second period, though all scores increased.

TIES BETWEEN FRONTAL SYMPTOMS AND ARTISTIC PRODUCTIONS

Some behavioral disorders associated with frontal damage may account for or parallel artistic expression, as suggested previously (Rankin et al., 2007; de Souza et al., 2010; Palmiero et al., 2012; Schott, 2012) and highlighted in our reported case. From a neurological point of view and based on the neuropsychological profile of our patient, we fist concluded that some frontal symptoms are possibly interfering with the drawings, while preserved visuospatial abilities enable their execution. The urge to draw on a daily basis and the huge amount of productions are possibly related to personality changes and compulsive behaviors provoked by frontal damage. Repetitive topics (plants, animals, people) and patterns (volcano, leaves) may be the manifestation of perseverations and stereotypies due to the frontal syndrome. Strange composition and infantile features may be explained by poor planning abilities (**Figure 4**).

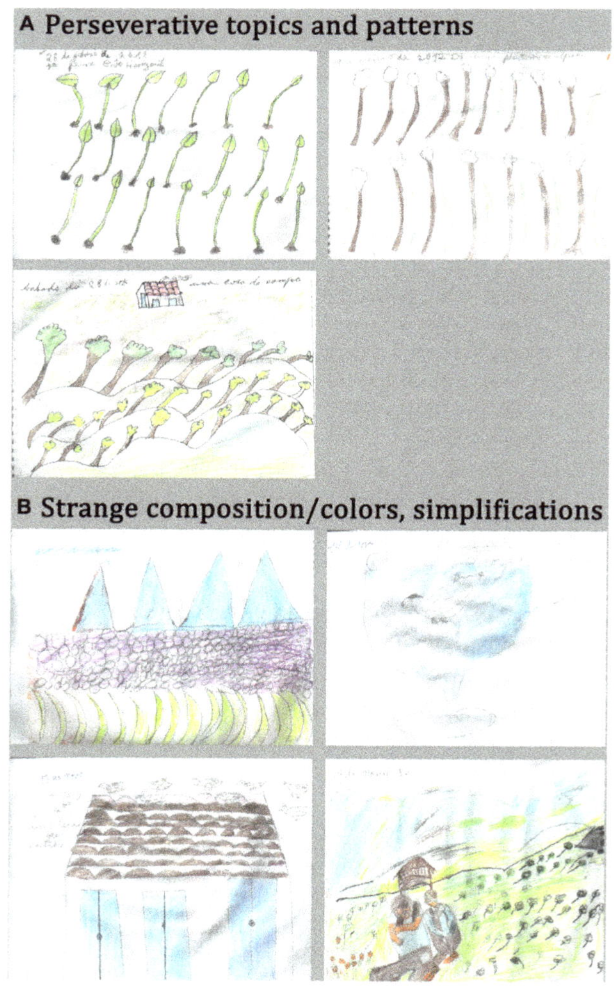

FIGURE 4 | Possible frontal manifestations expressed in the patient's drawings. (A) Perseverative topics and patterns. **(B)** Strange composition, color choices and simplifications.

Many patients with so called "artistic improvement" presented compulsive and/or obsessive behaviors (Finkelstein et al., 1991; Miller et al., 1998; Miller and Hou, 2004; Lythgoe et al., 2005; Serrano et al., 2005; Thomas-Anterion et al., 2010). As pointed by Schott (2012), in such patients, "a strong preference for a single art medium, a restricted focus on artistic themes, repetition, compulsion and seeking for perfection (...) enabled remarkable artistry to be achieved." The patient we report on also produced drawings in a compulsive manner; this may partly account for the acquisition of an artistic technique. The fact that her last drawings received higher scores than the first drawings (produced 3 years prior) supports this assumption. Compulsive and/or obsessive behaviors are a major symptom of bvFTD (Rascovsky et al., 2011). These behaviors are surprisingly in contrast with the apathy also frequently observed in bvFTD, as well as with the cognitive inertia associated with a poor fluency, as was the case in our patient. Compulsive behaviors are usually associated with severe disorders of social conduct. For example, the patient reported by Miller et al. (1998) developed new photographic skills during the course of FTD. Pictures were taken compulsively to obtain a "perfect image." However, at the same time, this compulsive demeanor also produced socially inappropriate behaviors, leading to severe social constraints, and ultimately to institutionalization. The patient we report also had ritualized behaviors that also led to social misconduct. In other words, the repetitive and ritualized behaviors related to frontal dysfunction may be expressed in the artistic domain, leading to new interests in making art or intense artistic activity with repetitive topics or productions. The reasons why some patients focus their compulsive behaviors on making art and others do not remain poorly understood.

Perseverations or patterning, which are also linked to frontal damage, were observed in our patient's drawings (trees and leaves, for instance). Surprisingly, our expert group remarked repetitions and made free comments about them but did not give especially high scores on the repetition criteria because they did not feel it was inappropriate or unaesthetic. A previous case-control study of creative production across bvFTD patients and normal controls (de Souza et al., 2010) showed that behavioral disorders, such as perseverations, may also partly explain the "originality" of some productions when frontal patients perform divergent thinking tests, but overall their originality score was impaired. Similarly, disinhibition, another cardinal symptom of frontal dysfunction, can interfere with creative activities, as also noted by de Souza et al. (2010); however this was not observed in the current case. Social disinhibition can lead to unexpected choices of topics, for instance with sexual content. The release of the inhibition exerted by frontal regions over the posterior regions may explain some unconventional or socially unusual aspects of creative productions as well as behaviors in frontal patients (Miller et al., 1996; Mell et al., 2003; Mendez, 2004; Miller and Hou, 2004; Drago et al., 2006b; Seeley et al., 2008).

In the cognitive sphere, some frontal lesions may help in overcoming knowledge constraints (Reverberi et al., 2005; Abraham, 2014). Patients with lateral prefrontal damage may experience a less sculpted (less constrained) response space in a given context than healthy subjects, enabling them to more easily consider any option, including those outside of contextual constraints (Reverberi et al., 2005). Overall, disinhibition or the loss of social conventions and associative knowledge may allow the emergence of creative productions (Miller et al., 1996, 2000; Miller and Hou, 2004; Liu et al., 2009). According to Rankin et al. (2007), productions from bvFTD patients may have an artistic value in the sense that they are freer from conventional representations and social conventions about art. It is more difficult to assume that this freeing from convention is an intentional and voluntary act.

Finally, our patient's drawings share other qualitative features that have been reported in previous FTD patients, especially with those described in Rankin and colleagues' study (Rankin et al., 2007) in which patient productions were assessed by scientists who had an interest in arts and not by professional artists. For instance, landscapes, people, animals and plants appear to be the preferred topics in frontal patient's productions. These preferred topics may be considered to be conventional and concrete but are often represented in an unusual way. The simplification of representations, judged as naïve or infantile, and unconventional or disordered composition with eccentricity of the subject, could be linked to a poor planning ability and lack of abstraction but could also contribute to the bizarreness and unusualness of the drawings.

Together, patient observations indicate that some clinical and behavioral symptoms of frontal dysfunction may facilitate the appearance of creative features in artistic products. This explanation cannot stand in the domain of creativity in which other frontal functions such as cognitive control, planning, mental manipulation, and abstraction are critical. Additionally, these observations raise the question of whether the artistic productions we observe reflect the same aspect of creative capacity and result from the same voluntary creative processes that are assessed in experimental creativity studies.

ARTISTIC AND NEUROSCIENTIFIC PERSPECTIVES

Patient studies and clinical observations may highlight the probable difference between creativity evaluated from an artistic point of view and creativity evaluated from a neuroscientific perspective. In the field of Art, aspects such as emotional or evocative impact, provocation and message, aesthetic value, or technical mastery may be more important than in other domains such as sciences and technology. These aspects are not captured by the consensual definition of creativity that focuses on originality and appropriateness. Within the frame of this definition, a difference may also be noted: originality may often be considered to be a predominant condition for creativity in the artistic field in which appropriateness is difficult to apprehend; however, in other domains such as science, appropriateness is a requirement. For example, patients studied in de Souza et al. (2010) were often inappropriate in their responses, while no control subjects were. The sexual content of their drawings may be regarded as inappropriate in an experimental testing context but is usually well accepted in artistic works. This suggests that each domain of creative expression differently prioritizes originality and appropriateness and makes different demands on the mental operations to achieve them.

It is also important to mention that experimental and neuroimaging approaches do not assess motivational, conative, or emotional factors affecting creative drive. However, these factors appear to be important in real life creativity, such as in the spontaneous productions of patients with an artistic preoccupation. As highlighted by Schott (2012), these patients are often described "as obsessive about their art, with an urge to create." It is then possible that emotional and motivational factors play an important role in real life creativity, including artistic creativity, but are poorly accounted for in experimental approaches of creativity. The latter are indeed based on cognitive theories of creative capacity with limited assessment of the emotional and conative aspects.

In our case, the score of evocative impact, which is intended to depend on the emotional expressiveness of the drawings, varied between the experts (0.3–9.8, with a mean value of 5.4). One method for analyzing the importance of emotional process in the artistic production of the patient would be to study the correlations between the scores on the CAT and objective measures of social-emotional cognition such as emotion recognition, empathy, and theory of mind. Unfortunately, these domains were not evaluated in our patient.

Finally, the difference between real life and experimental settings for measuring creativity is also in question. The evaluation of spontaneous patient productions was generally based on subjective assessments from authors, experts, or groups of judges. Our clinical case illustrates that subjective assessment, although framed by determined criteria and performed by experts in the field of visual arts, has a great inter-individual variability. Experimental theory-based approaches use more objective criteria to measure creative capacity, for instance fluency, flexibility, originality, or problem solving success. Several of these cognitive approaches have been used to study the neural basis of creativity in functional neuroimaging and in neurological patients. If theory-based approaches use more "objective" criteria, they are constrained by the hypothesis that they rely on. In other words, creativity tasks only assess the processes involved in creative capacity according to the cognitive model used. Each theory-based approach focuses on one or more aspects of the creative process, but none of them evaluates the creativity in all of its dimensions. In particular, theory-based creativity tasks do not necessarily capture artistic quality, even though they have been shown to be ecologically valid and statistically linked with artistic creativity (Kim, 2006; Plucker and Makel, 2010). On the contrary, theory-free creativity assessments, such as CAT, are not based on any particular theory of creativity, which means that their validity is not dependent upon the validity of any particular theory. Unfortunately, our patient was no longer able to perform experimental creativity tests at the time of the consultation; thus, we are not able to compare both approaches to creativity assessment in a case of artistic preoccupation.

Overall, the creativity attributed to patients preoccupied with arts during a frontal disease and creativity explored in experimental studies differ in several conceptual and experimental ways, and are probably affected differently by frontal symptoms.

OVERALL, CAN HYPOFRONTALITY FACILITATE CREATIVITY?

A common notion suggests that losing control, especially relaxing social and emotional inhibitions or conventions, may favor personal expression and creativity. The use of drugs such as alcohol may aim to approach this state. Several artistic streams are based on the spontaneous, non-controlled generation of ideas or objects, for instance using automatic writing or random painting. In the neuroscientific literature, some studies suggest that unconscious and uncontrolled processes facilitate divergent thinking and insight problem solving (Yaniv and Meyer, 1987; Dijksterhuis and Meurs, 2006; Dorfman et al., 2008; Zhong et al., 2008; Ritter and Dijksterhuis, 2014). Because control in behavioral, affective, social and cognitive spheres is largely associated with the functions of the PFC, the notion that hypofrontality could favor creativity may be valid. A recent theory (Chrysikou et al., 2013) also postulates that hypofrontality may enhance some aspects of creativity: the availability of bottom-up information that is usually filtered by the PFC may favor a breaking away from rule-based thinking. This is reinforced by the fact that some frontal patients appear to have abilities in some aspects of artistic expression.

The current review identified several clinical aspects of hypofrontality in the social, conative and cognitive domains that could explain some creative features of the patients' products. First, a social aspect related to the common view of hypofrontality is disinhibition. Social disinhibition can lead frontal patients to break with social conventions and propose unusual productions in creative (but also in uncreative) activities. Second, compulsive, repetitive or obsessive behaviors may lead to high productivity and improvements in technical skills. This obsessive-compulsive trait acts as a strong motivation toward a given activity. A third and more paradoxical aspect consists of a lower influence of habitual contextual associations in frontal patients. Patients with lateral PFC damage may be less constrained by learned rules, which may facilitate some problem-solving tasks (Reverberi et al., 2005). This aspect is paradoxical because it is in apparent opposition to the acknowledged role of the inferolateral PFC in overcoming prepotent responses [as observed in functional imaging and patient studies using Stroop tasks, no-go tasks or Hayling tasks (Aron et al., 2003; Brass et al., 2005; Picton et al., 2007; Volle et al., 2012), as well as in contextual control (Azuar et al., 2014)]. Overcoming prepotent responses and contextual control are both thought to play a role in creativity. Thus, whether highly creative people among the general population have more relaxed contextual constraints (as frontal patients may have) or increased abilities to intentionally overcome these constraints is an interesting topic for future research.

If hypofrontality generally evokes signs of disinhibition and poor control (usually associated with lateral and ventral portions of the PFC), we should also consider other roles of PFC in cognition that have been more recently highlighted. For instance, the medial PFC is part of the default network (Buckner et al., 2008), a set of functionally connected brain regions in which activity decreases when tasks require more focal attention, effort, or control. This network has been associated with spontaneous cognition and mind wandering (Gilbert et al., 2007; Mason et al., 2007; Christoff et al., 2009; Andrews-Hanna et al., 2010). This network can be distinguished from the set of regions functionally connected to lateral PFC (Gilbert et al., 2010). Some recent studies highlighted the role of the default network and of spontaneous cognition in creativity

(Takeuchi et al., 2012; Wise and Braga, 2014). Medial PFC is also involved in semantic processing (Buckner et al., 2008; Binder et al., 2009) and in semantic aspects of creativity (Green et al., 2012; Abraham, 2014). These data suggest that the lateral PFC is engaged in rule-based thinking, while the medial PFC appears to be involved in a more spontaneous mode of thinking such as associative thinking. The rostral PFC may act as a switch (Burgess et al., 2007) between these two modes. Both thinking modes are thought to be required for creativity, as suggested in several models (Vartanian et al., 2007; Gabora, 2010; Ward and Kolomyts, 2010; Ellamil et al., 2012). For instance, the uncontrolled association of ideas triggered by perceptual or emotional stimuli may favor unusual responses but may also lead to inappropriate responses if the control mode does not filter. How each mode is affected by frontal lesions and how it impacts creative capacity is poorly known. The consequences of damage to the rostromedial PFC on creativity may lead to poorer originality (de Souza et al., 2010; Shamay-Tsoory et al., 2011), but the mechanisms of this change and its relationship with the default network functions are unexplored.

Overall, the classical view in which PFC supports top-down controlled processing while subcortical and posterior brain regions are engaged in bottom-up uncontrolled processing may be more balanced regarding creativity. If the lateral PFC is largely associated with top-down control, some other PFC regions may be involved in the uncontrolled or bottom-up processing that is spontaneous cognition, including semantic associations and mind wandering. The interaction between controlled and spontaneous cognition *via* connectivity between the lateral and medial PFC networks (Spreng et al., 2010) may enable both original and appropriate ideas to emerge.

CONCLUSION

The functional and anatomical organization of the PFC supports different aspects of behavioral adaptation in humans, suggesting its role in the adaptive aspects of creativity as they are emphasized in its definition (i.e., creating something original and appropriate). Functional neuroimaging and experimental patient studies also suggest that the PFC, in particular the anterior PFC, may also play a critical role in originality aspects of creativity. Damage to the PFC may alter the intentional appropriateness and originality of patient productions by altering planning, fluency, mental flexibility, rule-based thinking, or abstraction. However, clinical observations of frontal damage patients suggest that some symptoms associated with frontal damage provoke cognitive, conative, and behavioral changes, including social disinhibition, compulsive behaviors, emotional distortions, and the relaxing of cognitive constraints, which can motivate and favor artistic productions. However, artistic production is not synonymous with creativity, because creativity refers to aspects such as emotional expression, evocative impact, aesthetic, and technical abilities, which are present in art but not necessarily in other domains of creativity. Art is thus difficult to capture using theory-based creativity tasks, and to our knowledge, patients with facilitation in the artistic domain have not been tested experimentally with such tasks. Therefore, whether these rare frontal patients increase their real creative capacity does not have a yes or no answer. Using theory-based creativity tasks, functional imaging and patient data suggest that distinct PFC subregions differently affect the different aspects of creativity. PFC cannot be considered as a unitary structure, and exploring its organization and interactions subserving different creativity processes, including controlled and spontaneous cognition, as well as social and affective aspects, may provide a more precise answer.

ACKNOWLEDGMENTS

This work was supported by the National Research Agency (ANR-09-RPDOC-004-01; Emmanuelle Volle) and by The National Council for Scientific and Technological Development (Brazil, CNPq—402853/2012-1; Leonardo C. de Souza). We thank our patient, Mrs. YCFZ, and her family for their willingness and interest in our research. We also thank all of the artists who evaluated the drawings of Mrs. YCFZ.

REFERENCES

Abraham, A. (2014). Creative thinking as orchestrated by semantic processing vs. cognitive control brain networks. *Front. Hum. Neurosci.* 8:95. doi: 10.3389/fnhum.2014.00095

Abraham, A., Beudt, S., Ott, D. V. M., and Yves von Cramon, D. (2012). Creative cognition and the brain: dissociations between frontal, parietal–temporal and basal ganglia groups. *Brain Res.* 1482, 55–70. doi: 10.1016/j.brainres.2012.09.007

Amabile, T. M. (1982). Social psychology of creativity: a consensual assessment technique. *J. Pers. Soc. Psychol.* 43, 997–1013. doi: 10.1037/0022-3514.43.5.997

Andrews-Hanna, J. R., Reidler, J. S., Huang, C., and Buckner, R. L. (2010). Evidence for the default network's role in spontaneous cognition. *J. Neurophysiol.* 104, 322–335. doi: 10.1152/jn.00830.2009

Annoni, J. M., Devuyst, G., Carota, A., Bruggimann, L., and Bogousslavsky, J. (2005). Changes in artistic style after minor posterior stroke. *J. Neurol. Neurosurg. Psychiatr.* 76, 797–803. doi: 10.1136/jnnp.2004.045492

Arden, R., Chavez, R. S., Grazioplene, R., and Jung, R. E. (2010). Neuroimaging creativity: a psychometric view. *Behav. Brain Res.* 214, 143–156. doi: 10.1016/j.bbr.2010.05.015

Aron, A. R., Fletcher, P. C., Bullmore, E. T., Sahakian, B. J., and Robbins, T. W. (2003). Stop-signal inhibition disrupted by damage to right inferior frontal gyrus in humans. *Nat. Neurosci.* 6, 115–116. doi: 10.1038/nn1003

Asari, T., Konishi, S., Jimura, K., Chikazoe, J., Nakamura, N., and Miyashita, Y. (2008). Right temporopolar activation associated with unique perception. *Neuroimage* 41, 145–152. doi: 10.1016/j.neuroimage.2008.01.059

Aziz-Zadeh, L., Kaplan, J. T., and Iacoboni, M. (2009). "Aha!": the neural correlates of verbal insight solutions. *Hum. Brain Mapp.* 30, 908–916. doi: 10.1002/hbm.20554

Aziz-Zadeh, L., Liew, S.-L., and Dandekar, F. (2012). Exploring the neural correlates of visual creativity. *Soc. Cogn. Affect. Neurosci.* 8, 475–480. doi: 10.1093/scan/nss021

Azuar, C., Reyes, P., Slachevsky, A., Volle, E., Kinkingnehun, S., Kouneiher, F., et al. (2014). Testing the model of caudo-rostral organization of cognitive control in the human with frontal lesions. *Neuroimage* 84, 1053–1060. doi: 10.1016/j.neuroimage.2013.09.031

Badre, D., and Wagner, A. D. (2007). Left ventrolateral prefrontal cortex and the cognitive control of memory. *Neuropsychologia* 45, 2883–2901. doi: 10.1016/j.neuropsychologia.2007.06.015

Bechtereva, N. P., Korotkov, A. D., Pakhomov, S. V., Roudas, M. S., Starchenko, M. G., and Medvedev, S. V. (2004). PET study of brain maintenance of verbal creative activity. *Int. J. Psychophysiol.* 53, 11–20. doi: 10.1016/j.ijpsycho.2004.01.001

Bengtsson, S. L., Csikszentmihalyi, M., and Ullen, F. (2007). Cortical regions involved in the generation of musical structures during improvisation in pianists. *J. Cogn. Neurosci.* 19, 830–842. doi: 10.1162/jocn.2007.19.5.830

Berkowitz, A. L., and Ansari, D. (2008). Generation of novel motor sequences: the neural correlates of musical improvisation. *Neuroimage* 41, 535–543. doi: 10.1016/j.neuroimage.2008.02.028

Bertolucci, P. H., Okamoto, I. H., Brucki, S. M., Siviero, M. O., Toniolo Neto, J., and Ramos, L. R. (2001). Applicability of the CERAD neuropsychological battery to Brazilian elderly. *Arq. Neuropsiquiatr.* 59, 532–536. doi: 10.1590/S0004-282X2001000400009

Binder, J. R., Desai, R. H., Graves, W. W., and Conant, L. L. (2009). Where is the semantic system? A critical review and meta-analysis of 120 functional neuroimaging studies. *Cereb. Cortex* 19, 2767–2796. doi: 10.1093/cercor/bhp055

Bogousslavsky, J. (2005). Artistic creativity, style and brain disorders. *Eur. Neurol.* 54, 103–111. doi: 10.1159/000088645

Brass, M., Derrfuss, J., Forstmann, B., and von Cramon, D. Y. (2005). The role of the inferior frontal junction area in cognitive control. *Trends Cogn. Sci.* 9, 314–316. doi: 10.1016/j.tics.2005.05.001

Buckner, R. L., Andrews-Hanna, J. R., and Schacter, D. L. (2008). The brain's default network: anatomy, function, and relevance to disease. *Ann. N.Y. Acad. Sci.* 1124, 1–38. doi: 10.1196/annals.1440.011

Budrys, V., Skullerud, K., Petroska, D., Lengveniene, J., and Kaubrys, G. (2007). Dementia and art: neuronal intermediate filament inclusion disease and dissolution of artistic creativity. *Eur. Neurol.* 57, 137–144. doi: 10.1159/000098464

Burgess, P. W., Alderman, N., Volle, E., Benoit, R. G., and Gilbert, S. J. (2009). Mesulam's frontal lobe mystery re-examined. *Restor. Neurol. Neurosci.* 27, 493–506. doi: 10.3233/RNN-2009-0511

Burgess, P. W., Dumontheil, I. I., and Gilbert, S. J. (2007). The gateway hypothesis of rostral prefrontal cortex (area 10) function. *Trends Cogn. Sci.* 11, 290–298. doi: 10.1016/j.tics.2007.05.004

Cardillo, E. R., Watson, C. E., Schmidt, G. L., Kranjec, A., and Chatterjee, A. (2012). From novel to familiar: tuning the brain for metaphors. *Neuroimage* 59, 3212–3221. doi: 10.1016/j.neuroimage.2011.11.079

Carlsson, I., Wendt, P. E., and Risberg, J. (2000). On the neurobiology of creativity. Differences in frontal activity between high and low creative subjects. *Neuropsychologia* 38, 873–885. doi: 10.1016/S0028-3932(99)00128-1

Catani, M., and Thiebaut de Schotten, M. (2012). *Atlas of Human Brain Connections.* New York, NY: Oxford University Press. doi: 10.1093/med/9780199541164.001.0001

Chakravarty, A. (2011). *De novo* development of artistic creativity in Alzheimer's disease. *Ann. Indian Acad. Neurol.* 14, 291–294. doi: 10.4103/0972-2327.91953

Changeux, J. (2005). "Creation, art and brain," *in Neurobiology of Human Values*, eds J.-P. Changeux, A. R. Damasio, W. Singer, and Y. Christen (Berlin; Heidelberg: Springer-Verlan), 1–11. doi: 10.1007/3-540-29803-7_1

Chatterjee, A., Bromberger, B., Smith, W. B. I. I., Sternschein, R., and Widick, P. (2011). Artistic production following brain damage: a study of three artists. *Leonardo* 44, 405–410. doi: 10.1162/LEON_a_00240

Chatterjee, A., Hamilton, R. H., and Amorapanth, P. X. (2006). Art produced by a patient with Parkinson's disease. *Behav. Neurol.* 17, 105–108. doi: 10.1155/2006/901832

Chavez-Eakle, R. A., Graff-Guerrero, A., Garcia-Reyna, J. C., Vaugier, V., and Cruz-Fuentes, C. (2007). Cerebral blood flow associated with creative performance: a comparative study. *Neuroimage* 38, 519–528. doi: 10.1016/j.neuroimage.2007.07.059

Christoff, K., Keramatian, K., Gordon, A. M., Smith, R., and Madler, B. (2009). Prefrontal organization of cognitive control according to levels of abstraction. *Brain Res.* 1286, 94–105. doi: 10.1016/j.brainres.2009.05.096

Christoff, K., Prabhakaran, V., Dorfman, J., Zhao, Z., Kroger, J. K., Holyoak, K. J., et al. (2001). Rostrolateral prefrontal cortex involvement in relational integration during reasoning. *Neuroimage* 14, 1136–1149. doi: 10.1006/nimg.2001.0922

Chrysikou, E. G., and Thompson-Schill, S. L. (2011). Dissociable brain states linked to common and creative object use. *Hum. Brain Mapp.* 32, 665–675. doi: 10.1002/hbm.21056

Chrysikou, E. G., Weber, M. J., and Thompson-Schill, S. L. (2013). A matched filter hypothesis for cognitive control. *Neuropsychologia.* doi: 10.1016/j.neuropsychologia.2013.10.021. [Epub ahead of print].

Cole, M. W., Reynolds, J. R., Power, J. D., Repovs, G., Anticevic, A., and Braver, T. S. (2013). Multi-task connectivity reveals flexible hubs for adaptive task control. *Nat. Neurosci.* 16, 1348–1355. doi: 10.1038/nn.3470

Crutch, S. J., Isaacs, R., and Rossor, M. N. (2001). Some workmen can blame their tools: artistic change in an individual with Alzheimer's disease. *Lancet* 357, 2129–2133. doi: 10.1016/S0140-6736(00)05187-4

Cummings, J. L., and Zarit, J. M. (1987). Probable Alzheimer's disease in an artist. *JAMA* 258, 2731–2734. doi: 10.1001/jama.1987.03400190113039

de Manzano, O., and Ullen, F. (2012). Goal-independent mechanisms for free response generation: creative and pseudo-random performance share neural substrates. *Neuroimage* 59, 772–780. doi: 10.1016/j.neuroimage.2011.07.016

de Souza, L. C., Volle, E., Bertoux, M., Czernecki, V., Funkiewiez, A., Allali, G., et al. (2010). Poor creativity in frontotemporal dementia: a window into the neural bases of the creative mind. *Neuropsychologia* 48, 3733–3742. doi: 10.1016/j.neuropsychologia.2010.09.010

Dietrich, A. (2004). The cognitive neuroscience of creativity. *Psychon. Bull. Rev.* 11, 1011–1026. doi: 10.3758/BF03196731

Dietrich, A., and Kanso, R. (2010). A review of EEG, ERP, and neuroimaging studies of creativity and insight. *Psychol. Bull.* 136, 822–848. doi: 10.1037/a0019749

Dijksterhuis, A., and Meurs, T. (2006). Where creativity resides: the generative power of unconscious thought. *Conscious. Cogn.* 15, 135–146. doi: 10.1016/j.concog.2005.04.007

Dorfman, L., Martindale, C., Gassimova, V., and Vartanian, O. (2008). Creativity and speed of information processing: a double dissociation involving elementary versus inhibitory cognitive tasks. *Pers. Individ. Dif.* 44, 1382–1390. doi: 10.1016/j.paid.2007.12.006

Drago, V., Crucian, G. P., Foster, P. S., Cheong, J., Finney, G. R., Pisani, F., et al. (2006a). Lewy body dementia and creativity: case report. *Neuropsychologia* 44, 3011–3015. doi: 10.1016/j.neuropsychologia.2006.05.030

Drago, V., Foster, P. S., Trifiletti, D., FitzGerald, D. B., Kluger, B. M., Crucian, G. P., et al. (2006b). What's inside the art? The influence of frontotemporal dementia in art production. *Neurology* 67, 1285–1287. doi: 10.1212/01.wnl.0000238439.77764.da

Dubois, B., Levy, R., Verin, M., Teixeira, C., Agid, Y., and Pillon, B. (1995). Experimental approach to prefrontal functions in humans. *Ann. N.Y. Acad. Sci.* 769, 41–60. doi: 10.1111/j.1749-6632.1995.tb38130.x

Edwards-Lee, T., Miller, B. L., Benson, D. F., Cummings, J. L., Russell, G. L., Boone, K., et al. (1997). The temporal variant of frontotemporal dementia. *Brain* 120(Pt 6), 1027–1040. doi: 10.1093/brain/120.6.1027

Eickhoff, S. B., Bzdok, D., Laird, A. R., Kurth, F., and Fox, P. T. (2012). Activation likelihood estimation meta-analysis revisited. *Neuroimage* 59, 2349–2361. doi: 10.1016/j.neuroimage.2011.09.017

Ellamil, M., Dobson, C., Beeman, M., and Christoff, K. (2012). Evaluative and generative modes of thought during the creative process. *Neuroimage* 59, 1783–1794. doi: 10.1016/j.neuroimage.2011.08.008

Espinel, C. H. (1996). de Kooning's late colours and forms: dementia, creativity, and the healing power of art. *Lancet* 347, 1096–1098. doi: 10.1016/S0140-6736(96)90285-8

Fellows, L. K. (2013). "Decision-making: executive functions meet motivation," in *Principles of Frontal Lobe Function, 2nd Edn.*, eds D. T. Stuss and R. T. Knight (New York, NY: Oxford University Press), 490–500.

Fink, A., Grabner, R. H., Benedek, M., Reishofer, G., Hauswirth, V., Fally, M., et al. (2009). The creative brain: investigation of brain activity during creative problem solving by means of EEG and FMRI. *Hum. Brain Mapp.* 30, 734–748. doi: 10.1002/hbm.20538

Fink, A., Grabner, R. H., Gebauer, D., Reishofer, G., Koschutnig, K., and Ebner, F. (2010). Enhancing creativity by means of cognitive stimulation: evidence from an fMRI study. *Neuroimage* 52, 1687–1695. doi: 10.1016/j.neuroimage.2010.05.072

Finkelstein, Y., Vardi, J., and Hod, I. (1991). Impulsive artistic creativity as a presentation of transient cognitive alterations. *Behav. Med.* 17, 91–94. doi: 10.1080/08964289.1991.9935164

Finney, G. R., and Heilman, K. M. (2007). Artwork before and after onset of progressive nonfluent aphasia. *Cogn. Behav. Neurol.* 20, 7–10. doi: 10.1097/WNN.0b013e31802b6c1f

Folstein, M. F., Folstein, S. E., and McHugh, P. R. (1975). "Mini-mental state." A practical method for grading the cognitive state of patients for the clinician. *J. Psychiatr. Res.* 12, 189–198. doi: 10.1016/0022-3956(75)90026-6

Fornazzari, L. R. (2005). Preserved painting creativity in an artist with Alzheimer's disease. *Eur. J. Neurol.* 12, 419–424. doi: 10.1111/j.1468-1331.2005.01128.x

Fuster, J. M., Bodner, M., and Kroger, J. K. (2000). Cross-modal and cross-temporal association in neurons of frontal cortex. *Nature* 405, 347–351. doi: 10.1038/35012613

Gabora, L. (2010). Revenge of the "Neurds": characterizing creative thought in terms of the structure and dynamics of memory. *Creat. Res. J.* 22, 1–13. doi: 10.1080/10400410903579494

Galarza, M., Isaac, C., Pellicer, O., Mayes, A., Broks, P., Montaldi, D., et al. (2014). Jazz, guitar, and neurosurgery: the Pat Martino case report. *World Neurosurg.* 81, 651.e1–e7. doi: 10.1016/j.wneu.2013.09.042

Gansler, D. A., Moore, D. W., Susmaras, T. M., Jerram, M. W., Sousa, J., and Heilman, K. M. (2011). Cortical morphology of visual creativity. *Neuropsychologia* 49, 2527–2532. doi: 10.1016/j.neuropsychologia.2011.05.001

Geake, J. G., and Hansen, P. C. (2005). Neural correlates of intelligence as revealed by fMRI of fluid analogies. *Neuroimage* 26, 555–564. doi: 10.1016/j.neuroimage.2005.01.035

Gilbert, S. J., Dumontheil, I., Simons, J. S., Frith, C. D., and Burgess, P. W. (2007). Comment on "Wandering minds: the default network and stimulus-independent thought." *Science* 317, 43; author reply 43. doi: 10.1126/science.1140801

Gilbert, S. J., Gonen-Yaacovi, G., Benoit, R. G., Volle, E., and Burgess, P. W. (2010). Distinct functional connectivity associated with lateral versus medial rostral prefrontal cortex: a meta-analysis. *Neuroimage* 53, 1359–1367. doi: 10.1016/j.neuroimage.2010.07.032

Godefroy, O. (2003). Frontal syndrome and disorders of executive functions. *J. Neurol.* 250, 1–6. doi: 10.1007/s00415-003-0918-2

Goel, V., and Vartanian, O. (2005). Dissociating the roles of right ventral lateral and dorsal lateral prefrontal cortex in generation and maintenance of hypotheses in set-shift problems. *Cereb. Cortex* 15, 1170–1177. doi: 10.1093/cercor/bhh217

Goldman-Rakic, P. S. (1995). Architecture of the prefrontal cortex and the central executive. *Ann. N.Y. Acad. Sci.* 769, 71–83. doi: 10.1111/j.1749-6632.1995.tb38132.x

Gonen-Yaacovi, G., de Souza, L. C., Levy, R., Urbanski, M., Josse, G., and Volle, E. (2013). Rostral and caudal prefrontal contribution to creativity: a meta-analysis of functional imaging data. *Front. Hum. Neurosci.* 7:465. doi: 10.3389/fnhum.2013.00465

Green, A. E., Kraemer, D. J. M., Fugelsang, J. A., Gray, J. R., and Dunbar, K. N. (2012). Neural correlates of creativity in analogical reasoning. *J. Exp. Psychol. Learn. Mem. Cogn.* 38, 264-272. doi: 10.1037/a0025764

Gretton, C., and ffytche, D. H. (2014). Art and the brain: a view from dementia. *Int. J. Geriatr. Psychiatry* 29, 111–126. doi: 10.1002/gps.3975

Howard-Jones, P. A., Blakemore, S. J., Samuel, E. A., Summers, I. R., and Claxton, G. (2005). Semantic divergence and creative story generation: an fMRI investigation. *Brain Res. Cogn. Brain Res.* 25, 240–250. doi: 10.1016/j.cogbrainres.2005.05.013

Huang, P., Qiu, L., Shen, L., Zhang, Y., Song, Z., Qi, Z., et al. (2013). Evidence for a left-over-right inhibitory mechanism during figural creative thinking in healthy nonartists. *Hum. Brain Mapp.* 34, 2724–2732. doi: 10.1002/hbm.22093

Jung, R. E. (2013). The structure of creative cognition in the human brain. *Front. Hum. Neurosci.* 7: 330. doi: 10.3389/fnhum.2013.00330

Jung, R. E., Grazioplene, R., Caprihan, A., Chavez, R. S., and Haier, R. J. (2010a). White matter integrity, creativity, and psychopathology: disentangling constructs with diffusion tensor imaging. *PLoS ONE* 5:e9818. doi: 10.1371/journal.pone.0009818

Jung, R. E., Segall, J. M., Jeremy Bockholt, H., Flores, R. A., Smith, S. M., Chavez, R. S., et al. (2010b). Neuroanatomy of creativity. *Hum. Brain Mapp.* 31, 398–409. doi: 10.1002/hbm.20874

Jung-Beeman, M., Bowden, E. M., Haberman, J., Frymiare, J. L., Arambel-Liu, S., Greenblatt, R., et al. (2004). Neural activity when people solve verbal problems with insight. *PLoS Biol.* 2:E97. doi: 10.1371/journal.pbio.0020097

Kapur, N. (1996). Paradoxical functional facilitation in brain-behaviour research. A critical review. *Brain* 119(Pt 5), 1775–90. doi: 10.1093/brain/119.5.1775

Kim, K. H. (2006). Can we trust creativity tests? A review of the torrance tests of creative thinking (TTCT). *Creat. Res. J.* 18, 3–14. doi: 10.1207/s15326934crj1801_2

Kleiner-Fisman, G., Black, S. E., and Lang, A. E. (2003). Neurodegenerative disease and the evolution of art: the effects of presumed corticobasal degeneration in a professional artist. *Mov. Disord.* 18, 294–302. doi: 10.1002/mds.10360

Koechlin, E., and Hyafil, A. (2007). Anterior prefrontal function and the limits of human decision-making. *Science* 318, 594–598. doi: 10.1126/science.1142995

Koechlin, E., Ody, C., and Kouneiher, F. (2003). The architecture of cognitive control in the human prefrontal cortex. *Science* 302, 1181–1185. doi: 10.1126/science.1088545

Kounios, J., Frymiare, J. L., Bowden, E. M., Fleck, J. I., Subramaniam, K., Parrish, T. B., et al. (2006). The prepared mind: neural activity prior to problem presentation predicts subsequent solution by sudden insight. *Psychol. Sci.* 17, 882–890. doi: 10.1111/j.1467-9280.2006.01798.x

Kowatari, Y., Lee, S. H., Yamamura, H., Nagamori, Y., Levy, P., Yamane, S., et al. (2009). Neural networks involved in artistic creativity. *Hum. Brain Mapp.* 30, 1678–1690. doi: 10.1002/hbm.20633

Kozbelt, A. (2011). "Theories of creativity," in *Encyclopedia of Creativity, 2nd Edn.*, eds M. A. Runco and S. R. Pritzker (San Diego, CA: Academic Press), 473–479. doi: 10.1016/B978-0-12-375038-9.00223-5

Kröger, S., Rutter, B., Stark, R., Windmann, S., Hermann, C., and Abraham, A. (2012). Using a shoe as a plant pot: neural correlates of passive conceptual expansion. *Brain Res.* 1430, 52–61. doi: 10.1016/j.brainres.2011.10.031

Levy, B. J., and Wagner, A. D. (2011). Cognitive control and right ventrolateral prefrontal cortex: reflexive reorienting, motor inhibition, and action updating. *Ann. N.Y. Acad. Sci.* 1224, 40–62. doi: 10.1111/j.1749-6632.2011.05958.x

Levy, R., and Volle, E. (2009). [The prefrontal cortex: composer and conductor of voluntary behaviors]. *Rev. Neurol. (Paris).* 165 Spec No 3, F159–F177.

Lhommée, E., Batir, A., Quesada, J. L., Ardouin, C., Fraix, V., Seigneuret, E., et al. (2014). Dopamine and the biology of creativity: lessons from Parkinson's disease. *Front. Neurol.* 5:55. doi: 10.3389/fneur.2014.00055

Limb, C. J., and Braun, A. R. (2008). Neural substrates of spontaneous musical performance: an fMRI study of jazz improvisation. *PLoS ONE* 3:e1679. doi: 10.1371/journal.pone.0001679

Liu, A., Werner, K., Roy, S., Trojanowski, J. Q., Morgan-Kane, U., Miller, B. L., et al. (2009). A case study of an emerging visual artist with frontotemporal lobar degeneration and amyotrophic lateral sclerosis. *Neurocase* 15, 235–247. doi: 10.1080/13554790802633213

Luo, J., Niki, K., and Phillips, S. (2004). Neural correlates of the 'Aha! reaction'. *Neuroreport* 15, 2013–2017. doi: 10.1097/00001756-200409150-00004

Lythgoe, M. F., Pollak, T. A., Kalmus, M., de Haan, M., and Chong, W. K. (2005). Obsessive, prolific artistic output following subarachnoid hemorrhage. *Neurology* 64, 397–398. doi: 10.1212/01.WNL.0000150526.09499.3E

Malloy-Diniz, L. F., Lasmar, V. A., Gazinelli Lde, S., Fuentes, D., and Salgado, J. V. (2007). The Rey Auditory-Verbal Learning Test: applicability for the Brazilian elderly population. *Rev. Bras. Psiquiatr.* 29, 324–329. doi: 10.1590/S1516-44462006005000053

Martin, R. C., and Cheng, Y. (2006). Selection demands versus association strength in the verb generation task. *Psychon. Bull. Rev.* 13, 396–401. doi: 10.3758/BF03193859

Mashal, N., Faust, M., Hendler, T., and Jung-Beeman, M. (2007). An fMRI investigation of the neural correlates underlying the processing of novel metaphoric expressions. *Brain Lang.* 100, 115–126. doi: 10.1016/j.bandl.2005.10.005

Mason, M. F., Norton, M. I., Van Horn, J. D., Wegner, D. M., Grafton, S. T., and Macrae, C. N. (2007). Wandering minds: the default network and stimulus-independent thought. *Science* 315, 393–395. doi: 10.1126/science.1131295

Maurer, K., and Prvulovic, D. (2004). Paintings of an artist with Alzheimer's disease: visuoconstructural deficits during dementia. *J. Neural. Transm.* 111, 235–245. doi: 10.1007/s00702-003-0046-2

Mednick, M. T., Mednick, S. A., and Jung, C. C. (1964). Continual association as a function of level of creativity and type of verbal stimulus. *J. Abnorm. Psychol.* 69, 511–515. doi: 10.1037/h0041086

Mednick, S. A. (1962). The associative basis of the creative process. *Psychol. Rev.* 69, 220–232. doi: 10.1037/h0048850

Mell, J. C., Howard, S. M., and Miller, B. L. (2003). Art and the brain: the influence of frontotemporal dementia on an accomplished artist. *Neurology* 60, 1707–1710. doi: 10.1212/01.WNL.0000064164.02891.12

Mendez, M. F. (2004). Dementia as a window to the neurology of art. *Med. Hypotheses* 63, 1–7. doi: 10.1016/j.mehy.2004.03.002

Mendez, M. F., and Perryman, K. M. (2003). Disrupted facial empathy in drawings from artists with frontotemporal dementia. *Neurocase* 9, 44–50. doi: 10.1076/neur.9.1.44.14375

Mesulam, M. M. (1998). From sensation to cognition. *Brain* 121(Pt 6), 1013–1052. doi: 10.1093/brain/121.6.1013

Midorikawa, A., Fukutake, T., and Kawamura, M. (2008). Dementia and painting in patients from different cultural backgrounds. *Eur. Neurol.* 60, 224–229. doi: 10.1159/000151697

Miller, B. L., Boone, K., Cummings, J. L., Read, S. L., and Mishkin, F. (2000). Functional correlates of musical and visual ability in frontotemporal dementia. *Br. J. Psychiatry* 176, 458–463. doi: 10.1192/bjp.176.5.458

Miller, B. L., Cummings, J., Mishkin, F., Boone, K., Prince, F., Ponton, M., et al. (1998). Emergence of artistic talent in frontotemporal dementia. *Neurology* 51, 978–982. doi: 10.1212/WNL.51.4.978

Miller, B. L., and Hou, C. E. (2004). Portraits of artists: emergence of visual creativity in dementia. *Arch. Neurol.* 61, 842–844. doi: 10.1001/archneur.61.6.842

Miller, B. L., Ponton, M., Benson, D. F., Cummings, J. L., and Mena, I. (1996). Enhanced artistic creativity with temporal lobe degeneration. *Lancet* 348, 1744–1745. doi: 10.1016/S0140-6736(05)65881-3

Miller, E. K., and Cohen, J. D. (2001). An integrative theory of prefrontal cortex function. *Annu. Rev. Neurosci.* 24, 167–202. doi: 10.1146/annurev.neuro.24.1.167

Nee, D. E., Jahn, A., and Brown, J. W. (2013). Prefrontal cortex organization: dissociating effects of temporal abstraction, relational abstraction, and integration with fMRI. *Cereb. Cortex.* doi: 10.1093/cercor/bht091. [Epub ahead of print].

Palmiero, M., Di Giacomo, D., and Passafiume, D. (2012). Creativity and dementia: a review. *Cogn. Process.* 13, 193–209. doi: 10.1007/s10339-012-0439-y

Pfeffer, R. I., Kurosaki, T. T., Harrah, C. H. Jr., Chance, J. M., and Filos, S. (1982). Measurement of functional activities in older adults in the community. *J. Gerontol.* 37, 323–329. doi: 10.1093/geronj/37.3.323

Picton, T. W., Stuss, D. T., Alexander, M. P., Shallice, T., Binns, M. A., and Gillingham, S. (2007). Effects of focal frontal lesions on response inhibition. *Cereb. Cortex* 17, 826–838. doi: 10.1093/cercor/bhk031

Plucker, J. A., and Makel, M. C. (2010). "Assessment of creativity," in *The Cambridge Handbook of Creativity*, eds J. C. Kaufman and R. J. Sternberg (Cambridge: Cambridge University Press), 48–73. doi: 10.1017/CBO9780511763205.005

Porto, C. S., Fichman, H. C., Caramelli, P., Bahia, V. S., and Nitrini, R. (2003). Brazilian version of the Mattis dementia rating scale: diagnosis of mild dementia in Alzheimer's disease. *Arq. Neuropsiquiatr.* 61, 339–345. doi: 10.1590/S0004-282X2003000300004

Qiu, J., Li, H., Jou, J., Liu, J., Luo, Y., Feng, T., et al. (2010). Neural correlates of the "Aha" experiences: evidence from an fMRI study of insight problem solving. *Cortex* 46, 397–403. doi: 10.1016/j.cortex.2009.06.006

Quental, N. B., Brucki, S. M., and Bueno, O. F. (2013). Visuospatial function in early Alzheimer's disease—the use of the Visual Object and Space Perception (VOSP) battery. *PLoS ONE* 8:e68398. doi: 10.1371/journal.pone.0068398

Ramnani, N., and Owen, A. M. (2004). Anterior prefrontal cortex: insights into function from anatomy and neuroimaging. *Nat. Rev. Neurosci.* 5, 184–194. doi: 10.1038/nrn1343

Rankin, K. P., Liu, A. A., Howard, S., Slama, H., Hou, C. E., Shuster, K., et al. (2007). A case-controlled study of altered visual art production in Alzheimer's and FTLD. *Cogn. Behav. Neurol.* 20, 48–61. doi: 10.1097/WNN.0b013e31803141dd

Rascovsky, K., Hodges, J. R., Knopman, D., Mendez, M. F., Kramer, J. H., Neuhaus, J., et al. (2011). Sensitivity of revised diagnostic criteria for the behavioural variant of frontotemporal dementia. *Brain* 134, 2456–2477. doi: 10.1093/brain/awr179

Reverberi, C., Toraldo, A., D'Agostini, S., and Skrap, M. (2005). Better without (lateral) frontal cortex? Insight problems solved by frontal patients. *Brain* 128, 2882–2890. doi: 10.1093/brain/awh577

Reynolds, J. R., McDermott, K. B., and Braver, T. S. (2006). A direct comparison of anterior prefrontal cortex involvement in episodic retrieval and integration. *Cereb. Cortex* 16, 519–528. doi: 10.1093/cercor/bhi131

Ritter, S. M., and Dijksterhuis, A. (2014). Creativity-the unconscious foundations of the incubation period. *Front. Hum. Neurosci.* 8:215. doi: 10.3389/fnhum.2014.00215

Runco, M. A. (2004). Creativity. *Annu. Rev. Psychol.* 55, 657–687. doi: 10.1146/annurev.psych.55.090902.141502

Runco, M. A., and Acar, S. (2012). Divergent thinking as an indicator of creative potential. *Creat. Res. J.* 24, 66–75. doi: 10.1080/10400419.2012.652929

Rutter, B., Kröger, S., Stark, R., Schweckendiek, J., Windmann, S., Hermann, C., et al. (2012). Can clouds dance? Neural correlates of passive conceptual expansion using a metaphor processing task: implications for creative cognition. *Brain Cogn.* 78, 114–122. doi: 10.1016/j.bandc.2011.11.002

Sahlas, D. J. (2003). Dementia with Lewy bodies and the neurobehavioral decline of Mervyn Peake. *Arch. Neurol.* 60, 889–892. doi: 10.1001/archneur.60.6.889

Schoenbaum, G., Roesch, M. R., Stalnaker, T. A., and Takahashi, Y. K. (2009). A new perspective on the role of the orbitofrontal cortex in adaptive behaviour. *Nat. Rev. Neurosci.* 10, 885–892. doi: 10.1038/nrn2753

Schott, G. D. (2012). Pictures as a neurological tool: lessons from enhanced and emergent artistry in brain disease. *Brain* 135, 1947–1963. doi: 10.1093/brain/awr314

Schrag, A., and Trimble, M. (2001). Poetic talent unmasked by treatment of Parkinson's disease. *Mov. Disord.* 16, 1175–1176. doi: 10.1002/mds.1239

Seeley, W. W., Matthews, B. R., Crawford, R. K., Gorno-Tempini, M. L., Foti, D., Mackenzie, I. R., et al. (2008). Unravelling Boléro: progressive aphasia, transmodal creativity and the right posterior neocortex. *Brain* 131, 39–49. doi: 10.1093/brain/awm270

Seger, C. A., Desmond, J. E., Glover, G. H., and Gabrieli, J. D. (2000). Functional magnetic resonance imaging evidence for right-hemisphere involvement in processing unusual semantic relationships. *Neuropsychology* 14, 361–369. doi: 10.1037/0894-4105.14.3.361

Serrano, C., Allegri, R. F., Martelli, M., Taragano, F., and Rinalli, P. (2005). [Visual art, creativity and dementia]. *Vertex* 16, 418–429.

Shah, C., Erhard, K., Ortheil, H.-J., Kaza, E., Kessler, C., and Lotze, M. (2013). Neural correlates of creative writing: an fMRI Study. *Hum. Brain Mapp.* 34, 1088–1101. doi: 10.1002/hbm.21493

Shallice, T., and Burgess, P. (1996). The domain of supervisory processes and temporal organization of behaviour. *Philos. Trans. R. Soc. Lond. B Biol. Sci.* 351, 1405–1411; discussion 1411–1412. doi: 10.1098/rstb.1996.0124

Shamay-Tsoory, S. G., Adler, N., Aharon-Peretz, J., Perry, D., and Mayseless, N. (2011). The origins of originality: the neural bases of creative thinking and originality. *Neuropsychologia* 49, 178–185. doi: 10.1016/j.neuropsychologia.2010.11.020

Siebörger, F. T., Ferstl, E. C., and von Cramon, D. Y. (2007). Making sense of nonsense: an fMRI study of task induced inference processes during discourse comprehension. *Brain Res.* 1166, 77–91. doi: 10.1016/j.brainres.2007.05.079

Simonton, D. K. (2010). Creative thought as blind-variation and selective-retention: combinatorial models of exceptional creativity. *Phys. Life Rev.* 7, 190–194. doi: 10.1016/j.plrev.2010.05.004

Spreng, R. N., Stevens, W. D., Chamberlain, J. P., Gilmore, A. W., and Schacter, D. L. (2010). Default network activity, coupled with the frontoparietal control network, supports goal-directed cognition. *Neuroimage* 53, 303-317. doi: 10.1016/j.neuroimage.2010.06.016

Sternberg, R. J. (2006). The nature of creativity. *Creat. Res. J.* 18, 87. doi: 10.1207/s15326934crj1801_10

Sternberg, R. J. L., and Lubart, T. (1999). "The concept of creativity: prospects and paradigms," in *Handbook of Creativity*, ed R. J. Sternberg (Cambridge: Cambridge University Press), 3–15.

Strenziok, M., Greenwood, P. M., Santa Cruz, S. A., Thompson, J. C., and Parasuraman, R. (2013). Differential contributions of dorso-ventral and rostro-caudal prefrontal white matter tracts to cognitive control in healthy older adults. *PLoS ONE* 8:e81410. doi: 10.1371/journal.pone.0081410

Takahata, K., Saito, F., Muramatsu, T., Yamada, M., Shirahase, J., Tabuchi, H., et al. (2014). Emergence of realism: enhanced visual artistry and high accuracy of visual numerosity representation after left prefrontal damage. *Neuropsychologia* 57, 38–49. doi: 10.1016/j.neuropsychologia.2014.02.022

Takeuchi, H., Taki, Y., Hashizume, H., Sassa, Y., Nagase, T., Nouchi, R., et al. (2012). The association between resting functional connectivity and creativity. *Cereb. Cortex* 22, 2921–2929. doi: 10.1093/cercor/bhr371

Takeuchi, H., Taki, Y., Sassa, Y., Hashizume, H., Sekiguchi, A., Fukushima, A., et al. (2010a). Regional gray matter volume of dopaminergic system associate with creativity: evidence from voxel-based morphometry. *Neuroimage* 51, 578–585. doi: 10.1016/j.neuroimage.2010.02.078

Takeuchi, H., Taki, Y., Sassa, Y., Hashizume, H., Sekiguchi, A., Fukushima, A., et al. (2010b). White matter structures associated with creativity: evidence from diffusion tensor imaging. *Neuroimage* 51, 11–18. doi: 10.1016/j.neuroimage.2010.02.035

Thomas-Anterion, C. (2009). Emergence of artist talent and neurology: three cases. *Rev. Neuropsychol.* 1, 221–228. doi: 10.1684/nrp.2009.0029

Thomas-Anterion, C., Creac'h, C., Dionet, E., Borg, C., Extier, C., Faillenot, I., et al. (2010). De novo artistic activity following insular–SII ischemia. *Pain* 150, 121–127. doi: 10.1016/j.pain.2010.04.010

Thomas-Anterion, C., Honore-Masson, S., Dirson, S., and Laurent, B. (2002). Lonely cowboy's thoughts. *Neurology* 59, 1812–1813. doi: 10.1212/01.WNL.0000035637.48621.68

Thompson-Schill, S. L., and Botvinick, M. M. (2006). Resolving conflict: a response to Martin and Cheng (2006). *Psychon. Bull. Rev.* 13, 402–408; discussion: 09–11.

Tian, F., Tu, S., Qiu, J., Lv, J. Y., Wei, D. T., Su, Y. H., et al. (2011). Neural correlates of mental preparation for successful insight problem solving. *Behav. Brain Res.* 216, 626–630. doi: 10.1016/j.bbr.2010.09.005

Torrance, E. P. (2004). Un résumé historique du développement des tests de pensée créative de Torrance. *Rev. Eur. Psychol. Appl.* 54, 57–63. doi: 10.1016/j.erap.2004.01.003

van Buren, B., Bromberger, B., Potts, D., Miller, B., and Chatterjee, A. (2013). Changes in painting styles of two artists with Alzheimer's disease. *Psychol. Aesthet. Creat. Arts* 7, 89–94. doi: 10.1037/a0029332

Vartanian, O., and Goel, V. (2005). Task constraints modulate activation in right ventral lateral prefrontal cortex. *Neuroimage* 27, 927–933. doi: 10.1016/j.neuroimage.2005.05.016

Vartanian, O., Martindale, C., and Kwiatkowski, J. (2007). Creative potential, attention, and speed of information processing. *Pers. Individ. Dif.* 43, 1470–1480. doi: 10.1016/j.paid.2007.04.027

Volle, E., de Lacy Costello, A., Coates, L. M., McGuire, C., Towgood, K., Gilbert, S., et al. (2012). Dissociation between verbal response initiation and suppression after prefrontal lesions. *Cereb. Cortex* 22, 2428–2440. doi: 10.1093/cercor/bhr322

Volle, E., Gilbert, S. J., Benoit, R. G., and Burgess, P. W. (2010). Specialization of the rostral prefrontal cortex for distinct analogy processes. *Cereb. Cortex* 20, 2647–2659. doi: 10.1093/cercor/bhq012

Volle, E., Levy, R., and Burgess, P. W. (2013). "A new era for lesion-behavior mapping of prefrontal functions," in *Principles of Frontal Lobe Function, 2nd edn.*, eds D. T. Stuss and R. T. Knight (New York, NY: Oxford University Press), 500–523.

Ward, T. B., and Kolomyts, Y. (2010). "Cognition and creativity," in *The Cambridge Handbook of Creativity*, eds J. C. Kaufman and R. J. Sternberg (Cambridge: Cambridge University Press), 93–112. doi: 10.1017/CBO9780511763205.008

Warrington, E. K., and James, M. (1991). *Visual Object and Space Perception Battery*. Bury St Edmunds: Thames Valley Test Company

Wise, R. J., and Braga, R. M. (2014). Default mode network: the seat of literary creativity? *Trends Cogn. Sci.* 18, 116–117. doi: 10.1016/j.tics.2013.11.001

Wu, T. Q., Miller, Z. A., Adhimoolam, B., Zackey, D. D., Khan, B. K., Ketelle, R., et al. (2013). Verbal creativity in semantic variant primary progressive aphasia. *Neurocase*. doi: 10.1080/13554794.2013.860179. [Epub ahead of print].

Yaniv, I., and Meyer, D. E. (1987). Activation and metacognition of inaccessible stored information: potential bases for incubation effects in problem solving. *J. Exp. Psychol. Learn. Mem. Cogn.* 13, 187–205. doi: 10.1037/0278-7393.13.2.187

Yeterian, E. H., Pandya, D. N., Tomaiuolo, F., and Petrides, M. (2012). The cortical connectivity of the prefrontal cortex in the monkey brain. *Cortex* 48, 58–81. doi: 10.1016/j.cortex.2011.03.004

Zhong, C. B., Dijksterhuis, A., and Galinsky, A. D. (2008). The merits of unconscious thought in creativity. *Psychol. Sci.* 19, 912–918. doi: 10.1111/j.1467-9280.2008.02176.x

22

Caloric vestibular stimulation as a treatment for conversion disorder: a case report and medical hypothesis

Michael Noll-Hussong[1]*, Sabrina Holzapfel[2], Dan Pokorny[1] and Simone Herberger[3]

[1] Klinik und Poliklinik fuer Psychosomatische Medizin und Psychotherapie des Universitaetsklinikums Ulm, Ulm, Germany
[2] Hals-Nasen-Ohrenklinik und Poliklinik, Klinikum rechts der Isar, Technische Universitaet Muenchen, Muenchen, Germany
[3] Klinik fuer Psychosomatische Medizin und Psychotherapie des Klinikums Muenchen-Harlaching, Muenchen, Germany

Edited by:
Ripu D. Jindal, University of Pittsburgh School of Medicine, USA

Reviewed by:
Tariq Munshi, Queen's University, Canada
Casimiro Cabrera Abreu, Queen's University, Canada

***Correspondence:**
Michael Noll-Hussong, Department of Psychosomatic Medicine and Psychotherapy, University of Ulm, Albert-Einstein-Allee 23, Ulm D-89081, Germany
e-mail: minohu@gmx.net

Conversion disorder is a medical condition in which a person has paralysis, blindness, or other neurological symptoms that cannot be clearly explained physiologically. To date, there is neither specific nor conclusive treatment. In this paper, we draw together a number of disparate pieces of knowledge to propose a novel intervention to provide transient alleviation for this condition. As caloric vestibular stimulation has been demonstrated to modulate a variety of cognitive functions associated with brain activations, especially in the temporal–parietal cortex, anterior cingulate cortex, and insular cortex, there is evidence to assume an effect in specific mental disorders. Therefore, we go on to hypothesize that lateralized cold vestibular caloric stimulation will be effective in treating conversion disorder and we present provisional evidence from one patient that supports this conclusion. If our hypothesis is correct, this will be the first time in psychiatry and neurology that a clinically well-known mental disorder, long considered difficult to understand and to treat, is relieved by a simple or common, non-invasive medical procedure.

Keywords: conversion disorder, vestibular stimulation, case report, medical hypothesis

"[...]that mysterious leap from the soul to the body."
Sigmund Freud, Vorlesungen zur Einführung in die Psychoanalyse, 1916–1917

... and about 100 years later:
"Perhaps the most chastening lesson [...] is the striking lack of specificity of any of the findings so far described. Although we might predict that a patient describing bodily disturbance of "some kind" will exhibit abnormalities of certain candidate brain regions, we would have great difficulty modifying their diagnosis or treatment on the basis of the results of brain scanning."
Sean A. Spence, 2006 (1)

INTRODUCTION

Conversion disorder (2) as defined in DSM-IV (3) describes symptoms such as weakness, paralysis, seizures, or abnormal movements that are not attributable to a general medical condition or to feigning, and that are judged to be associated with psychological factors (4). It has been estimated that 10% of all mental disorders and 30% of neurological inpatients suffer from conversion disorder (2, 5, 6). However, as diagnosis is not easy (7), there are few evidence-based treatments for conversion disorder (8, 9). The name "conversion disorder" refers both to a hypothesis based on psychoanalytic etiology and to a long history of a multitude of disorders formerly named "hysteria" (10–12). Follow-up data of patients, especially those with psychogenic movement disorders revealed a persistence in abnormal movements in more than 90% of subjects. Prevalence rates of mental illness in excess of those found in the general population and in neurological disorders, plus an inability to acknowledge the essentially psychological nature of their condition characterize the outcome picture and lead to a poor longer-term prognosis in these patients (13). In special cases, the clinical phenomenology resembles the "alien hand sign" first described by Brion and Jedynak as a "feeling of estrangement between the patient and one of his hands" (14). This may, on the one hand, indicate the lack of awareness of the origin of their symptoms in conversion disorder patients as a possible result from suppression of brain activity normally related to self-agency (15), and, on the other hand, the frequent clinical impression that the symptoms are often accompanied by an affective state traditionally named "*belle indifférence*" – a condition in which the person is unconcerned with symptoms (16).

Although long dominant, the conversion hypothesis is now just one of many competing etiological hypotheses and has little supportive empirical evidence (17). Furthermore, the name "conversion disorder" has not been widely accepted by either non-psychiatrists or patients (18–20). Low education, presence of a personality disorder, and high Hamilton depression score were found to be significantly associated with conversion disorder (21). As there are many similarities between the symptoms of conversion, hysteria, and phenomena produced in hypnotic contexts, a model has been proposed that develops the idea of a central executive structure, similar to the notion of a supervisory attentional system, acting outside self-awareness but at a late stage of information processing, which can be directly influenced by both internal and external sources to produce the relevant phenomena (22). Thus, as conversion disorder, pain disorder, and dissociation disorders appear to be linked by a common mechanism, they could be classified together under the heading of "auto-suggestive disorder"

(22). Altogether, the notion that the etiology of these symptoms is wholly psychological may be scientifically incorrect. For example, functional brain imaging studies that demonstrated contralateral thalamic hypoactivity in hemisensory conversion encourage us to understand conversion symptoms from a non-dualistic brain as well as mind perspective (23–27).

Caloric vestibular stimulation (CVS) is a physiological technique demonstrated to modulate tactile perception in healthy subjects after left ear CVS (28). Moreover, it has been shown that CVS is helpful, amongst others, in some patients with central pain like Dejerine–Roussy syndrome (thalamic pain syndrome) (29, 30), central post-stroke pain (31), aphasia (32), and spatial neglect (33), right-sided central pain following transverse myelitis of the cervical spinal cord (34), and post-stroke tactile allodynia (35). On the other hand, it has been shown that CVS has no effect on tinnitus (36).

Interestingly, CVS could also transiently improve hemianesthesia in right brain-damaged patients (37–39). Recent studies suggest that these effects are based on the anatomical overlap between vestibular and tactile projections (37) in the human brain. For example, in a right brain-damaged patient with neglect, this symptom was improved especially following left CVS, and worsened following right CVS. No modification of neglect was observed after bilateral vestibular stimulation (40).

The first case of transitory attenuation of neglect phenomena during CVS was documented by Silberpfennig (41) in 1941. The finding has been confirmed by Rubens by testing unilateral neglect on tasks requiring visual exploration of extrapersonal space in a series of patients (42). Cappa et al. demonstrated the positive effects of vestibular stimulation on personal and extrapersonal neglect, respectively, and on awareness of disease in four patients with severe neglect and anosognosia, and speculated about a possible role of vestibular stimulation in hemispheric brain activation (43). The effects of vestibular stimulation on somatophrenic delusion were investigated by Bisiach et al. in a patient suffering from fronto-temporo-parietal infarction located in the right hemisphere (44). They could show that transitory remission of the patient's delusional belief was consistently observed during unilateral vestibular activation, achieved by cold-water irrigation of the contralesional ear (43). Ramachandran replicated these results in one patient with anosognosia in parietal lobe syndrome (45), and recently – as there may be a unitary mechanism underlying both anosognosia (46) and unrealistic optimism – it has been shown that left-sided cold-water CVS attenuates unrealistic optimism in healthy adults (47).

Altogether, and focusing on mental disorders in particular, it has recently been shown that a single-session CVS may have short-lived beneficial effects in mania and perhaps in other types of psychoses (48). Recently, the beneficial effects of CVS on denial of illness and manic delusions in schizoaffective disorder have been shown in a case series of three patients (48). Body integrity image disorder (BIID) is characterized by a feeling of mismatch between the internal feeling of how one's body should be and the physical reality of how it actually is. Patients with this condition have an often-overwhelming desire for amputation of a specific limb at a specific level. Such patients are not psychotic or delusional; however, they do express an inexplicable emotional abhorrence to the limb they wish removed. It is also known that such patients show a left-sided preponderance for their desired amputation – conversion disorders are also prevalent on the left side, especially in women (49). Often, BIID patients take drastic action to be rid of the offending limb. Given the left-sided bias, emotional rejection, and specificity of desired amputation, we suggest that there are clear similarities to be drawn between BIID and somatoparaphrenia. In this rare condition, which follows a right parietal stroke, the patient rejects (usually) his left arm as "alien" (50). Ramachandran et al. go on to hypothesize that a dysfunction of the right parietal lobe is also the cause of BIID and suggest that this leads to an uncoupling of the construct of one's body image in the right parietal lobe from how one's body physically is (50, 51). Recently, and interestingly in healthy subjects, it has been shown that CVS, depending on the side of stimulation, has a modulating effect on mood and affective control (52).

Taking all the disparate pieces of the mentioned knowledge together, there is reason to speculate about the positive effects of CVS in special mental disorders like conversion disorder, somatoform (pain) disorders, dissociative disorder, and even posttraumatic stress disorder (PTSD) in terms of a "functional neglect" that shares a lot of the above-mentioned symptoms like unclear functional losses, perturbed affective states, and emotional peculiarities. In this pilot study, we tested for the first time, in one patient, the idea that single-session CVS by application of cold-water to the left ear induces a clinically significant, short-lived beneficial effect on conversion disorder.

CASE REPORT

We have provisional data from one 26-year-old right-handed male patient with conversion disorder or psychogenic movement disorder diagnosed using Fahn and Williams' criteria (53) in terms of a hyperkinetic disturbance of voluntary motor function (54), especially of his arms and, varying, the upper part of the body (e.g., involuntary "bowings"), with more than 2 years' duration. The German patient had received many different medical treatments with no longer lasting improvement, resulting in a significant burden for the patient and his family. In some cases, physical activity alleviated the symptoms, as has been described elsewhere (55), as (interpersonal) "stress" could trigger the symptoms.

BEHAVIORAL INSTRUMENTS

Patient burden was controlled at the beginning using "The Symptom Checklist-90-R (SCL-90-R)" (56, 57), the scales for emotion experience (SEE), emotional competence questionnaire (EKF), Beck's depression inventory (BDI), and temperament and character inventory (TCI). According to the homepage of the publishing house Pearson Assessments (58), "the symptom checklist-90-R (SCL-90-R) instrument helps evaluate a broad range of psychological problems and symptoms of psychopathology. The instrument is also useful in measuring patient progress or treatment outcomes." The 90 items of the self-assessment checklist are scaled from 0 to 4 and is associated with the problems the patient has been suffering during the last 7 days. The summarizing global severity index (GSI) is a *de facto* standard for psychotherapy clinical practice and research, and serves as a kind of "symptom severity thermometer." The nine specific subscales of the GSI provide an overview of the spectrum of patient complaints.

The SEE (59) assesses individual emotional experiences as well as appraisal and regulation of emotions on a five-point Likert scale including "1 = not true at all," "2 = hardly true," "3 = moderate true," "4 = fairly true," and "5 = absolute true." The questionnaire comprises 42 items, which constitute seven subscales: (1) acceptance of emotions assesses a positive appreciation of one's own feelings; (2) experience of emotion flooding describes the experience of too many concurrent feelings; (3) experience of emotion deficit contains items describing individuals who perceive few emotions and feel cut off from their body; (4) body-related symbolization of emotions refers to bodily sensations that denote mental processes and feelings; (5) imaginative symbolization of emotions contains items that see fantasies and dreams as helpful for coping with diverse problems; (6) experience of emotion regulation refers to the ability to regulate emotions and moods by calming oneself or getting into a lively mood; and (7) experience of self-control assesses the ability to appear outwardly controlled and self-possessed (60).

The EKF (61) comprises 62 items and participants rate on a five-point Likert-type scale the extent to which they agree (ranging from strongly agree to strongly disagree) with the statements depicted. The questionnaire consists of four subscales measuring the constructs recognizing and understanding one's own emotions, recognizing and understanding the emotions of others, the ability to regulate and control one's own emotions, and emotional expressiveness. The total score reflects a person's self-rated emotional competence as a subdomain of their self-concept (62).

The applied BDI-II is a 21-item self-report instrument that measures cognitive and endogenous aspects of depression on four-point scales ranging from 0 to 3. The standard cut-offs are as follows: 0–9 indicates no depression; 10–18 a mild depression; 19–29 a moderate depression; and >29 a severe depression. This questionnaire has undergone extensive reliability and validation studies (63, 64).

The German version (65) of the TCI consists of seven factors: four dimensions of temperament (novelty seeking, harm avoidance, reward dependence, and persistence) and three dimensions of character (self-directedness, cooperativeness, and self-transcendence). It is a self-assessment tool with 240 true/false items (66). The temperament subdimensions can be divided into the following parts: (1) novelty seeking NS (subscales: exploratory excitability, impulsiveness, extravagance, and disorderliness); (2) harm avoidance HS (anticipatory worry, fear of uncertainty, shyness, and fatigability); (3) reward dependence RD (sentimentality, attachment, and dependence); and (4) persistence (P).

The character subdimensions can be divided into the following parts: (5) self-directedness SD (responsibility, purpose, resourcefulness, self-acceptance, and enlightened second nature); (6) cooperativeness C (social acceptance, empathy, helpfulness, compassion, and pure-hearted conscience); and (7) self-transcendence ST (self-forgetfulness, transpersonal identification, and spiritual acceptance).

The gray-shaded area between standardized T-scores 40 and 60 shown in **Figures 1** and **2** corresponds roughly to the middle 68.3% proportion of the German population. Interestingly, all of the psychometric results of the patient were almost in this "normal" range. Being compared with the population, the scale values of the patient were neither too high, nor too low.

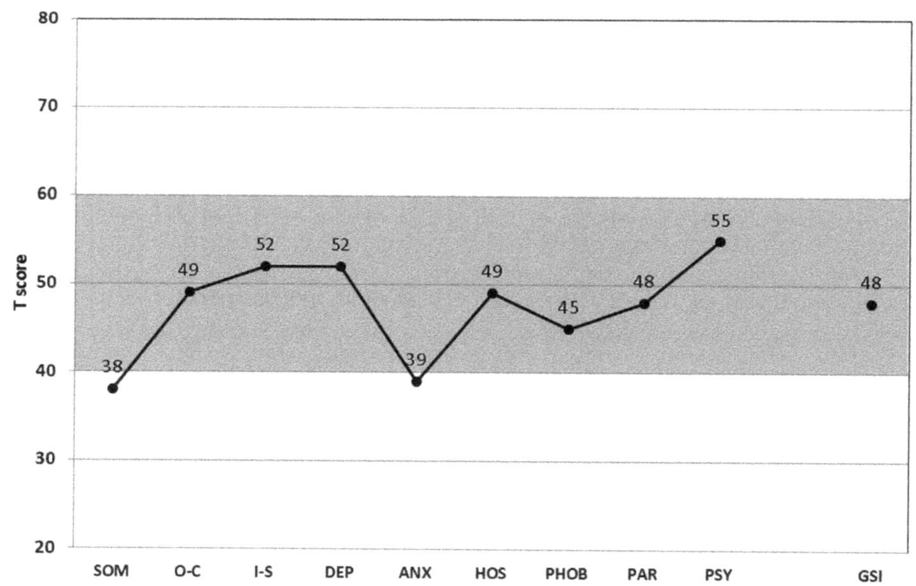

FIGURE 1 | Score *Profile* of the symptom checklist-90-R (SCL-90-R). All nine subscales (SOM, somatization; O–C, obsessive–compulsive; I-S, interpersonal sensitivity; DEP, depression; ANS, anxiety; HOS, hostility; PHOB, phobic anxiety; PAR, paranoid ideation; PSY, psychoticism), and the GSI (global severity index) are presented (67). (T50, T60, T70: thresholds for the standard male German population. T60 is considered "clinically suspicious" and T70 "clinically relevant." For the GSI, T60 is already considered "clinically relevant." Gray-shaded area depicts the normal range.)

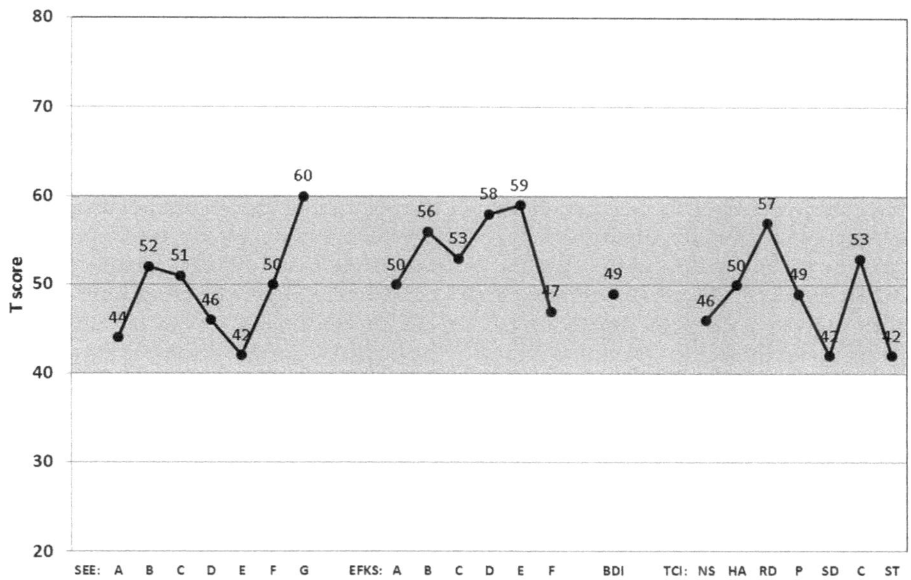

FIGURE 2 | Score *Profiles* of the scales for emotion experience (SEE), emotional competence questionnaire (EKF), Beck's depression inventory (BDI), and temperament and character inventory (TCI). All relevant subscales of the SEE (A, acceptance of one's emotions; B, experience of emotion flooding; C, experience of emotion deficiency; D, body-related symbolization of emotions; E, imaginative symbolization of emotions; F, experience of emotion regulation; G, experience of self-control), EKF (A, recognizing and understanding one's emotions; B, recognizing emotions in others; C, regulation and control of one's emotions; D, emotional expressivity; E, regulation of the feelings of others; F, adjustment to feelings), BDI-II, and TCI (NS, novelty seeking; HS, harm avoidance; RD, reward dependence; P, persistence; SD, self-directedness; C, cooperativeness; ST, self-transcendence) are presented. (Gray-shaded area depicts the normal range.)

In fact, it happens rather rarely that all results of relevant subscales lay in the "main stream field." Hence, from the psychometric point of view (despite the clinical and subjective impression of the sufferer), the patient seems to be "suspiciously healthy." Last not least (and "*primum nil nocere*"), no adverse reactions were reported.

PATIENT REPORTS (EXCERPTS, IN ENGLISH TRANSLATION)

- First trial, 30°C water, 20 s, left CVS:

> "[...]I had slight symptoms when I went to the otolaryngology department. The ladies there were very nice. The treatment itself was unproblematic. Only the left ear was exposed to "cold" water. My sense of balance was minimally disturbed when I was lying down. This was over after about 2 minutes. I was walking down the hall back to the ward again at 8:39. I of course tried to evoke symptoms by repeating "I remember..." – but to no avail. No symptoms appeared when I attempted to consciously evoke them. I just couldn't really do it. That is, I was able to think the thought through. I'll try explaining it better next week. I didn't want to get too euphoric, though. And unfortunately, rightly so. Today, shortly after 8 p.m., I was back at square one. I had just finished showering and was once again trying my "I remember...," and since then, the usual "rules of the game" from before the otolaryngological checkup have applied. I'll describe this situation in words better next week as well."

- Second trial, 1 week later, 20°C water, 30 s, left CVS:

> "I went to the otolaryngology department today. There were some technical problems at first [that lasted for an hour], then the stimulation was conducted. The desired results were unfortunately not achieved. The symptoms could not be interrupted. I can of course only speculate why it didn't work out this time. I was "stressed" about an appointment I had at 9:00, which I would be late to [because of the technical problems mentioned above]. A symptom-triggering situation unintentionally crossed my mind during the stimulation. The interruption last time was a coincidence. Which I find difficult to imagine, however."

- Third and final trial, 1 week later, 20°C water, 60 s, left CVS:

> "My expectations today were very limited. [...] I have virtually no symptoms at the moment, i.e., I am not reacting very strongly. I definitely do, however, have enough symptoms to be able to assess the effects of a stimulation. Now about the stimulation: it again had the effect that I could talk about the "handshaking situation" or similar situations or to consciously evoke them without developing any symptoms. "Stress" and "minor allegations" don't seem to be causing me any problems so far. I just took a chance and arrived nearly 10 minutes late to my relational care appointment. Whether this would have also been possible without the stimulation is not determinable. I had a slight relapse, however, at 13:44, which was prompted by the relational counseling session.

A terse allegation, which has nothing to do with the above, but it occurred when the relational counseling session came to an end. I wished my counselor a nice vacation, even though I'll see her again next week for the nightshift. So, too soon (minor allegation). It all came back to me again when I was in my room at 13:44 and triggered slight symptoms. That's when I thought to myself "there goes the stimulation's effect," since I was briefly confronted with recollections again from that point on, a bit stronger than before the stimulation. But I was already used to it from the first stimulation, when the "effect" began to diminish after 36 h. I wanted to write you a mail thereafter. But after 2 min, I was no longer responding to recollections of movements and therefore waited until now. I have not had any further movement disorders so far. Not even when the content of this mail briefly disappeared;). I am curious how long it'll last. I don't plan to force the issue, though."

3 days later:

"I have not noticed any further real movement disorders so far. There were only some very slight indications, expressed more internally through minimal tension or a very slowed and inhibited movement disorder which only manifests itself very rarely, i.e., 2–3 times since Friday. I am less prone to "stress," i.e., stressful situations are no longer accompanied by movement disorders, which allows you to act in a completely different mode."

DISCUSSION

In our patient, left caloric irrigation caused an immediate and sustained relief from his functional disability that has so far lasted at least for hours. It has been stated that the vestibular system is unique among the senses because of the entirely multisensory nature of its cortical projections (68) and its overlapping with other neural networks, e.g., emotional circuits (69). In this context, it has recently been hypothesized that the human vestibular cortex may be crucial for bodily self-consciousness (70).

Neuroanatomical and neuroimaging studies have shown that vestibular stimulation activates somatosensory areas, and particularly the so-called parieto-insular vestibular cortex in the monkey, while deactivating visual areas (68). Further, recent psychophysical studies have shown that vestibular stimulation facilitates detection of electrocutaneous stimuli, suggesting a vestibular–somatosensory perceptual interaction (68, 71). While several recent reports have described the capacity of CVS to transiently improve or reverse a wide range of attentional, cognitive, and motor impairments, e.g., in mentally retarded, emotionally disturbed, and learning-disabled individuals (72) or autistic children (73), most examples are in right hemisphere-damaged patients with long-standing brain injury (37–39). Typically, patients have been tested several months or years after the onset of the deficit. A possible mechanism for the temporary reintegration of multiple cognitive functions is that vestibular stimulation activates thalamocortical mechanisms that reintegrate impaired cortical regions (74). In this context, it has been hypothesized that the essential aspect leading to neglect in brain-damaged patients is a disturbance of those cortical structures that are crucial for transforming the sensory input coordinates from the peripheral sensory organs into an egocentric, body-centered coordinate frame of reference (75), supporting a "representational theory of neglect" (76, 77). Furthermore, it has been shown that caloric stimulation impairs performance in a high-resolution mental imagery and mental rotation task, respectively, but not another cognitive task (78), and one may consequently speculate about the special power of mental imagery – and derived psychotherapeutic procedures – in some mental disorders. Last but not least, an *in vivo* microdialysis study has shown that vestibular stimulation with ice water increases acetylcholine release from rat hippocampus to 160% compared with the basal rate (79), which could reflect one facet of memory facilitation in the mentioned mental disorders (like conversion disorder, but perhaps also PTSD). However and as a limitation – but in all fairness, not unique for CVS – one has to consider placebo effects (80–83).

Finally, at least two related, also unspecific neural stimulation techniques and their published benefits should be mentioned. First, as the experiments of Alessandro Volta were amongst the first to indicate that visuo-spatial function can be altered by stimulating the vestibular nerves with galvanic current, it has recently been shown that Galvanic vestibular stimulation speeds visual memory recall (84). Second, transcranial magnetic stimulation (TMS) is a method of non-invasive brain stimulation that affects the cerebral cortex but not deep structures (85). In patients with movement disorders, the most common application of TMS has been to test the excitability of connections within and among motor areas of the cortex, which has provided useful information on pathophysiology; however, inter-individual variability in the responses has resulted in difficulties in translating this method into a clinically applicable diagnostic use (85). Repeated stimulation (e.g., 1 Hz for 20 min) can result in long-term plastic changes in the motor system, which has led to increased interest in possible therapeutic applications (85). As there is no agreement on the most effective therapy for motor conversion symptoms, functional electric stimulation has also been successfully used to reverse conversion paralysis (86–89). Moreover, it has been speculated that a decrease of motor excitability during motor imagery is the electrophysiological correlate of a disturbed voluntary control in motor conversion disorder (90, 91). Remarkably, these results further indicate that this abnormality is not restricted to the clinically affected body part. One may speculate that, amongst others, vestibular stimulation (92), TMS, and even the central effects of acupuncture (93) share some features that could reintegrate the neural circuits (94) underlying affective or movement initiation and control.

CONCLUSION

If our hypothesis is shown to be correct, this will be the first time in neurology and psychiatry that a potentially chronic mental disorder, long considered difficult to treat, can be transiently relieved by a simple non-invasive, conventional medical procedure. It would offer at least a new therapeutic approach to pseudoneurological syndromes and insights in their etiology. It would also, again, demonstrate the astonishing and rapid plasticity of the brain, especially in relation to psychomotor phenomena and unconscious integration of body schema (95, 96). Altogether, psychogenic movement disorders represent a unique opportunity for medical and scientific specialties to collaborate in the care of a potentially curable but significantly disabling illness (97).

REFERENCES

Spence SA. All in the mind? The neural correlates of unexplained physical symptoms. *Adv Psychiatr Treat* (2006) 12(5):349–58. doi:10.1192/apt.12.5.349

Noll-Hussong M, Henningsen P. Zur Neuro-Psychosomatik der Konversion. *Schweiz Arch Neurol Psychiatr* (2009) 160:356–61. doi:10.1111/j.1439-0388.1993.tb00716.x

American Psychiatric Association. *Diagnostic and Statistic Manual of Mental Disorders (Text Revision)*. 4th ed. Washington, DC: American Psychiatric Pub- lishing, Inc (2000).

Stone J, LaFrance WC Jr, Levenson JL, Sharpe M. Issues for DSM-5: conversion disorder. *Am J Psychiatry* (2010) 167(6):626–7. doi:10.1176/appi.ajp.2010. 09101440

Carson AJ, Best S, Postma K, Stone J, Warlow C, Sharpe M. The outcome of neu- rology outpatients with medically unexplained symptoms: a prospective cohort study. *J Neurol Neurosurg Psychiatry* (2003) 74(7):897–900. doi:10.1136/jnnp. 74.7.897

Nimnuan C, Hotopf M, Wessely S. Medically unexplained symptoms: an epidemiological study in seven specialities. *J Psychosom Res* (2001) 51(1):361–7. doi:10.1016/S0022-3999(01)00223-9

Morgante F, Edwards MJ, Espay AJ, Fasano A, Mir P, Martino D, et al. Diagnos- tic agreement in patients with psychogenic movement disorders. *Mov Disord* (2012) 27(4):548–52. doi:10.1002/mds.24903

Stone J, Carson A, Sharpe M. Functional symptoms in neurology: management. *J Neurol Neurosurg Psychiatry* (2005) 76(Suppl 1):i13–21. doi:10.1136/jnnp.2004.061655

Ruddy R, House A. Psychosocial interventions for conversion disorder. *Cochrane Database Syst Rev* (2005) (4):CD005331.

Bogousslavsky J. Hysteria after Charcot: back to the future. *Front Neurol Neurosci* (2011) 29:137–61. doi:10.1159/000321783

Mai FM. "Hysteria" in clinical neurology. *Can J Neurol Sci* (1995) 22(2):101–10.

Gould R, Miller BL, Goldberg MA, Benson DF. The validity of hysterical signs and symptoms. *J Nerv Ment Dis* (1986) 174(10):593–7. doi:10.1097/00005053-198610000-00003

Feinstein A, Stergiopoulos V, Fine J, Lang AE. Psychiatric outcome in patients with a psychogenic movement disorder: a prospective study. *Neuropsychiatry Neuropsychol Behav Neurol* (2001) 14(3):169–76.

Goldberg G, Bloom KK. The alien hand sign. Localization, lateralization and recovery. *Am J Phys Med Rehabil* (1990) 69(5):228–38. doi:10.1097/00002060-199010000-00002

Blakemore RL, Hyland BI, Hammond-Tooke GD, Anson JG. Distinct modulation of event-related potentials during motor preparation in patients with motor conversion disorder. *PLoS One* (2013) 8(4):e62539. doi:10.1371/journal.pone. 0062539

Stone J, Smyth R, Carson A, Warlow C, Sharpe M. La belle indifference in con- ver- sion symptoms and hysteria: systematic review. *Br J Psychiatry* (2006) 188:204–9. doi:10.1192/bjp.188.3.204

Nicholson TR, Stone J, Kanaan RA. Conversion disorder: a problematic diagnosis. *J Neurol Neurosurg Psychiatry* (2011) 82(11):1267–73. doi:10.1136/jnnp. 2008.171306

Espay AJ, Goldenhar LM, Voon V, Schrag A, Burton N, Lang AE. Opinions and clinical practices related to diagnosing and managing patients with psychogenic movement disorders: an international survey of movement disorder society members. *Mov Disord* (2009) 24(9):1366–74. doi:10.1002/mds. 22618

Friedman JH, LaFrance WC Jr. Psychogenic disorders: the need to speak plainly. *Arch Neurol* (2010) 67(6):753–5. doi:10.1001/archneurol.2010.91

Kanaan R, Armstrong D, Barnes P, Wessely S. In the psychiatrist's chair: how neurologists understand conversion disorder. *Brain* (2009) 132(Pt 10):2889–96. doi:10.1093/brain/awp060

Binzer M, Andersen PM, Kullgren G. Clinical characteristics of patients with motor disability due to conversion disorder: a prospective control group study. *J Neurol Neurosurg Psychiatry* (1997) 63(1):83–8. doi:10.1136/jnnp.63.1.83

Oakley DA. Hypnosis and conversion hysteria: a unifying model. *Cogn Neuropsychiatry* (1999) 4(3):243–65. doi:10.1080/135468099395954

Vuilleumier P, Chicherio C, Assal F, Schwartz S, Slosman D, Landis T. Functional neuroanatomical correlates of hysterical sensorimotor loss. *Brain* (2001) 124(Pt 6):1077–90. doi:10.1093/brain/124.6.1077

Ellenstein A, Kranick SM, Hallett M. An update on psychogenic movement dis- orders. *Curr Neurol Neurosci Rep* (2011) 11(4):396–403. doi:10.1007/s11910- 011-0205-z

Lang AE, Voon V. Psychogenic movement disorders: past developments, current status, and future directions. *Mov Disord* (2011) 26(6):1175–86. doi:10.1002/ mds.23571

Edwards MJ, Bhatia KP. Functional (psychogenic) movement disorders: merging mind and brain. *Lancet Neurol* (2012) 11(3):250–60. doi:10.1016/S1474-4422(11)70310-6

Nowak DA, Fink GR. Psychogenic movement disorders: aetiology, phenomenology, neuroanatomical correlates and therapeutic approaches. *Neuroimage* (2009) 47(3):1015–25. doi:10.1016/j.neuroimage.2009.04.082

Ferre ER, Sedda A, Gandola M, Bottini G. How the vestibular system modulates tactile perception in normal subjects: a behavioural and physiological study. *Exp Brain Res* (2011) 208(1):29–38. doi:10.1007/s00221-010-2450-9

Ramachandran VS, McGeoch PD, Williams L, Arcilla G. Rapid relief of tha- la- mic pain syndrome induced by vestibular caloric stimulation. *Neurocase* (2007) 13(3):185–8. doi:10.1080/13554790701450446

Ramachandran VS, McGeoch PD, Williams L. Can vestibular caloric stimulation be used to treat Dejerine-Roussy syndrome? *Med Hypotheses* (2007) 69(3):486–8. doi:10.1016/j.mehy.2006.12.013

McGeoch PD, Williams LE, Lee RR, Ramachandran VS. Behavioural evi- dence for vestibular stimulation as a treatment for central post-stroke pain. *J Neurol Neurosurg Psychiatry* (2008) 79(11):1298–301. doi:10.1136/jnnp.2008. 146738

Wilkinson D, Morris R, Milberg W, Sakel M. Caloric vestibular stimulation in aphasic syndrome. *Front Integr Neurosci* (2013) 7:99. doi:10.3389/fnint.2013. 00099

Sturt R, David Punt T. Caloric vestibular stimulation and postural control in patients with spatial neglect following stroke. *Neuropsychol Rehabil* (2013) 23(2):299–316. doi:10.1080/09602011.2012.755831

McGeoch PD, Ramachandran VS. Vestibular stimulation can relieve central pain of spinal origin. *Spinal Cord* (2008) 46(11):756–7. doi:10.1038/sc.2008.47

McGeoch PD, Williams LE, Song T, Lee RR, Huang M, Ramachandran VS. Post-stroke tactile allodynia and its modulation by vestibular stimulation: a MEG case study. *Acta Neurol Scand* (2009) 119(6):404–9. doi:10.1111/j.1600-0404.2008.01106.x

Baguley DM, Knight R, Bradshaw L. Does caloric vestibular stimulation mod- ulate tinnitus? *Neurosci Lett* (2011) 492(1):52–4. doi:10.1016/j.neulet.2011.01. 052

Bottini G, Paulesu E, Sterzi R, Warburton E, Wise RJ, Vallar G, et al. Modulation of conscious experience by peripheral sensory stimuli. *Nature* (1995) 376(6543):778–81. doi:10.1038/376778a0

Bottini G, Paulesu E, Gandola M, Loffredo S, Scarpa P, Sterzi R, et al. Left caloric vestibular stimulation ameliorates right hemianesthesia. *Neurology* (2005) 65(8):1278–83. doi:10.1212/01.wnl.0000182398.14088.e8

Bottini G, Sterzi R, Paulesu E, Vallar G, Cappa SF, Erminio F, et al. Identification of the central vestibular projections in man: a positron emission tomography activation study. *Exp Brain Res* (1994) 99(1):164–9. doi:10.1007/BF00241421

Rode G, Tilikete C, Luaute J, Rossetti Y, Vighetto A, Boisson D. Bilateral vestibu- lar stimulation does not improve visual hemineglect. *Neuropsychologia* (2002) 40(7):1104–6. doi:10.1016/S0028-3932(01)00187-7

Silberpfennig J. Contributions to the problems of eye movement. *Confin Neurol* (1941) 4:1–13. doi:10.1159/000106147

Rubens AB. Caloric stimulation and unilateral visual neglect. *Neurology* (1985) 35(7):1019–24. doi:10.1212/WNL.35.7.1019

Cappa S, Sterzi R, Vallar G, Bisiach E. Remission of hemineglect and anosognosia during vestibular stimulation. *Neuropsychologia* (1987) 25(5):775–82. doi:10.1016/0028-3932(87)90115-1

Bisiach E, Rusconi ML, Vallar G. Remission of somatoparaphrenic delu- sion through vestibular stimulation. *Neuropsychologia* (1991) 29(10):1029–31. doi:10.1016/0028-3932(91)90066-H

Ramachandran VS. Anosognosia in parietal lobe syndrome. *Conscious Cogn* (1995) 4(1):22–51. doi:10.1006/ccog.1995.1002

Ronchi R, Rode G, Cotton F, Farne A, Rossetti Y, Jacquin-Courtois S. Remission of anosognosia for right hemiplegia and neglect after caloric vestibular stimulation. *Restor Neurol Neurosci* (2013) 31(1):19–24. doi:10.3233/RNN- 120236

McKay R, Tamagni C, Palla A, Krummenacher P, Hegemann SC, Straumann D, et al. Vestibular stimulation attenuates unrealistic optimism. *Cortex* (2013) 49(8):2272–5. doi:10.1016/j.cortex.2013.04.005

Levine J, Toder D, Geller V, Kraus M, Gauchman T, Puterman M, et al. Beneficial effects of caloric vestibular stimulation on denial of illness and manic delu- sions in schizoaffective disorder: a case report. *Brain Stimul* (2011) 5(3):267–73. doi:10.1016/j.brs.2011.03.004

Smokler IA, Shevrin H. Cerebral lateralization and personality style. *Arch Gen Psychiatry* (1979) 36(9):949–54. doi:10.1001/archpsyc.1979.01780090035004

Ramachandran VS, McGeoch P. Can vestibular caloric stimulation be used to treat apotemnophilia? *Med Hypotheses* (2007) 69(2):250–2. doi:10.1016/j.mehy. 2006.12.013

McGeoch PD, Brang D, Song T, Lee RR, Huang M, Ramachandran VS. Xenomelia: a new right parietal lobe syndrome. *J Neurol Neurosurg Psychiatry* (2011) 82(12):1314–9. doi:10.1136/jnnp-2011-300224

Preuss N, Hasler G, Mast FW. Caloric vestibular stimulation modulates affective control and mood. *Brain Stimul* (2014) 7(1):133–40. doi:10.1016/j.brs.2013.09. 003

Fahn S, Williams DT. Psychogenic dystonia. *Adv Neurol* (1988) 50:431–55.

Reich SG. Pearls: hyperkinetic movement disorders. *Semin Neurol* (2010) 30(1):15–22. doi:10.1055/s-0029-1245005

Dallocchio C, Arbasino C, Klersy C, Marchioni E. The effects of physical activity on psychogenic movement disorders. *Mov Disord* (2010) 25(4):421–5. doi:10.1002/mds.22952

Derogatis LR, Cleary PA. Confirmation of the dimensional structure of the SCL-90: a study in construct validation. *J Clin Psychol* (1977) 33:981–9. doi:10.1002/1097-4679(197710)33:4<981::AID-JCLP2270330412>3.0.CO;2-0

Marcelissen TA, Leong RK, Nieman FH, van Lankveld JJ, van Kerrebroeck PE, de Wachter SG. Psychological and psychiatric factors as predictors for success in sacral neuromodulation treatment. *BJU Int* (2011) 108(11):1834–8. doi:10.1111/j.1464-410X.2011.10205.x

Available from: http://psychcorp.pearsonassessments.com/HAIWEB/Cultures/en-us/Productdetail.htm?Pid=PAg514

Behr M, Becker M. *SEE – Skalen zum Erleben von Emotionen (Scales for Emotion Experience)*. Göttingen: Hogrefe (2004).

Werner NS, Duschek S, Schandry R. Relationships between affective states and decision-making. *Int J Psychophysiol* (2009) 74(3):259–65. doi:10.1016/j. ijpsycho.2009.09.010

Rindermann H. *EKF – Emotionale-Kompetenz-Fragebogen – Einschätzung emo- tionaler Kompetenzen und emotionaler Intelligenz aus Selbst- und Fremdsicht*. Göttingen: Hogrefe (2009).

Lemenager T, Gwodz A, Richter A, Reinhard I, Kammerer N, Sell M, et al. Self-concept deficits in massively multiplayer online role-playing games addiction. *Eur Addict Res* (2013) 19(5):227–34. doi:10.1159/000345458

Hautzinger M. The Beck depression inventory in clinical practice. *Nervenarzt* (1991) 62(11):689–96.

Otti A, Guendel H, Wohlschlager A, Zimmer C, Noll-Hussong M. Frequency shifts in the anterior default mode network and the salience network in chronic pain disorder. *BMC Psychiatry* (2013) 13:84. doi:10.1186/1471-244X-13-84

Richter J, Eisemann M, Richter G, Cloninger C. *Das Temperament- und Charakter-Inventar (TCI). Deutsche Übersetzung und Bearbeitung*. Frankfurt: Swets (1999).

Cloninger CR. *The Temperament and Character Inventory (TCI): A Guide to its Development and Use*. St. Louis, MO: Center for Psychobiology of Personality, Washington University (1994).

Noll-Hussong M, Autenrieth M, Pokorny D, Herberger S, Huber D. The subject, its biology, and the chronic recurrent cystitis. *Case Rep Psychiatry* (2012) 2012:601705. doi:10.1155/2012/601705

Ferre ER, Bottini G, Haggard P. Vestibular inputs modulate somatosensory cor- tical processing. *Brain Struct Funct* (2012) 217(4):859–64. doi:10.1007/s00429- 012-0404-7

Preuss N, Mast FW, Hasler G. Purchase decision-making is modulated by vestibular stimulation. *Front Behav Neurosci* (2014) 8:51. doi:10.3389/fnbeh. 2014.00051

Lopez C. A neuroscientific account of how vestibular disorders impair bodily self-consciousness. *Front Integr Neurosci* (2013) 7:91. doi:10.3389/fnint.2013. 00091

Bottini G, Gandola M, Sedda A, Ferre ER. Caloric vestibular stimulation: interaction between somatosensory system and vestibular apparatus. *Front Integr Neurosci* (2013) 7:66. doi:10.3389/fnint.2013.00066

Weeks ZR. Effects of the vestibular system on human development, part 2: effects of vestibular stimulation on mentally retarded, emotionally disturbed, and learning-disabled individuals. *Am J Occup Ther* (1979) 33(7):450–7.

Freeman BJ, Frankel F, Ritvo ER. The effects of response contingent vestibular stimulation on the behavior of autistic and retarded children. *J Autism Child Schizophr* (1976) 6(4):353–8. doi:10.1007/BF01537912

Schiff ND, Pulver M. Does vestibular stimulation activate thalamocortical mechanisms that reintegrate impaired cortical regions? *Proc Biol Sci* (1999) 266(1417):421–3. doi:10.1098/rspb.1999.0654

Karnath HO. Subjective body orientation in neglect and the interactive contri- bution of neck muscle proprioception and vestibular stimulation. *Brain* (1994) 117(Pt 5):1001–12. doi:10.1093/brain/117.5.1001

Rode G, Perenin MT. Temporary remission of representational hemineglect through vestibular stimulation. *Neuroreport* (1994) 5(8):869–72. doi:10.1097/ 00001756-199404000-00004

Geminiani G, Bottini G. Mental representation and temporary recovery from unilateral neglect after vestibular stimulation. *J Neurol Neurosurg Psychiatry* (1992) 55(4):332–3. doi:10.1136/jnnp.55.4.332-a

Mast FW, Merfeld DM, Kosslyn SM. Visual mental imagery during caloric vestibular stimulation. *Neuropsychologia* (2006) 44(1):101–9. doi:10.1016/j.neuropsychologia.2005.04.005

Horii A, Takeda N, Mochizuki T, Okakura-Mochizuki K, Yamamoto Y, Yamatodani A. Effects of vestibular stimulation on acetylcholine release from rat hippocampus: an in vivo microdialysis study. *J Neurophysiol* (1994) 72(2):605–11.

Miller FG, Colloca L, Kaptchuk TJ. The placebo effect: illness and interpersonal healing. *Perspect Biol Med* (2009) 52(4):518–39. doi:10.1353/pbm.0.0115

Hrobjartsson A, Gotzsche PC. Placebo interventions for all clinical condi- tions. *Cochrane Database Syst Rev* (2004) (3):CD003974. doi:10.1002/14651858.CD003974.pub2

Enck P, Benedetti F, Schedlowski M. New insights into the placebo and nocebo responses. *Neuron* (2008) 59(2):195–206. doi:10.1016/j.neuron.2008.06.030

Baik JS, Han SW, Park JH, Lee MS. Psychogenic paroxysmal dyskinesia: the roleof placebo in the diagnosis and management. *Mov Disord* (2009) 24(8):1244–5. doi:10.1002/mds.22509

Wilkinson D, Nicholls S, Pattenden C, Kilduff P, Milberg W. Galvanic vestibular stimulation speeds visual memory recall. *Exp Brain Res* (2008) 189(2):243–8. doi:10.1007/s00221-008-1463-0

Edwards MJ, Talelli P, Rothwell JC. Clinical applications of transcranial magnetic stimulation in patients with movement disorders. *Lancet Neurol* (2008) 7(9):827–40. doi:10.1016/S1474-4422(08)70190-X

Chastan N, Parain D, Verin E, Weber J, Faure MA, Marie JP. Psychogenic aphonia: spectacular recovery after motor cortex transcranial magnetic stimulation. *J Neurol Neurosurg Psychiatry* (2009) 80(1):94. doi:10.1136/jnnp.2008.154302

Feinstein A. Psychogenic aphonia: spectacular recovery after motor cortex tran- scranial magnetic stimulation. *J Neurol Neurosurg Psychiatry* (2009) 80(1):4. doi:10.1136/jnnp.2008.162842

Schonfeldt-Lecuona C, Connemann BJ, Spitzer M, Herwig U. Transcranial mag- netic stimulation in the reversal of motor conversion disorder. *Psychother Psy- chosom* (2003) 72(5):286–8. doi:10.1159/000071900

Schonfeldt-Lecuona C, Connemann BJ, Viviani R, Spitzer M, Herwig U. Tran- scranial magnetic stimulation in motor conversion disorder: a short case series. *J Clin Neurophysiol* (2006) 23(5):472–5. doi:10.1097/01.wnp.0000219004. 69158.1e

Liepert J, Hassa T, Tuscher O, Schmidt R. Abnormal motor excitability in patients with psychogenic paresis. A TMS study. *J Neurol* (2009) 256(1):121–6. doi:10.1007/s00415-009-0090-4

Liepert J, Hassa T, Tuscher O, Schmidt R. Electrophysiological correlates of motor conversion disorder. *Mov Disord* (2008) 23(15):2171–6. doi:10.1002/mds. 21994

Lopez C, Blanke O, Mast FW. The human vestibular cortex revealed by coordinate-based activation likelihood estimation meta-analysis. *Neuroscience* (2012) 212:159–79. doi:10.1016/j.neuroscience.2012.03.028

Van Nuenen BF, Wohlgemuth M, Wong Chung RE, Abdo WF, Bloem BR. Acupuncture for psychogenic movement disorders: treatment or diagnostic tool? *Mov Disord* (2007) 22(9):1353–5. doi:10.1002/mds.21467

Klingner CM, Volk GF, Flatz C, Brodoehl S, Dieterich M, Witte OW, et al. Components of vestibular cortical function. *Behav Brain Res* (2013) 236(1):194–9. doi:10.1016/j.bbr.2012.08.049

Rode G, Vallar G, Revol P, Tilikete C, Jacquin-Courtois S, Rossetti Y, et al. Facial macrosomatognosia and pain in a case of Wallenberg's syndrome: selective effects of vestibular and transcutaneous stimulations. *Neuropsychologia* (2012) 50(2):245–53. doi:10.1016/j.neuropsychologia.2011.11.018

Lopez C, Schreyer HM, Preuss N, Mast FW. Vestibular stimulation modi- fies the body schema. *Neuropsychologia* (2012) 50(8):1830–7. doi:10.1016/j.neuropsychologia.2012.04.008

Kranick SM, Gorrindo T, Hallett M. Psychogenic movement disorders and motor conversion: a roadmap for collaboration between neurology and psychiatry. *Psychosomatics* (2011) 52(2):109–16. doi:10.1016/j.psym.2010. 12.017

23

Resistive and reactive changes to the impedance of intracortical microelectrodes can be mitigated with polyethylene glycol under acute *in vitro* and *in vivo* settings

Salah Sommakia[1,2], Janak Gaire[3], Jenna L. Rickus[1,2,4] and Kevin J. Otto[1,3]*

[1] Weldon School of Biomedical Engineering, Purdue University, West Lafayette, IN, USA
[2] Physiological Sensing Facility at the Bindley Bioscience Center and Birck Nanotechnology Center, Purdue University, West Lafayette, IN, USA
[3] Department of Biological Sciences, Purdue University, West Lafayette, IN, USA
[4] Department of Agricultural and Biological Engineering, Purdue University, West Lafayette, IN, USA

Edited by:
Ulrich G. Hofmann, Albert-Ludwigs-University Freiburg, Germany

Reviewed by:
Xuefeng F. Wei, The College of New Jersey, USA
Abhishek Prasad, University of Miami, USA

***Correspondence:**
Kevin J. Otto, Weldon School of Biomedical Engineering, Purdue University, 206 S. Martin Jischke Drive, West Lafayette, IN 47907, USA
e-mail: kotto@purdue.edu

The reactive response of brain tissue to implantable intracortical microelectrodes is thought to negatively affect their recordable signal quality and impedance, resulting in unreliable longitudinal performance. The relationship between the progression of the reactive tissue into a glial scar and the decline in device performance is unclear. We show that exposure to a model protein solution *in vitro* and acute implantation result in both resistive and capacitive changes to electrode impedance, rather than purely resistive changes. We also show that applying 4000 MW polyethylene glycol (PEG) prevents impedance increases *in vitro*, and reduces the percent change in impedance *in vivo* following implantation. Our results highlight the importance of considering the contributions of non-cellular components to the decline in neural microelectrode performance, and present a proof of concept for using a simple dip-coated PEG film to modulate changes in microelectrode impedance.

Keywords: intracortical microelectrodes, foreign-body reaction, impedance spectroscopy, polyethylene glycols, dip coating

INTRODUCTION

Failure of intracortical microelectrodes typically manifests as increased impedance and decreased signal to noise ratio, and is thought to be associated with the formation of a dense glial scar and loss of neuronal density. *In vivo* impedance monitoring is a common tool to assess the functionality of implanted intracortical microelectrodes, and has been used to infer the progression of the reactive tissue response to implanted intracortical microelectrodes (Williams et al., 1999, 2007; Vetter et al., 2004). Recent research shows that changes in electrical properties monitored by impedance spectroscopy do not always perfectly correlate with cellular responses (Prasad et al., 2012; Prasad and Sanchez, 2012), implicating additional biotic and abiotic factors. *In vitro* testing in 3D gel constructs reveal that different glial cells adhered to the surface of a microelectrode have different impedance profiles (Frampton et al., 2010). One factor that has not been well investigated is the adsorption of proteins and other biomolecules. While adsorbed proteins have been implicated in the biological response (Leung et al., 2008), their effects on the electrical impedance of intracortical microelectrodes have not been previously described with impedance spectroscopy. Prevalent electrical circuit models of the tissue electrode interface assume that adsorbed proteins result in purely resistive impedance changes (Johnson et al., 2005; Otto et al., 2006; Williams et al., 2007), but there is not sufficient empirical verification of this assumption. To the best of the authors' knowledge, there are no reports in the literature on the effects of adsorbed proteins or non-cellular components on the impedance of intracortical microelectrodes.

Another aspect to the problem of biomolecule adsorption is the question of preventing detrimental changes to the electrical characteristics of intracortical microelectrodes using simple and cost effective approaches. For implantable devices in other biological systems, protein-resistant or anti-fouling treatments are commonplace (Salacinski et al., 2001; Bluestein et al., 2010; Li and Henry, 2011). One of the most common materials used to enhance the biocompatibility of biomedical implants is polyethylene glycol (PEG). Due to its hydrophilic nature, PEG prevents the adsorption of proteins by reducing access to the more hydrophobic surface onto which proteins prefer to bind (Michel et al., 2005). Typically, PEG is chemically grafted onto a substrate and reliably reduces protein adsorption (Sharma et al., 2004a,b; Muthusubramaniam et al., 2011). In the context of intracortical microelectrodes, PEG has traditionally been used as a scaffold for thick drug eluting hydrogels (Winter et al., 2007; Rao et al., 2012), the size scale of which might exacerbate neuronal displacement. Thinner conformal microgel coatings which incorporate PEG as a cross linker have been investigated, but do not significantly improve the chronic tissue response (Gutowski et al., 2014).

Free-floating PEG injected intravenously has been reported to improve cellular and behavioral recovery following traumatic brain injury (Koob et al., 2005, 2008; Koob and Borgens, 2006). Because of the complexity of the reactive tissue response of the brain to implanted microelectrodes, and the fact that the cause of the majority of chronic microelectrode failures are unknown (Barrese et al., 2013), the long-term effects of a simply applied anti-fouling coating on the tissue response cannot be confidently predicted. In the short-term, however, it is possible that such a simply applied anti-fouling coating might improve the electrical properties of acutely implanted neural microelectrodes, which, in turn, might improve the accuracy of impedance monitoring as a predictive tool for the progression of the tissue response. The authors are not aware of any reports in the literature that examine the effects of a simple dip-coated PEG film on the electrical properties of neural microelectrodes under acute *in vitro* or *in vivo* settings.

The primary objective of this paper is to quantify the acute effects on microelectrode impedance of adsorbed proteins *in vitro*, and non-cellular molecular components *in vivo*. A secondary objective is to present a proof of concept on the use of an aqueous dip-coated PEG film in preventing impedance changes to neural microelectrodes during acute timescales. For this proof of concept experiment, a molecular weight of 4000 Da was chosen according to literature reports demonstrating optimal antifouling properties at this molecular weight (Su et al., 2009). We first present an analysis of changes in intracortical microelectrode impedance following immersion in a model protein solution mimicking *in vivo* brain protein concentration. Total impedance, resistance, and reactance are analyzed at different frequency values to quantify the contribution of adsorbed proteins to the impedance changes affecting electrode performance. We show that a dip-coated film of a relatively high molecular weight PEG prevents changes in impedance upon immersion in protein solution. We then demonstrate in an acute *in vivo* experiment that increases in microelectrode impedance after insertion into the cortex can be reduced by applying the same PEG treatment to the electrode shank and implantation site.

MATERIALS AND METHODS

IN VITRO STUDY WITH MODEL PROTEIN SOLUTION

Electrochemical measurements of 16-channel single shank Michigan electrode arrays (CNCT, Ann Arbor, MI) were made using an Autolab potentiostat PG-STAT12 with a built-in frequency response analyzer (EcoChemie, Utrecht, The Netherlands). For this study, a three-electrode cell configuration was used with the microelectrode site functioning as the working electrode, a large-area Pt wire functioning as the counter electrode, and an Accumet, gel-filled, KCl saturated calomel electrode (Thermo Fischer Scientific, Fair Lawn, NJ) functioning as the reference electrode. This three-electrode setup was chosen for this study because of its ability to isolate the electrode/solution interface impedance component.

For each electrode array, cyclic voltammetry (CV) was performed by sweeping the applied voltage from −0.6 to +0.8 V at a scanning rate of 1 V/s to determine sites with broken or poor connections, designated as those sites exhibiting a maximum current below 1 nA. These sites were discarded from the analysis, thus yielding a total of 30 functional sites on three different electrode arrays.

Electrochemical impedance spectroscopy (EIS), using the PGSTAT12, was used to measure the impedance of the electrode sites with the application of 15 sequentially applied sinusoidal waves at logarithmically spaced frequencies ranging from 46 Hz to 10 kHz, with an amplitude of 25 mVRMS. For each electrode, impedance spectroscopy was performed in PBS following each of three different treatments: (a) no treatment; (b) immersion in a 10% solution of bovine serum albumin (BSA) (Sigma-Aldrich, St. Louis, MO) in PBS, the concentration of which was chosen to mimic protein concentration in rat cerebral cortex (Banay-Schwartz et al., 1992); and (c) immersion in a 20% solution of 4000 MW PEG (Alfa-Aesar, Ward Hill, MA), air-drying for 1 min, then immersion in BSA. Immersion and subsequent removal from the described solutions was done at a controlled velocity using a micro-manipulator. An additional volume of 100 μl of PEG was further applied directly onto the microelectrode shank as it was immersed in BSA to mimic a topical application. Electrodes were rinsed with deionized water and anodically cleaned between the different treatments using 10-s long DC pulses, as described previously (Sommakia et al., 2009). Bode and Nyquist plots were generated for all treatment groups. Comparisons of the resistance, reactance and total impedance were done at 50 Hz, 100 Hz, 1 kHz, and 10 kHz.

ACUTE *IN VIVO* STUDY

The laboratory animal protocol for this work was approved through the Purdue Animal Care and Use Committee (West Lafayette, IN, USA), and conforms to the guidelines of the US National Institutes of Health. Three Sprague Dawley rats (Harlan Laboratories, Indianapolis, IN) were used for this study. Each rat was anesthetized with 2% isofluorane, then transferred to a stereotactic frame and maintained with 0.5–1% isofluorane delivered through a nose cone. The head was shaved and swabbed with alternating washes of betadine and alcohol, and an eye lubricating ointment applied. Lidocaine was injected subcutaneously at multiple positions in the head, and then a midline incision approximately 2 cm long was made along the cranium with a scalpel. The underlying pericranium was removed to expose the skull. A single burr hole was made with a dental drill towards the back of the head, slightly anterior to the ears, and a stainless steel bone screw attached to a segment of platinum wire was threaded into it to serve as a counter electrode. Bilateral craniotomies about 2.5 mm in diameter were made with a dental drill, approximately 2.5 mm anterior to Bregma and 2 mm lateral to the midline. For each craniotomy, a slit was made in the dura using surgical microscissors. One craniotomy serving as a control was wetted with 0.9% sterile saline before electrode insertion, while the other craniotomy was wetted with 20% w/v solution of 4000 MW PEG in MilliQ water prior to electrode insertion.

16-channel single-shank Michigan probes were also used for this study. Because of the difficulty of achieving a three-electrode setup in a surgical setting, a two-electrode setup was chosen instead. Prior to insertion into the cortex, baseline impedance was established *in vitro* by performing the same EIS procedure described above, but in a two-electrode setup. The electrode was then manually inserted into the exposed cortex of the control craniotomy using a magnet-stabilized micromanipulator, and EIS was measured 5 min after insertion. The electrode was then removed, rinsed with MilliQ water, and cleaned by applying a DC bias of 1.5 V for 10 s in PBS, as described previously (Sommakia et al., 2009). After verifying the return of the 1 kHz impedance to baseline, the electrode was dip-coated at a controlled velocity using a micromanipulator in a 20% solution of 4000 MW PEG in MilliQ water for 1 min and allowed to dry for 2 min. The PEG-coated electrode was then inserted using the micromanipulator into the other craniotomy wetted with PEG, and EIS was performed again.

STATISTICAL ANALYSIS

Statistical analysis was performed using the SAS 9.3 statistical package (SAS Institute, Cary, NC). A general linear model (GLM) procedure was used to perform a one way ANOVA with block to remove variations between the different electrodes by treating electrodes as a statistical block. Tukey *post-hoc* tests were used to identify statistically significant differences between the groups at a significance level of $\alpha = 0.05$. Plots were generated using MATLAB (The MathWorks Inc., Natick, MA).

RESULTS

ANALYSIS OF IMPEDANCE CHANGES WITH MODEL PROTEIN SOLUTION AND PEG *IN VITRO*

An examination of Bode plots reveals that the gain for electrodes immersed into is higher than for uncoated controls for all frequencies, indicating an overall increase in impedance. Electrodes treated with PEG prior to BSA immersion show more congruence with the gain of uncoated electrodes (**Figure 1A**). The phase for non-PEG treated electrodes immersed in BSA exhibits lower angles at the lower end of the frequency spectrum, and the difference is most pronounced in the middle of the spectrum between 200–500 Hz (**Figure 1B**). In **Figure 2**, the Nyquist plot for non-PEG treated electrodes immersed in BSA reveal a shift up and the right compared to the controls, indicating both increased resistance and reactance, with the most pronounced divergence occurring toward the middle of the plot. In contrast, the plot for electrodes pretreated with PEG shows more congruence with uncoated controls in the middle of the plot and slight divergence at the lower end of the plot, corresponding to the higher frequencies. To better understand the details of these changes and their potential implication for mitigation attempts, we examined the percent changes in resistance, reactance, and total impedance at various points across the frequency spectrum.

Figure 3A shows percent changes in the real component of the impedance, i.e., resistance, relative to the control at four frequency values across the spectrum. Electrodes immersed in BSA without PEG pretreatment exhibited statistically significant increases in the resistance compared to the uncoated control at examined frequencies. The highest resistance increase relative to control was in the middle of the frequency spectrum, specifically at 1 kHz, with a 30.7% increase in resistance. At 50 Hz, the increase in resistance for the BSA coated electrodes without PEG pretreatment was 14.5%, at 100 Hz, the resistance increase was 23.9%, and 10 kHz, the resistance increase was 17%. The electrodes pretreated with PEG prior to BSA immersion, on the other hand, did not exhibit any significant differences in resistance compared to the uncoated controls at all examined frequencies.

Figure 3B shows percent changes in the imaginary component of the impedance, i.e., reactance, relative to the control at four frequency values. For electrodes not pretreated with PEG prior to immersion in BSA, no significant increase in reactance was observed at 50 Hz or 100 Hz, while increases of 12% and 15% were observed at 1 kHz and 10 kHz, respectively. In contrast, electrodes pretreated with PEG prior to immersion in BSA exhibited modest decreases in the reactance relative to control at all frequencies (−6.3% at 50 Hz, −6.3% at 100 Hz, −4.2 at 1 kHz, and −4.8% at 10 kHz). **Figure 3C** shows the percent changes in total impedance relative to the control at four frequency values. For electrodes not pretreated with PEG prior to BSA immersion, no significant difference in total impedance was observed at 50 Hz, but progressive increases in the impedance were observed at the higher frequencies (4.5% at 100 Hz, 13.5% at 1 kHz, 15.3% at 10 kHz). For electrodes pretreated with PEG prior to BSA immersion, modest decreases in total impedance were observed at the lower frequencies (−5.8% at 50 Hz, −5.6% at 100 Hz, −3.9 at 1 kHz), while no significant difference in the total impedance compared to the control was observed 10 kHz.

ANALYSIS OF IMPEDANCE CHANGES *IN VIVO* WITH AND WITHOUT PEG

Figure 4A shows the percent increase of the real component of the impedance, i.e., resistance, between the *in vitro* baseline and the *in vivo* measurement at four frequency values across the spectrum. In both cases of no treatment and PEG treatment, the resistance exhibited a significant increase when measured *in vivo* compared to the *in vitro* baseline. Insertion into the cortex without PEG treatment, however, resulted in a larger increase from the *in vitro* baseline at all frequencies compared to insertion with PEG treatment. The percent change in resistance was also frequency-dependent. For the no treatment condition, the percent increase from baseline was as follows: 71.8 ± 2.99% at 50 Hz, 89.8 ± 3.77% at 100 Hz, 209.5 ± 9.1% at 1 kHz, and 290.5 ± 13.7% at 10 kHz; while for the PEG treatment condition, the percent increase from baseline was: 44.6 ± 3% at 50 Hz, 58 ± 3.9% at 100 Hz, 149.5 ± 9.3% at 1 kHz, and 223.3 ± 14% at 10 kHz. The percent increase in resistance from baseline for the no treatment condition was significantly different from the percent increase in resistance from baseline for the PEG treatment at all frequencies.

Figure 4B shows the percent increase of the imaginary component of the impedance, i.e., reactance, between the *in vitro* baseline and the *in vivo* measurement at four frequency values across the spectrum. In both cases of PEG treatment or no treatment, the reactance increased significantly when measured *in vivo* compared to the *in vitro* baseline. Insertion into the cortex without PEG treatment, however, resulted in a larger increase in reactance from baseline compared to insertion with PEG treatment. The percent change in reactance was also frequency-dependent. For the no treatment condition, the percent increase from baseline was as follows: 45.4 ± 1.6% at 50 Hz, 48.1 ± 2%

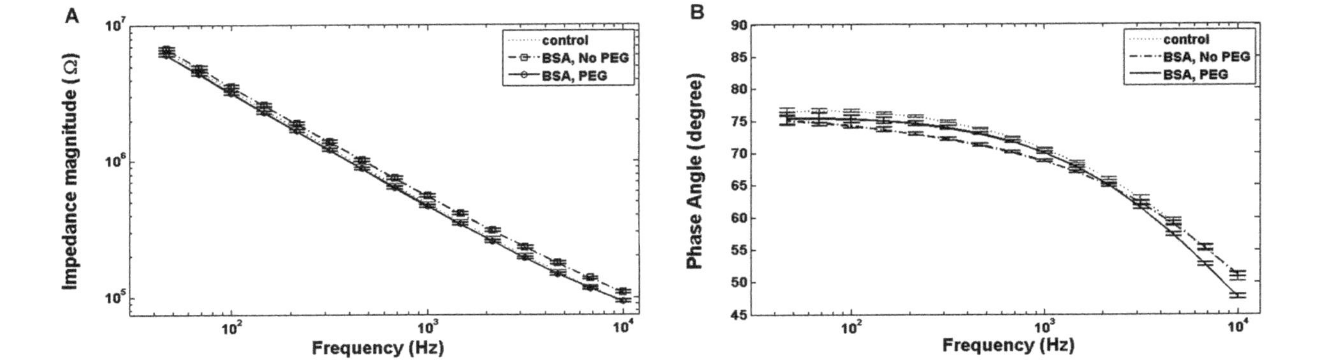

FIGURE 1 | Bode plots. **(A)** For electrodes immersed in BSA with no PEG coating, the total impedance magnitude plot is higher than the control, while electrodes coated with PEG prior to BSA immersion show an impedance magnitude plot indistinguishable from control. **(B)** Electrodes immersed in BSA with no PEG coating show lower phase angles at lower and intermediate frequencies compared to the control, while the phase angle for electrodes coated with PEG prior to immersion in BSA exhibit smaller phase angles at all frequencies.

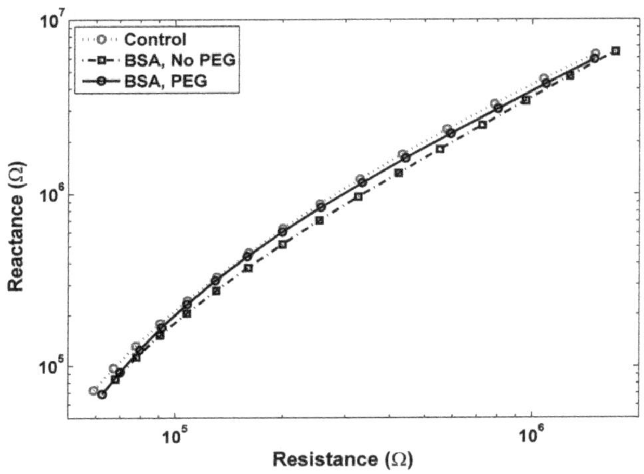

FIGURE 2 | Nyquist plot for electrodes pretreated with PEG prior to immersion in BSA is close to the control plot, with a slight shift to the left at lower frequencies, indicating a decrease in resistance. Nyquist plot for electrodes not pretreated with PEG before BSA shows a shift up and to the right, indicating increases in both resistance and reactance.

at 100 Hz, 66.4 ± 2.3% at 1 kHz, and 146.8 ± 6.2% at 10 kHz; while for the PEG treatment condition, the percent increase from baseline was: 30.8 ± 1.6% at 50 Hz, 31.4 ± 2% at 100 Hz, 41 ± 2.4% at 1 kHz, and 97.1 ± 6.4% at 10 kHz. The percent increase in reactance from baseline for the no treatment condition was significantly different from the percent increase in resistance from baseline for the PEG treatment at all frequencies. The amount of percent change in reactance is lower than the amount of percent change in resistance at each respective frequency. **Figure 4C** shows the percent increase in total impedance between the *in vitro* baseline and *in vivo* measurement at four frequency values across the spectrum. In both cases of PEG treatment or no treatment, the total impedance increased significantly when measured *in vivo* compared to the *in vitro* baseline. Insertion into the cortex without PEG treatment, however, resulted in a larger increase from baseline compared to insertion with PEG treatment. The percent change in total impedance was also frequency-dependent. For the no treatment condition, the percent increase in total impedance from baseline was as follows: 47.4 ± 1.7% at 50 Hz, 52.2 ± 2.1% at 100 Hz, 88.62 ± 2.9% at 1 kHz, and 214.5 ± 9.8% at 10 kHz; while for the PEG treatment condition, the percent increase in total impedance from baseline was: 33.6 ± 1.6% at 50 Hz, 33.5 ± 2.1% at 100 Hz, 57.1 ± 3% at 1 kHz, and 162 ± 10% at 10 kHz. The percent increase in total impedance from baseline for the no treatment condition was significantly different from the percent increase in total impedance from baseline for the PEG treatment at all frequencies.

DISCUSSION

RATIONALE

The prevalent narrative in the literature suggests that the *in vivo* reactive tissue response is an aggregate of amplified biological processes that begin with device insertion and accompanying trauma. The indwelling implant acts as a sink for various proinflammatory proteins, as well as a substrate for cell attachment (Leung et al., 2008). To the best of the authors' knowledge, the impedance changes resulting from protein adhesion onto neural microelectrodes have not been previously quantified, nor have the effects of anti-fouling treatments on impedance of neural microelectrodes. Most current efforts towards mitigating the reactive tissue response focus on targeting and quantifying the cellular component of the reactive tissue response. Recent findings, however, indicate that strong cellular responses to implanted microelectrodes do not necessarily correspond to similar changes in electrode impedance (Prasad and Sanchez, 2012). We posit that extracellular components of the reactive tissue response might be more instrumental in altering the electrical properties of implanted electrodes, and thus offer an attractive alternative for quantification and mitigation. The primary objective of this paper was to identify non-cellular components as potential modulators of impedance changes in neural microelectrodes, and to quantify the effects of a specific type of non-cellular component *in vitro*

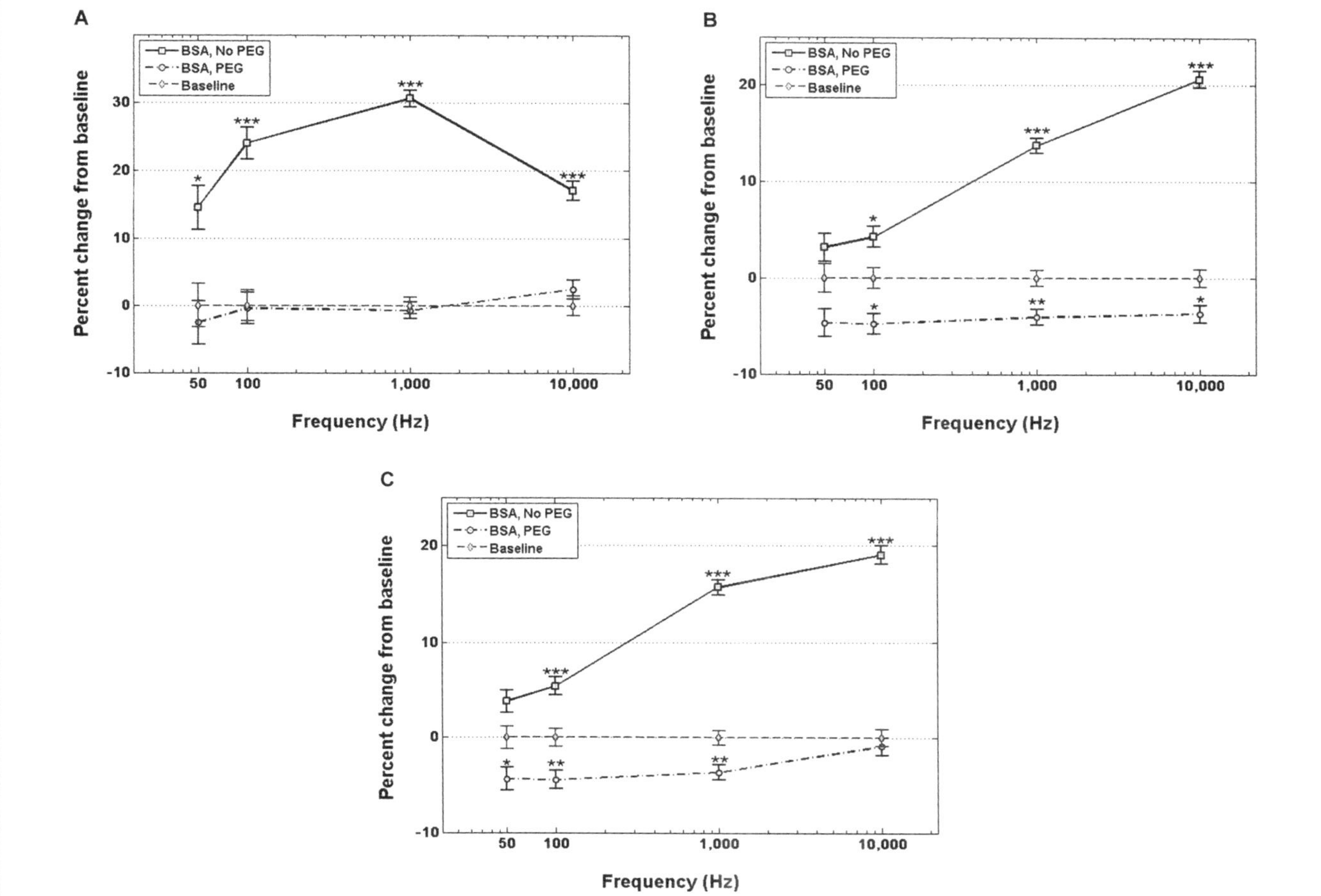

FIGURE 3 | Changes in electrode impedance following immersion in BSA, without and with PEG treatment. (A) Resistance of electrodes immersed in BSA with no PEG treatment exhibits significant increases compared to control at all observed frequencies, notably an increase in resistance of 30.7% compared to control at 1 kHz. Electrodes treated with PEG prior to immersion in BSA exhibit no significant changes in resistance compared to control. **(B)** Reactance of electrodes immersed in BSA with no PEG treatment exhibit significant increases at frequencies greater than 50 Hz, with the highest increase observed at 10 kHz. PEG treatment prior to immersion in BSA resulted in minor, but significant decreases at frequencies greater than 50 Hz. **(C)** Changes in total impedance closely match changes in reactance. Error bars represent the standard error of the means. Single asterisks (*) respresent $p < 0.05$, double asterisks (**) represent $p < 0.001$, triple asterisks (***) represent $p < 0.0001$.

(proteins). The secondary objective was to demonstrate a proof of concept at acute time scales for using PEG applied via a simple dip-coating process to prevent impedance changes caused by non-cellular components both *in vitro* and *in vivo*.

EXPLANATION OF RESULTS

For the *in vitro* study with the model protein solution, a three-electrode setup was chosen for its ability to isolate the electrode/solution interface impedance. Changes in impedance measured using this three-electrode setup indicate changes only at the electrode/solution interface (Bard and Faulkner, 2001). Because of the combination of low currents, short timescales, micro-scale working electrodes, and a large area counter, it was assumed that very minimal changes could have occurred at the recording surface. Using this measurement paradigm, our first finding was that significant increases in resistance at all examined frequencies occur immediately upon exposure to a model protein solution with a concentration mimicking *in vivo* concentrations. Furthermore, significant increases in the reactance are observed at higher frequencies, including the physiologically relevant 1 kHz. The aggregate impedance effect is that of a significant increase at frequencies higher than 50 Hz. These observed *in vitro* changes in impedance might not exactly match *in vivo* changes, given the difference in protein composition in the brain, and the presence of additional biomolecules with widely varying degrees of hydrophobicity, such as lipids and polysaccharides (O'Brien and Sampson, 1965; Pease, 1966; Margolis and Margolis, 1974; Norton et al., 1975). This finding of changes in both resistive and capacitive components following protein adsorption challenges current assumptions inherent in prevalent electrical circuit models of the device tissue interface. Such models typically assume that protein adsorption causes purely resistive changes in impedance (Johnson et al., 2005; Otto et al., 2006; Williams et al., 2007). We demonstrate that the exposure of microelectrodes to a protein solution

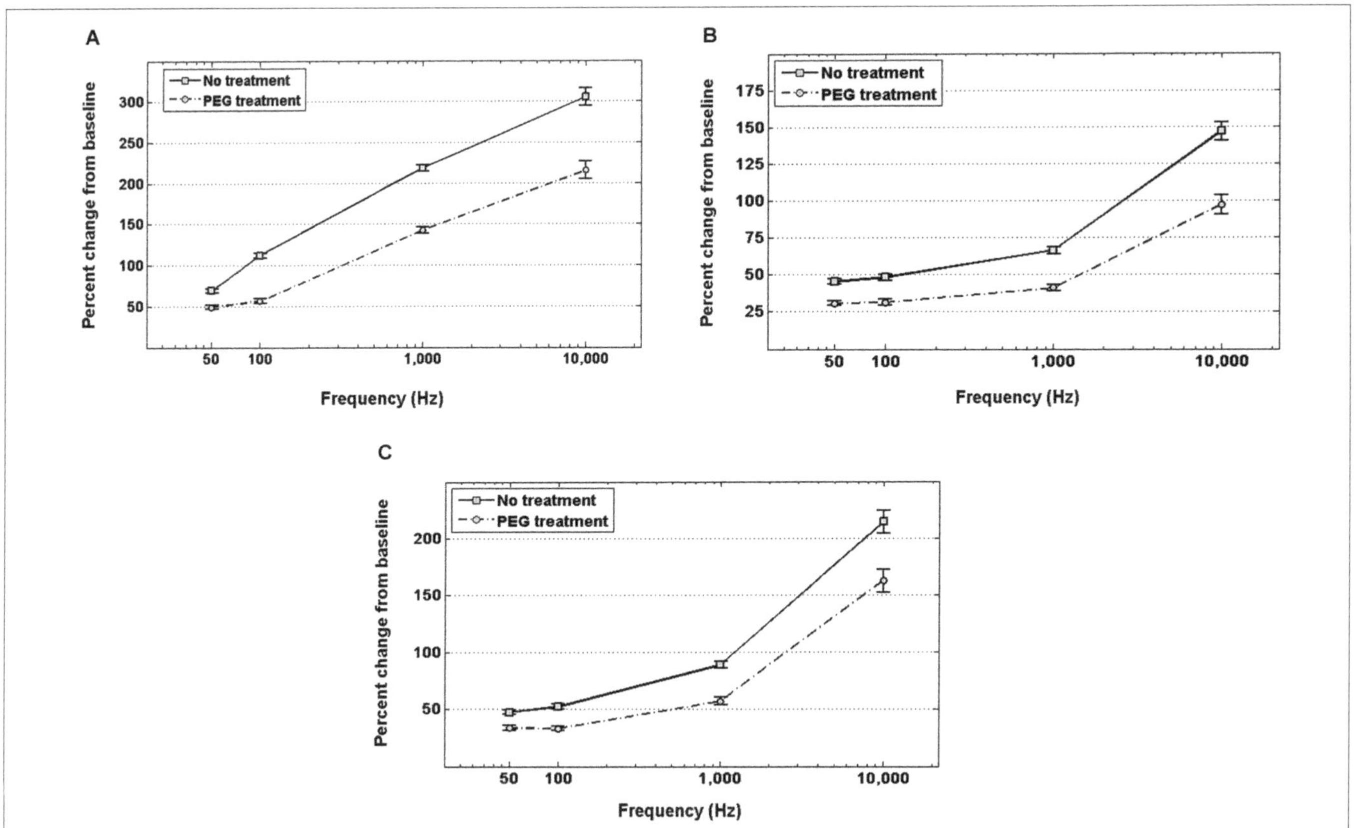

FIGURE 4 | *In vivo* increase in resistance (A), reactance (B), and total impedance (C) from *in vitro* baseline, with and without PEG treatment. For either treatment condition, a significant increase in impedance (both resistance and reactance) from the *in vitro* baseline is observed at all frequencies ($p < 0.05$). For electrodes with no treatment, the percent increase in impedance (both resistance and reactance) from baseline was significantly higher ($p < 0.05$) than the percent increase with PEG treatment at all frequencies.

results in both resistive and capacitive changes in impedance, rather than purely resistive changes. These findings suggest a need for the reexamination of assumptions upon which prevalent electrical circuit models for the tissue electrode interface are built. More accurate or representative equivalent circuit models might improve the utility of impedance monitoring to accurately deduce the progression of the reactive tissue response.

Our study further demonstrates that treating electrodes with a PEG film via dip coating prior to immersion in a protein solution negates these increases in impedance at physiologically relevant frequencies. That electrodes pretreated with PEG exhibit slight decreases in reactance supports our working hypothesis that the PEG film forms a hydrated layer close to the electrode surface that prevents proteins from accessing the surface of the electrode, while simultaneously avoiding detrimental effects on charge transfer at the electrode-electrolyte layer.

For the acute *in vivo* study, a two-electrode setup was used due to the difficulty of implementing a three-electrode setup within a surgical setting. The use of a two-electrode setup means that the impedance of the tissue/electrode interface and the impedance of the tissue are lumped into a single impedance source. The expected contribution of the tissue impedance component is confirmed by the considerable increase observed in both the resistance and capacitance following the insertion of the electrode into the rat brain. For this study, we wanted to examine the contribution of non-cellular components to the change in impedance, and therefore chose a short time scale during which no tissue remodeling occurs. Since cellular responses in the brain following electrode implantation are not observed until several hours post implantation (Kozai et al., 2012), our impedance measurement needed to be conducted within that time frame. We chose an arbitrary time point of 5 min post-insertion to minimize the exposure of the animals to unnecessary anesthesia, but it is possible for impedance changes to be time sensitive.

The application of an aqueous solution of a higher molecular weight PEG by dip-coating onto the microelectrode and directly into the craniotomy resulted in a reduction in the magnitude of the increase from the *in vitro* baseline impedance. Because the tissue impedance component is presumed not to change within this short time frame, we can assume that the difference in impedance with PEG treatment compared to the no treatment condition is due primarily to the modulation of the electrode/tissue interface impedance component. In the control craniotomy, we posit that a considerable portion of the immediate impedance increase comes from hydrophobic biomolecules that come into contact with the electrode surface and hinder charge transfer. The application of free-floating high molecular weight PEG appears to confer some degree of protection from the effects of aforementioned biomolecules, and results in lower impedance. With this simple method of applying PEG via dip-coating, there are concerns about the uniformity of coatings between electrodes. While we did not directly quantify the morphology of our dip-coated PEG films, we did attempt to control the deposition process to minimize variability. Since the dip-coating velocity is a major contributing factor to the uniformity of dip-coated films (Scriven, 1988), we controlled our dip-coating velocity by using a micromanipulator. Because we did observe statistically significant changes in impedance in response to our dip coatings, we did not make further attempts to identify and reduce individual contributors to inter-electrode variations.

Much more research needs to be conducted into the use of PEG to understand its potential long-term effects on the functional longevity of implantable intracortical microelectrodes. While prior research in the field has found that conformal microgel PEG coatings that do prevent cellular adhesion *in vitro* do not result in significant improvement to the cellular composition of the chronic electrode tissue interface (Gutowski et al., 2014), the effects of such PEG-containing coatings on the electrical properties of functional electrodes have not been tested. It is possible that significant protective effects using grafted coatings have not been observed due to the use of lower molecular weights. For our proof of concept demonstration for PEG, we used a molecular weight of 4000 Da, which has been shown to be optimal for reducing biofouling in comparison with lower molecular weights (Su et al., 2009). With biopolymers, there are concerns about degradability which might limit the long-term potential for such coatings to modulate the reactive tissue response. PEG, however, is generally not considered easily degradable in physiological conditions, and degradable PEG hydrogels generally need to be engineered with special cleavage sites to facilitate biodegradability (Drury and Mooney, 2003). On the other hand, the effects of long-term presence of large polymeric molecules in the brain should be considered before employing such molecules as neurointegrative coatings.

These complex considerations surrounding such antifouling coatings present an attractive research area. While chemically immobilized coatings are a commonplace choice for neurointegrative coatings, there might be additional merits to weakly attached PEG films. For example, intravenous treatment with higher molecular weight PEG has been shown to improve cellular and behavioral recovery in traumatic brain injury (Koob et al., 2005, 2008; Koob and Borgens, 2006), due to its fusogen properties which allow it to induce membrane sealing of damaged cells and tissue (Shi, 2013). It is possible that these properties of higher molecular weight PEG can be similarly effective in disrupting deposition of proteins and other molecules at the electrode vicinity, in addition to mitigating chronic blood-brain barrier damage, a major factor in chronic device failure (Saxena et al., 2013). Before dip-coated PEG films can be prescribed as a long-term solution for preventing the reactive tissue response and increase the functional longevity of implantable neural microelectrodes, more extensive parametric studies need to be conducted. These studies should consider the molecular weight of the PEG used, in addition to the morphological characteristics of the applied films, such as roughness and thickness, and related properties such as degradation kinetics. The delivery method of PEG films is also an open question. It might be necessary to combine multiple delivery methods; for example, concurrently immobilizing PEG onto the electrode surface and applying free-floating PEG. One potential approach under investigation is the use of thin-film silica sol-gel coatings, which have the potential to incorporate released and immobilized molecules, and do not adversely affect electrical properties (Pierce et al., 2009). Such future experiments with PEG should combine impedance monitoring with histological analysis of the reactive tissue response on a chronic time scale. Our findings provide a first step by highlighting the potential contribution of non-cellular molecular components to impedance changes, and offer a proof of concept for dip-coated PEG films as a potential component within a holistic neurointegrative strategy.

ACKNOWLEDGMENTS

Funding for this research was provided by the Purdue Research Foundation, the Indiana Spinal Cord and Brain Injury Research Grant Program (Fund # 00015115), and the Defense Advanced Research Projects Agency (DARPA) Microsystems Technology Office (MTO), under the auspices of Dr. Jack W. Judy (jack.judy@darpa.mil) and Dr. Doug Weber (douglas.weber@darpa.mil) as part of the Reliable Neural Technology Program, through the Space and Naval Warfare Systems Command (SPAWAR) Systems Center (SSC) Pacific grant No. N66001-11-1-4013. Thanks to members of the Neuroprostheses Research Laboratory for feedback on the manuscript.

REFERENCES

Banay-Schwartz, M., Kenessey, A., DeGuzman, T., Lajtha, A., and Palkovits, M. (1992). Protein content of various regions of rat brain and adult and aging human brain. *Age (Omaha)* 15, 51–54. doi: 10.1007/bf02435024

Bard, A. J., and Faulkner, L. R. (2001). *Electrochemical Methods: Fundamentals and Applications.* 2nd Edn. Hoboken, NJ: Wiley Sons.

Barrese, J. C., Rao, N., Paroo, K., Triebwasser, C., Vargas-Irwin, C., Franquemont, L., et al. (2013). Failure mode analysis of silicon-based intracortical microelectrode arrays in non-human primates. *J. Neural Eng.* 10:066014. doi: 10.1088/1741-2560/10/6/066014

Bluestein, D., Chandran, K. B., and Manning, K. B. (2010). Towards non-thrombogenic performance of blood recirculating devices. *Ann. Biomed. Eng.* 38, 1236–1256. doi: 10.1007/s10439-010-9905-9

Drury, J. L., and Mooney, D. J. (2003). Hydrogels for tissue engineering: scaffold design variables and applications. *Biomaterials* 24, 4337–4351. doi: 10.1016/s0142-9612(03)00340-5

Frampton, J. P., Hynd, M. R., Shuler, M. L., and Shain, W. (2010). Effects of glial cells on electrode impedance recorded from neural prosthetic devices *in vitro*. *Ann. Biomed. Eng.* 38, 1031–1047. doi: 10.1007/s10439-010-9911-y

Gutowski, S. M., Templeman, K. L., South, A. B., Gaulding, J. C., Shoemaker, J. T., LaPlaca, M. C., et al. (2014). Host response to microgel coatings on neural electrodes implanted in the brain. *J. Biomed. Mater. Res. A* 102, 1486–1499. doi: 10.1002/jbm.a.34799

Johnson, M. D., Otto, K. J., and Kipke, D. R. (2005). Repeated voltage biasing improves unit recordings by reducing resistive tissue impedances. *IEEE Trans. Neural Syst. Rehabil. Eng.* 13, 160–165. doi: 10.1109/tnsre.2005.847373

Koob, A. O., and Borgens, R. B. (2006). Polyethylene glycol treatment after traumatic brain injury reduces beta-amyloid precursor protein accumulation in degenerating axons. *J. Neurosci. Res.* 83, 1558–1563. doi: 10.1002/jnr.20837

Koob, A. O., Colby, J. M., and Borgens, R. B. (2008). Behavioral recovery from traumatic brain injury after membrane reconstruction using polyethylene glycol. *J. Biol. Eng.* 2:9. doi: 10.1186/1754-1611-2-9

Koob, A. O., Duerstock, B. S., Babbs, C. F., Sun, Y., and Borgens, R. B. (2005). Intravenous polyethylene glycol inhibits the loss of cerebral cells after brain injury. *J. Neurotrauma* 22, 1092–1111. doi: 10.1089/neu.2005.22.1092

Kozai, T. D. Y., Vazquez, A. L., Weaver, C. L., Kim, S.-G., and Cui, X. T. (2012). *In vivo* two-photon microscopy reveals immediate microglial reaction to implantation of microelectrode through extension of processes. *J. Neural Eng.* 9:066001. doi: 10.1088/1741-2560/9/6/066001

Leung, B. K., Biran, R., Underwood, C. J., and Tresco, P. A. (2008). Characterization of microglial attachment and cytokine release on biomaterials of differing surface chemistry. *Biomaterials* 29, 3289–3297. doi: 10.1016/j.biomaterials.2008.03.045

Li, S., and Henry, J. J. (2011). Nonthrombogenic approaches to cardiovascular bioengineering. *Annu. Rev. Biomed. Eng.* 13, 451–475. doi: 10.1146/annurev-bioeng-071910-124733

Margolis, R. U., and Margolis, R. K. (1974). Distribution and metabolism of mucopolysaccharides and glycoproteins in neuronal perikarya, astrocytes and oligodendroglia. *Biochemistry* 13, 2849–2852. doi: 10.1021/bi00711a011

Michel, R., Pasche, S., Textor, M., and Castner, D. G. (2005). Influence of PEG architecture on protein adsorption and conformation. *Langmuir* 21, 12327–12332. doi: 10.1021/la051726h

Muthusubramaniam, L., Lowe, R., Fissell, W. H., Li, L., Marchant, R. E., Desai, T. A., et al. (2011). Hemocompatibility of silicon-based substrates for biomedical implant applications. *Ann. Biomed. Eng.* 39, 1296–1305. doi: 10.1007/s10439-011-0256-y

Norton, W. T., Abe, T., Poduslo, S. E., and DeVries, G. H. (1975). The lipid composition of isolated brain cells and axons. *J. Neurosci. Res.* 1, 57–75. doi: 10.1002/jnr.490010106

O'Brien, J. S., and Sampson, E. L. (1965). Lipid composition of the normal human brain: gray matter, white matter and myelin. *J. Lipid Res.* 6, 537–544.

Otto, K. J., Johnson, M. D., and Kipke, D. R. (2006). Voltage pulses change neural interface properties and improve unit recordings with chronically implanted microelectrodes. *IEEE Trans. Biomed. Eng.* 53, 333–340. doi: 10.1109/tbme.2005.862530

Pease, D. C. (1966). Polysaccharides associated with the exterior surface of epithelial cells: kidney, intestine, brain. *J. Ultrastruct. Res.* 15, 555–588. doi: 10.1016/s0022-5320(66)80128-4

Pierce, A. L., Sommakia, S., Rickus, J. L., and Otto, K. J. (2009). Thin-film silica sol-gel coatings for neural microelectrodes. *J. Neurosci. Methods* 180, 106–110. doi: 10.1016/j.jneumeth.2009.02.008

Prasad, A., and Sanchez, J. C. (2012). Quantifying long-term microelectrode array functionality using chronic *in vivo* impedance testing. *J. Neural Eng.* 9:026028. doi: 10.1088/1741-2560/9/2/026028

Prasad, A., Xue, Q.-S., Sankar, V., Nishida, T., Shaw, G., Streit, W. J., et al. (2012). Comprehensive characterization and failure modes of tungsten microwire arrays in chronic neural implants. *J. Neural Eng.* 9:056015. doi: 10.1088/1741-2560/9/5/056015

Rao, L., Zhou, H., Li, T., Li, C., and Duan, Y. Y. (2012). Polyethylene glycol-containing polyurethane hydrogel coatings for improving the biocompatibility of neural electrodes. *Acta Biomater.* 8, 2233–2242. doi: 10.1016/j.actbio.2012.03.001

Salacinski, H. J., Goldner, S., Giudiceandrea, A., Hamilton, G., Seifalian, A. M., Edwards, A., et al. (2001). The mechanical behavior of vascular grafts: a review. *J. Biomater. Appl.* 15, 241–278. doi: 10.1106/na5t-j57a-jtdd-fd04

Saxena, T., Karumbaiah, L., Gaupp, E. A., Patkar, R., Patil, K., Betancur, M., et al. (2013). The impact of chronic blood–brain barrier breach on intracortical electrode function. *Biomaterials* 34, 4703–4713. doi: 10.1016/j.biomaterials.2013.03.007

Scriven, L. E. (1988). Physics and applications of dip coating and spin coating. *MRS Proc.* 121, 717–729. doi: 10.1557/proc-121-717

Sharma, S., Johnson, R. W., and Desai, T. A. (2004a). Evaluation of the stability of nonfouling ultrathin poly(ethylene glycol) films for silicon-based microdevices. *Langmuir* 20, 348–356. doi: 10.1021/la034753l

Sharma, S., Johnson, R. W., and Desai, T. A. (2004b). XPS and AFM analysis of antifouling PEG interfaces for microfabricated silicon biosensors. *Biosens. Bioelectron.* 20, 227–239. doi: 10.1016/j.bios.2004.01.034

Shi, R. (2013). Polyethylene glycol repairs membrane damage and enhances functional recovery: a tissue engineering approach to spinal cord injury. *Neurosci. Bull.* 29, 460–466. doi: 10.1007/s12264-013-1364-5

Sommakia, S., Rickus, J. L., and Otto, K. J. (2009). Effects of adsorbed proteins, an antifouling agent and long-duration DC voltage pulses on the impedance of silicon-based neural microelectrodes. *Conf. Proc. IEEE Eng. Med. Biol. Soc.* 2009, 7139–7142. doi: 10.1109/IEMBS.2009.5332456

Su, Y.-L., Cheng, W., Li, C., and Jiang, Z. (2009). Preparation of antifouling ultrafiltration membranes with poly (ethylene glycol)-*graft*-polyacrylonitrile copolymers. *J. Memb. Sci.* 329, 246–252. doi: 10.1016/j.memsci.2009.01.002

Vetter, R. J., Williams, J. C., Hetke, J. F., Nunamaker, E. A., and Kipke, D. R. (2004). Chronic neural recording using silicon-substrate microelectrode arrays implanted in cerebral cortex. *IEEE Trans. Biomed. Eng.* 51, 896–904. doi: 10.1109/tbme.2004.826680

Williams, J. C., Hippensteel, J. A., Dilgen, J., Shain, W., and Kipke, D. R. (2007). Complex impedance spectroscopy for monitoring tissue responses to inserted neural implants. *J. Neural Eng.* 4, 410–423. doi: 10.1088/1741-2560/4/4/007

Williams, J. C., Rennaker, R. L., and Kipke, D. R. (1999). Long-term neural recording characteristics of wire microelectrode arrays implanted in cerebral cortex. *Brain Res. Brain Res. Protoc.* 4, 303–313. doi: 10.1016/s1385-299x(99)00034-3

Winter, J. O., Cogan, S. F., and Rizzo, J. F. (2007). Neurotrophin-eluting hydrogel coatings for neural stimulating electrodes. *J. Biomed. Mater. Res. B Appl. Biomater.* 81, 551–563. doi: 10.1002/jbm.b.30696

24

Neurogenic and non-neurogenic functions of endogenous neural stem cells

Erica Butti, Melania Cusimano, Marco Bacigaluppi* and Gianvito Martino*

Neuroimmunology Unit, Division of Neuroscience, Institute of Experimental Neurology, San Raffaele Scientific Institute, Milan, Italy

Edited by:
Luca Bonfanti, University of Turin, Italy

Reviewed by:
Joanne C. Conover, University of Connecticut, USA
Michael Chopp, Henry Ford Health System/Henry Ford Hospital, USA

****Correspondence:***
Marco Bacigaluppi and Gianvito Martino, Neuroimmunology Unit, Division of Neuroscience, Institute of Experimental Neurology, San Raffaele Scientific Institute, Via Olgettina 58, 20132 Milan, Italy
e-mail: bacigaluppi.marco@hsr.it; martino.gianvito@hsr.it

Adult neurogenesis is a lifelong process that occurs in two main neurogenic niches of the brain, namely in the subventricular zone (SVZ) of the lateral ventricles and in the subgranular zone (SGZ) of the dentate gyrus (DG) in the hippocampus. In the 1960s, studies on adult neurogenesis have been hampered by the lack of established phenotypic markers. The precise tracing of neural stem/progenitor cells (NPCs) was therefore, not properly feasible. After the (partial) identification of those markers, it was the lack of specific tools that hindered a proper experimental elimination and tracing of those cells to demonstrate their terminal fate and commitment. Nowadays, irradiation, cytotoxic drugs as well as genetic tracing/ablation procedures have moved the field forward and increased our understanding of neurogenesis processes in both physiological and pathological conditions. Newly formed NPC progeny from the SVZ can replace granule cells in the olfactory bulbs of rodents, thus contributing to orchestrate sophisticated odor behavior. SGZ-derived new granule cells, instead, integrate within the DG where they play an essential role in memory functions. Furthermore, converging evidence claim that endogenous NPCs not only exert neurogenic functions, but might also have non-neurogenic homeostatic functions by the release of different types of neuroprotective molecules. Remarkably, these non-neurogenic homeostatic functions seem to be necessary, both in healthy and diseased conditions, for example for preventing or limiting tissue damage. In this review, we will discuss the neurogenic and the non-neurogenic functions of adult NPCs both in physiological and pathological conditions.

Keywords: neural stem cells, neurogenesis, inflammation, transplantation, germinal niches, bystander effect

INTRODUCTION

In 1913 Santiago Ramón y Cajal established that neurons of the brain are only generated during the neurodevelopmental phase, thus setting the so called "no new neurons" doctrine (Ramon Y Cajal, 1913). However, he soon reconsidered his conclusions when evaluating the results of an experiment performed a couple of years before by his younger assistant Francisco Tello. This experiment, in fact, showed that regenerating fibers growing from the stump of a transected optic nerve could suture with a "regenerating" peripheral sciatic nerve (Tello, 1907).

Nevertheless, despite this initial hint, the existence of dividing cells of neural origin in the central nervous system (CNS) was still debated (Hamilton, 1901; Allen, 1912) and could not be formally demonstrated until the beginning of the'60 when Smart (1961) and Altman (Altman and Das, 1965) demonstrated the effective presence of proliferating neural cells—i.e., neurogenesis—in the adult rodent brain. However, this finding would have been indisputably confirmed only 20 years later, namely when Fernando Nottebohm showed that neurogenesis in the ventricular zone is a phenomenon that normally occurs in intact adult female canaries (Nottebohm, 1981; Goldman and Nottebohm, 1983). Few years' later, adult neural stem/precursor cells (NPCs) were identified as a source of new neurons also in the brain of non-human primates and humans (Kukekov et al., 1999; Ming and Song, 2005). Later on, *in vitro* stable culturing systems either for rodent and human NPCs were established (Reynolds and Weiss, 1992).

Nowadays, we know that neurogenesis in the adult brain occurs in physiological conditions in specific neurogenic niches that have particular anatomical and functional characteristics. The role of neurogenesis after injury however still needs to be fully clarified. While there is substantial evidence that active, and latent, neurogenic niches might contribute to the formation of new cells upon CNS tissue damage, the precise role of these newly formed cells has not been yet completely understood. Here we review the possibility that endogenous NPCs exert functional roles not directly related to the production of new cells (the so called "non-neurogenic functions").

NEUROGENESIS IN THE ADULT BRAIN: FROM CELLS TO FUNCTIONS

THE ADULT RODENT BRAIN

Neurogenesis in the adult rodent brain occurs during adulthood in two main neurogenic niches, namely in the subgranular zone (SGZ) of the dentate gyrus (DG) in the hippocampus and in the subventricular zone (SVZ) of the lateral ventricles.

The SGZ is a thin layer of cells located between the two DG layers of granule and hilus cells. The primary role of SGZ is to generate new cells capable to functionally integrate within the long term potentiation (LTP) (Kitamura et al., 2009). They also showed that decreased neurogenesis is accompanied by a prolonged hippocampus-dependent period of associative fear memory: this mechanism has been proposed to play a role in clearing disused old memories to preserve the learning capacity of the hippocampus (Willshaw and Buckingham, 1990). Animals exposed to an environmental enrichment showed enhanced hippocampal neurogenesis (Kempermann et al., 1997).

The functional role of NPCs residing within the SVZ is certainly more controversial. As said before, newly formed NPCs in the rodent SVZ migrate along the RMS to the OB where they integrate as interneurons within the granule and glomerular cell layers; a process considered important in maintaining and reorganizing the OB system (Imayoshi et al., 2008). The integration of the new neurons in the OB and DG is varied: in the OB, neurogenesis contributes to the maintenance and reorganization of the whole system while in the DG new neurons are added to modulate and refine the existing neuronal circuits (Imayoshi et al., 2008). While SVZ neurogenesis in the adult brain seems not to exert a role in retaining the memory of spontaneous odor discrimination and innate olfactory preference (Imayoshi et al., 2008), it seems to be involved in consolidating long-lasting olfactory traces (Gheusi et al., 2000; Lazarini et al., 2009). Indeed, the increased survival of new-born granule cells observed after the enrichment is necessary for the increased inhibitory activity in the OB and leads to a better discrimination of highly similar odorants (Moreno et al., 2009). Recent studies have confirmed these data and assessed that while easy odor tasks (Mandairon et al., 2006)—e.g., the habituation-dishabituation test—do not need neurogenesis (Kageyama et al., 2012), more difficult odor tasks, instead, do require modulation of the new-born neuron survival (Mandairon et al., 2006).

Besides the role in smell recognition, the instinctive response to pheromones is also processed by the main and accessory olfactory systems; SVZ neurogenesis plays an essential role in this context (Kageyama et al., 2012). For example, olfactory activities are very important for the maintenance of pregnancy (Bruce, 1959; Kaba et al., 1994): pregnancy induces biphasic stimulation of neurogenesis in the SVZ, leading to a biphasic increase in the production of both granule cells and periglomerular cells in the OB (Shingo et al., 2003). Neurogenesis in females is also induced by dominant male pheromones and seems to be important for sexual behaviors (Mak et al., 2007). Also in male, paternal-offspring recognition behaviors seem to rely on postnatal offspring interaction and are coupled to increased neurogenesis in the paternal OB and hippocampus (Mak and Weiss, 2010; Kageyama et al., 2012). Finally, SVZ neurogenesis might be required for predator avoidance and sex-specific responses that are olfaction dependent and innately programmed (Sakamoto et al., 2011).

NON-NEUROGENIC FUNCTIONS

In the last few years, other non-neurogenic functions of NPCs in the brain have been unraveled. NPCs are in fact able to produce and secrete a wide variety of factors that regulate and drive complex functions of the brain. A recent report showed that neuroblasts derived from both neurogenic niches (the SVZ and SGZ) exert a physiological phagocytic activity in clearing apoptotic neuronal precursors, and that this phagocytic activity is critically important in maintaining neurogenesis in the brain. Interestingly, NPC phagocytosis requires the intracellular engulfment protein ELMO1 to promote Rac activation downstream of phagocytic receptors (Lu et al., 2011).

Moreover, recent evidence supports the importance of non-neurogenic functions of NPCs. Sierra et al. demonstrated in fact that apoptotic new-born cells are rapidly cleared out through phagocytosis by unchallenged microglia present in the adult SGZ niche and that microglia is important in maintaining the homeostasis of the baseline neurogenic cascade (Sierra et al., 2010). Mosher et al. expanded this finding by demonstrating that NPCs are able, through the secretion of vascular endothelial growth factor (VEGF), to modulate microglial activation, proliferation and phagocytosis (Mosher et al., 2012). Furthermore, a bilateral cross-talk between NPCs and microglia seems to take place (Mosher et al., 2012).

Another "homeostatic" function coupled to NPCs has been recently described. Despite not having classical features of a neurogenic niche, median eminence tanycytes may also generate new-born neurons (Kokoeva et al., 2005; Lee et al., 2012). After a first study supporting the idea that hypothalamic neurogenesis in adult mice has a role in the control of energy-balance, including the capacity of regulating leptin-induced phosphorylation of signal transducer and activator of transcription 3 (STAT3) (Kokoeva et al., 2005), another recent work showed that median eminence tanycytes have a role in regulating the weight and metabolic activity of adult mice (Lee et al., 2012).

Moreover, newly generated neuroblasts residing within the SGZ seem to be able to dynamically regulate stress reactivity at both the endocrine and behavioral levels by buffering stress responses, through the regulation of the hypothalamic–pituitary–adrenal axis (Snyder et al., 2011). In fact, neurogenesis-deficient mice also showed increased food avoidance after acute stress, increased behavioral despair in the forced swim test, and decreased sucrose preference, a measure of anhedonia (Snyder et al., 2011). It would be interesting to understand whether the observed alterations can be attributed to an alteration of median eminence tancytes (and vice versa), given that the models used for ablation of NPCs in this work did not exclusively target a single NPC subpopulation.

These data altogether support the concept that NPCs might exert, besides pure neurogenic functions, also a broad spectrum of "bystander" non-neurogenic functions aimed at maintaining the homeostasis of the brain (**Figure 1**) (Martino and Pluchino, 2006).

ROLE OF ENDOGENOUS NPCs DURING CNS PATHOLOGY

NEUROGENIC FUNCTIONS

Different types of brain damage—such as stroke, epileptic seizures, trauma—induce the proliferation of NPCs in neurogenic areas, i.e., the SGZ and the SVZ (Riquelme et al., 2008). The majority of neurons formed in SGZ after an insult become dentate granule cells, similar to what occurs in the intact brain, while in the SVZ newly generated cells often migrate, away from the RMS, toward the lesion site (Jin et al., 2001).

Adult brain reacts to an ischemic injury by a long-lasting generation of neuroblasts from the SVZ; SDF-1a/CXCR4 signaling

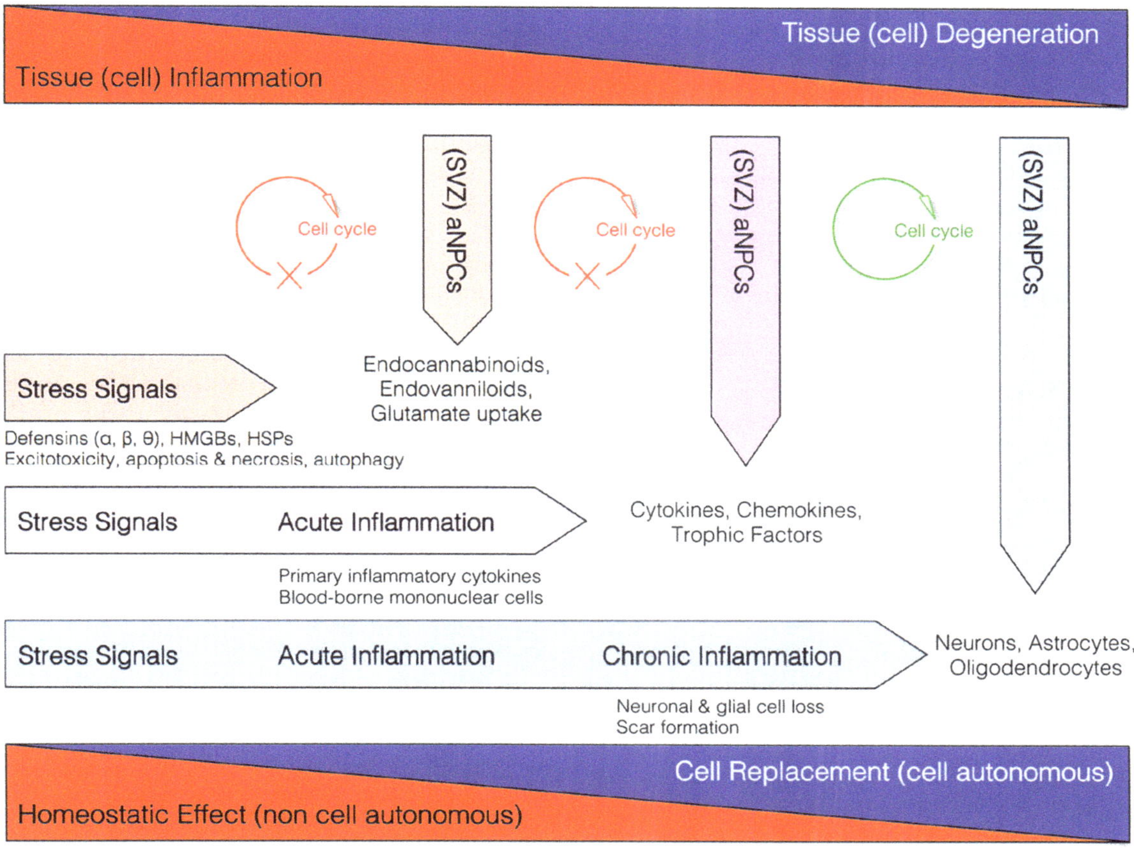

FIGURE 1 | Homeostatic multi-step actions exerted by endogenous NPCs: from maladaptive (stressful) conditions to pathological chronic tissue damage. Endogenous NPCs adapt their homeostatic functions to the needs of the tissue. In order to reduce excitotoxicity so to prevent reactive inflammation, endogenous NPCs release neuroprotective molecules (i.e., endocannabinoids, endovanilloids) and increase glutamate uptake as soon as the occurrence of early stress signals. If this barrier fails and acute inflammation occurs, endogenous NPCs release different neuroprotective and anti-inflammatory molecules (e.g., cytokines, chemokines, and trophic factors) that, in turn, restrain the CNS infiltration of blood-borne inflammatory cells and the acute inflammatory reaction. This latter second-step process is also finalized to reduce the secondary tissue damage. Finally, during chronic inflammatory conditions when tissue architecture is already compromised, NPCs might differentiate into new cellular elements in order to replace endogenous cells lost.

regulates the migration of new striatal neurons generated from endogenous NPCs toward the ischemic damage (Imitola et al., 2004). Within these newly formed peri-infarct neurovascular niches, newly-born immature neurons interact with the remodeling vasculature thanks to their production of stromal-derived factor 1 (SDF1) and angiopoietin 1 (Ang1) (Ohab et al., 2006). Interestingly neurogenesis and angiogenesis, another important reparative process taking place in the peri-ischemic tissue, are tightly coupled after stroke by VEGF that stimulates cell genesis (Teng et al., 2008).

A long-lasting neurogenic response reactive to ischemic injury has been observed not only in animal models but also in stroke patients (Marti-Fabregas et al., 2010). Interestingly, the enhanced neurogenic response is paralleled by increased microglia recruitment, probably due to a stroke-induced up regulation of CXCL10 in the SVZ; this chemokine might act as chemoattractant of CXCR3-expressing microglia (Rappert et al., 2004; Thored et al., 2009). About 80–90% of newly formed striatal neurons that potentially could replace the dead neurons will eventually die (Arvidsson et al., 2002; Thored et al., 2006, 2007). In fact, only a small portion of SVZ-derived cells migrated into striatum does assume features of mature neurons with action potentials in a rodent model of ischemic stroke (Arvidsson et al., 2002).

Similarly to stroke, also epilepsy is associated with an increased level of progenitor proliferation paralleled with an accelerated maturation and integration of only few newly generated neurons (Rotheneichner et al., 2013). Neurons formed in the DG, after an epileptic insult, undergo caspase-mediated apoptotic death, similarly to NPCs isolated from the adult SVZ (Ekdahl et al., 2001). In animal models of epilepsy, the initial rise in neurogenesis is then followed by a long-lasting reduction of neurogenesis (Hattiangady et al., 2004). Reduced cell proliferation has been also observed in the hippocampus of children during the chronic phase of a frequent seizure convulsive disorder (Mathern et al., 2002; Rotheneichner et al., 2013). In experimental epilepsy, SVZ-derived cells migrate toward the hippocampus and differentiate terminally into glial but not neuronal cells (Parent et al., 2006). Newly born neurons might exacerbate chronically epileptic hippocampus if they aberrantly migrate and incorporate in the dentate hilus (Hattiangady and Shetty, 2008). Interestingly, inflammation might influence the functional integration of adult-born hippocampal neurons as a high degree of synaptic plasticity of the new neurons has been reported in an inflammatory environment. This effect seems to be finalized to counteract inflammation-induced increase of excitatory input (Jakubs et al., 2008). However, the extent to which seizure-induced neurogenesis might contribute to the formation of newly formed neurons destined to integrate into the damaged epileptic hippocampus still need to be clarified.

NON-NEUROGENIC FUNCTIONS

As said above, there is an increased reactive neurogenesis followed by a scarce integration of newly formed neurons into neuronal damaged circuits. This chain of events appears to be paradoxical. Several hypotheses have been proposed. One of these states that NPCs might exert tissue protective functions by deviating from their neuronal default into a glial differentiation pathway or remaining undifferentiated and secrete neuroprotective molecules in a bystander fashion.

Instead of differentiating into the neuronal default pattern, NPCs (from both SVZ and SGZ) may turn into both astroglial and oligodendroglial cells—a gliogenic rather than a neurogenic response—in order to constrain and/or prevent tissue damage. Several recent evidence supports this NPC-mediated phenomenon reacting to a CNS injury.

Localized photothrombotic/ischemic cortical injury triggers the production of BBB stabilizing astrocytes from the postnatal SVZ niche; an event controlled by the Notch modulator thrombospondin 4 (Thbs4). Indeed, knockout mice for Thbs4 had a distorted neuroblast-astrocyte production, an abnormal glial scar formation, and a significant delayed increase of perilesional microvascular hemorrhages (Benner et al., 2013).

In demyelinating diseases, such as multiple sclerosis (MS), NPCs in the rodent SVZ niche become activated, upon demyelination, and provide a potential source of myelinating oligodendrocytes. SVZ-derived cells expand and migrate to the lesions, undergo oligodendrogenesis (Nait-Oumesmar et al., 1999), acquire morphology of myelinating cells, and express myelin proteins (Menn et al., 2006).

Using genetic fate mapping, it has been shown that, after a spinal cord injury (SCI), ependymal cells lining the central canal of the spinal cord have neurogenic potential. Indeed, in mice undergoing SCI, ependymal cell progeny starts migrating from the ependymal layer toward the injury site within 3 days after the injury; once within the lesion site, proliferating cells predominately differentiate into scar-forming astrocytes (Barnabe-Heider et al., 2010). In fact the glial scar that forms after SCI is composed by resident astrocytes and, in its central part, by ependymal cell–derived astrocytes (Barnabe-Heider et al., 2010). Ependymal cell–derived astrocytes might thus contribute to reinforce the injured spinal cord thus avoiding the expansion of the cystic cavity (Barnabe-Heider et al., 2010). Finally, cells recruited by the SCI not only produce scar-forming glial cells, but also, to a lesser degree, oligodendrocytes (Meletis et al., 2008).

The production of new neuronal or glial cells seems not to be the prevailing and sole mechanism of reactive neurogenesis occurring in response to tissue damage.

In stroke, not integrating newly formed SVZ-derived cells seem to protect from tissue injury through the secretion of neurotrophic factors (Jin et al., 2010; Wang et al., 2012; Sun et al., 2013). In a recent work SVZ NPCs were indeed shown to protect striatal neurons from glutamatergic excitotoxicity (as that occurring in the early phase of ischemic stroke and epilepsy) by releasing endogenous endocannabinoids (AEA and 2-AG) capable of binding to their specific receptors (CB1 and CB2) (Butti et al., 2012). Interestingly endovanilloids secreted by SVZ NPCs were found to suppress the growth of high-grade astrocytomas (HGA). NPCs by releasing endovanilloids activate the transient receptor potential vanilloid subfamily member-1 (TRPV1) on HGA cells that, in turn, triggers tumor cell death and prolongs overall survival time of the mice (Stock et al., 2012).

Also in another CNS injury model, SCI, scar stabilizing NPC-derived astrocytes do not only restrict secondary enlargement of the lesion and further axonal loss (Sabelström et al., 2013), but also exert a non-neurogenic action via the secretion of growth factors acting as neuroprotectant to enhance the survival of neurons adjacent to the traumatic lesion.

As previously pointed out, whether a homeostatic function of the endogenous NPCs might occur, the SVZ zone seems to be the more appropriate area. In fact, as stated before, SVZ NPCs are in close communication with two different microenvironments being tightly apposed to blood vessels and in contact with the CSF, and also very close to crucial areas of the midbrain containing GABAergic neurons. A further confirmation of this working hypothesis came from a recent work showing that dendritic cell (DC) traffic within the CNS—from the choroid plexus to the cervical lymph nodes—along the RMS in order to modulate CNS-infiltrating regulatory T cell (Treg) function. This migration of DC seems to dampen experimental CNS auto-inflammatory diseases, thus suggesting that it ultimately prevents pathogenic T-cells from entering the CNS (Mohammad et al., 2014).

NEUROGENIC vs. NON-NEUROGENIC FUNCTIONS

Another important, but so far only partially solved issue, concerns how of NPCs can determine their fate between neurogenic and non-neurogenic functions in pathological conditions. The predominant view, supported by NPC transplantation studies, but confirmed to be valid also for endogenous NPCs as well, is that inflammation is in part responsible for the fate decision of newly formed NPCs.

Inflammation, as process occurring as a consequence of autoimmunity and/or traumatic and ischemic injuries, alter endogenous NPC proliferation and differentiation characteristics in a non-cell autonomous fashion (Pluchino et al., 2005). When inflammation fades away and neurodegeneration prevails, endogenous NPCs tend to differentiate into multiple neuronal lineages, depending on the situation, partially capable of integrating into damaged neuronal circuits (Kokaia et al., 2012).

However, in acute inflammatory conditions, while remaining undifferentiated, transplanted SVZ-derived NPCs might promote CNS tissue healing via the secretion of immunomodulatory and neuroprotective molecules, capable of reducing detrimental tissue responses. Instead, in chronic inflammatory conditions NPCs seem to be driven toward cell replacement (Martino and Pluchino, 2006).

TRANSPLANTATION OF NPCs IN INFLAMMATORY CNS DISEASES

As underlined before, NPC replacement-based studies allow to investigate the multimodal—neurogenic vs. non-neurogenic functions—mechanism of action of endogenous NPCs (Pluchino et al., 2005).

Whatever the therapeutic action exerted, transplanted NPCs show a certain degree of pathotropism toward inflammatory foci. This is due to the fact that such cells constitutively express an armamentarium of chemokines and chemokine receptors (e.g., CCR1, CCR5, CXCR3 and CXCR4), cell adhesion molecules (e.g., CD44) (Rampon et al., 2008) and integrins (e.g., VLA4) (Campos et al., 2004, 2006; Leone et al., 2008). Transplanted NPCs, very similarly to endogenous NPCs, have the characteristic to be able to follow and reach chemoattractant foci both when intraparenchymally and/or systemically injected (Ji et al., 2004; Pluchino et al., 2005).

When transplanted in acute or chronic inflammatory diseases (e.g., stroke, SCI, or MS), the majority of NPCs survive close to perivascular inflammatory foci (i.e., the atypical ectopic niche) where they interact with many other cell types such as CNS-infiltrating blood-borne inflammatory cells, endothelial cells and CNS-resident astrocytes and microglia. Within these ectopic niches, inflammatory molecules [e.g., interferon (IFN)γ, tumor necrosis factor (TNFα)] inhibit NPCs differentiation by blocking their cell cycle by up regulating the expression of cell cycle dependent kinase inhibitors (Pluchino et al., 2008). As undifferentiated cells, NPCs can produce a wide array of both secreted and transmembrane molecules which, in turn, exert both immunomodulatory and neurotrophic factors (Irvin et al., 2004; Pluchino et al., 2005; Seifert et al., 2005; Martino and Pluchino, 2006; Bacigaluppi et al., 2009; Cusimano et al., 2012).

In relapsing-remitting experimental autoimmune encephalomyelitis (EAE), the experimental model of MS, intravenously (i.v.) transplanted NPCs promote the apoptosis of encephalitogenic T cells either via the expression of death receptor ligands (for example, FasL, Trail and Apo3L) or the production of soluble mediators—i.e., NO synthase (iNOS), IFNγ—involved in mitochondrial-mediated apoptosis (Einstein et al., 2003, 2006; Pluchino et al., 2005). In the post-acute phase of ischemic or haemorrhagic stroke, i.v. transplantation of NPCs reduced activation of macrophage/microglia cells and CNS recruitment of blood-borne inflammatory cells (Lee et al., 2008; Bacigaluppi et al., 2009). Similarly, in the immediate time points following SCI, intrathecally (i.c.) as well as intralesionally transplanted NPCs modulate the local T cell, the microglial response (Ziv et al., 2006) and the recruitment of CNS infiltrating classically activated pro-inflammatory macrophages (Cusimano et al., 2012). Interestingly, it has been recently shown that also embryonic like induced pluripotent stem cell (iPSC)-derived NPCs—once transplanted intrathecally into mice with EAE—protect oligodendrocytes and OPCs from cell death. This transplantation promotes myelin tissue reconstruction via the selective production of leukemia inhibiting factor (LIF), and this production is guided by the inflammatory microenvironment (Laterza et al., 2013).

NPCs are therefore able to prevent inflammation-induced neuronal programmed cell death and glial scar formation—occurring, for example, in EAE, SCI, stroke—mainly via the paracrine secretion of the nerve growth factor (NGF), brain-derived neurotrophic factor (BDNF), ciliary neurotrophic factor (CNTF), and glial-derived neurotrophic factor (GDNF) (Teng et al., 2002; Lu et al., 2003; Pluchino et al., 2003, 2005; Chu et al., 2004; Ryu et al., 2004; Ziv et al., 2006; Redmond et al., 2007; Bacigaluppi et al., 2009).

Another bystander effect exerted by transplanted NPCs is to directly modulate neuronal circuit plasticity (Zhang and Chopp, 2009). In an experimental model of ischemic stroke human foetal NPCs significantly improved functional outcomes by promoting neuronal dendritic arborization in both hemispheres and axonal projections within the corticostriatal and corticospinal pathways. These effects have been attributed to the capacity of transplanted NPCs to re-express developmental molecules such as guidance molecules (i.e., slit, thrombospondin 1 and 2) but also trophic factor such as VEGF (Andres et al., 2011).

CONCLUSIONS

NPCs in the adult brain exert an important homeostatic role either by producing new cells (neuronogenic or gliogenic function) or by orchestrating important processes (non-neurogenic functions): both actions are pivotal for the maintenance of the proper functioning of the CNS. Those neurogenic and non-neurogenic functions are in part NPC autonomous but are also driven by the microenvironment that might foster, according to the tissue needs, one of these functions. Our understanding of the complex interplay between neuronal, macroglial, and microglial cells in physiological and pathological conditions is continuously evolving, and we have now to consider NPCs as integral part of this interplay. New techniques of molecular biology and genetics will allow us to further understand the neurogenic vs. non-neurogenic functions of endogenous NPCs, and this knowledge would certainly help the scientific community to design efficacious stem cell-based treatment for still incurable neurological disorders.

ACKNOWLEDGMENTS

This work has been in part supported by the National Multiple Sclerosis Society (NMSS), Fondazione Italiana Sclerosi Multipla (FISM), MIUR Regione Lombardia (NetLips Project), ELA Foundation, TargetBrain (EU Framework 7 project HEALTH-F2-2012-279017) and NEUROKINE ITN network (EU project). We acknowledge the help of Dr. Stefano Sandrone.

REFERENCES

Abbracchio, M. P., Burnstock, G., Verkhratsky, A., and Zimmermann, H. (2009). Purinergic signalling in the nervous system: an overview. *Trends Neurosci.* 32, 19–29. doi: 10.1016/j.tins.2008.10.001

Allen, E. (1912). The cessation of mitosis in the central nervous system of albino rat. *J. Comp. Neurol.* 22, 547–568.

Altman, J., and Das, G. D. (1965). Autoradiographic and histological evidence of postnatal hippocampal neurogenesis in rats. *J. Comp. Neurol.* 124, 319–335. doi: 10.1002/cne.901240303

Alvarez-Buylla, A., and Lim, D. A. (2004). For the long run: maintaining germinal niches in the adult brain. *Neuron* 41, 683–686. doi: 10.1016/S0896-6273(04)00111-4

Andres, R. H., Horie, N., Slikker, W., Keren-Gill, H., Zhan, K., Sun, G., et al. (2011). Human neural stem cells enhance structural plasticity and axonal transport in the ischaemic brain. *Brain* 134, 1777–1789. doi: 10.1093/brain/awr094

Arvidsson, A., Collin, T., Kirik, D., Kokaia, Z., and Lindvall, O. (2002). Neuronal replacement from endogenous precursors in the adult brain after stroke. *Nat. Med.* 8, 963–970. doi: 10.1038/nm747

Bacigaluppi, M., Pluchino, S., Peruzzotti-Jametti, L., Kilic, E., Kilic, U., Salani, G., et al. (2009). Delayed post-ischaemic neuroprotection following systemic neural stem cell transplantation involves multiple mechanisms. *Brain* 132, 2239–2251. doi: 10.1093/brain/awp174

Barnabe-Heider, F., Goritz, C., Sabelstrom, H., Takebayashi, H., Pfrieger, F. W., Meletis, K., et al. (2010). Origin of new glial cells in intact and injured adult spinal cord. *Cell Stem Cell* 7, 470–482. doi: 10.1016/j.stem.2010.07.014

Belluzzi, O., Benedusi, M., Ackman, J., and Loturco, J. J. (2003). Electrophysiological differentiation of new neurons in the olfactory bulb. *J. Neurosci.* 23, 10411–10418.

Benner, E. J., Luciano, D., Jo, R., Abdi, K., Paez-Gonzalez, P., Sheng, H., et al. (2013). Protective astrogenesis from the SVZ niche after injury is controlled by Notch modulator Thbs4. *Nature* 497, 369–373. doi: 10.1038/nature12069

Bergmann, O., Liebl, J., Bernard, S., Alkass, K., Yeung, M. S., Steier, P., et al. (2012). The age of olfactory bulb neurons in humans. *Neuron* 74, 634–639. doi: 10.1016/j.neuron.2012.03.030

Bruce, H. M. (1959). An exteroceptive block to pregnancy in the mouse. *Nature* 184, 105. doi: 10.1038/184105a0

Butti, E., Bacigaluppi, M., Rossi, S., Cambiaghi, M., Bari, M., Cebrian Silla, A., et al. (2012). Subventricular zone neural progenitors protect striatal neurons from glutamatergic excitotoxicity. *Brain* 135, 3320–3335. doi: 10.1093/brain/aws194

Campos, L. S., Decker, L., Taylor, V., and Skarnes, W. (2006). Notch, epidermal growth factor receptor, and beta1-integrin pathways are coordinated in neural stem cells. *J. Biol. Chem.* 281, 5300–5309. doi: 10.1074/jbc.M511886200

Campos, L. S., Leone, D. P., Relvas, J. B., Brakebusch, C., Fassler, R., Suter, U., et al. (2004). Beta1 integrins activate a MAPK signalling pathway in neural stem cells that contributes to their maintenance. *Development* 131, 3433–3444. doi: 10.1242/dev.01199

Chu, K., Kim, M., Park, K. I., Jeong, S. W., Park, H. K., Jung, K. H., et al. (2004). Human neural stem cells improve sensorimotor deficits in the adult rat brain with experimental focal ischaemia. *Brain Res.* 1016, 145–153. doi: 10.1016/j.brainres.2004.04.038

Cooper-Kuhn, C. M., Winkler, J., and Kuhn, H. G. (2004). Decreased neurogenesis after cholinergic forebrain lesion in the adult rat. *J. Neurosci. Res.* 77, 155–165. doi: 10.1002/jnr.20116

Curtis, M. A., Eriksson, P. S., and Faull, R. L. (2007a). Progenitor cells and adult neurogenesis in neurodegenerative diseases and injuries of the basal ganglia. *Clin. Exp. Pharmacol. Physiol.* 34, 528–532. doi: 10.1111/j.1440-1681.2007.04609.x

Curtis, M. A., Kam, M., Nannmark, U., Anderson, M. F., Axell, M. Z., Wikkelso, C., et al. (2007b). Human neuroblasts migrate to the olfactory bulb via a lateral ventricular extension. *Science* 315, 1243–1249. doi: 10.1126/science.1136281

Cusimano, M., Biziato, D., Brambilla, E., Alfaro-Cervello, C., Snider, S., Donegà, M., et al. (2012). Transplanted NPCs instruct phagocytes to remodel the injured spinal cord tissue. *Brain* 135, 447–460. doi: 10.1093/brain/awr339

Diaz, D., Valero, J., Airado, C., Baltanas, F. C., Weruaga, E., and Alonso, J. R. (2009). Sexual dimorphic stages affect both proliferation and serotonergic innervation in the adult rostral migratory stream. *Exp. Neurol.* 216, 357–364. doi: 10.1016/j.expneurol.2008.12.013

Doetsch, F., Caille, I., Lim, D. A., Garcia-Verdugo, J. M., and Alvarez-Buylla, A. (1999). Subventricular zone astrocytes are neural stem cells in the adult mammalian brain. *Cell* 97, 703–716. doi: 10.1016/S0092-8674(00)80783-7

Einstein, O., Grigoriadis, N., Mizrachi-Kol, R., Reinhartz, E., Polyzoidou, E., Lavon, I., et al. (2006). Transplanted neural precursor cells reduce brain inflammation to attenuate chronic experimental autoimmune encephalomyelitis. *Exp. Neurol.* 198, 275–284. doi: 10.1016/j.expneurol.2005.11.007

Einstein, O., Karussis, D., Grigoriadis, N., Mizrachi-Kol, R., Reinhartz, E., Abramsky, O., et al. (2003). Intraventricular transplantation of neural precursor cell spheres attenuates acute experimental allergic encephalomyelitis. *Mol. Cell. Neurosci.* 24, 1074–1082. doi: 10.1016/j.mcn.2003.08.009

Ekdahl, C. T., Mohapel, P., Elmer, E., and Lindvall, O. (2001). Caspase inhibitors increase short-term survival of progenitor-cell progeny in the adult rat dentate gyrus following status epilepticus. *Eur. J. Neurosci.* 14, 937–945. doi: 10.1046/j.0953-816x.2001.01713.x

Encinas, J. M., Vaahtokari, A., and Enikolopov, G. (2006). Fluoxetine targets early progenitor cells in the adult brain. *Proc. Natl. Acad. Sci. U.S.A.* 103, 8233–8238. doi: 10.1073/pnas.0601992103

Eriksson, P. S., Perfilieva, E., Bjork-Eriksson, T., Alborn, A. M., Nordborg, C., Peterson, D. A., et al. (1998). Neurogenesis in the adult human hippocampus. *Nat. Med.* 4, 1313–1317. doi: 10.1038/3305

Filippov, V., Kronenberg, G., Pivneva, T., Reuter, K., Steiner, B., Wang, L. P., et al. (2003). Subpopulation of nestin-expressing progenitor cells in the adult murine hippocampus shows electrophysiological and morphological characteristics of astrocytes. *Mol. Cell. Neurosci.* 23, 373–382. doi: 10.1016/S1044-7431(03)00060-5

Fuentealba, L. C., Obernier, K., and Alvarez-Buylla, A. (2012). Adult neural stem cells bridge their niche. *Cell Stem Cell* 10, 698–708. doi: 10.1016/j.stem.2012.05.012

Fukuda, S., Kato, F., Tozuka, Y., Yamaguchi, M., Miyamoto, Y., and Hisatsune, T. (2003). Two distinct subpopulations of nestin-positive cells in adult mouse dentate gyrus. *J. Neurosci.* 23, 9357–9366.

Garcia, A. D., Doan, N. B., Imura, T., Bush, T. G., and Sofroniew, M. V. (2004). GFAP-expressing progenitors are the principal source of constitutive neurogenesis in adult mouse forebrain. *Nat. Neurosci.* 7, 1233–1241. doi: 10.1038/nn1340

Gheusi, G., Cremer, H., McLean, H., Chazal, G., Vincent, J. D., and Lledo, P. M. (2000). Importance of newly generated neurons in the adult olfactory bulb for odor discrimination. *Proc. Natl. Acad. Sci. U.S.A.* 97, 1823–1828. doi: 10.1073/pnas.97.4.1823

Goldman, S. A., and Nottebohm, F. (1983). Neuronal production, migration, and differentiation in a vocal control nucleus of the adult female canary brain. *Proc. Natl. Acad. Sci. U.S.A.* 80, 2390–2394. doi: 10.1073/pnas.80.8.2390

Hamilton, A. (1901). The division of differentiated cells in the central nervous system of the white rat. *J. Comp. Neurol.* 11, 297–320. doi: 10.1002/cne.910110403

Hattiangady, B., Rao, M. S., and Shetty, A. K. (2004). Chronic temporal lobe epilepsy is associated with severely declined dentate neurogenesis in the adult hippocampus. *Neurobiol. Dis.* 17, 473–490. doi: 10.1016/j.nbd.2004.08.008

Hattiangady, B., and Shetty, A. K. (2008). Implications of decreased hippocampal neurogenesis in chronic temporal lobe epilepsy. *Epilepsia* 49 (Suppl. 5), 26–41. doi: 10.1111/j.1528-1167.2008.01635.x

Hoglinger, G. U., Rizk, P., Muriel, M. P., Duyckaerts, C., Oertel, W. H., Caille, I., et al. (2004). Dopamine depletion impairs precursor cell proliferation in Parkinson disease. *Nat. Neurosci.* 7, 726–735. doi: 10.1038/nn1265

Imayoshi, I., Sakamoto, M., Ohtsuka, T., Takao, K., Miyakawa, T., Yamaguchi, M., et al. (2008). Roles of continuous neurogenesis in the structural and functional integrity of the adult forebrain. *Nat. Neurosci.* 11, 1153–1161. doi: 10.1038/nn.2185

Imitola, J., Raddassi, K., Park, K. I., Mueller, F. J., Nieto, M., Teng, Y. D., et al. (2004). Directed migration of neural stem cells to sites of CNS injury by the stromal cell-derived factor 1alpha/CXC chemokine receptor 4 pathway. *Proc. Natl. Acad. Sci. U.S.A.* 101, 18117–18122. doi: 10.1073/pnas.0408258102

Irvin, D. K., Nakano, I., Paucar, A., and Kornblum, H. I. (2004). Patterns of Jagged1, Jagged2, Delta-like 1 and Delta-like 3 expression during late embryonic and postnatal brain development suggest multiple functional roles in progenitors and differentiated cells. *J. Neurosci. Res.* 75, 330–343. doi: 10.1002/jnr.10843

Jakubs, K., Bonde, S., Iosif, R. E., Ekdahl, C. T., Kokaia, Z., Kokaia, M., et al. (2008). Inflammation regulates functional integration of neurons born in adult brain. *J. Neurosci.* 28, 12477–12488. doi: 10.1523/JNEUROSCI.3240-08.2008

Ji, J. F., He, B. P., Dheen, S. T., and Tay, S. S. (2004). Expression of chemokine receptors CXCR4, CCR2, CCR5 and CX3CR1 in neural progenitor cells isolated from the subventricular zone of the adult rat brain. *Neurosci. Lett.* 355, 236–240. doi: 10.1016/j.neulet.2003.11.024

Jin, K., Minami, M., Lan, J. Q., Mao, X. O., Batteur, S., Simon, R. P., et al. (2001). Neurogenesis in dentate subgranular zone and rostral subventricular zone after focal cerebral ischaemia in the rat. *Proc. Natl. Acad. Sci. U.S.A.* 98, 4710–4715. doi: 10.1073/pnas.081011098

Jin, K., Wang, X., Xie, L., Mao, X. O., and Greenberg, D. A. (2010). Transgenic ablation of doublecortin-expressing cells suppresses adult neurogenesis and worsens stroke outcome in mice. *Proc. Natl. Acad. Sci. U.S.A.* 107, 7993–7998. doi: 10.1073/pnas.1000154107

Kaba, H., Hayashi, Y., Higuchi, T., and Nakanishi, S. (1994). Induction of an olfactory memory by the activation of a metabotropic glutamate receptor. *Science* 265, 262–264. doi: 10.1126/science.8023145

Kageyama, R., Imayoshi, I., and Sakamoto, M. (2012). The role of neurogenesis in olfaction-dependent behaviors. *Behav. Brain Res.* 227, 459–463. doi: 10.1016/j.bbr.2011.04.038

Kazanis, I. (2009). The subependymal zone neurogenic niche: a beating heart in the centre of the brain: how plastic is adult neurogenesis? Opportunities for therapy and questions to be addressed. *Brain* 132, 2909–2921. doi: 10.1093/brain/awp237

Kempermann, G., Kuhn, H. G., and Gage, F. H. (1997). More hippocampal neurons in adult mice living in an enriched environment. *Nature* 386, 493–495. doi: 10.1038/386493a0

Kitamura, T., Saitoh, Y., Takashima, N., Murayama, A., Niibori, Y., Ageta, H., et al. (2009). Adult neurogenesis modulates the hippocampus-dependent period of associative fear memory. *Cell* 139, 814–827. doi: 10.1016/j.cell.2009.10.020

Knoth, R., Singec, I., Ditter, M., Pantazis, G., Capetian, P., Meyer, R. P., et al. (2010). Murine features of neurogenesis in the human hippocampus across the lifespan from 0 to 100 years. *PLoS ONE* 5:e8809. doi: 10.1371/journal.pone.0008809

Kokaia, Z., Martino, G., Schwartz, M., and Lindvall, O. (2012). Cross-talk between neural stem cells and immune cells: the key to better brain repair? *Nat. Neurosci.* 15, 1078–1087. doi: 10.1038/nn.3163

Kokoeva, M. V., Yin, H., and Flier, J. S. (2005). Neurogenesis in the hypothalamus of adult mice: potential role in energy balance. *Science* 310, 679–683. doi: 10.1126/science.1115360

Koos, T., and Tepper, J. M. (1999). Inhibitory control of neostriatal projection neurons by GABAergic interneurons. *Nat. Neurosci.* 2, 467–472. doi: 10.1038/8138

Kukekov, V. G., Laywell, E. D., Suslov, O., Davies, K., Scheffler, B., Thomas, L. B., et al. (1999). Multipotent stem/progenitor cells with similar properties arise from two neurogenic regions of adult human brain. *Exp. Neurol.* 156, 333–344. doi: 10.1006/exnr.1999.7028

Laterza, C., Merlini, A., De Feo, D., Ruffini, F., Menon, R., Onorati, M., et al. (2013). iPSC-derived neural precursors exert a neuroprotective role in immune-mediated demyelination via the secretion of LIF. *Nat. Commun.* 4, 2597. doi: 10.1038/ncomms3597

Lazarini, F., Mouthon, M. A., Gheusi, G., De Chaumont, F., Olivo-Marin, J. C., Lamarque, S., et al. (2009). Cellular and behavioral effects of cranial irradiation of the subventricular zone in adult mice. *PLoS ONE* 4:e7017. doi: 10.1371/journal.pone.0007017

Lee, D. A., Bedont, J. L., Pak, T., Wang, H., Song, J., Miranda-Angulo, A., et al. (2012). Tanycytes of the hypothalamic median eminence form a diet-responsive neurogenic niche. *Nat. Neurosci.* 15, 700–702. doi: 10.1038/nn.3079

Lee, S. T., Chu, K., Jung, K. H., Kim, S. J., Kim, D. H., Kang, K. M., et al. (2008). Anti-inflammatory mechanism of intravascular neural stem cell transplantation in haemorrhagic stroke. *Brain* 131, 616–629. doi: 10.1093/brain/awm306

Leone, S., Mutti, C., Kazantsev, A., Sturlese, M., Moro, S., Cattaneo, E., et al. (2008). SAR and QSAR study on 2-aminothiazole derivatives, modulators of transcriptional repression in Huntington's disease. *Bioorg. Med. Chem.* 16, 5695–5703. doi: 10.1016/j.bmc.2008.03.067

Lois, C., and Alvarez-Buylla, A. (1994). Long-distance neuronal migration in the adult mammalian brain. *Science* 264, 1145–1148. doi: 10.1126/science.8178174

Lu, P., Jones, L. L., Snyder, E. Y., and Tuszynski, M. H. (2003). Neural stem cells constitutively secrete neurotrophic factors and promote extensive host axonal growth after spinal cord injury. *Exp. Neurol.* 181, 115–129. doi: 10.1016/S0014-4886(03)00037-2

Lu, Z., Elliott, M. R., Chen, Y., Walsh, J. T., Klibanov, A. L., Ravichandran, K. S., et al. (2011). Phagocytic activity of neuronal progenitors regulates adult neurogenesis. *Nat. Cell Biol.* 13, 1076–1083. doi: 10.1038/ncb2299

Mak, G. K., Enwere, E. K., Gregg, C., Pakarainen, T., Poutanen, M., Huhtaniemi, I., et al. (2007). Male pheromone-stimulated neurogenesis in the adult female brain: possible role in mating behavior. *Nat. Neurosci.* 10, 1003–1011. doi: 10.1038/nn1928

Mak, G. K., and Weiss, S. (2010). Paternal recognition of adult offspring mediated by newly generated CNS neurons. *Nat. Neurosci.* 13, 753–758. doi: 10.1038/nn.2550

Mandairon, N., Sacquet, J., Garcia, S., Ravel, N., Jourdan, F., and Didier, A. (2006). Neurogenic correlates of an olfactory discrimination task in the adult olfactory bulb. *Eur. J. Neurosci.* 24, 3578–3588. doi: 10.1111/j.1460-9568.2006.05235.x

Marti-Fabregas, J., Romaguera-Ros, M., Gomez-Pinedo, U., Martinez-Ramirez, S., Jimenez-Xarrie, E., Marin, R., et al. (2010). Proliferation in the human ipsilateral subventricular zone after ischaemic stroke. *Neurology* 74, 357–365. doi: 10.1212/WNL.0b013e3181cbccec

Martino, G., and Pluchino, S. (2006). The therapeutic potential of neural stem cells. *Nat. Rev. Neurosci.* 7, 395–406. doi: 10.1038/nrn1908

Mathern, G. W., Leiphart, J. L., De Vera, A., Adelson, P. D., Seki, T., Neder, L., et al. (2002). Seizures decrease postnatal neurogenesis and granule cell development in the human fascia dentata. *Epilepsia* 43(Suppl. 5), 68–73. doi: 10.1046/j.1528-1157.43.s.5.28.x

Meletis, K., Barnabe-Heider, F., Carlen, M., Evergren, E., Tomilin, N., Shupliakov, O., et al. (2008). Spinal cord injury reveals multilineage differentiation of ependymal cells. *PLoS Biol.* 6:e182. doi: 10.1371/journal.pbio.0060182

Menn, B., Garcia-Verdugo, J. M., Yaschine, C., Gonzalez-Perez, O., Rowitch, D., and Alvarez-Buylla, A. (2006). Origin of oligodendrocytes in the subventricular zone of the adult brain. *J. Neurosci.* 26, 7907–7918. doi: 10.1523/JNEUROSCI.1299-06.2006

Ming, G. L., and Song, H. (2005). Adult neurogenesis in the mammalian central nervous system. *Annu. Rev. Neurosci.* 28, 223–250. doi: 10.1146/annurev.neuro.28.051804.101459

Mirzadeh, Z., Merkle, F. T., Soriano-Navarro, M., Garcia-Verdugo, J. M., and Alvarez-Buylla, A. (2008). Neural stem cells confer unique pinwheel architecture to the ventricular surface in neurogenic regions of the adult brain. *Cell Stem Cell* 3, 265–278. doi: 10.1016/j.stem.2008.07.004

Mohammad, M. G., Tsai, V. W., Ruitenberg, M. J., Hassanpour, M., Li, H., Hart, P. H., et al. (2014). Immune cell trafficking from the brain maintains CNS immune tolerance. *J. Clin. Invest.* 124, 1228–1241. doi: 10.1172/JCI71544

Monje, M. L., Toda, H., and Palmer, T. D. (2003). Inflammatory blockade restores adult hippocampal neurogenesis. *Science* 302, 1760–1765. doi: 10.1126/science.1088417

Moreno, M. M., Linster, C., Escanilla, O., Sacquet, J., Didier, A., and Mandairon, N. (2009). Olfactory perceptual learning requires adult neurogenesis. *Proc. Natl. Acad. Sci. U.S.A.* 106, 17980–17985. doi: 10.1073/pnas.0907063106

Mosher, K. I., Andres, R. H., Fukuhara, T., Bieri, G., Hasegawa-Moriyama, M., He, Y., et al. (2012). Neural progenitor cells regulate microglia functions and activity. *Nat. Neurosci.* 15, 1485–1487. doi: 10.1038/nn.3233

Nait-Oumesmar, B., Decker, L., Lachapelle, F., Avellana-Adalid, V., Bachelin, C., and Baron-Van Evercooren, A. (1999). Progenitor cells of the adult mouse subventricular zone proliferate, migrate and differentiate into oligodendrocytes after demyelination. *Eur. J. Neurosci.* 11, 4357–4366. doi: 10.1046/j.1460-9568.1999.00873.x

Nottebohm, F. (1981). A brain for all seasons: cyclical anatomical changes in song control nuclei of the canary brain. *Science* 214, 1368–1370. doi: 10.1126/science.7313697

Ohab, J. J., Fleming, S., Blesch, A., and Carmichael, S. T. (2006). A neurovascular niche for neurogenesis after stroke. *J. Neurosci.* 26, 13007–13016. doi: 10.1523/JNEUROSCI.4323-06.2006

Palmer, T. D., Willhoite, A. R., and Gage, F. H. (2000). Vascular niche for adult hippocampal neurogenesis. *J. Comp. Neurol.* 425, 479–494. doi: 10.1002/1096-9861(20001002)425:4%3C479::AID-CNE2%3E3.0.CO;2-3

Parent, J. M., Von Dem Bussche, N., and Lowenstein, D. H. (2006). Prolonged seizures recruit caudal subventricular zone glial progenitors into the injured hippocampus. *Hippocampus* 16, 321–328. doi: 10.1002/hipo.20166

Platel, J. C., Dave, K. A., and Bordey, A. (2008). Control of neuroblast production and migration by converging GABA and glutamate signals in the postnatal forebrain. *J. Physiol.* 586, 3739–3743. doi: 10.1113/jphysiol.2008.155325

Platel, J. C., Dave, K. A., Gordon, V., Lacar, B., Rubio, M. E., and Bordey, A. (2010). NMDA receptors activated by subventricular zone astrocytic glutamate are critical for neuroblast survival prior to entering a synaptic network. *Neuron* 65, 859–872. doi: 10.1016/j.neuron.2010.03.009

Pluchino, S., Muzio, L., Imitola, J., Deleidi, M., Alfaro-Cervello, C., Salani, G., et al. (2008). Persistent inflammation alters the function of the endogenous brain stem cell compartment. *Brain* 131, 2564–2578. doi: 10.1093/brain/awn198

Pluchino, S., Quattrini, A., Brambilla, E., Gritti, A., Salani, G., Dina, G., et al. (2003). Injection of adult neurospheres induces recovery in a chronic model of multiple sclerosis. *Nature* 422, 688–694. doi: 10.1038/nature01552

Pluchino, S., Zanotti, L., Rossi, B., Brambilla, E., Ottoboni, L., Salani, G., et al. (2005). Neurosphere-derived multipotent precursors promote neuroprotection by an immunomodulatory mechanism. *Nature* 436, 266–271. doi: 10.1038/nature03889

Ramon Y Cajal, S. (1913). *Degeneration and Regeneration of the Nervous System*. London: Oxford Univ. Press.

Rampon, C., Weiss, N., Deboux, C., Chaverot, N., Miller, F., Buchet, D., et al. (2008). Molecular mechanism of systemic delivery of neural precursor cells to the brain: assembly of brain endothelial apical cups and control of transmigration by CD44. *Stem Cells* 26, 1673–1682. doi: 10.1634/stemcells.2008-0122

Rappert, A., Bechmann, I., Pivneva, T., Mahlo, J., Biber, K., Nolte, C., et al. (2004). CXCR3-dependent microglial recruitment is essential for dendrite loss after brain lesion. *J. Neurosci.* 24, 8500–8509. doi: 10.1523/JNEUROSCI.2451-04.2004

Redmond, D. E. Jr., Bjugstad, K. B., Teng, Y. D., Ourednik, V., Ourednik, J., Wakeman, D. R., et al. (2007). Behavioral improvement in a primate Parkinson's model is associated with multiple homeostatic effects of human neural stem cells. *Proc. Natl. Acad. Sci. U.S.A.* 104, 12175–12180. doi: 10.1073/pnas.0704091104

Reynolds, B. A., and Weiss, S. (1992). Generation of neurons and astrocytes from isolated cells of the adult mammalian central nervous system. *Science* 255, 1707–1710. doi: 10.1126/science.1553558

Riquelme, P. A., Drapeau, E., and Doetsch, F. (2008). Brain micro-ecologies: neural stem cell niches in the adult mammalian brain. *Philos. Trans. R. Soc. Lond. B Biol. Sci.* 363, 123–137. doi: 10.1098/rstb.2006.2016

Rotheneichner, P., Marschallinger, J., Couillard-Despres, S., and Aigner, L. (2013). Neurogenesis and neuronal regeneration in status epilepticus. *Epilepsia* 54(Suppl. 6), 40–42. doi: 10.1111/epi.12274

Ryu, J. K., Kim, J., Cho, S. J., Hatori, K., Nagai, A., Choi, H. B., et al. (2004). Proactive transplantation of human neural stem cells prevents degeneration of striatal neurons in a rat model of Huntington disease. *Neurobiol. Dis.* 16, 68–77. doi: 10.1016/j.nbd.2004.01.016

Sabelström, H., Stenudd, M., Reu, P., Dias, D. O., Elfineh, M., Zdunek, S., et al. (2013). Resident neural stem cells restrict tissue damage and neuronal loss after spinal cord injury in mice. *Science* 342, 637–640. doi: 10.1126/science.1242576

Sahay, A., Scobie, K. N., Hill, A. S., O'carroll, C. M., Kheirbek, M. A., Burghardt, N. S., et al. (2011). Increasing adult hippocampal neurogenesis is sufficient to improve pattern separation. *Nature* 472, 466–470. doi: 10.1038/nature09817

Sakamoto, M., Imayoshi, I., Ohtsuka, T., Yamaguchi, M., Mori, K., and Kageyama, R. (2011). Continuous neurogenesis in the adult forebrain is required for innate olfactory responses. *Proc. Natl. Acad. Sci. U.S.A.* 108, 8479–8484. doi: 10.1073/pnas.1018782108

Sanai, N., Berger, M. S., Garcia-Verdugo, J. M., and Alvarez-Buylla, A. (2007). Comment on "Human neuroblasts migrate to the olfactory bulb via a lateral ventricular extension". *Science* 318, 393. doi: 10.1126/science.1145011

Sanai, N., Nguyen, T., Ihrie, R. A., Mirzadeh, Z., Tsai, H. H., Wong, M., et al. (2011). Corridors of migrating neurons in the human brain and their decline during infancy. *Nature* 478, 382–386. doi: 10.1038/nature10487

Sanai, N., Tramontin, A. D., Quinones-Hinojosa, A., Barbaro, N. M., Gupta, N., Kunwar, S., et al. (2004). Unique astrocyte ribbon in adult human brain contains neural stem cells but lacks chain migration. *Nature* 427, 740–744. doi: 10.1038/nature02301

Sawamoto, K., Wichterle, H., Gonzalez-Perez, O., Cholfin, J. A., Yamada, M., Spassky, N., et al. (2006). New neurons follow the flow of cerebrospinal fluid in the adult brain. *Science* 311, 629–632. doi: 10.1126/science.1119133

Seifert, T., Bauer, J., Weissert, R., Fazekas, F., and Storch, M. K. (2005). Differential expression of sonic hedgehog immunoreactivity during lesion evolution in autoimmune encephalomyelitis. *J. Neuropathol. Exp. Neurol.* 64, 404–411.

Shingo, T., Gregg, C., Enwere, E., Fujikawa, H., Hassam, R., Geary, C., et al. (2003). Pregnancy-stimulated neurogenesis in the adult female forebrain mediated by prolactin. *Science* 299, 117–120. doi: 10.1126/science.1076647

Shors, T. J., Townsend, D. A., Zhao, M., Kozorovitskiy, Y., and Gould, E. (2002). Neurogenesis may relate to some but not all types of hippocampal-dependent learning. *Hippocampus* 12, 578–584. doi: 10.1002/hipo.10103

Sierra, A., Encinas, J. M., Deudero, J. J., Chancey, J. H., Enikolopov, G., Overstreet-Wadiche, L. S., et al. (2010). Microglia shape adult hippocampal neurogenesis through apoptosis-coupled phagocytosis. *Cell Stem Cell* 7, 483–495. doi: 10.1016/j.stem.2010.08.014

Singer, B. H., Jutkiewicz, E. M., Fuller, C. L., Lichtenwalner, R. J., Zhang, H., Velander, A. J., et al. (2009). Conditional ablation and recovery of forebrain neurogenesis in the mouse. *J. Comp. Neurol.* 514, 567–582. doi: 10.1002/cne.22052

Smart, I. (1961). The subependymal layer of the mouse brain and its cell production as shown by autography after [H3]-thymidine injection. *J. Comp. Neurol.* 116, 325–327. doi: 10.1002/cne.901160306

Snyder, J. S., Hong, N. S., McDonald, R. J., and Wojtowicz, J. M. (2005). A role for adult neurogenesis in spatial long-term memory. *Neuroscience* 130, 843–852. doi: 10.1016/j.neuroscience.2004.10.009

Snyder, J. S., Soumier, A., Brewer, M., Pickel, J., and Cameron, H. A. (2011). Adult hippocampal neurogenesis buffers stress responses and depressive behaviour. *Nature* 476, 458–461. doi: 10.1038/nature10287

Spalding, K. L., Bergmann, O., Alkass, K., Bernard, S., Salehpour, M., Huttner, H. B., et al. (2013). Dynamics of hippocampal neurogenesis in adult humans. *Cell* 153, 1219–1227. doi: 10.1016/j.cell.2013.05.002

Stock, K., Kumar, J., Synowitz, M., Petrosino, S., Imperatore, R., Smith, E. S., et al. (2012). Neural precursor cells induce cell death of high-grade astrocytomas through stimulation of TRPV1. *Nat. Med.* 18, 1232–1238. doi: 10.1038/nm.2827

Sun, C., Sun, H., Wu, S., Lee, C. C., Akamatsu, Y., Wang, R. K., et al. (2013). Conditional ablation of neuroprogenitor cells in adult mice impedes recovery of poststroke cognitive function and reduces synaptic connectivity in the perforant pathway. *J. Neurosci.* 33, 17314–17325. doi: 10.1523/JNEUROSCI.2129-13.2013

Tavazoie, M., Van Der Veken, L., Silva-Vargas, V., Louissaint, M., Colonna, L., Zaidi, B., et al. (2008). A specialized vascular niche for adult neural stem cells. *Cell Stem Cell* 3, 279–288. doi: 10.1016/j.stem.2008.07.025

Tello, J. F. (1907). *La Regeneration dans les Voies Optiques*. Madrid: Trab Lab Invest Biol Univ Madr.

Teng, H., Zhang, Z. G., Wang, L., Zhang, R. L., Zhang, L., Morris, D., et al. (2008). Coupling of angiogenesis and neurogenesis in cultured endothelial cells and neural progenitor cells after stroke. *J. Cereb. Blood Flow Metab.* 28, 764–771. doi: 10.1038/sj.jcbfm.9600573

Teng, Y. D., Lavik, E. B., Qu, X., Park, K. I., Ourednik, J., Zurakowski, D., et al. (2002). Functional recovery following traumatic spinal cord injury mediated by a unique polymer scaffold seeded with neural stem cells. *Proc. Natl. Acad. Sci. U.S.A.* 99, 3024–3029. doi: 10.1073/pnas.052678899

Thored, P., Arvidsson, A., Cacci, E., Ahlenius, H., Kallur, T., Darsalia, V., et al. (2006). Persistent production of neurons from adult brain stem cells during recovery after stroke. *Stem Cells* 24, 739–747. doi: 10.1634/stemcells.2005-0281

Thored, P., Heldmann, U., Gomes-Leal, W., Gisler, R., Darsalia, V., Taneera, J., et al. (2009). Long-term accumulation of microglia with proneurogenic phenotype concomitant with persistent neurogenesis in adult subventricular zone after stroke. *Glia* 57, 835–849. doi: 10.1002/glia.20810

Thored, P., Wood, J., Arvidsson, A., Cammenga, J., Kokaia, Z., and Lindvall, O. (2007). Long-term neuroblast migration along blood vessels in an area with transient angiogenesis and increased vascularization after stroke. *Stroke* 38, 3032–3039. doi: 10.1161/STROKEAHA.107.488445

Tong, C. K., Chen, J., Cebrian-Silla, A., Mirzadeh, Z., Obernier, K., Guinto, C. D., et al. (2014). Axonal control of the adult neural stem cell niche. *Cell Stem Cell* 14, 500–511. doi: 10.1016/j.stem.2014.01.014

Villeda, S. A., Luo, J., Mosher, K. I., Zou, B., Britschgi, M., Bieri, G., et al. (2011). The ageing systemic milieu negatively regulates neurogenesis and cognitive function. *Nature* 477, 90–94. doi: 10.1038/nature10357

Wang, X., Mao, X., Xie, L., Sun, F., Greenberg, D. A., and Jin, K. (2012). Conditional depletion of neurogenesis inhibits long-term recovery after experimental stroke in mice. *PLoS ONE* 7:e38932. doi: 10.1371/journal.pone.0038932

Willshaw, D. J., and Buckingham, J. T. (1990). An assessment of Marr's theory of the hippocampus as a temporary memory store. *Philos. Trans. R. Soc. Lond. B Biol. Sci.* 329, 205–215. doi: 10.1098/rstb.1990.0165

Young, S. Z., Taylor, M. M., and Bordey, A. (2011). Neurotransmitters couple brain activity to subventricular zone neurogenesis. *Eur. J. Neurosci.* 33, 1123–1132. doi: 10.1111/j.1460-9568.2011.07611.x

Zhang, Z. G., and Chopp, M. (2009). Neurorestorative therapies for stroke: underlying mechanisms and translation to the clinic. *Lancet Neurol.* 8, 491–500. doi: 10.1016/S1474-4422(09)70061-4

Zhao, C., Deng, W., and Gage, F. H. (2008). Mechanisms and functional implications of adult neurogenesis. *Cell* 132, 645–660. doi: 10.1016/j.cell.2008.01.033

Ziv, Y., Avidan, H., Pluchino, S., Martino, G., and Schwartz, M. (2006). Synergy between immune cells and adult neural stem/progenitor cells promotes functional recovery from spinal cord injury. *Proc. Natl. Acad. Sci. U.S.A.* 103, 13174–13179. doi: 10.1073/pnas.0603747103

Conflict of Interest Statement: The authors declare that the research was conducted in the absence of any commercial or financial relationships that could be construed as a potential conflict of interest.

Permissions

All chapters in this book were first published in BGBABMTEFNDH, by Frontiers; hereby published with permission under the Creative Commons Attribution License or equivalent. Every chapter published in this book has been scrutinized by our experts. Their significance has been extensively debated. The topics covered herein carry significant findings which will fuel the growth of the discipline. They may even be implemented as practical applications or may be referred to as a beginning point for another development.

The contributors of this book come from diverse backgrounds, making this book a truly international effort. This book will bring forth new frontiers with its revolutionizing research information and detailed analysis of the nascent developments around the world.

We would like to thank all the contributing authors for lending their expertise to make the book truly unique.

They have played a crucial role in the development of this book. Without their invaluable contributions this book wouldn't have been possible. They have made vital efforts to compile up to date information on the varied aspects of this subject to make this book a valuable addition to the collection of many professionals and students.

This book was conceptualized with the vision of imparting up-to-date information and advanced data in this field. To ensure the same, a matchless editorial board was set up. Every individual on the board went through rigorous rounds of assessment to prove their worth. After which they invested a large part of their time researching and compiling the most relevant data for our readers.

The editorial board has been involved in producing this book since its inception. They have spent rigorous hours researching and exploring the diverse topics which have resulted in the successful publishing of this book. They have passed on their knowledge of decades through this book. To expedite this challenging task, the publisher supported the team at every step. A small team of assistant editors was also appointed to further simplify the editing procedure and attain best results for the readers.

Apart from the editorial board, the designing team has also invested a significant amount of their time in understanding the subject and creating the most relevant covers. They scrutinized every image to scout for the most suitable representation of the subject and create an appropriate cover for the book.

The publishing team has been an ardent support to the editorial, designing and production team. Their endless efforts to recruit the best for this project, has resulted in the accomplishment of this book. They are a veteran in the field of academics and their pool of knowledge is as vast as their experience in printing. Their expertise and guidance has proved useful at every step. Their uncompromising quality standards have made this book an exceptional effort. Their encouragement from time to time has been an inspiration for everyone.

The publisher and the editorial board hope that this book will prove to be a valuable piece of knowledge for researchers, students, practitioners and scholars across the globe.

List of Contributors

Vanessa Raymont
Vietnam Head Injury Study, Henry M. Jackson Foundation, National Naval Medical Center, Bethesda, MD, USA
Cognitive Neuroscience Section, National Institute of Neurological Disorders and Stroke, National Institutes of Health, Bethesda, MD, USA
Department of Radiology, Johns Hopkins University, Baltimore, MD, USA

Andres M. Salazar and Frank Krueger
Cognitive Neuroscience Section, National Institute of Neurological Disorders and Stroke, National Institutes of Health, Bethesda, MD, USA

Jordan Grafman
Cognitive Neuroscience Section, National Institute of Neurological Disorders and Stroke, National Institutes of Health, Bethesda, MD, USA
Traumatic Brain Injury Research Laboratory, Kessler Foundation, West Orange, NJ, USA

Silke Schicktanz
Department of Medical Ethicsand History of Medicine, University Medical Center Göttingen, Göttingen, Germany

Mark Schweda
Department of Medical Ethicsand History of Medicine, University Medical Center Göttingen, Göttingen, Germany
Lichtenberg Kolleg, University of Göttingen, Göttingen, Germany

Jesse F. Ballenger
Health Administration Department, Drexel University, Philadelphia, PA, USA

Patrick J. Fox
Institute for Health & Aging, University of California, San Francisco, San Francisco, CA, USA

Jodi Halpern and Guy Micco
UC Berkeley-UCSF Joint Medical Program, School of Public Health, University of California, Berkeley, Berkeley, CA, USA

Joel H. Kramer
Memory and Aging Center, Sandler Neurosciences Center, University of California, San Francisco, San Francisco, CA, USA

Stephen G. Post
Compassionate Care & Bioethics, Stony Brook Medicine, Stony Brook, NY, USA

Charis Thompson
Department of Gender and Women's Studies, University of California, Berkeley, Berkeley, CA, USA
Department of Sociology, London School of Economics, London, UK

Robert T. Knight
Department of Psychology, University of California, Berkeley, Berkeley, CA, USA
Helen Wills Neuroscience Institute, University of California, Berkeley, Berkeley, CA, USA

William J. Jagust
UC Berkeley-UCSF Joint Medical Program, School of Public Health, University of California, Berkeley, Berkeley, CA, USA
Helen Wills Neuroscience Institute, University of California, Berkeley, Berkeley, CA, USA

Ann M. Turnley, Harleen S. Basrai and Kimberly J. Christie
Department of Anatomy and Neuroscience, The University of Melbourne, Parkville, VIC, Australia

Antonio Luchicchi, John Noel M.Viaña and Huibert D. Mansvelder
Department of Integrative Neurophysiology, Center for Neurogenomics and Cognitive Research, Neuroscience Campus Amsterdam, Vrije Universiteit, Amsterdam, Netherlands

Bernard Bloem
Department of Integrative Neurophysiology, Center for Neurogenomics and Cognitive Research, Neuroscience Campus Amsterdam, Vrije Universiteit, Amsterdam, Netherlands
Mc Govern Institute for Brain Research, Massachusetts Institute of Technology, Cambridge, MA, USA

Lorna W. Role
Department of Neurobiology and Behavior, Stony Brook University, Stony Brook, NY, USA

A. Rory McQuiston
Department of Anatomy and Neurobiology, Virginia Common wealth University, Richmond, VA, USA

Livio Oboti
Children's National Health System, Center for Neuroscience Research, Washington, DC, USA

Paolo Peretto
Department of Life Sciences and Systems Biology, Neuroscience Institute Cavalieri Ottolenghi, University of Torino, Orbassano, Italy

Sean Austin O.Lim
Committee on Neurobiology, University of Chicago, Chicago, IL, USA

Un Jung Kang
Department of Neurology, Columbia University, NewYork, NY, USA

Daniel S. McGehee
Committee on Neurobiology, University of Chicago, Chicago, IL, USA
Department of Anesthesia and Critical Care, University of Chicago, Chicago, IL, USA

Claudio Giachino and Verdon Taylor
Department of Biomedicine, University of Basel, Basel, Switzerland

Ninah Koolen, Vladimir Matic and Sabine VanHuffel
Division STADIUS, Department of Electrical Engineering (ESAT), University of Leuven, Leuven, Belgium
iMinds-KU Leuven Medical ITD epartment, Leuven, Belgium

Anneleen Dereymaeker, Katrien Jansen, Jan Vervisch and Gunnar Naulaers
Department of Development and Regeneration, University of Leuven, Leuven, Belgium

Okko Räsänen
Department of Signal Processing and Acoustics, Aalto University, Espoo, Finland

Maarten De Vos
Department of Psychology, University of Oldenburg, Oldenburg, Germany
Department of Engineering Science, Institute of Biomedical Engineering, University of Oxford, Oxford, UK

Sampsa Vanhatalo
Department of Children's Clinical Neurophysiology, HUS Medical Imaging Centerand Children's Hospital, Helsinki University Central Hospital and University of Helsinki, Helsinki, Finland

Kirsten Obernier, Cheuk Ka Tong and Arturo Alvarez-Buylla
Department of Neurological Surgery, The Eli and Edythe Broad Center of Regeneration Medicine and Stem Cell Research, University of California, San Francisco, San Francisco, CA, USA

Dionisio A. Amodeo, Julia Yi, and Michael E. Ragozzino
Laboratory of Integrative Neuroscience, Department of Psychology, University of Illinois at Chicago, Chicago, IL, USA

John A. Sweeney
Department of Psychiatry, University of Texas Southwestern Medical Center, Dallas, TX, USA

Dirk Hoyer, Alexander Schmidt, FlorianTetschke, Samuel Nowack, Liviu Moraru, Theresa Götz and Otto W. Witte
Biomagnetic Center, Hans Berger Department of Neurology, Jena University Hospital, Friedrich Schiller University, Jena, Germany

Jens Haueisen
Institute of Biomedical Engineering and Informatics, Ilmenau University of Technology, Ilmenau, Germany

Eva-Maria Kowalski
Biomagnetic Center, Hans Berger Department of Neurology, Jena University Hospital, Friedrich Schiller University, Jena, Germany
Institute of Biomedical Engineering and Informatics, Ilmenau University of Technology, Ilmenau, Germany

Anja Rudolph, Ulrike Wallwitz, Isabelle Kynass, Franziska Bode, JanineTegtmeyer and Kathrin Kumm
Biomagnetic Center, Hans Berger Department of Neurology, Jena University Hospital, Friedrich Schiller University, Jena, Germany
Department of Obstetrics, Jena University Hospital, Friedrich Schiller University, Jena, Germany

Ekkehard Schleußner and Uwe Schneider
Department of Obstetrics, Jena University Hospital, Friedrich Schiller University, Jena, Germany

Abhishek Prasad
Department of Biomedical Engineering, University of Miami, Coral Gables, FL, USA

Qing-Shan Xue and Wolfgang J. Streit
Department of Neuroscience, University of Florida, Gainesville, FL,USA

Robert Dieme, Viswanath Sankar and Toshikazu Nishida
Department of Electrical and Computer Engineering, University of Florida, Gainesville, FL, USA

Roxanne C. Mayrand
Department of Neuroscience, University of Miami, Coral Gables, FL, USA

Justin C. Sanchez
Department of Biomedical Engineering, University of Miami, Coral Gables, FL, USA
Department of Neuroscience, University of Miami, Coral Gables, FL, USA

Miami Project to Cure Paralysis, University of Miami, Miami, FL, USA

Ibolja Cernak
Biomedicine Business Area, National Security Technology Department, Johns Hopkins University Applied Physics Laboratory, Laurel, MD, USA

Talin Babikian and Robert F. Asarnow
Psychiatry and Biobehavioral Sciences, University of California Los Angeles David Geffen School of Medicine, Los Angeles, CA, USA

Fabienne Cazalis
Psychiatry and Biobehavioral Sciences, University of California Los Angeles David Geffen School of Medicine, Los Angeles, CA, USA
Department of Anatomy, Ross University School of Medicine, Roseau, Commonwealth of Dominica

Christopher Giza, Sarah Copeland and David Hovda
Department of Neurosurgery, University of California Los Angeles David Geffen School of Medicine, Los Angeles, CA, USA

Elisa Castagnola, Alberto Ansaldo, Emma Maggiolini and Davide Ricci
Robotics, Brain and Cognitive Sciences Department, Istituto Italiano di Tecnologia, Genoa, Italy

Tamara Ius and Miran Skrap
Struttura Complessa di Neurochirurgia, Azienda Ospedaliero-Universitaria Santa Maria della Misericordia, Udine, Italy

Luciano Fadiga
Robotics, Brain and Cognitive Sciences Department, Istituto Italiano di Tecnologia, Genoa, Italy
Section of Human Physiology, Department of Biomedical Sciences, University of Ferrara, Ferrara, Italy

Fleur A. Camfferman and Filip Cools
Department of Neonatology, Universitair Ziekenhuis Brussel, Vrije Universiteit Brussel, Brussels, Belgium

Ginette M. Ecury-Goossen and Jhuresy E. LaRoche
Department of Neonatology, Erasmus Medical Centre, Rotterdam, Netherlands

Willem van't Leven
Department of Biomedical Engineering, Erasmus Medical Centre, Rotterdam, Netherlands

Nicode Jong and Hendrik J. Vos
Department of Biomedical Engineering, Erasmus Medical Centre, Rotterdam, Netherlands
Department of Imaging Physics, Delft University of Technology, Delft, Netherlands

Martin D. Verweij
Department of Imaging Physics, Delft University of Technology, Delft, Netherlands

Kazem Nasserinejad
Department of Biostatistics, Erasmus Medical Centre, Rotterdam, Netherlands

Paul Govaert
Department of Neonatology, Universitair Ziekenhuis Brussel, Vrije Universiteit Brussel, Brussels, Belgium
Department of Neonatology, Erasmus Medical Centre, Rotterdam, Netherlands

Jeroen Dudink
Department of Neonatology, Erasmus Medical Centre, Rotterdam, Netherlands
Department of Radiology, Erasmus Medical Centre, Rotterdam, Netherlands

VeronikaSchöpf, GregorKasprian, RamonaWoitek, DanielaPrayer
Division of Neuro-and Musculos keletal Radiology, Department of Biomedical Imaging and Image-guided Therapy, Medical University of Vienna, Vienna, Austria

ThomasSchleg, AndrasJakab
Computation al Imaging Research Laboratory, Department of Biomedical Imaging and Image-guided Therapy, Medical University of Vienna, Vienna, Austria

Enrica Boda and Annalisa Buffo
Department of Neuroscience Rita Levi-Montalcini, Neuroscience Institute Cavalieri Ottolenghi, University of Turin, Turin, Italy

GeorgLangs
Computation al Imaging Research Laboratory, Department of Biomedical Imaging and Image-guided Therapy, Medical University of Vienna, Vienna, Austria
Computer Science and Artificia lIntelligence Lab, Massachusetts Institute of Technology, Cambridge, MA, USA

Sook-Kyung C. Kwon, Erzsebet Kovesdi, Andrea B. Gyorgy, Daniel Wingo, Alaa Kamnaksh, John Walker and Denes V. Agoston
Department of Anatomy, Physiology and Genetics, School of Medicine, Uniformed Services University, Bethesda, MD, USA

Joseph B. Long
Division of Military Casualty Research, Walter Reed Army Institute of Research, Silver Spring, MD, USA

Leonardo C. deSouza, Henrique C. Guimarães, Antônio L.Teixeira and Paulo Caramelli
Neuropsychiatric Branch, Neurology Division, University Hospital, Universidade Federal de Minas Gerais, Belo Horizonte, Brazil

Richard Levy
Inserm, U1127, ICMF rontlab, Paris, France
CNRS, UMR7225, ICMF rontlab, Paris, France
Sorbonne Universités, UPMC UnivParis06, UMRS1127, Paris, France
Institut du Cerveauet de la Moelle épinière, ICMF rontlab, Paris, France
AP-HP, HôpitalSaint-Antoine, Servicede Neurologie, Paris, France

Bruno Dubois
Inserm, U1127, ICMF rontlab, Paris, France
CNRS, UMR7225, ICMF rontlab, Paris, France
Sorbonne Universités, UPMC UnivParis06, UMRS1127, Paris, France
Institut du Cerveauet de la Moelle épinière, ICMF rontlab, Paris, France
AP-HP, HôpitalSaint-Antoine, Servicede Neurologie, Paris, France
AP-HP, Hôpital de la Salpétrière, Neurology Department, Institut de la Mémoire etdela Maladied' Alzheimer, Paris, France

Emmanuelle Volle
Inserm, U1127, ICMF rontlab, Paris, France
CNRS, UMR7225, ICMF rontlab, Paris, France
Sorbonne Universités, UPMC UnivParis06, UMRS1127, Paris, France
Institut du Cerveauet de la Moelle épinière, ICMF rontlab, Paris, France

Michael Noll-Hussong and Dan Pokorny
Klinik und Poliklinik fuer Psychosomatische Medizin und Psychotherapie des Universitaetsklinikums Ulm, Ulm, Germany

Sabrina Holzapfel
Hals-Nasen-Ohrenklinik und Poliklinik, Klinikum rechts der Isar, Technische UniversitaetMuenchen, Muenchen, Germany

Simone Herberger
Klinik fuer Psychosomatische Medizin und Psychotherapie des Klinikums Muenchen-Harlaching, Muenchen, Germany

Salah Sommakia
Weldon School o fBiomedical Engineering, Purdue University, West Lafayette, IN, USA
Physiological Sensing Facility at the Bindley Bioscience Center and Birck Nanotechnology Center, Purdue University, West Lafayette, IN, USA

Janak Gaire
Department of Biological Sciences, Purdue University, West Lafayette, IN, USA

Jenna L. Rickus
Weldon School of Biomedical Engineering, Purdue University, West Lafayette, IN, USA
Physiological Sensing Facility at the Bindley Bioscience Center and Birck Nanotechnology Center, Purdue University, West Lafayette, IN, USA
Department ofAgricultural and Biological Engineering, Purdue University, West Lafayette,IN, USA

Kevin J. Otto
Weldon School o fBiomedical Engineering, Purdue University, West Lafayette, IN, USA
Department of Biological Sciences, Purdue University, West Lafayette, IN, USA

Erica Butti, Melania Cusimano, Marco Bacigaluppi and Gianvito Martino
Neuroimmunology Unit, Division of Neuroscience, Institute of Experimental Neurology, San Raffaele Scientific Institute, Milan, Italy

Index

O

P

R

S

T

V

CPSIA information can be obtained
at www.ICGtesting.com
Printed in the USA
LVHW062010100122
708212LV00002B/157

9 781639 874859